Eugene N. Myers · Robert L. Ferris (Eds.)

Salivary Gland Disorders

Eugene N. Myers · Robert L. Ferris (Eds.)

Salivary Gland Disorders

With 449 Figures and 50 Tables

Springer

Eugene N. Myers, MD, FACS, FRCS Edin (Hon)
Distinguished Professor and Emeritus Chair
Department of Otolaryngology
University of Pittsburgh, School of Medicine
The Eye & Ear Institute, Suite 519
200 Lothrop Street
Pittsburgh, PA 15213
USA

Robert L. Ferris, MD, PhD, FACS
Associate Professor and Chief
Department of Otolaryngology and of Immunology
University of Pittsburgh, School of Medicine
Co-Leader, Cancer Immunology Program
University of Pittsburgh Cancer Institute
200 Lothrop Street, Suite 500
Pittsburgh, PA 15213
USA

Library of Congress Control Number: 2007923957

ISBN 978-3-540-47070-0 Springer Berlin Heidelberg New York

Springer is a part of Springer Science+Business Media

springer.com

Editor: Marion Philipp, Heidelberg, Germany
Desk Editor: Irmela Bohn, Heidelberg, Germany
Reproduction, typesetting and production: LE-TEX Jelonek, Schmidt & Vöckler GbR, Leipzig, Germany
Cover design: Frido Steinen-Broo, EStudio, Calamar, Spain
Illustrations (Chapter 1): Joe Bloch, BlochArt, Inc., Brooklyn, NY, USA

Printed on acid-free paper 24/3180/YL 5 4 3 2 1 0

Dedication

We dedicate this book to the patients afflicted with disorders of the salivary glands so that the information presented here may be used to alleviate their suffering. We also dedicate it to our devoted wives, Barbara L. Myers and Laura Ferris, for their patience and support throughout its conception and completion.

Eugene N. Myers, MD
Robert L. Ferris, MD, PhD

Preface

The management of salivary disorders encompasses a broad array of both benign and malignant diseases. We felt that a detailed text addressing this topic has been needed for some time. The book begins with chapters such as diagnostic approaches based on clinical, radiographic, and pathologic assessment of salivary gland disorders. We have featured the role of sialendoscopy, a recently developed technique for diagnosis and treatment of obstructive diseases of the salivary glands. The benign aspects of salivary diseases in addition to the approach to management of salivary malignancies are then addressed. The problems of a unique cluster of salivary gland disorders in children are also included.

The main strength of this book is the group of internationally known authorities who have contributed their expertise and experience in authoring definitive chapters on salivary gland disorders. Photographs and sketches are included to illustrate both the disorders and surgical techniques described. We believe this to be the most comprehensive textbook available.

We hope this book will serve as a useful reference and a practical manual for the clinicians of many specialties who treat patients with salivary gland disorders. Whether used as an introductory or advanced referenced text, we hope the readers will find that this book contributes to their practice.

We are indebted to our editorial coordinator, Mary Jo Tutchko, for her untiring commitment and dedication to the organization and completion of this book. We also thank Charmaine D. Woods for her valuable assistance. We appreciate the foresight and support of Springer, our publisher, for enabling this text to be published in the form we envisioned. Marion M. Philipp, Senior Editor Clinical Medicine, and Irmela Bohn, Desk Editor Clinical Medicine, both of Springer, have been very helpful, patient, and supportive during this project and we offer our appreciation to them.

Eugene N. Myers, MD
Robert L. Ferris, MD, PhD

Contents

List of Contributors

Ahmed Afifi, MD
Clinical Instructor
Division of Plastic Surgery
University of Pittsburgh Medical Center
3705 5th Avenue
Pittsburgh, PA 15213
USA
E-mail: ahafifi@yahoo.com

Athanassios Argiris, MD, FACP
Medical Oncologist
Associate Professor of Medicine
University of Pittsburgh School of Medicine
Co-Director, Head and Neck Cancer Program
University of Pittsburgh Cancer Institute
5150 Center Avenue
Pittsburgh, PA 152132
USA
E-mail: argirisae@upmc.edu

Moisés A. Arriaga, MD, FACS
Clinical Professor of Otolaryngology
Louisiana State University Health Science Center
New Orleans, Louisiana
Pittsburgh Ear Associates, Allegheny General Hospital
420 East North Avenue, Suite 402
Pittsburgh, PA 15212
USA
E-mail: tec8lote@aol.com

Ioli-Ioanna Artopoulou, DDS, MS
Postgraduate Student
Department of Dental Biomaterials
National and Kapodistrian University
of Athens School of Dentistry
81 Kythirion str.
17456 Alimos, Athens
Greece
E-mail: iartopoulou@gmail.com

Patrick J. Bradley, MBA, FRCS
Consultant Head and Neck Oncologic Surgeon
Department of Otorhinolaryngology, Head and Neck
Surgery, University Hospital
Queens Medical Centre
Nottingham, NG7 2UH
UK
E-mail: pjbradley@zoo.co.uk

Michael T. Brennan DDS, MHS
Oral Medicine Residency Director
Director, Sjögren's Syndrome and Salivary Disorders
Center, Department of Oral Medicine
Carolinas Medical Center
PO Box 32861
Charlotte, NC 28232
USA
E-mail: mike.brennan@carolinas.org

Andre G. Brun, DMD
Resident
Department of Oral Medicine
Carolinas Medical Center
PO Box 32861
Charlotte, NC 28232
USA
E-mail: andre.brun@carolinas.org

Lisa Buckmiller, MD
Clinical Director, Vascular Anomalies Program
Department of Otolaryngology – Head and Neck
Surgery, Arkansas Children's Hospital
800 Marshall Street, Slot 668
Little Rock, AR 72202-3591
USA
E-mail: buckmillerlisam@uams.edu

Dana Thuy Bui, BA
Research Associate
Department of Head and Neck Surgery
University of Texas MD Anderson Cancer Center
Student
The University of Texas Medical School at Houston
1515 Holcombe Blvd # 441
Houston, TX 77030-4009
USA
Email: dana.t.bui@uth.tmc.edu

Claudio Cernea, MD
Alameda Franca
267-cjto 21
Sao Paulo, SP 01422-000
Brazil
E-mail: cerneamd@uol.com.br

Mark S. Chambers, DMD, MS
Associate Professor, Director of Clinical Research
Department of Head and Neck Surgery
University of Texas M.D. Anderson Cancer Center
1515 Holcombe Boulevard
Houston, TX 77030-4009
USA
E-mail: mchamber@mdanderson.org

William L. Chung, DDS, MD
Assistant Professor
Department of Oral & Maxillofacial Surgery
University of Pittsburgh Medical Center
3459 5th Ave., Suite 202 South
Pittsburgh, PA 15213
USA
E-mail: chungwl@upmc.edu

Jonathan Clark, MBBS (Hons), BSc, FRACS
Head and Neck Surgeon
Sydney Head and Neck Cancer Institute
Royal Prince Alfred Hospital
PO Box M142
Missenden Road
Camperdown, NSW 2050
Australia
E-mail: jcjc@tpg.com.au

Hugh D. Curtin, MD
Professor of Radiology
Harvard Medical School
Chief of Radiology
Massachusetts Eye and Ear Infirmary
243 Charles Street
Boston, MA 02114
USA
Email: hdcurtin@meei.harvard.edu

Frederic W.-B. Deleyiannis MD, MPhil, MPH
Assistant Professor
Division of Plastic Surgery
Departments of Surgery and Otolaryngology
University of Pittsburgh Medical Center
Suite 6b Scaife Hall
3550 Terrace Street
Pittsburgh, PA 15261
USA
E-mail: deleyiannisfw@msx.upmc.edu

Fernando Luiz Dias, MD, PhD
Av Alexandre Ferreira 190
Lagoa
Rio de Janeiro, RJ 2270-220
Brazil
E-mail: fdias@inca.gov.br

Pavel Dulguerov, MD, PhD
Department of Oto-Rhino-Laryngology –
Head & Neck Surgery
University Hospital of Geneva, Switzerland
24, rue Micheli-du-Crest
CH-1211 Geneva 14
Switzerland
E-mail: pavel.dulguerov@hcuge.ch

David W. Eisele, MD, FACS
Professor and Chairman, Director
Division of Head and Neck Surgery
Department of Otolaryngology – Head and Neck
Surgery
University of California, San Francisco
400 Parnassus Avenue, Suite A-730
San Francisco, CA 94143-0342
USA
E-mail: deisele@ohns.ucsf.edu

Robert L. Ferris, MD, PhD, FACS
Associate Professor and Chief
Department of Otolaryngology and of Immunology
University of Pittsburgh, School of Medicine
Co-Leader, Cancer Immunology Program
University of Pittsburgh Cancer Institute
200 Lothrop Street, Suite 500
Pittsburgh, PA 15213
USA
E-mail: ferrisrl@upmc.edu

Philip C. Fox, DDS
6509 Seven Locks Road
Cabin John, MD 20818
USA
E-mail: pcfox@comcast.net

Adam S. Garden, MD
Professor and Section Chief, Head and Neck Radiation Oncology
Department of Radiation Oncology #97
University of Texas M.D. Anderson Cancer Center
1515 Holcombe Boulevard
Houston, TX 77030
USA
E-mail: agarden@mdanderson.org

Kristin B. Gendron, MD
Visiting Instructor
Department of Otolaryngology
University of Pittsburgh, School of Medicine
200 Lothrop Street
The Eye & Ear Institute, Suite 500
Pittsburgh, PA 15213
USA
E-mail: kristingendron@hotmail.com

Christian Hall, MD
Resident in Otolaryngology
Clinical Professor of Otolaryngology
Louisiana State University Health Science Center
533 Bolivar Street, Fl 5
New Orleans, LA 70112-1349
USA
E-mail: chall@lsuhsc.edu

F. Christopher Holsinger, MD, FACS
Assistant Professor
Department of Head and Neck Surgery
University of Texas MD Anderson Cancer Center
1515 Holcombe Blvd # 441
Houston, TX 77030-4009
USA
Email: holsinger@mdanderson.org

Catherine H. Hong BDS, MS
Section Head of Pediatric Dentistry
Department of Oral Medicine
Carolinas Medical Center
P.O. Box 32861
Charlotte, NC 28232
USA
E-mail: catherine.hong@carolinas.org

Paul D. Kim, MD
Assistant Professor of Surgery
Department of Otolaryngology-Head Neck Surgery
Loma Linda University School of Medicine
11234 Anderson Street, Suite 2584
Loma Linda, CA 92354
USA
E-mail: kimpaul46@gmail.com

Melda Kunduk, PhD
Assistant Professor, School of Allied Health
Clinical Professor of Otolaryngology
Louisiana State University Health Science Center
533 Bolivar Street, Fl 5
New Orleans, LA 70112-1349
USA
E-mail: mkundu@lsuhsc.edu

George E. Laramore, PhD, MD
Department of Radiation Oncology
PO Box 356043
University of Washington Medical Center
Seattle, WA 98195-6043
USA
E-mail: georgel@u.washington.edu

Scott A. Laurie, MD, FRCPC
Medical Oncologist
The Ottawa Hospital Regional Cancer Centre
Assistant Professor
University of Ottawa
501 Smyth Road
Ottawa, ON, Canada K1H 1C4
E-mail: slaurie@ottawahospital.on.ca

Roberto Lima, MD
Avenida Armando Lombardi, 1000 Blc2 107
Barra da Tijuca
Rio de Janeiro, RJ 22641-003
Brazil
E-mail: rlimamd@uol.com.br

David L. Mandell, MD, FAAP
Assistant Professor
Department of Otolaryngology
University of Pittsburgh School of Medicine
Director, Pediatric Airway Center
Children's Hospital of Pittsburgh
3705 Fifth Avenue
Pittsburgh, PA 15213
USA
E-mail: david.mandell@chp.edu

Francis Marchal, MD
Sialendoscopy Unit
Department Otolaryngology, Head and Neck Surgery
University Hospital of Geneva
24, rue Micheli du Crest
1205 Geneva
Switzerland
E-mail: francis.marchal@bluewin.ch

Eric J. Moore, MD
Assistant Professor of Otolaryngology
Department of Otorhinolaryngology
Mayo Clinic
200 First Street, SW
Rochester, MN 55905-0001
USA
E-mail: Moore.Eric@mayo.edu

Eugene N. Myers, MD, FACS, FRCS Edin (Hon)
Distinguished Professor and Emeritus Chair
Department of Otolaryngology
University of Pittsburgh, School of Medicine
The Eye & Ear Institute, Suite 519
200 Lothrop Street
Pittsburgh, PA 15213
USA
E-mail: myersen@upmc.edu

Daniel Nuss, MD, FACS
Clinical Professor of Otolaryngology
Chairman, Department of Otolaryngology
Louisiana State University Health Science Center
533 Bolivar Street, Fl 5
New Orleans, LA 70112-1349
USA
E-mail: DNuss@lsuhsc.edu

Christopher J. O'Brien, AM, MB, BS, MS, FRACS
Professor, Director of Cancer Services
Sydney South West Area Health Service
Director, Sydney Head and Neck Cancer Institute
Royal Prince Alfred Hospital
PO Box M142
Missenden Road
Camperdown, NSW 2050
Australia
E-mail: headandneck@email.cs.nsw.gov.au

Kerry D. Olsen, MD
Professor of Otolaryngology
Department of Otorhinolaryngology
Mayo Clinic
200 First Street, SW
Rochester, MN 55905-0001
USA
E-mail: Olsen.Kerry@mayo.edu

Robert L. Peel, MD
Associate Professor
Department of Pathology and Laboratory Medicine
University of Pittsburgh School of Medicine
A616.1 Presbyterian University Hospital
200 Lothrop Street
Pittsburgh, PA 15213
USA
E-mail: peelrl@upmc.edu

Raja R. Seethala, MD
Assistant Professor
Department of Pathology and Laboratory Medicine
University of Pittsburgh School of Medicine
A616.3 Presbyterian University Hospital
200 Lothrop Street
Pittsburgh, PA 15213
USA
E-mail: seethalarr@upmc.edu

Alfred A. Simental Jr, MD
Associate Professor and Chief
Department of Otolaryngology – Head and Neck Surgery
Loma Linda University
11234 Anderson Street, Suite 2586
Loma Linda, CA 92350
USA
E-mail: asimenta@ahs.llumc.edu

Lorna Sneddon, FRCS Edin
Head and Neck Fellow
Sydney Head and Neck Cancer Institute
Royal Prince Alfred Hospital
PO Box M142
Missenden Road
Camperdown, NSW 2050
Australia
E-mail: headandneck@email.cs.nsw.gov.au

Brendan C. Stack Jr, MD, FACS, FACE
Department of Otolaryngology
University of Arkansas for Medical Sciences
4301 W Markham Street, #543
Little Rock, AR 72205-7199
USA
E-mail: bstack@uams.edu

Eberhard Stennert, MD
Professor
Jean-Uhrmacher-Institut,
Geibelstrasse 29–31
50931 Cologne
Germany
E-mail: eberhard.stennert@uni-koeln.de

James Y. Suen, MD, FACS
Professor and Chair
Department of Otolaryngology
University of Arkansas for Medical Sciences
4301 W Markham Street, #543
Little Rock, AR 72205-7199
USA
E-mail: suenjamesy@uams.edu

Yoav P. Talmi, MD, FACS
Clinical Professor and Chief
Department of Otolaryngology
Head and Neck Service
The Chaim Sheba Medical Center
Tel Hashomer, 52621
Israel
E-mail: yoav.talmi@sheba.health.gov.il

Rohan R. Walvekar, MD, DNB(ENT), DORL
Clinical Assistant Professor
Department of Otolaryngology
University of Pittsburgh School of Medicine
200 Lothrop Street
The Eye & Ear Institute, Suite 500
Pittsburgh, PA 15213
USA
E-mail: walvekarrr@upmc.edu

Steven J. Wang, MD, FACS
Assistant Professor
Otolaryngology Section Chief, San Francisco VA Medical Center
Department of Otolaryngology – Head and Neck Surgery
University of California, San Francisco
400 Parnassus Avenue, Suite A-730
San Francisco, CA 94143-0342
USA
E-mail: swang@ohns.ucsf.edu

Grace C.H. Yang, MD, FIAC
Professor of Clinical Pathology and Laboratory Medicine
Papanicolaou Cytology Laboratory
New York Presbyterian Hospital-Weill Cornell Medical Center
525 East 68 St., F-766D
New York, NY 10021
USA
E-Mail: gry2001@med.cornell.edu

Chapter 1

Anatomy, Function, and Evaluation of the Salivary Glands

1

F. Christopher Holsinger and Dana T. Bui

Contents

Core Features

- Embryology of the salivary glands and their associated structures
- Detailed anatomy of the parotid, submandibular, sublingual, and minor salivary glands, including nervous innervation, arterial supply, and venous and lymphatic drainage
- Histology and organization of the acini and duct systems within the salivary glands
- Physiology and function of the glands with respect to the production of saliva
- Considerations when taking a patient's history
- The intra- and extraoral aspects of inspection and palpation during a physical examination

Introduction

The human salivary gland system can be divided into two distinct exocrine groups. The *major salivary glands* include the paired parotid, submandibular, and sublingual glands. Additionally, the mucosa of the upper aerodigestive tract is lined by hundreds of small, *minor salivary glands*. The major function of the salivary glands is to secrete saliva, which plays a significant role in lubrication, digestion, immunity, and the overall maintenance of homeostasis within the human body.

Developmental Anatomy

In the last 15 years, significant improvement has been made in our understanding of the molecular basis of salivary gland development, supplanting and expanding classical teaching in the embryology and developmental anatomy.

Early work suggests that development of the salivary glands begins during the sixth to eighth embryonic week when oral ectodermal outpouchings extend into the adjacent mesoderm and serve as the site of origin for major salivary gland growth. The development of major salivary glands is thought to consist of three main stages [1, 8]. The first stage is marked by the presence of a primordial anlage (from the German verb *anlagen*, meaning to lay a foundation or to prepare) and the formation of branched duct buds due to repeated epithelial cleft and bud development. Ciliated epithelial cells form the lining of the lumina, while external surfaces are lined by ectodermal myoepithelial cells [2]. The early appearance of lobules and duct canalization occur during the second stage. Primitive acini and distal duct regions, both containing myoepithelial cells, form within the seventh month of embryonic life. The third stage is marked by maturation of the acini and intercalated ducts, as well as the diminishing prominence of interstitial connective tissue.

The first of the glands to appear, during the sixth gestational week, is the primordial *parotid gland*. It develops from the posterior stomodeum, which laterally elongates into solid cords across the developing masseter muscle. The cords then canalize to form ducts, and acini are formed at the distal ends. A capsule formed from the ambient mesenchyme surrounds the gland and associated lymph nodes [14]. Small buds appear in the floor of the mouth lateral to the tongue during the sixth week of embryonic life and extend posteriorly around the mylohyoid muscle into the submandibular triangle. These buds eventually develop into the *submandibular glands*. A capsule from the surrounding mesenchyme is fully developed around the gland by the third gestational month [8]. During the ninth embryonic month, the *sublingual gland* anlage is formed from multiple endodermal epithelial buds in the paralingual sulcus of the floor of the mouth. Absence of a capsule is due to infiltration of the glands by sublingual connective tissue. Intraglandular lymph nodes and major ducts also do not generally develop within sublingual glands. Upper respiratory ectoderm gives rise to simple tubuloacinar units. They develop into the *minor salivary glands* during the 12th intrauterine week [17].

Recent work using murine models has shown the complexity of the underlying molecular events orchestrating classical embryological findings. Development of the salivary glands is an example of branching morphogenesis, a process fundamental to many developing organs, including lung, mammary gland, pancreas, and kidney [12]. Branching organs develop a complex arborization and morphology through a program of repetitive, self-similar branching forks to create new epithelial outgrowths. The developmental growth of a multicellular organ such as a salivary gland is based on a set of interdependent mechanisms and signaling pathways. The resulting expression of these pathways is dynamic, organized, and changes correspondingly with each developmental stage. The sonic hedgehog (Shh) signaling plays an essential role during craniofacial development [13]. Other pathways, including the fibroblast growth factor family of receptors and associated ligands, have also been shown to play a crucial role [28].

Parotid Gland

Anatomy

The paired parotid glands are the largest of the major salivary glands and weigh, on average, 15–30 g. Located in the preauricular region and along the posterior surface of the mandible, each parotid gland is divided by the facial nerve into a superficial lobe and a deep lobe (Fig. 1.1). The *superficial lobe*, overlying the lateral surface of the masseter, is defined as the part of the gland lateral to the facial nerve. The *deep lobe* is medial to the facial nerve and located between the mastoid process of the temporal

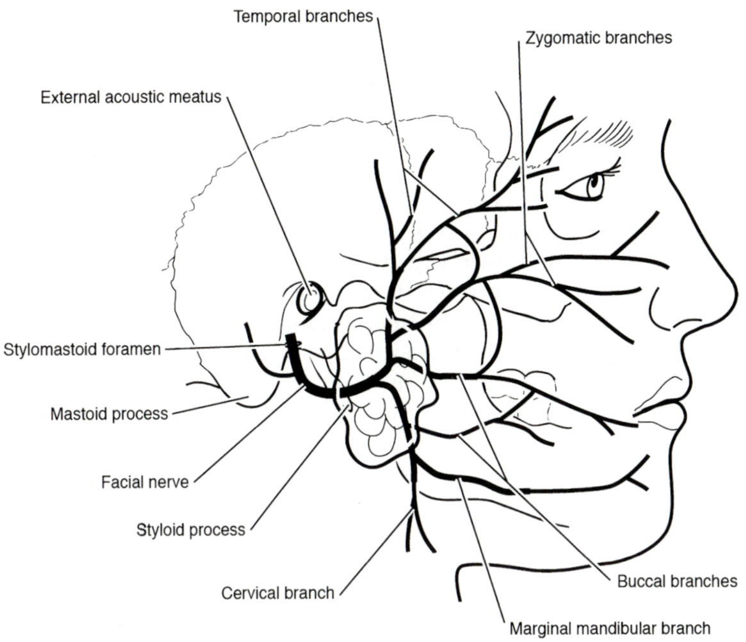

Fig. 1.1: The parotid gland and the facial nerve branching

bone and the ramus of the mandible. Most benign neoplasms are found within the superficial lobe and can be removed by a superficial parotidectomy. Tumors arising in the deep lobe of the parotid gland can grow and extend laterally, displacing the overlying superficial lobe without direct involvement. These parapharyngeal tumors can grow into "dumbbell-shaped" tumors, because their growth is directed through the stylomandibular tunnel [5].

The parotid gland is bounded superiorly by the zygomatic arch. Inferiorly, the tail of the parotid gland extends down and abuts the anteromedial margin of the sternocleidomastoid muscle. This tail of the parotid gland extends posteriorly over the superior border of the sternocleidomastoid muscle toward the mastoid tip. The deep lobe of the parotid lies within the parapharyngeal space [10].

An *accessory parotid gland* may also be present lying anteriorly over the masseter muscle between the parotid duct and zygoma. Its ducts empty directly into the parotid duct through one tributary. Accessory glandular tissue is histologically distinct from parotid tissue in that it may contain mucinous acinar cells in addition to the serous acinar cells [6].

Fascia

The deep cervical fascia continues superiorly to form the parotid fascia, which is split into superficial and deep layers to enclose the parotid gland. The thicker superficial fascia is extended superiorly from the masseter and sternocleidomastoid muscles to the zygomatic arch. The deep layer extends to the *stylomandibular ligament (or membrane)*, which separates the superficial and deep lobes of the parotid gland. The stylomandibular ligament is an important surgical landmark when considering the resection of deep lobe tumors. In fact, stylomandibular tenotomy [22] can be a crucial maneuver in providing exposure for en bloc resections of deep-lobe parotid or other parapharyngeal space tumors. The parotid fascia forms a dense inelastic capsule and, because it also covers the masseter muscle deeply, can sometimes be referred to as the *parotid masseteric fascia.*

Stensen's Duct

The parotid duct, also known as Stensen's duct, secretes a serous saliva into the vestibule of the oral cavity. From the anterior border of the gland, it travels parallel to the zygoma, approximately 1 cm below it, in an anterior direction across the masseter muscle. It then turns sharply to pierce the buccinator muscle and enters the oral cavity opposite the second upper molar tooth.

Neural Anatomy

The facial nerve (CN VII) exits the skull base via the stylomastoid foramen, which is slightly posterolateral to the styloid process and anteromedial to the mastoid process. Before entering the posterior portion of the parotid gland, three motor branches are given off to innervate the posterior belly of the digastric muscle, the stylohyoid muscle, and the postauricular muscles.

The main trunk of the facial nerve then passes through the parotid gland and, at the *pes anserinus* (Latin: goose's foot), divides into the temporofacial and lower cervicofacial divisions approximately 1.3 cm from the stylomastoid foramen. The upper *temporofacial division* forms the frontal, temporal, zygomatic, and buccal branches. The lower *cervicofacial division* forms the marginal mandibular and cervical branches. Branches from the major upper and lower branches often anastomose to create the diverse network of midfacial buccal branches.

The *temporal branch* traverses parallel to the superficial temporal vessels across the zygoma to supply the frontal belly of the occipitofrontalis muscle, the orbicularis oculi, the corrugator supercilii, and the anterior and superior auricular muscles. The *zygomatic branch* travels directly over the periosteum of the zygomatic arch to innervate the zygomatic, orbital, and infraorbital muscles. The *buccal branch* travels with Stensen's duct anteriorly over the masseter muscle to supply the buccinator, upper lip, and nostril muscles. Buccal branches can either arise from the upper temporofacial or the lower cervicofacial division. The *marginal mandibular branch* courses along the inferior border of the parotid gland to innervate the lower lip and chin muscles. It lies superficial to the posterior facial vein and retromandibular veins in the plane of the deep cervical fascia directly beneath the platysma muscle. The *cervical branch* supplies the platysma muscle. Like the marginal mandibular branch, it is located within the plane of the deep cervical fascia direct underneath the platysma.

Small connections can exist among the temporal, zygomatic, and buccal branches, and anatomic variations in facial nerve branching patterns occur commonly. Each terminal branch can be located distally and traced retrograde across the parotid gland to the main trunk of the facial nerve. The facial nerve can also be identified at the stylomastoid foramen by performing a mastoidectomy if identification by the usual landmarks is not possible [5, 10, 23].

The great auricular nerve is a sensory branch of the cervical plexus, particularly C2 and C3, and innervates the posterior portion of the pinna and the lobule. The nerve parallels the external jugular vein along the lateral surface of the sternocleidomastoid muscle to the tail of the parotid gland, where it splits into anterior and posterior branches. The great auricular nerve is often injured during parotidectomy, which can result in long-term sensory loss in the lobule. Harvesting of this nerve can be used for facial nerve grafting in certain cases.

The auriculotemporal nerve is a branch of the mandibular nerve, the third inferior subdivision of the trigeminal nerve (V_3). After exiting the foramen ovale, the nerve traverses superiorly to innervate the skin and scalp immediately anterior to the ear. Its course runs parallel to the superficial temporal vessels and anterior to the external auditory canal.

Autonomic Nerve Innervation

The glossopharyngeal nerve (CN IX) provides visceral secretory innervation to the parotid gland. The nerve carries preganglionic parasympathetic fibers from the inferior salivatory nucleus in the medulla through the jugular foramen (Fig. 1.2). Distal to the inferior ganglion, a small branch of CN IX (*Jacobsen's nerve*) reenters the skull through the inferior tympanic canaliculus and into the middle ear to form the *tympanic plexus*. The preganglionic fibers then course along as the lesser petrosal nerve into the middle cranial fossa and out the foramen ovale to synapse in the *otic ganglion*. Postganglionic parasympathetic fibers exit the otic ganglion beneath the mandibular nerve to join the auriculotemporal nerve in the infratemporal fossa. These fibers innervate the parotid gland for the secretion of saliva. Postganglionic sympathetic fibers innervate salivary glands, sweat glands, and cutaneous blood vessels through the external carotid plexus from the *superior cervical ganglion*. Acetylcholine serves as the neurotransmitter for both postganglionic sympathetic and parasympathetic fibers [10]. This physiologic coincidence allows for the development of "gustatory sweating" (also known as Frey's syndrome)

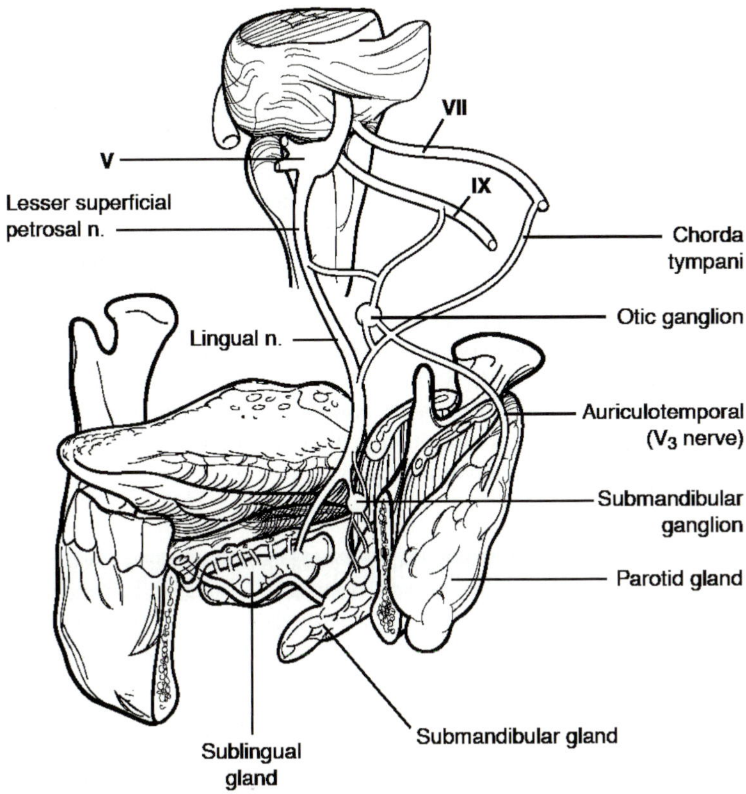

Fig. 1.2: Parasympathetic supply to the major salivary glands

following parotidectomy [19, 26]. Patients develop sweating and flushing of the skin overlying the parotid region during eating due to aberrant autonomic reinnervation of the sweat glands by the regenerating parasympathetic fibers from any residual parotid gland. Frey's syndrome may occur in as many as 25–60% of patients postoperatively. The risk for Frey's syndrome can be minimized first by complete and meticulous superficial parotidectomy. Second, by developing skin flaps of appropriate thickness, exposed apocrine glands of the skin are protected from ingrowth and stimulation by the severed branches of the auriculotemporal nerve and their parasympathetic stimulation during meals. There are numerous nonsurgical and surgical treatments for persistent Frey's syndrome following parotidectomy (see Chapter 5, Treatment of Frey's Syndrome).

Arterial Supply

The blood supply to the parotid gland is from branches of the *external carotid artery*, which courses superiorly from the carotid bifurcation and parallel to the mandible under the posterior belly of the digastric muscle. The artery then travels medial to the parotid gland and splits into two terminal branches. The *superficial temporal artery* runs superiorly from the superior portion of the parotid gland to the scalp within the superior pretragal region. The *maxillary artery* leaves the medial portion of the parotid and supplies the infratemporal fossa and the pterygopalatine fossa. During radical parotidectomy, this vessel must be controlled especially when marginal or segmental mandibulectomy is required. The *transverse facial artery* branches off the superficial temporal artery and runs anteriorly between the zygoma and parotid duct to supply the parotid gland, parotid duct, and the masseter muscle [10].

Venous Drainage

The *retromandibular vein*, formed by the union of the maxillary vein and the superficial temporal vein, runs through the parotid gland just deep to the facial nerve to join the external jugular vein. There is substantial variation in the surgical anatomy of the retromandibular vein, which may bifurcate into an anterior and posterior branch. The *anterior branch* can unite with the posterior facial vein, forming the common facial vein. The posterior facial *vein* lies immediately deep to the marginal mandibular branch of the facial nerve and is therefore often used as a landmark for identification of the nerve branch, especially at the antegonial notch of the mandible where the nerve dips inferiorly [3]. The *posterior branch of the retromandibular vein* may combine with the post-auricular vein above the sternocleidomastoid muscle and drain into the external jugular vein.

Lymphatic Drainage

Contrary to the lymphatic drainage of the other salivary glands, there is a high density of lymph nodes within and around the parotid gland. The parotid is the only salivary gland with two nodal layers, both of which drain into the superficial and deep cervical lymph systems. Approximately 90% of the nodes are located in the superficial layer between the glandular tissue and its capsule. The parotid gland, external auditory canal, pinna, scalp, eyelids, and lacrimal glands are all drained by these superficial nodes. The deep layer of nodes drains the gland, external auditory canal, middle ear, nasopharynx, and soft palate [7].

Parapharyngeal Space

Tumors of the deep parotid lobe often extend medially into the parapharyngeal space (PPS). This space just posterior to the infratemporal fossa is shaped like an inverted pyramid. The greater cornu of the hyoid bone serves as the apex and the petrous bone of the skull base acts as the pyramidal base. The PPS is bound medially by the *lateral pharyngeal wall*, which consists of the superior constrictor muscles, the buccopharyngeal fascia and the tensor veli palatine. The ramus of the mandible and the medial pterygoid muscle make up the lateral border. The parapharyngeal space is bordered anteriorly by the pterygoid fascia and the pterygomandibular raphe. The posterior border is lined by the carotid sheath and prevertebral fascia.

A line from the styloid process to the medial portion of the medial pterygoid plate divides the parapharyngeal space into two compartments. The *prestyloid compartment* contains the deep lobe of the parotid gland, minor salivary glands, as well as neurovascular structures, including the internal maxillary artery, ascending pharyngeal artery, the inferior alveolar nerve, the lingual nerve, and the auriculotemporal nerve. The *poststyloid compartment* contains the internal jugular vein, carotid artery and vagus nerve within the carotid sheath, as well as cranial nerves IX, X, XI, and XII and the cervical sympathetic chain. Neurogenic tumors or paragangliomas from the cervical sympathetics or cranial nerves can thus arise in this compartment [4].

Submandibular Gland

Anatomy

The submandibular gland (in older texts, this gland was sometimes referred to as "the submaxillary gland") is the second largest major salivary gland and weighs 7–16 g (Fig. 1.3). The gland is located in the *submandibular triangle*, which has a superior boundary formed by the inferior edge of the mandible and inferior boundaries formed by the anterior and posterior bellies of the digastric muscle. Also lying within the triangle are the submandibular lymph nodes, facial artery and vein, mylohyoid muscle, and the lingual, hypoglossal, and mylohyoid nerves. Most of the submandibular gland lies posterolateral to the mylohyoid muscle. During neck dissection or submandibular gland excision, this mylohyoid muscle must be gently retracted anteriorly to expose the lingual nerve and submandibular ganglion. Often, smaller, tongue-like projections of the gland follow the duct, as it ascends toward the oral cavity, deep to the mylohyoid muscle [29]. However, these projections should be distinguished from the sublingual gland which lies superior to the mylohyloid muscle. (For more detail, see Chapter 21, Management of Tumors of the Submandibular and Sublingual Glands.)

Fascia

The middle layer of the deep cervical fascia encloses the submandibular gland. This fascia is clinically relevant be-

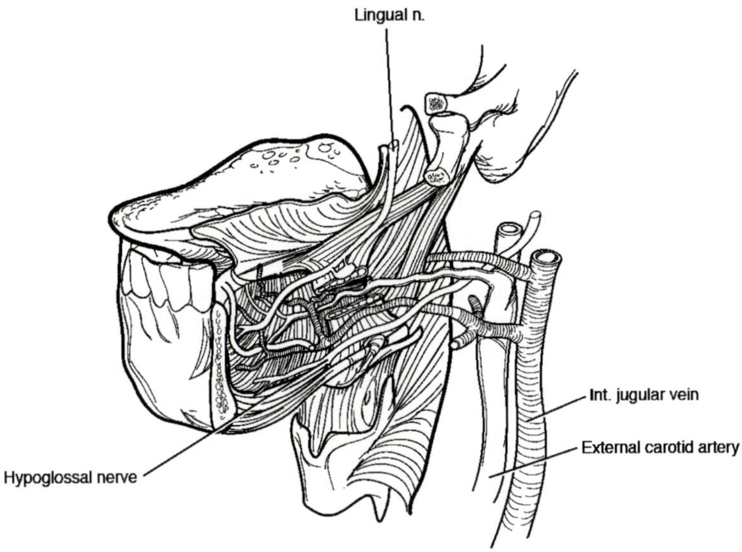

Fig. 1.3: The submandibular gland and important anatomic landmarks

cause the marginal mandibular branch of the facial nerve is superficial to it, and care must be taken to preserve the nerve during surgery in the submandibular region. Thus, division of the submandibular gland fascia, when oncologically appropriate, is a reliable method of preserving and protecting the marginal mandibular branch of the facial nerve during neck dissection and/or submandibular gland resection.

Wharton's Duct

The submandibular gland has both mucous and serous cells that empty into ductules, which in turn empty into the *submandibular duct*. The duct exits anteriorly from the sublingual aspect of the gland, coursing deep to the lingual nerve and medial to the sublingual gland. It eventually forms Wharton's duct between the hyoglossus and mylohyoid muscles on the genioglossus muscle. Wharton's duct, the main excretory duct of the submandibular gland, is approximately 4–5 cm long, running superior to the hypoglossal nerve while inferior to the lingual nerve. It empties lateral to the lingual frenulum through a papilla in the floor of the mouth behind the lower incisor tooth. The openings for the sublingual gland, or the *sublingual caruncles*, are located near the midline of the sublingual fold in the ventral tongue.

Neural Anatomy

Both the submandibular and the sublingual glands are innervated by the secretomotor fibers of the facial nerve (CN VII). Parasympathetic innervation from the *superior salivatory nucleus* in the pons passes through the nervus intermedius and into the internal auditory canal to join the facial nerve. The fibers are next conveyed by the *chorda tympani nerve* in the mastoid segment of CN VII, which travels through the middle ear and petrotympanic fissure to the infratemporal fossa. The *lingual nerve*, a branch of the marginal mandibular division of the fifth cranial nerve (CN V), then carries the presynaptic fibers to the *submandibular ganglion*. The postsynaptic nerve leaves the ganglion to innervate both the submandibular and sublingual glands to secrete watery saliva. As in the parotid gland, sympathetic innervation from the *superior cervical ganglion* accompanies the lingual artery to the submandibular tissue and causes glandular production of mucoid saliva instead [5].

The *lingual nerve* branches off the mandibular division of the trigeminal nerve (V_3) in the infratemporal fossa to supply general sensation and taste to the anterior two thirds of the tongue. The nerve courses laterally between the medial pterygoid muscle and ramus of the mandible and enters the oral cavity at the lower third molar to then travel across the hyoglossus along the floor of the mouth in a submucosal plane. Beneath the mandible, a small motor nerve branches off and travels posteriorly from the lingual nerve to innervate the mylohyoid muscle. These fibers are usually sacrificed during surgical removal of the submandibular gland. Parasympathetic fibers are carried via the lingual nerve to the submandibular ganglion, and postsynaptic fibers exit along the course of the submandibular duct to innervate the gland.

The hypoglossal nerve (CN XII) supplies motor innervation to all extrinsic and intrinsic muscles of the tongue except for the palatoglossus muscle. From the hypoglossal canal at the base of the skull, the nerve is pulled inferiorly during embryonic development down into the neck by the occipital branch of the external carotid artery. From here, the hypoglossal nerve travels just deep to the posterior belly of the digastric muscle and common tendon until it reaches the submandibular triangle. Here CN XII lies deep in the triangle covered by a thin layer of fascia. Its location is anterior, deep and medial relative to the submandibular gland. Typically the nerve has a close relationship to the anterior belly of the digastric muscle. It then ascends anterior to the lingual nerve and its genu deep to the mylohyoid muscle. Extreme care should be taken to preserve this important nerve during head and neck surgery.

Arterial Supply

Both the submandibular and sublingual glands are supplied by the *submental* and *sublingual arteries*, branches of the lingual and facial arteries. The *facial artery*, the tortuous branch of the external carotid artery, is the main arterial blood supply of the submandibular gland. It runs medial to the posterior belly of the digastric muscle and then hooks over to course superiorly deep to the gland. The artery exits at the superior border of the gland and the inferior aspect of the mandible known as the *facial notch*. It then runs superiorly and adjacent to the inferior branches of the facial nerve into the face. During submandibular gland resection, the artery must be sacrificed twice, first at the inferior border of the mandible and again just superior to the posterior belly of the digastric muscle. The *lingual artery* branches inferior to or with the facial artery off the external carotid artery. It runs deep to the digastric muscle along the lateral surface of the middle constrictor and then courses anterior and medial to the hyoglossus muscle.

Venous Drainage

The submandibular gland is mainly drained by the *anterior facial vein*, which is in close approximation to the facial artery as it runs inferiorly and posteriorly from the face to the inferior aspect of the mandible. Because it lies just deep to the marginal mandibular division of the facial nerve, ligation and superior retraction of the anterior facial vein can help preserve this branch of the facial nerve during submandibular gland surgery. It forms extensive anastomoses with the infraorbital and superior ophthalmic veins. The *common facial vein* is formed by the union of the anterior and posterior facial veins over the middle aspect of the gland. The common facial vein then courses lateral to the gland and exits the submandibular triangle to join the internal jugular vein.

Lymphatic Drainage

The prevascular and postvascular lymph nodes draining the submandibular gland are located between the gland and its fascia, but are not embedded in the glandular tissue. They lie in close approximation to the facial artery and vein at the superior aspect of the gland and empty into the deep cervical and jugular chains. These nodes are frequently associated with cancers in the oral cavity, especially in the buccal mucosa and the floor of the mouth. Thus, when ligating the facial artery and its associated plexus of veins, greater care must be taken not only to resect all associated lymphoadipose tissue, but also to preserve the marginal mandibular branch of the facial nerve, which runs in close proximity to these structures.

Sublingual Gland

The smallest of the major salivary glands is the sublingual gland, weighing 2–4 g. Consisting mainly of mucous acinar cells, it lies as a flat structure in a submucosal plane within the anterior floor of the mouth, superior to the mylohyoid muscle and deep to the sublingual folds opposite the lingual frenulum [11]. Lateral to it are the mandible and genioglossus muscle. There is no true fascial capsule surrounding the gland, which is instead covered by oral mucosa on its superior aspect. Several ducts (*of Rivinus*) from the superior portion of the sublingual gland either secrete directly into the floor of mouth, or empty into *Bartholin's duct* that then continues into Wharton's duct.

Both the sympathetic and parasympathetic nervous systems innervate the sublingual gland. The presynaptic parasympathetic (secretomotor) fibers of the *facial nerve* are carried by the chorda tympani nerve to synapse in the submandibular ganglion. Postganglionic fibers then exit the *submandibular ganglion* and join the lingual nerve to supply the sublingual gland. Sympathetic nerves innervating the gland travel from the *cervical ganglion* with the facial artery [5].

Blood is supplied to the sublingual gland by the *submental* and *sublingual arteries*, branches of the lingual and facial arteries, respectively. The venous drainage parallels the corresponding arterial supply. The sublingual gland is mainly drained by the submandibular lymph nodes.

Ranulas are cysts or mucoceles of the sublingual gland, and they can exist either simply within the sublingual space or plunging posteriorly to the mylohyoid muscle into the neck. A simple ranula will most commonly present as a bluish, nontender mass in the floor of the mouth and may either be a retention cyst or an extravasation pseudocyst. A plunging ranula will present as a soft, painless cervical mass and is always an extravasation pseudocyst (see Chapter 10, Management of Mucocele and Ranula).

Minor Salivary Glands

About 600 to 1,000 minor salivary glands, ranging in size from 1 to 5 mm, line the oral cavity and oropharynx. The greatest number of these glands are in the lips, tongue, buccal mucosa, and palate, although they can also be found along the tonsils, supraglottis, and paranasal sinuses. Each gland has a single duct which secretes, directly into the oral cavity, saliva which can be either serous, mucous, or mixed.

Postganglionic parasympathetic innervation arises mainly from the *lingual nerve*. The palatine nerves, however, exit the sphenopalatine ganglion to innervate the superior palatal glands. The oral cavity region itself determines the blood supply and venous and lymphatic drainage of the glands. Any of these sites can also be the source of glandular tumors [11].

Histology

All glands in general are derived from epithelial cells and consist of *parenchyma* (the secretory unit and associated ducts) and *stroma* (the surrounding connective tissue that penetrates and divides the gland into lobules). Secretory products are synthesized intracellularly and subsequently released from secretory granules by various mechanisms. Glands are usually classified into two main groups. *Endocrine glands* contain no ducts, and the secretory products are released directly into the bloodstream or lymphatic system. In contrast, *exocrine glands* secrete their products through a duct system that connects them to the adjacent external or internal epithelial surfaces. Salivary glands are classified as exocrine glands that secrete saliva through ducts from a flask-like, blind-ended secretory structure called *the salivary acinus.*

The acinus itself can be divided into three main types. *Serous acini* in salivary glands are roughly spherical and release via exocytosis a watery protein secretion that is minimally glycosylated or nonglycosylated from secretory (or zymogen) granules. The acinar cells comprising the acinus are pyramidal, with basally located nuclei surrounded by dense cytoplasm and secretory granules that are most abundant in the apex. *Mucinous acini* store a viscous, slimy glycoprotein (*mucin*) within secretory granules that become hydrated when released to form *mucus.* Mucinous acinar cells are commonly simple columnar cells with flattened, basally situated nuclei and water-soluble granules that make the intracellular cytoplasm appear clear. *Mixed*, or *seromucous, acini* contain components of both types, but one type of secretory unit may dominate. Mixed secretory units are commonly observed as serous *demilunes* (or half-moons) capping mucinous acini.

Between the epithelial cells and basal lamina of the acinus, flat *myoepithelial cells* (or basket cells) form a latticework and possess cytoplasmic filaments on their basal side to aid in contraction, and thus forced secretion, of the acinus. Myoepithelial cells are also observed around intercalated ducts, but here they are more spindle shaped [16].

Electrolyte modification and transportation of saliva are carried out by the different segments of the salivary gland's duct system (Fig. 1.4). The acini first secrete through small canaliculi into the intercalated ducts, which in turn empty into striated ducts within the glandular lobule. The intercalated duct is comprised of an irregular myoepithelial cell layer lined with squamous or low cuboidal epithelium. Bicarbonate is secreted into while chloride is absorbed from the acinar product within the intercalated duct segment. Striated ducts have distinguishing basal striations due to membrane invagination and mitochondria and are lined by a simple columnar

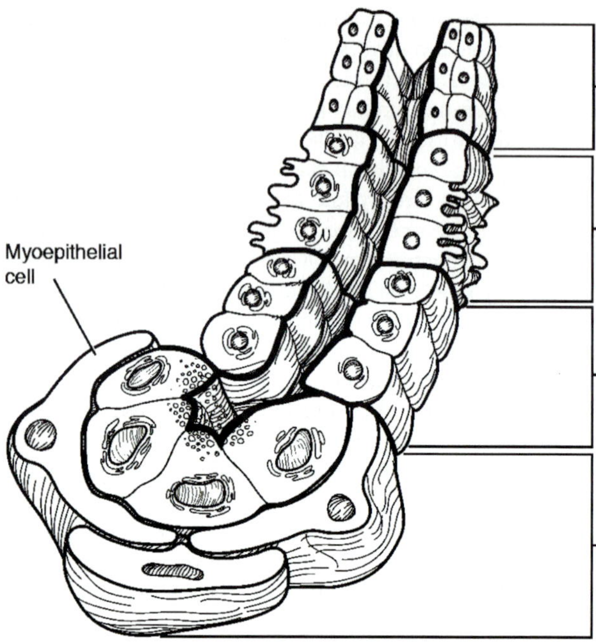

Fig. 1.4: Functional histology of the salivon

epithelium. These ducts are involved with the reabsorption of sodium from the primary secretion and the concomitant secretion of potassium into the product. The abundant presence of mitochondria is necessary for the ducts' transport of both water and electrolytes. The acinus, intercalated duct, and striated duct are collectively known as a single secretory unit called a *salivon* [15].

The next segment of the duct system is marked by the appearance of the interlobular excretory ducts within the connective tissue of the glandular septae. The epithelial lining is comprised of sparse goblet cells interspersed among the pseudostratified columnar cells. As the diameter of the duct increases, the composition of the epithelial lining transitions to stratified columnar, and then to nonkeratinized stratified squamous cells, within the oral cavity [16].

The arterial blood flow received by the salivary glands is high relative to their weight and is opposite the flow of saliva within the duct system. The acini and ductules are supplied by separate parallel capillary beds. The high permeability of these vessels permits rapid transfer of molecules across their basement membranes. The high volume of saliva produced by the salivary glands relative to their weight is partly due to the high blood flow rate through the glandular tissue.

The serous acini that make up the *parotid gland* are roughly spherical, and they are comprised of pyramidal epithelial cells surrounded by a distinct basement membrane. Merocrine secretion by the epithelial cells releases a secretory mixture containing amylase, lysozyme, an IgA secretory piece, and lactoferrin into the central lumen of the acinus. The main excretory duct is also known as *Stensen's duct* and empties into the oral cavity opposite the second upper molar tooth.

The *submandibular gland* is classified as a mixed gland that is predominantly serous with tubular acini. The majority of acinar cells are serous with very granular eosinophilic cytoplasm. Only approximately 10% of the acini are mucinous, with large, triangular acinar cells containing central nuclei and clear cytoplasmic mucin vacuoles ranging in size. The mucinous cells are capped by demilunes, which are crescent-shaped formations of serous cells. The intercalated ducts of the submandibular gland are longer than those of the parotid gland, while striated ducts are shorter by comparison. *Wharton's duct* serves as the main excretory duct and empties into the floor of the mouth.

Like the submandibular gland, the *sublingual gland* has mixed acini with observable serous demilunes within the glandular tissue. Unlike the submandibular gland, however, the sublingual gland is predominantly mucinous. The main duct empties into the submandibular duct and is also known as *Bartholin's duct*. Several smaller ducts (*of Rivinus*) also directly secrete into the floor of the mouth.

The *minor salivary glands* are found throughout the oral cavity, with the greatest density in the buccal and labial mucosa, the posterior hard palate, and tongue base. They are not as often observed, however, in the attached gingiva and closely associated anterior hard palatal mucosa. The majority of these glands are either mucinous or seromucinous, except for the serous *Ebner's glands* on the posterior aspect of the tongue. These deep posterior salivary glands of the tongue are also marked by the presence of ciliated cells, especially within the distal segments of the excretory ducts. The minor salivary gland duct system is simpler than that of the major salivary glands, where the intercalated ducts are longer and the striated ducts are either less developed or not present [15].

Physiology of Salivary Glands

Saliva production, the main function of the salivary glands, is crucial in the processes of digestion, lubrication, and protection in the body. Saliva is actively produced in high volumes relative to the mass of the salivary glands, and it is almost completely controlled extrinsically by both the parasympathetic and sympathetic divisions of the autonomic nervous system.

Saliva plays a crucial role in the digestion of carbohydrates and fats through two main enzymes. *Ptyalin* is an α-amylase in saliva that cleaves the internal α-1,4-glycosidic bonds of starches to yield maltose, maltotriose, and α-limit dextrins. This enzyme functions at an optimal pH of 7, but rapidly denatures when exposed to a pH less than 4, such as when in contact with the acidic secretions of the stomach. Up to 75% of the carbohydrate content in a meal, however, is broken down by the enzyme within the stomach. This is due to the fact that a significant portion of an ingested meal remains unmixed within the oral region, and thus there is a delay in the mixture of gastric juices with the food bolus. Starch digestion is not slowed in the absence of ptyalin because pancreatic amylase is identical to salivary amylase and is thus able to break down all carbohydrates when in the small intestine. The salivary glands of the tongue produce *lingual lipase*, which functions to break down triglycerides. Unlike ptyalin, this enzyme is functional within the acidic stomach and proximal duodenum because it is optimally active at a low pH. Saliva also serves to dissolve and transport food particles away from taste buds to increase taste sensitivity.

The mucus constituent of saliva facilitates the lubrication of food particles during the act of chewing, which serves to mix the food with saliva. Lubrication eases the processes of swallowing and of the bolus traveling down the esophagus. Salivary lubrication is also crucial for speech.

The antibacterial properties of saliva are due to its many protective organic constituents. The binding glycoprotein for immunoglobulin A (IgA), known as the *secretory piece*, forms a complex with IgA that is immunologically active against viruses and bacteria. *Lysozyme* causes bacterial agglutination and autolysin activation to degrade bacterial cell walls. *Lactoferrin* inhibits the growth of bacteria that need iron by chelating with the element. Saliva also serves as a protective buffer for the mouth by diluting harmful substances and lowering the temperature of solutions that are too hot. It washes out foul-tasting substances from the mouth and neutralizes gastric juice to protect the oral cavity and esophagus. *Xerostomia*, or dry mouth, due to lack of salivation, can lead to chronic buccal mucosal infections or dental caries.

Comprised of both inorganic and organic compounds, saliva is distinguished by its high volume compared to salivary gland weight, high potassium concentration, and low osmolarity (Fig. 1.5). The large relative volume of saliva production is due to its high secretion rate, which can go up to 1 ml per gram of salivary gland per minute. Saliva is mostly hypotonic to plasma, but its osmolarity increases with increasing rate of secretion, and at its highest rate saliva approaches isotonicity. The concentration of electrolytes in saliva also changes with varying secretion rates.

Within the salivary gland, potassium (K^+) concentration is always high while sodium (Na^+) concentration is low compared to that found in plasma. With increasing flow rates, however, Na^+ concentration increases, while K^+ concentration initially decreases slightly and then levels off to a constant level. Chloride (Cl^-) concentrations follow the same general pattern as Na^+ concentrations. In other words, Na^+ and Cl^- are generally secreted and then slowly reabsorbed along the course of the salivary system, from acinus to duct. The salivary concentration of bicarbonate (HCO_3^-) is hypertonic compared to in plasma except at lower rates of secretion.

Initially within the salivon, the acini first produce a primary secretion that is relatively isotonic to plasma. As the saliva travels through the ducts, Na^+ and Cl^- are

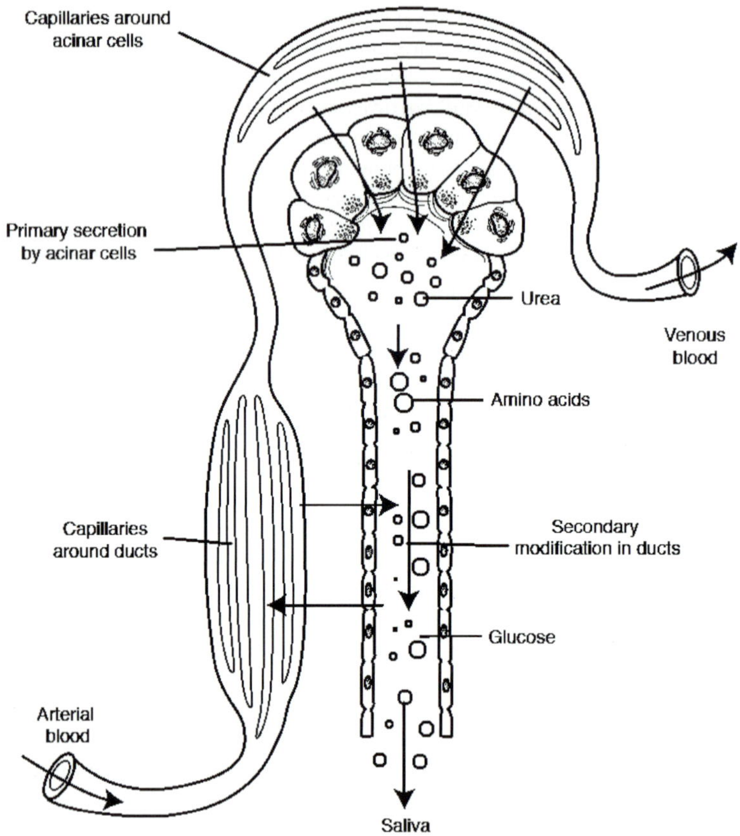

Fig. 1.5: Electrolyte secretion by the acinar and ductal cells

reabsorbed, while K^+ and HCO_3^- are secreted into the fluid. Less time is available for the movement of these electrolytes when the flow rate of saliva is higher. At high flow rates, therefore, plasma and saliva are similar in concentration. At lower secretion rates, K^+ concentration is higher in the saliva, while Na^+ and Cl^- concentrations are significantly lower. Bicarbonate concentrates remains fairly hypertonic relative to in plasma even with higher flow rates due to its secretory stimulation by most salivary gland agonists. Saliva is mostly hypotonic to plasma due to the fact that reabsorption of Na^+ and Cl^- is greater than the secretion of K^+ and HCO_3^- within the salivary ducts.

Several organic compounds present in saliva have already been discussed: α-amylase, lingual lipase, mucus, lysozymes, glycoproteins, lactoferrin, and the IgA secretory piece. Saliva is also comprised of the organic *blood group antigens* A, B, AB, and O. *Kallikrein* is secreted by the salivary glands during increased metabolic activity. Kallikrein enzymatically converts plasma protein into bradykinin, a vasodilator, in order to increase blood flow to the glands. Saliva contains approximately one tenth the total amount of protein as that found in plasma.

The secretion, blood flow, and growth of salivary glands are mostly controlled by both branches of the autonomic nervous system. Even though the parasympathetic nervous system has more influence on the secretion rate of the salivary glands than the sympathetic system, secretion is *stimulated* by both branches.

Parasympathetic innervation of the major salivary glands follows branches of the facial and glossopharyngeal nerves. Parasympathetic stimulation activates both acinar activity and ductal transport mechanisms, leading to glandular vasodilation as well as myoepithelial cell contraction. *Acetylcholine* (ACh) serves as the parasympathetic neurotransmitter that acts on the muscarinic receptors of the salivary glands. The subsequent formation of inositol trisphosphate leads to increased Ca^{2+} concentrations within the cell, released from either intracellular Ca^{2+} stores or from the plasma. This second messenger significantly effects salivary volume secretion. Glandular secretion is sustained by *acetylcholinesterases*, which inhibit the breakdown of ACh. The muscarinic antagonist *atropine*, however, decreases salivation by competing with ACh for the salivary receptor site.

The sympathetic supply to the salivary gland is mainly from the thoracic spinal nerves of the superior cervical ganglion. Like parasympathetic innervation, myoepithelial cell contraction also results. Changes in blood flow, however, are biphasic: vasoconstriction due to α-adrenergic receptor activation is followed by vasodilation due to buildup of vasodilator metabolites. Binding of the neurotransmitter *norepinephrine* to α-adrenergic receptor results in formation of 3',5'-cyclic adenosine monophosphate (cAMP), which then leads to phosphorylation of various proteins and activation of different enzymes. Increases in cAMP result in increased salivary enzyme and mucus content.

Within saliva, K^+ concentrations increase while Na^+ concentrations decrease in the presence of antidiuretic hormone (ADH) or aldosterone. Unlike other digestive glands, however, these two hormones do not affect salivary gland secretion rate.

About 1 l of saliva is secreted by a normal adult each day. During unstimulated salivation, 69% of saliva is contributed by the submandibular glands, 26% by the parotid, and 5% by the sublingual glands. The relative amounts supplied by the parotid and submandibular glands, however, are switched during stimulation, where two thirds of secretion is then from the parotid gland. Of total flow, 7–8% is due to the minor salivary glands regardless of stimulation. The presence of food in the mouth, the act of chewing, and nausea all stimulate salivation, while sleep, fatigue, dehydration, and fear inhibit it. Salivary secretion rates are not dependent on age, and flow rates remain constant despite the degeneration of acinar cells during the aging process. Medication side effects or systemic disease are more likely to be responsible for hypofunction of salivary glands in elderly patients [15, 17].

Evaluation of the Salivary Glands

Symptoms indicative of salivary gland disorders are limited in number and generally nonspecific. Patients usually complain of swelling, pain, xerostomia, foul taste, and sometimes *sialorrhea*, or excessive salivation. Despite the prevalence of modern technology in the identification of salivary gland disorders, a detailed history and thorough physical examination still play significant roles in the clinical diagnosis of the patient, and great care should be taken during these initial steps of evaluation.

History

When taking a patient's history, the practiced skills of attentive listening and patience are required for subsequent diagnosis and proper treatment most fitting to the patient's expectations and needs. The medical profile of the patient can provide helpful clues to the current condition of the salivary glands, for dysfunction of these glands is often associated with certain systemic disorders such as diabetes mellitus, arteriosclerosis, hormonal imbalances, and neurologic disorders. Either xerostomia or sialorrhea, for instance, may be due to factors affecting the medullary salivary center, autonomic outflow pathway, salivary gland function itself, or fluid and electrolyte balance.

The factors of age group and gender are also important, for several diseases are often related to age or gender. The autoimmune disorder known as *Sjögren's syndrome*, for example, is common in menopausal women, while *mumps*, parotid swelling due to paramyxoviral infection, usually occurs in children between the ages of 4 and 10 years.

Drug history of the patient should also be considered, for salivary function is often affected by drug usage. Xerostomia is often due to the use of diuretics and other antihypertensive drugs [9, 18].

A careful dietary and nutrition history should be obtained. Patients who are dehydrated chronically from bulimia or anorexia or during chemotherapy are at risk for parotitis. Swelling and pain during meals followed by a reduction in symptoms after meals may indicate partial ductal stenosis.

Xerostomia is a debilitating consequence of radiation therapy to the head and neck and a history of prior radiation should be sought.

Physical Examination

The superficial location of the salivary glands allows thorough inspection and palpation for a complete physical examination. Initial inspection involves the careful examination of the head and neck regions, both intraorally and extraorally, and should be carried out in a systematic way so as to not miss any crucial signs.

During the initial *extraoral inspection*, the patient should stand three to four feet away and directly facing in front of the examiner. The examiner should inspect symmetry, color, possible pulsation and discharging of sinuses on both sides of the patient. Enlargement of major or minor salivary glands, most commonly the parotid or submandibular, may occur on one or both sides. *Parotitis* typically presents as preauricular swelling, but may not be visible if deep in the parotid tail or within the substance of the gland. *Submandibular swelling* presents just medial and inferior to the angle of the mandible. Salivary gland swelling can generally be differentiated from those of lymphatic origin as being single, larger, and smoother, but the two types are often easily confused. Significant neurologic deficits should be examined as well. Facial nerve paralysis in conjunction with a parotid mass, for example, should remind us of a *malignant* parotid neoplasm, although it does occur rarely with benign neoplasms as well.

In addition to signs of possible asymmetry, discoloration, or pulsation, *intraoral inspection* also includes assessment of the duct orifices and possible obstructions. The proper lighting with a headlight should always be used when inspecting within the oral cavity and pharynx. The openings of Stensen's and Wharton's ducts can be inspected intraorally opposite the second upper molar and at the root of the tongue, respectively. Drying off the mucosa around the ducts with an air blower and then pressing on the corresponding glands will allow the examiner to assess the flow or lack of flow of saliva. Sialolithiasis can sometimes be found by careful intraoral palpation. Dental hygiene and the presence of periodontal disease should also be noted since deficient oral maintenance is a major predisposing factor to various infectious diseases.

Size, consistency, and other qualities of the salivary glands and associated masses can be evaluated through extraoral and intraoral palpation. Bimanual assessment should be performed whenever possible with the palmar aspect of the fingertips.

During *extraoral palpation* of the face and neck, the patient's head is inclined forward to maximally expose the parotid and submandibular gland regions. The examiner may stand in front of or behind the patient. It should be noted that observable salivary or lymphatic gland swellings do not rise with swallowing, while swellings associated with the thyroid gland and larynx do elevate.

Finally, bimanual palpation (extraoral with one hand, introral with the other) must be performed to examine the parotid and submandibular glands. One or two gloved fingers should be inserted within the oral cavity to palpate the glands and main excretory ducts internally, while using the other hand to externally support the head and neck. By rolling the hands over the glands both internally and externally, subtle mass lesions can be identified. In the submandibular gland, lymph nodes extrinsic to the gland can often be distinguished from pathology within the gland itself using this technique. The neck should then also be carefully examined for lymphadenopathy.

Finally, a careful survey of minor salivary gland tissue should be performed, especially in the anterior labial, buccal, and posterior palatal mucosa. Increased salivation from the duct orifices due to pressure externally applied to the glands may indicate inflammation [9, 18]. Finally, rare clinical entities, such as hemangiomas and other vascular anomalies, may be identified by auscultation.

Radiologic and Endoscopic Examination of the Salivary Glands

Although a thorough history and complete physical examination are crucial steps in the diagnosis and eventual treatment of any salivary gland disorder, patients occasionally provide little more than vague complaints of pain and/or swelling. For patients with these unclear symptoms and no physical signs, radiographic diagnostic studies, such as sialography, plain-film radiography, computed tomography, and magnetic resonance imaging, can play in important role in clarifying the etiology of such nonspecific symptoms. For patients with known disease, imaging can assist in treatment selection and planning. This final section will provide a brief introduction to these various techniques, which will then be covered in greater detail in subsequent chapters.

Sialography relies on the injection of contrast medium into glandular ducts so that the pathway of salivary flow can be visualized by plain-film radiographs. Correct exposure and positioning is achieved by taking preliminary plain radiographs prior to the injection of a radiopaque medium [9]. The most common indication for sialography is the presence of a salivary calculus, which is a deposit of mostly calcium salts that can block flow of saliva and cause pain, swelling, and inflammation or lead to infection. Patients with calculi usually complain of a recurrent and acute onset of pain and swelling during eating. Often, sialographic examination is unnecessary if the preliminary radiographs detect the calculus beforehand. Other indications for sialography include gradual or chronic glandular enlargement (which can be due to sarcoidosis, infection, sialosis, Sjögren's syndrome, benign lymphoepithelial lesion, or a neoplasm), a clinically palpable mass in one of the glandular regions (possible tumor, cyst, or focal inflammation), recurrent sialadenitis, or dryness of the mouth.

Although conventional sialography can be clinically useful in the diagnosis and the determination of treatment for various salivary disorders, its effectiveness remains arguable while its rate of usage is highly variable [25, 30]. This method should not be performed when the patient has an acute salivary gland infection, has a known sensitivity to iodine-containing compounds, or is anticipating thyroid function tests. Thus, other methods of radiographic diagnosis are currently preferred and have largely replaced sialographic examination.

Computed tomography (CT) is now more widely used to assess the parotid and submandibular glands. The advantage of CT imaging is the two-dimensional view of the salivary glands, which can elucidate relationships to adjacent vital structures as well as to assess the draining cervical lymphatics. The parotid gland has low attenuation due to its high fat content and is therefore easily discernible by CT scanning. The submandibular gland has a lower fat content and higher density compared to the parotid gland and thus has a much higher attenuation, although extrinsic and intrinsic mass differentiation is easier to evaluate. Although stones can be identified, salivary gland inflammation is not generally an indication for CT. While CT is often utilized as a primary screening tool for the detection of parotid and submandibular gland abnormalities, in difficult cases, a higher-sensitivity approach using both CT and sialography (CT-sialography) can be used [24]. Differences between intrinsic and extrinsic parotid gland masses, however, are often difficult to assess especially when present in the parapharyngeal space [27].

Magnetic resonance imaging (MRI) is more often used for assessment of parapharyngeal space abnormalities. MRI provides better contrast resolution, exposes the patient to less harmful radiation, and yields detailed images on several different planes without patient repositioning. This technique therefore is preferred in the evaluation of parapharyngeal space masses, especially in discriminating between deep lobe parotid tumors and other pathology, such as schwannoma and/or glomus vagale. MRI, however, is inferior to CT scanning for the detection of calcifications and early bone erosion. Chronic inflammation of the salivary glands and calculi are not indications for MRI.

Sialendoscopy is a minimally invasive technique that inspects the salivary glands using narrow-diameter, rigid fiberoptic endoscopes [20]. Endoscopic visualization of ductal and glandular pathology provides an excellent alternative to the indirect diagnostic techniques described above. As such, sialendoscopy has opened up a new frontier for both evaluation and treatment of salivary gland disease [21]. Lacrimal probes are used to gently dilate the ductal orifice and then the endoscope is introduced under direct visualization. During lavage of the glandular duct of interest, direct inspection of the duct and hilum of the gland is performed. Thus, in one setting, at the time of diagnosis, treatment and therapy for benign lesions can be performed (see Chapter 6, Sialendoscopy). Through a CO_2-laser papillotomy, sialolithectomy can be easily performed [21]. Pharmacotherapy and laser-ablation can also be performed. Sialendoscopy has also been shown to have a significantly low complication rate and is generally well-tolerated [31]. This relatively new technique has shown much promise in the diagnosis and treatment of chronic obstructive sialadenitis (COS), sialolithiasis, and other obstructive diseases of the salivary glands.

Take Home Messages

- Salivary gland development is the result of branching morphogenesis. Molecular biology is beginning to unravel signaling pathways implicated in both craniofacial development and salivary gland histogenesis, including the sonic hedgehog (Shh) and the fibroblast growth factor family.
- Human saliva is not only important for lubrication in the oral cavity, but plays a crucial role in digestive and protective processes.
- Both visual inspection with optimal lighting and bimanual palpation is crucial in the precise physical examination of the major and minor salivary glands.
- Sialendoscopy is a novel modality for diagnostic evaluation as well as therapeutic intervention for disorders of the salivary glands.

References

1. Arey LB (1974) Developmental anatomy; a textbook and laboratory manual of embryology. Revised 7th ed. W.B. Saunders, Inc., Philadelphia
2. Bernfield M, Banerjee S, Cohn R (1972) Dependence of salivary epithelial morphology and branching morphogenesis upon acid mucopolysaccharide-protein (proteoglycan) at the epithelial surface. J Cell Biol 52:674–689
3. Bhattacharyya N, Varvares M (1999) Anomalous relationship of the facial nerve and the retromandibular vein: a case report. J Oral Maxillofac Surg 57:75–76
4. Carrau RL, Johnson JT, Myers EN (1997) Management of tumors of the parapharyngeal space. Oncology (Williston Park) 11:633–640; discussion 640, 642
5. Davis RA, Anson BJ, Budinger JM, et al. (1956) Surgical anatomy of the facial nerve and parotid gland based upon a study of 350 cervicofacial halves. Surg Gynecol Obstet 102: 385–412
6. Frommer J (1977) The human accessory parotid gland: its incidence, nature, and significance. Oral Surg Oral Med Oral Pathol 43: 671–676
7. Garatea-Crelgo J, Gay-Escoda C, Bermejo B, et al. (1993) Morphological study of the parotid lymph nodes. J Craniomaxillofac Surg 21:207–209
8. Gibson MH (1983) The prenatal human submandibular gland: a histological, histochemical and ultrastructural study. Anat Anz 153:91–105
9. Graamans K, von der Akker HP (1991) History and physical examination. In: Graamans AK (ed) Diagnosis of Salivary Gland Disorders. Kluwer Academic Publishers, Dordrecht, Germany, pp 1-3
10. Grant J (1972) An Atlas of Anatomy, Sixth edn. Williams & Wilkins, Baltimore
11. Hollinshead WH (1982) Anatomy for Surgeons: Volume I, The Head and Neck, Third ed. J.B. Lippincott Company, Philadelphia
12. Jaskoll T, Melnick M (1999) Submandibular gland morphogenesis: stage-specific expression of TGF-alpha/EGF, IGF, TGF-beta, TNF, and IL-6 signal transduction in normal embryonic mice and the phenotypic effects of TGF-beta2, TGF-beta3, and EGF-r null mutations. Anat Rec 256:252–268
13. Jaskoll T, Leo T, Witcher D, et al. (2004) Sonic hedgehog signaling plays an essential role during embryonic salivary gland epithelial branching morphogenesis. Dev Dyn 229: 722–732
14. Johns M (1977) The salivary glands: anatomy & embryology. Otolaryngol Clin North Am 10:261
15. Johnson LR (ed) (2003) Secretion. Elsevier, Amsterdam
16. Junqueria L, Carneiro J (2003) Basic Histology: Text & Atlas., Tenth edn. McGraw-Hill, New York
17. Kontis TC, Johns ME (2001) Anatomy and Physiology of the Salivary Glands. In: Bailey BJ (ed) Head and Neck Surgery – Otolaryngology. Lippincott Williams & Wilkins, Philadelphia
18. Mason D, Chisholm D (1975) Salivary Glands in Health and Disease. WB Saunders, London
19. Myers EN, Conley J (1970) Gustatory sweating after radical neck dissection. Arch Otolaryngol 91:534–542
20. Nahlieli O, Baruchin AM (1997) Sialoendoscopy: three years' experience as a diagnostic and treatment modality. J Oral Maxillofac Surg 55:912–918; discussion 919–920
21. Nahlieli O, Baruchin AM (2000) Long-term experience with endoscopic diagnosis and treatment of salivary gland inflammatory diseases. Laryngoscope 110:988–993
22. Orabi AA, Riad MA, O'Regan MB (2002) Stylomandibular tenotomy in the transcervical removal of large benign parapharyngeal tumours. Br J Oral Maxillofac Surg 40: 313–316
23. Pogrel M, Schmidt B, Ammar A (1996) The relationship of the buccal branch of the facial nerve to the parotid duct. J Oral Maxillofac Surg 54:71–73
24. Quinn HJ Jr. (1976) Symposium: management of tumors of the parotid gland. II. Diagnosis of parotid gland swelling. Laryngoscope 86:22–24
25. Rabinov K, Weber AL (1985) Radiology of the Salivary Glands. G.K. Hall Medical Publishers, Boston
26. Roark DT, Sessions RB, Alford BR (1975) Frey's syndrome-a technical remedy. Ann Otol Rhinol Laryngol 84:734–739
27. Som PM, Biller HF (1979) The combined computerized tomography-sialogram. A technique to differentiate deep lobe parotid tumors from extraparotid pharyngomaxillary space tumors. Ann Otol Rhinol Laryngol 88:590–595
28. Uehara T (2006) Localization of FGF-6 and FGFR-4 during prenatal and early postnatal development of the mouse sublingual gland. J Oral Sci 48:9–14
29. Woodburne RT, Burkel WE (1988) Essentials of Human Anatomy, Eighth edn. Oxford University Press, New York, Oxford
30. Yune H (1977) Sialography and dacrocystography. In: Miller R, Skucas J (eds) Radiographic contrast agents. University Park Press, Baltimore, pp 485–492
31. Ziegler CM, Hedemark A, Brevik B, et al. (2003) Endoscopy as minimal invasive routine treatment for sialolithiasis. Acta Odontol Scand 61:137–140

Chapter 2

Imaging of the Salivary Glands

2

Hugh D. Curtin

Contents

Core Features

- This chapter discusses the various imaging modalities emphasizing the strengths and weaknesses of each.
- For tumor evaluation, predicting the precise diagnosis is less important than defining the anatomy of the tumor. Particular emphasis is placed on characterization of the margin and evaluation of possible perineural spread.
- Various fat pads close to the skull base serve as markers for detection or exclusion of perineural spread. These include the fat in the stylomastoid foramen, the fat just below foramen ovale, and the fat in the pterygopalatine fossa.
- Several imaging approaches to inflammation can be effective but only if the strengths and limitations of each are considered.

Introduction

Many different imaging modalities are useful in the evaluation of the salivary glands [7, 15, 18, 21]. In some instances, one imaging technique is clearly preferable but in many situations the information can be gathered using one of a number of approaches. This chapter will briefly describe the imaging techniques most frequently applied to diseases of the salivary glands. Then approaches to the two major clinical entities for which imaging is requested, palpable masses and recurrent swelling, will be covered. There are special considerations in each of these situations and there are also variations depending upon the specific gland being assessed. Abnormalities of the parotid, submandibular, and sublingual glands all require slightly different imaging considerations as do lesions arising in the minor salivary glands. In some cases, imaging can give a fairly accurate determination of the exact identity of a lesion but in many situations, particularly in tumor evaluation, demonstration of the anatomy of the abnormality is more important. The chapter will emphasize the imaging information that is most important to practical clinical planning.

Imaging Modalities

Plain films, computed tomography (CT), magnetic resonance imaging (MRI), and ultrasound are all commonly used in evaluation of salivary gland pathology. Sialography is done less frequently but can still provide useful information in particular circumstances. Nuclear medicine provides very specific information regarding certain lesions as well.

Plain films can detect calculi but their effectiveness is limited by superimposition of bone on the areas of interest. Specialized obliquities are required to project the region of a particular gland away from obscuring osseous structures. In many institutions, plain films have been almost completely replaced by computed tomography for detection of calculi. Combining plain films with injection of contrast into the salivary ducts for sialography does give an excellent demonstration of ductal anatomy and is very sensitive for identification of obstructing lesions. Sialography can assess perforations or interruption of a duct in trauma cases.

Computed tomography is superb at detecting small calcifications or calculi and does a reasonable job evaluating mass lesions. The density of fat is very different from that of bordering muscles so computed tomography can show the anatomy of the salivary glands and bordering soft tissues. The fat planes around the various glands allow definition of tumors and, as importantly, allow demonstration of extension of neoplasm away from a gland. This information is important in assessing aggressive malignancies, particularly those with perineural spread. There are, however, some instances where tumors can be invisible to computed tomography and so MRI is therefore usually preferred for assessment of tumors. Computed tomography does have a major advantage in speed of the examination compared to MRI. The CT study can be done in less than thirty seconds on modern scanners rather than the minimum of twenty to thirty minutes required for MRI and so many patients with palpable masses are imaged with computed tomography. As long as the limitations are considered, this approach can be reliable.

Magnetic resonance imaging is preferred by most radiologists for evaluation of tumors of the salivary glands. The varying sequences can almost always precisely define the margins of the tumor. The T1-weighted sequence for instance shows high or bright signal from the fat where as the T2-weighted sequence shows high signal from fluid. Different specialized sequences can indicate flow or can separate cysts from solids. Perineural spread toward or into the skull base is more reliably defined by MRI with gadolinium. However, no imaging finding has been proven reliable enough to avoid biopsy in most situations. Some patients cannot tolerate MRI because of claustrophobia or because of the length of time required. There are also contraindications such as pacemakers and various implants. MR sialography uses specialized sequences that show the ductal anatomy in cases of suspected obstruction.

Ultrasound can also evaluate many salivary gland pathologies [2, 8]. Ultrasound provides information about superficial lesions. This modality is limited by bone reflectivity so cannot assess some of the deeper structures such as the parapharyngeal extension of the parotid gland. If the abnormality is accessible to the ultrasound probe, this examination can separate cysts from solids and can identify a dilated duct in calculus obstruction. Often the particular calculus can be identified by acoustic "shadowing" contributing to the evaluation. Newer ultrasound machines take advantage of Doppler effects to determine flow within a lesion and to identify blood vessels. The effectiveness of ultrasound of the neck is considered to be dependent on the operator's experience but can be very valuable.

Nuclear medicine has very specific applications. A Tc-99m pertechnetate scan shows high radionuclide uptake in Warthin's tumor and in oncocytoma. Positron emission tomography (PET) shows metabolically active tissue. The normal salivary gland can show activity on PET scans but highly metabolic tumors of appreciable size can be identified [12, 13, 19]. Unfortunately PET cannot consistently separate benign from malignant tumors. Warthin's tumors are particularly active and pleomorphic adenomas frequently show increased metabolic activity [19].

Evaluation of Masses (Tumors and Cysts)

General

Most salivary gland masses are palpable. Some are found incidentally at imaging done for some unrelated reason. One cannot reliably define that a lesion is benign but there are some strong indicators of malignancy. An irregular margin or apparent extension along a nerve strongly indicates malignancy (Fig. 2.1). Smooth sharp margins can be seen in various benign lesions but also in malignancies, particularly those which are of low grade histology. Various signal changes on MRI have been considered suggestive of malignancy but these have not proven reliable [1, 16, 17]. For instance, low signal on T2-weighted imaging, was considered suggestive of malignancy but now is thought to occur in any cellular tumor. Most head and neck radiologists feel that there is simply too much overlap to make a prediction based on the signal appearance alone.

Because of its frequency, the imaging appearance of the pleomorphic adenoma (benign mixed tumor) deserves special attention. This tumor virtually always has a sharp margin without irregular extension into the surrounding soft tissues (Figs. 2.2, 2.3). Following the line of least resistance, the pleomorphic adenoma can extend through the stylomandibular tunnel forming a dumbbell-shaped tumor with a component in the more lateral parotid gland and a significant mass in the prestyloid parapharyngeal

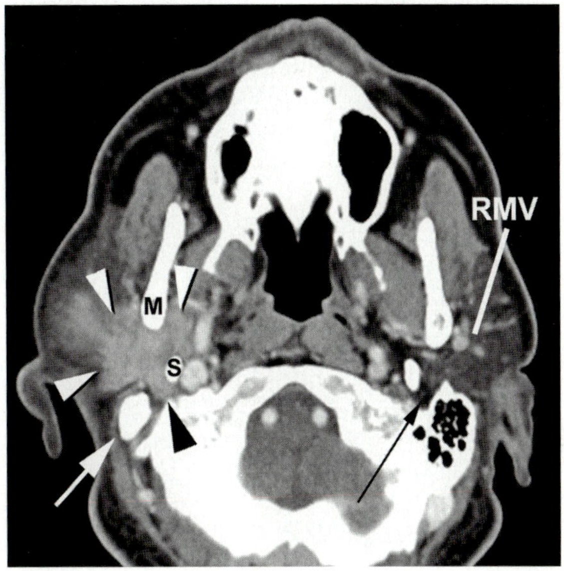

Fig. 2.1: Malignant tumor of the parotid. The malignancy (*white arrowheads*) has an unsharp irregular margin. Tumor extends through the stylomandibular tunnel between the styloid process (*S*) and the posterior edge of the mandible (*M*) into the parapharyngeal space. Tumor extends into the fat (*black arrowhead*) of the stylomastoid foramen. Styloid (*S*), mastoid tip (*white arrow*), fat in the normal stylomastoid foramen (*black arrow*), retromandibular vein (*RMV*)

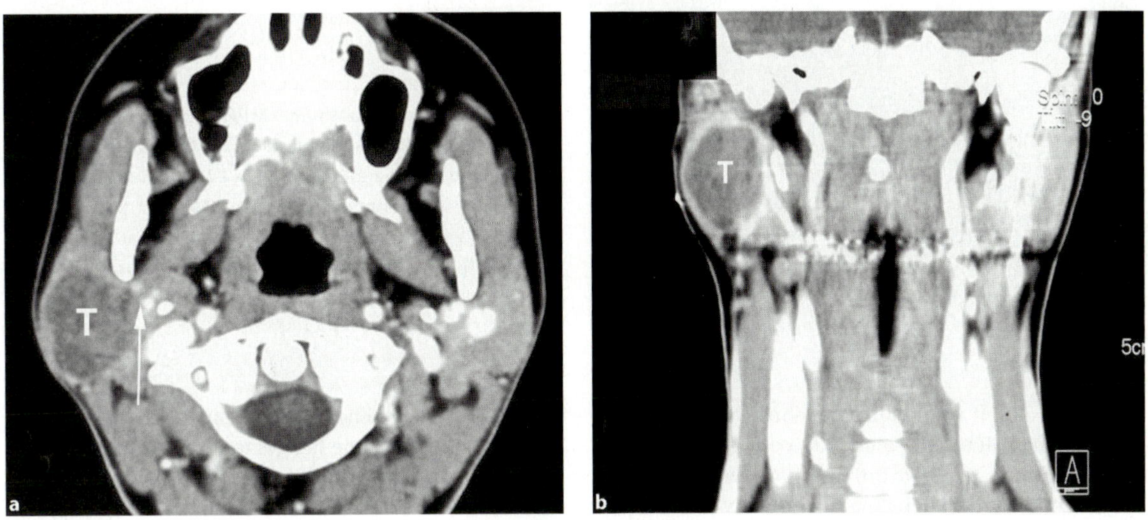

Fig. 2.2: Pleomorphic adenoma contrast enhanced CT. **a** Axial plane. The tumor (*T*) has a sharp slightly undulating or bosselated margin. The retromandibular vein (*arrow*) is displaced medially. **b** Coronal plane shows the sharp margin of the tumor (*T*)

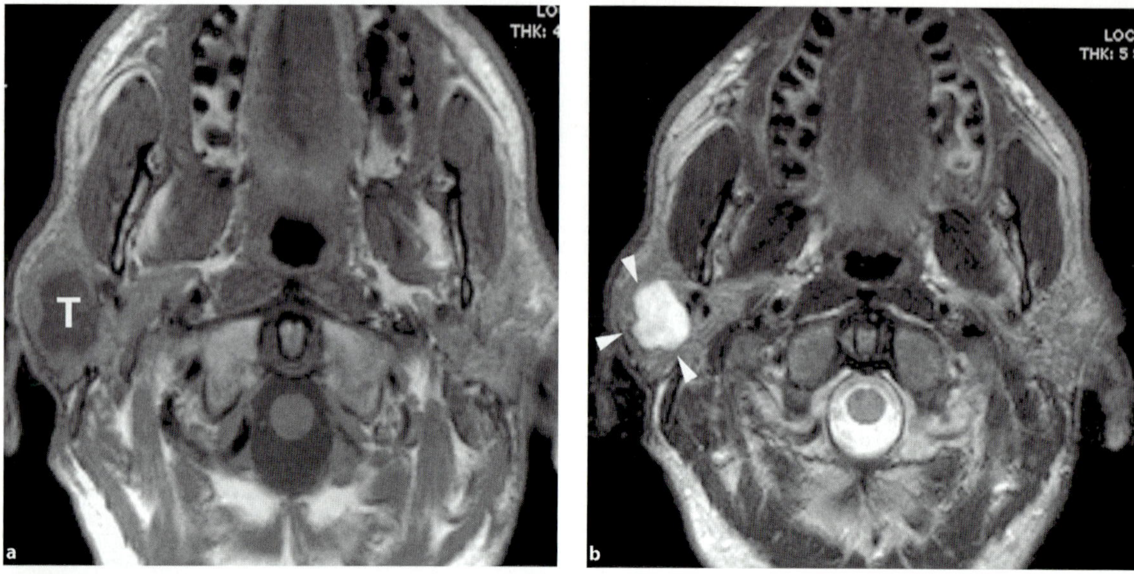

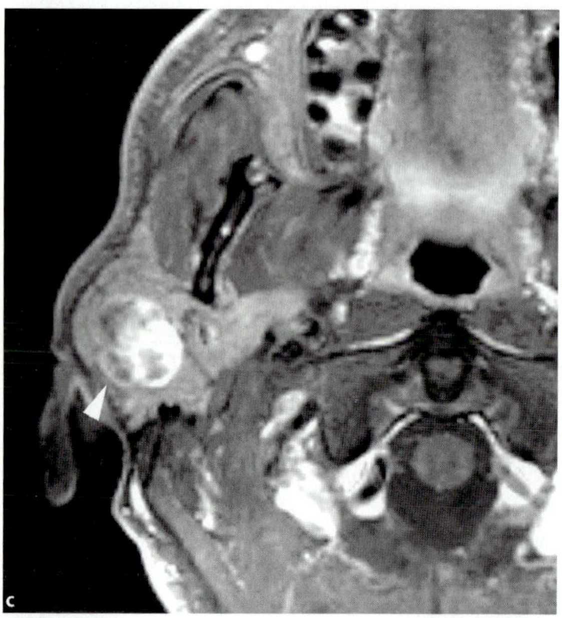

Fig. 2.3: Pleomorphic adenoma, MRI. **a** Axial T1-weighted image, no contrast, shows the tumor (*T*) in the superficial parotid lateral to the retromandibular vein. **b** T2-weighted image shows high signal in the tumor. The lesion has slight protuberances or bosselations (*arrowheads*). **c** Postcontrast axial T1-weighted image with fat suppression. The lesion shows characteristic enhancement and demonstrates the bosselation (*arrowhead*) of the lesion

space (Fig. 2.4). It will not extend along the nerves. As it expands, the lesion can remodel the contiguous bone but does not invade in a more infiltrative manner.

Not truly lobulated, the margin of many pleomorphic adenomas is slightly undulating or shows several slight bulges or surface eminences (Figs. 2.2, 2.3). The term "bosselated" has been applied to this appearance and when seen is strongly suggestive of the diagnosis.

Pleomorphic adenomas frequently show gradual enhancement [10]. If one images too quickly after intravenous contrast is injected, the lesion may actually be almost invisible on CT scan. A delayed scan frequently will show the delayed enhancement typical of this tumor and demonstrate the margin (Fig. 2.5). This has actually become more of a problem with the most modern CT scan technology. Many scanning protocols attempt to empha-

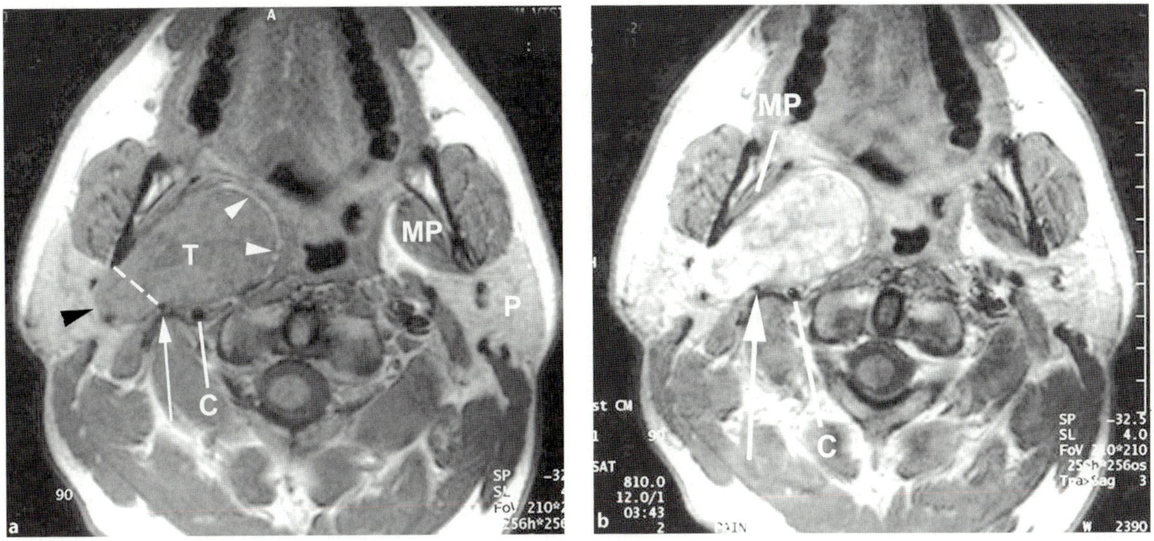

Fig. 2.4: Pleomorphic adenoma arising in the prestyloid parapharyngeal space, MRI. **a** T1-weighted image without contrast. The tumor (*T*) fills the prestyloid parapharyngeal space. The tumor pushes the parapharyngeal fat anteromedially (*white arrowheads*). Laterally the lesion pushes beyond the plane of the stylomandibular tunnel (*dashed line*). The lateral margin (*black arrowhead*) displaces the retromandibular vein laterally. The key landmarks in identifying a lesion as arising in the prestyloid space are the carotid artery (*C*) the styloid process (*arrow*), the medial pterygoid muscle (*MP*) and the posterior margin of the mandible. Note the normal appearance of the parotid gland (*P*) on the left. **b** Axial T1-weighted image postcontrast. The lesion shows enhancement typical of pleomorphic adenoma. Carotid (*C*), styloid process (*arrow*), compressed and displaced medial pterygoid muscle (*MP*)

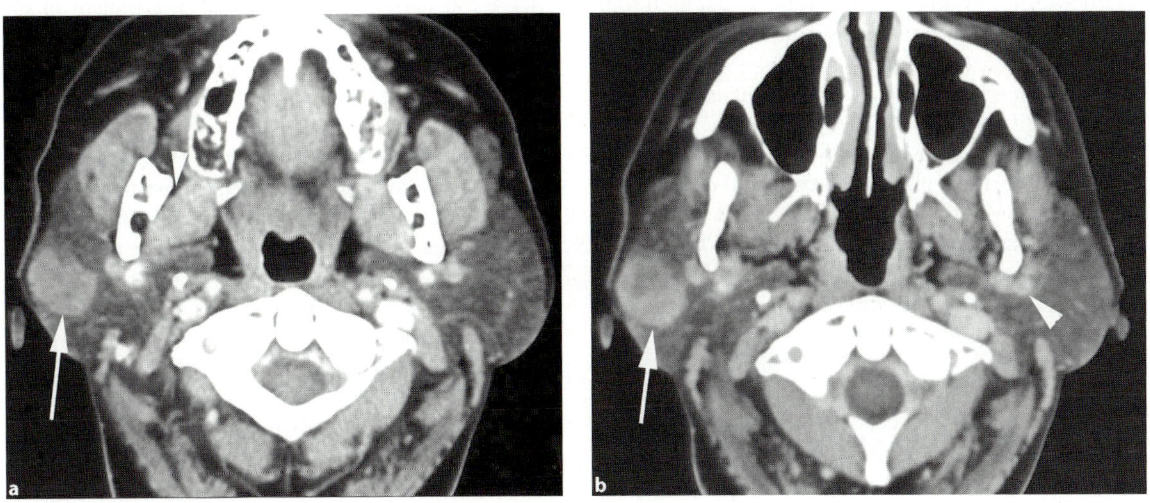

Fig. 2.5: Pleomorphic adenoma. CT showing gradual enhancement after injection of contrast. **a** Initial axial image. This image was taken immediately after the injection of contrast. The tumor (*arrow*) can barely be seen in the superficial parotid gland. Position of the lingual nerve (*arrowhead*). **b** Delayed image. After several minutes there is gradual enhancement of the tumor (*arrow*). This is typical of a pleomorphic adenoma. Retromandibular vein (*arrowhead*)

size visualization of the arteries and veins and so the scan is done as the contrast is being injected and at that time the tumor may not be visible against the background of the normal parotid gland. Late visualization is another good indicator of the diagnosis of pleomorphic adenoma. The delayed enhancement phenomenon does not tend to be a problem with MRI. The multiple sequences used with MRI will almost always be sufficient to visualize the tumor. Also, several sequences are done after the injection of intravenous contrast so there would be time for gradual enhancement to occur. Consistent reliable visualization of lesions is the primary reason that most head and neck radiologists prefer MRI to CT for investigation of salivary gland tumors.

Pleomorphic adenomas are almost always solitary neoplasms. Tumors that are multiple occur almost exclusively in the parotid gland. Warthin's tumors, oncocytomas, lymph nodes, and the lymphoepithelial cysts associated with HIV infection can all be multiple. Similarly primary epithelial salivary gland malignancies present as single lesions within the gland rather than multiple tumors though there can be lymphadenopathy in the lower neck.

Not all "tumors" or space occupying lesions are solid tumors. Various cystic lesions are also considered. Sialoceles, branchial cleft cysts, and ranulas all occur in the region of the salivary glands. Lymphoepithelial cysts can occur in HIV-positive patients frequently with associated lymphadenopathy. There can be cystic lesions (usually small) associated with Sjögren's disease. In addition some lesions such as Warthin's tumor and others can have a substantial cystic component.

Finally, an obstructed duct can present as a "mass" as the gland enlarges. Usually there is pain but if the condition is chronic, pain may not be a major complaint. If the main duct of a gland is obstructed then the entire gland tends to be large. If the entire gland is large and no normal gland is seen around a visualized "mass," then neoplasm is very unlikely. Obstruction of a branch duct however can give a more confusing picture as the entire gland is not enlarged.

Specific Locations

The likelihood of a tumor having a certain histology varies with the gland involved. Even the rate of malignancy varies. For instance, a tumor in the submandibular gland is more likely malignant than one identified in the parotid gland. Thus the gland of origin is important in predicting the most likely identity of the tumor. Biopsy either by needle or by excision is usually needed for the final determination. Once a mass is identified, imaging defines the extent of the disease as exactly as possible emphasizing the course of major nerves that serve as potential pathways for perineural tumor spread. Landmarks that are crucial to therapy planning are dependent on the gland in question. The likely pathways for perineural spread vary with the gland involved.

Parotid Gland

The majority of lesions in the parotid gland are benign. Pleomorphic adenoma is the most frequent benign tumor encountered. Mucoepidermoid carcinoma is the most common malignancy but there are others as described elsewhere in this volume. No finding is considered to be specific in separating these lesions. The diagnosis of adenoid cystic carcinoma is particularly important because of the likelihood of perineural spread. If there are multiple lesions, Warthin's tumors, lymphoepithelial cysts, lymph nodes, and oncocytomas should be considered though most of these can present as a single lesion as well. Enlarged nodes within the parotid gland can be the result of lymphoma, chronic lymphocytic leukemia (CLL), sarcoid, and several other pathologies. Sjögren's disease can present with mass-like enlargement of the glands. The findings are usually bilateral and the entire gland is affected. Schwannoma of the facial nerve should be considered if the lesion is along the course of the facial nerve.

The relationship of a parotid tumor to the facial nerve and to the stylomandibular tunnel is important for surgical planning. The facial nerve is occasionally visible but not consistently seen. The stylomandibular tunnel is always visible.

The landmarks to determine the approximate location of the facial nerve as it traverses the parotid gland are the stylomastoid foramen and the retromandibular vein (Fig. 2.1). There is normally fat in the stylomastoid foramen as the nerve exits between the styloid process and the mastoid tip. Small "dots" within the fat represent either the nerve or the stylomastoid artery, a branch usually from the occipital artery. A line drawn from the foramen to the lateral margin of the retromandibular gland approximates the position of the facial nerve.

The styloid process and the posterior edge of mandible form the margins of the stylomandibular tunnel (Fig. 2.4). These osseous structures can be clearly demonstrated at computed tomography. MRI demonstrates the posterior margin of the mandible but the styloid process may not be obvious. The muscles attached to the styloid process are outlined by fat and may help identify this important landmark.

If one can establish that a tumor is in the prestyloid parapharyngeal space (PPS), then the lesion is almost certainly of salivary gland origin and most commonly is arising from the parotid gland. The imaging findings of such a lesion are very typical [4]. A lesion arising in the PPS pushes the fat medially and anteriorly. The fat usually outlines the margin of the lesion (Fig. 2.4). The residual fat is compressed against the constrictor ring of the pharynx. The wall of the pharynx bulges medially in larger tumors. The most important landmarks for establishing the location in the PPS are the carotid artery, the styloid process, the posterior margin of the mandible, and the medial pterygoid muscle (Fig. 2.4). Lesions that are posterior to the margin of the mandible and the medial pterygoid muscle and are anterior to the carotid artery and the styloid process are within the prestyloid space and thus almost certainly of salivary derivation. As a tumor in the PPS enlarges, it will bulge laterally through the stylomandibular tunnel toward the facial nerve and more superficial parotid. In the normal case, imaging identifies the parapharyngeal process bulging variably through the stylomandibular tunnel on the side opposite to the tumor.

Lesions located posterior to the carotid artery and that with lateral growth appear to bulge behind the styloid process are in the poststyloid or retrostyloid parapharyngeal space and are not of parotid origin. These are more likely tumors arising from the neural structures that accompany the carotid artery and are usually nerve sheath tumors or paragangliomas. The parapharyngeal fat deviates anteriorly and laterally away from these tumors. Masticator space lesions arise anterior to the prestyloid PPS and obliterate the fat between the pterygoid muscles pushing the parapharyngeal fat posteriorly and medially. Such lesions can arise from bone, dental structures, nerves (third division, trigeminal nerve), the temporomandibular joint, or other various mesenchymal structures but are not of parotid origin.

Perineural spread of tumor is one of the most important considerations in any salivary gland abnormality particularly with adenoid cystic carcinoma. Even if the lesion is clearly benign, one should carefully examine the major pathways by which tumor can follow a nerve away from the primary tumor. In the parotid gland, there are two major routes toward the skull base. These are the facial nerve and the auriculotemporal nerve, a small branch of the third division of the trigeminal nerve.

The facial nerve is the classic route of perineural spread associated with parotid tumors. The facial nerve passes through the fat in the stylomastoid foramen as it enters the temporal bone. A nerve enlarged by perineural spread will obliterate the fat in the foramen (Fig. 2.1). This effect can be seen on CT or MRI as fat is very evident on T1-weighted MRI or on CT. As tumor extends upward along the nerve within the temporal bone, the facial nerve canal is usually enlarged. CT can detect this change. MRI relies on the enhancement of the involved nerve as it passes through the temporal bone but high resolution scans can detect the enlargement as well. The entire nerve should be assessed all the way through the temporal bone to the internal auditory canal even if there is no clinical facial paralysis.

The second pathway, following the auriculotemporal branch of the trigeminal nerve, can carry tumor around the posterior edge of the mandible and upward toward the foramen ovale. Approaching the skull base the nerve passes into the masticator space traveling through a small fat pad along the medial aspect of the lateral pterygoid muscle and just inferior to the foramen ovale (Fig. 2.6). Again an enlarged nerve will obliterate the fat normally seen in this location. Normally the nerve can be seen within the fat fairly consistently. If the fat and nerve are normal then perineural spread is extremely unlikely. If the tumor does pass into the skull base through the foramen ovale, the gasserian ganglion at the inferior lateral aspect of Meckel's cave becomes the next target, so a normal appearance should be verified in every case of parotid tumor (Fig. 2.6). If perineural tumor does reach the gasserian ganglion then the preganglionic segment of the trigeminal nerve passing toward the pons and the second division of the trigeminal nerve passing through the foramen rotundum should be assessed for further extension of tumor.

Magnetic resonance imaging is considered the preferred modality in evaluating possible perineural spread into the skull base. MRI visualizes the enlarged nerve, the obliterated fat, or the enlarged ganglion. Often there is atrophy of the masticator muscles, masseter and pterygoids, innervated by V_3. Some imagers use fat suppressed

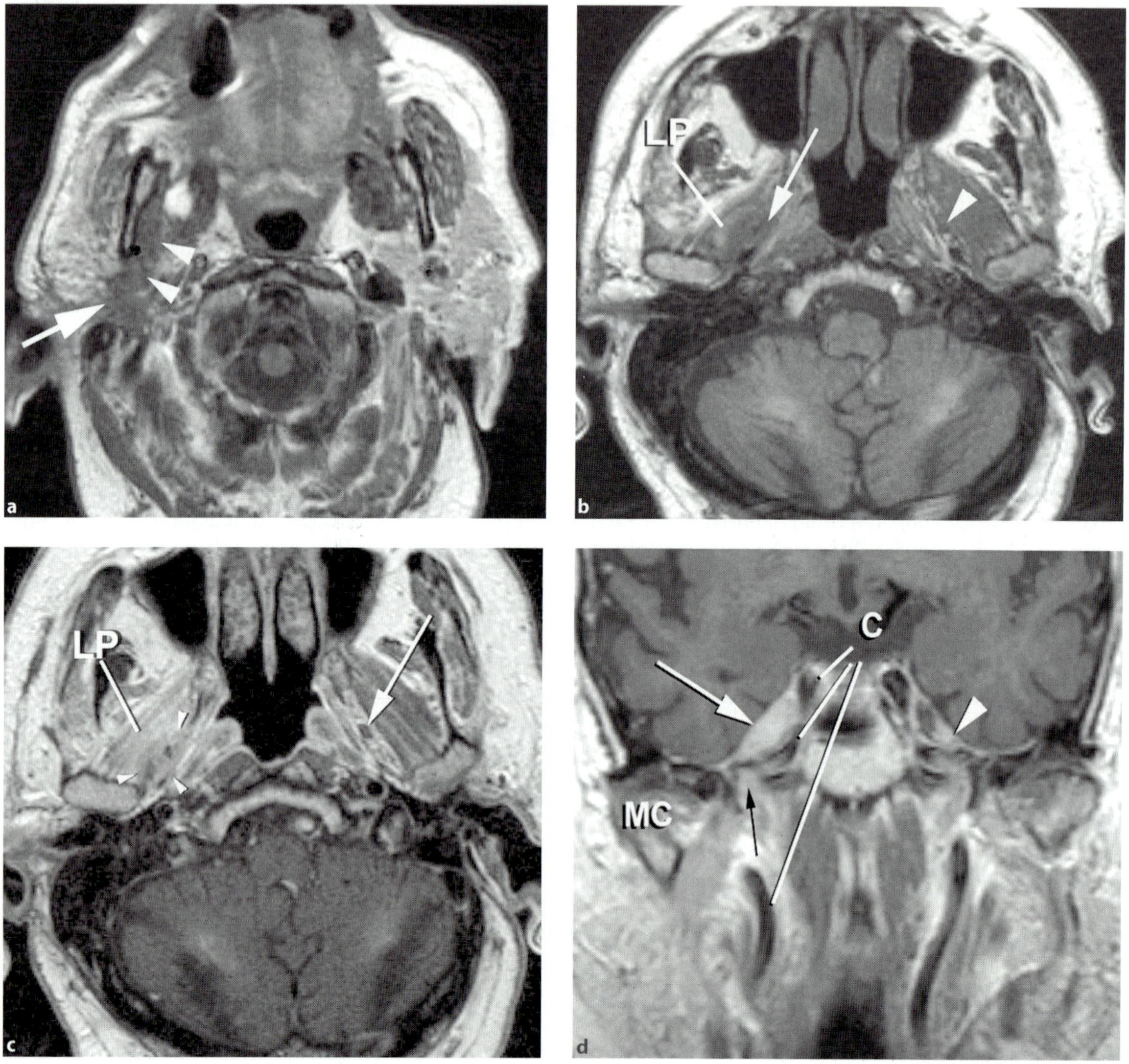

Fig. 2.6: Carcinoma of the parotid gland with perineural spread along the auriculotemporal nerve of the trigeminal nerve through the foramen ovale to the gasserian ganglion and Meckel's cave, MRI. **a** Axial T1-weighted image without contrast shows the infiltrative tumor in the parotid gland (*arrow*). There had been previous surgery. There is tumor (*arrowheads*) extending along the auriculotemporal nerve into the masticator space toward the main branches of the third division of the trigeminal nerve. **b** Axial T1-weighted image without contrast just inferior to foramen ovale. The tumor enlarges the nerve just beneath foramen ovale obliterating the important fat plane (*arrow*) along the medial margin of the lateral pterygoid muscle (*LP*). The lateral pterygoid muscle has atrophied slightly due to denervation. Note the normal trigeminal nerve third division (*arrowhead*) on the opposite side along the medial margin of a normal lateral pterygoid muscle. **c** Postcontrast T1-weighted image at the same level as **b**. Denervated lateral pterygoid (*LP*) muscle shows slight enhancement. The tumor (*arrowheads*) extending along the trigeminal nerve is better defined within the fat just inferior to foramen ovale. Note the appearance of the normal nerve (*arrow*) on the opposite side. **d** Coronal image through Meckel's cave. The tumor (*white arrow*) having followed the trigeminal nerve through foramen ovale obliterates the gasserian ganglion and the cerebrospinal fluid in Meckel's cave. Compare to the gasserian ganglion area (*arrowhead*) on the opposite side. Tumor just beneath foramen ovale (*black arrow*), mandibular condyle (*MC*), carotid artery (*C*)

imaging while others prefer very high resolution post-contrast imaging without fat suppression for this evaluation. As long as the nerves can be precisely defined and a determination can be made about their involvement, either strategy can be effective.

Submandibular Gland

Tumors of the submandibular gland are less common but when present are more likely malignant than are those in the parotid gland. When a patient presents with a palpable mass in the submandibular region, the goals of imaging are to determine the origin of the lesion and assess the extent.

The first task for imaging is to determine whether the lesion is arising within the submandibular gland or is actually contiguous to it (Fig. 2.7). The most common mass to be confused with a submandibular gland tumor is an enlarged lymph node. This is an important distinction as such lesions are frequently treated much differently than tumors of the submandibular gland. If the abnormality is an enlarged lymph node, a fat plane can usually be seen between the node and the submandibular gland. If the node is very large the gland can be compressed and deformed. The radiologist tries to estimate whether the gland is of normal size in an effort to make the distinction between an intrinsic and an extrinsic mass.

A neoplasm arising in the submandibular gland will not replace the entire gland. Some amount of normal gland almost always remains bordering the tumor. If this is not identified and the entire gland appears abnormal then enlargement from obstruction is more likely and the course of the submandibular duct is carefully examined for calculus or, less likely, some other obstructing lesion.

Perineural spread from a submandibular gland neoplasm is unusual. We have seen spread along the lingual nerve reaching this pathway via small branches connecting the gland to the nerve. In every case of tumor of the submandibular gland, the course of the nerve should be assessed. The nerve courses between the anterior margin of the medial pterygoid muscle and the anterior edge of the ramus of the mandible (Fig. 2.5). More superiorly the nerve joins the remainder of the third division of the trigeminal nerve and passes through the previously mentioned small fat pad just inferior to the foramen ovale, along the medial margin of the lateral pterygoid muscle. The final destination is the gasserian ganglion at the lower lateral margin of Meckel's cave.

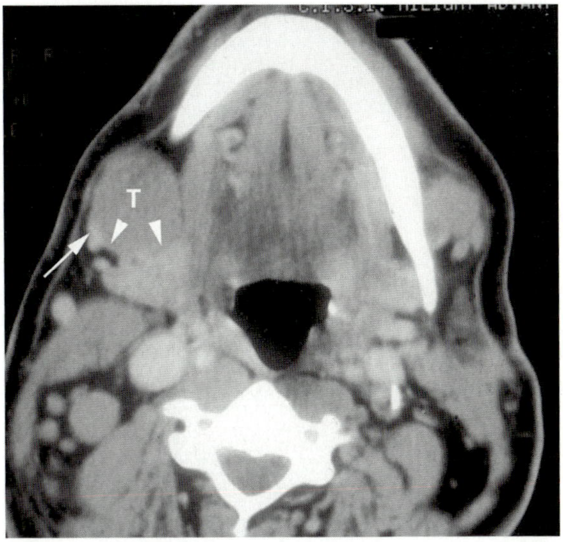

Fig. 2.7: Tumor of the submandibular gland. The tumor (*T*), which is partially imbedded into the submandibular gland, has a sharp margin (*arrowheads*). The lesion cannot be separated from the gland. A small amount of submandibular gland tissue (*arrow*) molds along the margin of the lesion

Sublingual Gland

The sublingual gland lies in the sublingual space tucked beneath the mucosa of the floor of the mouth and between the mylohyoid muscle and the geniohyoid/genioglossus muscle complex. The important landmarks for any lesion are the muscular boundaries of the space. Lesions can exit the space posteriorly via the gap between the hyoglossus muscle and the posterior margin of the mylohyoid muscle. This is the same gap through which the submandibular duct courses. Alternatively lesions can pass directly through the muscle following a small defect in the muscle through which a vessel passes. Herniation of the gland through the muscle itself can be mistaken for a submandibular region mass at imaging but the appearance is so similar to that of the gland that the diagnosis can usually be made.

Tumors of the sublingual gland are somewhat rare. The ranula is a more common cause of a "bulge" in the floor of the mouth (Fig. 2.8). The ranula has a characteristic appearance as a cyst filling the sublingual space [3].

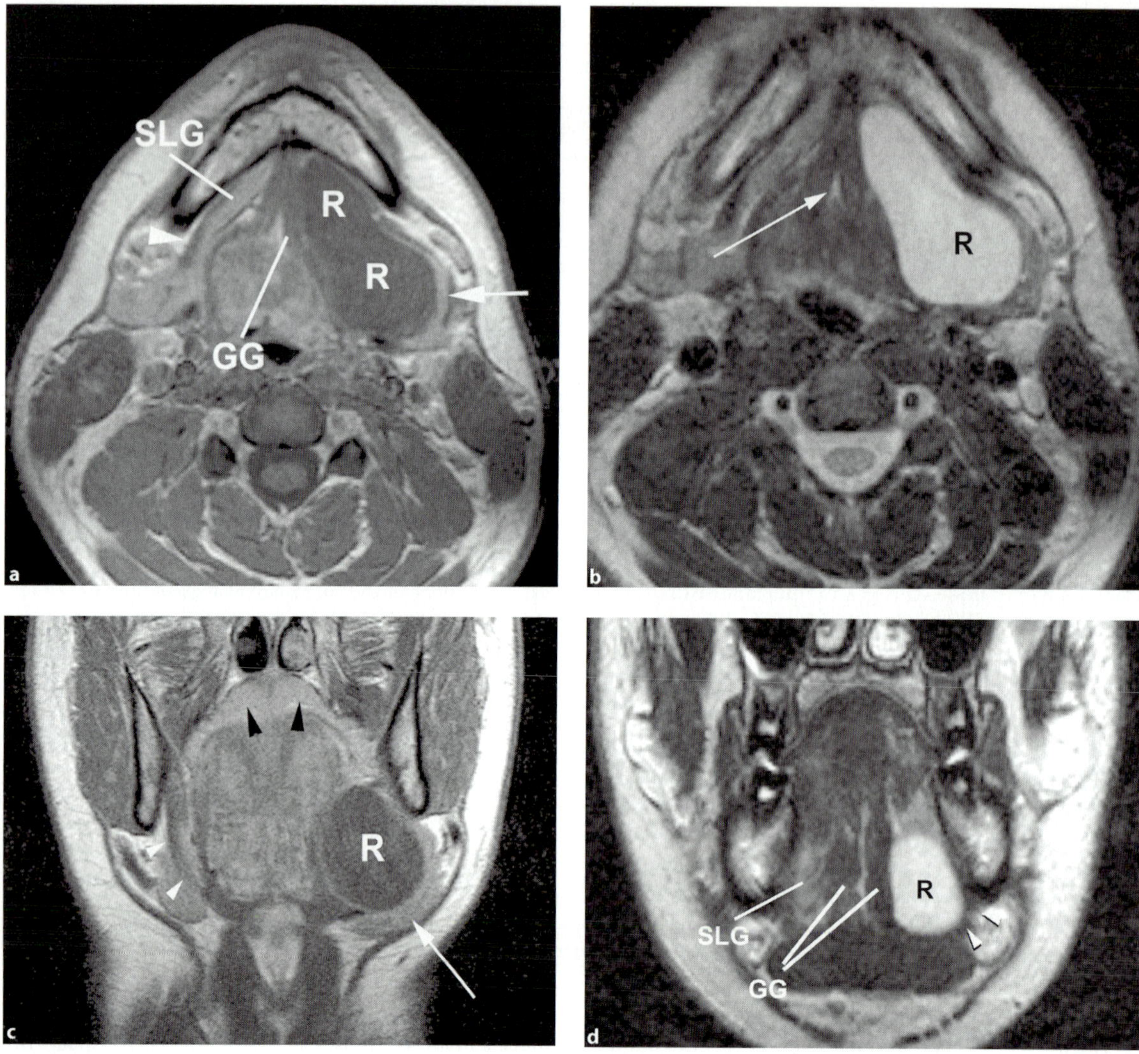

Fig. 2.8: Ranula, MRI. **a** Axial T1-weighted image after contrast. The ranula (*R*) fills the sublingual space and protrudes beyond the mylohyoid muscle into the submandibular space indenting the submandibular gland (*arrow*). Genioglossus muscle (*GG*), normal sublingual gland on the opposite side (*SLG*), mylohyoid on the normal side (*arrowhead*). **b** T2-weighted images axial plane. The ranula (*R*) is clearly defined by the high signal. Midline fatty raphae of the tongue (*arrow*). **c** Coronal T1-weighted image after contrast. The ranula (*R*) fills the sublingual space and displaces the submandibular gland (*arrow*). Normal mylohyoid on the opposite side (*white arrowheads*), minor salivary glands along the roof of the mouth (*black arrowheads*). **d** Coronal T2-weighted image. The ranula (*R*) shows high signal and is found between the genioglossus muscle (*GG*) and the mylohyoid muscle (*arrowheads*) in the sublingual space. Normal sublingual gland (*SLG*) on the opposite side

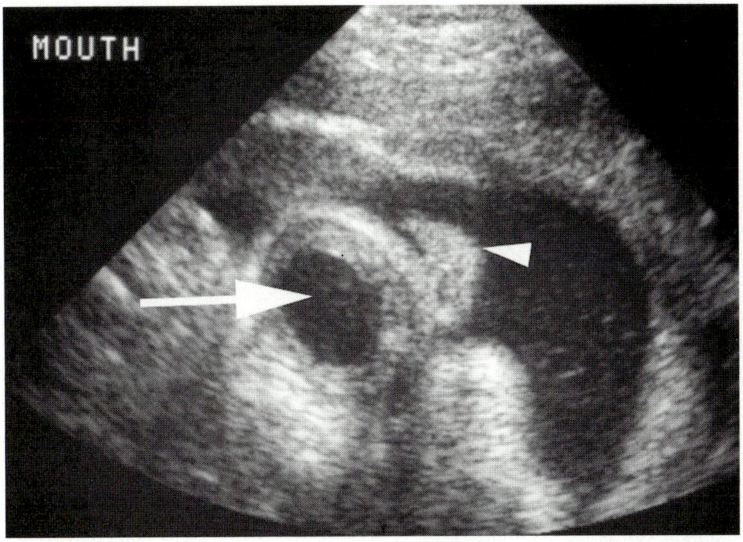

Fig. 2.9: Prenatal ultrasound of salivary cyst of oral cavity. Coronal plane. The salivary cyst (*arrow*) is the hypoechoic area spreading the lips outward preventing mouth closure. Tip of nose (*arrowhead*). With permission from Doubilet PM, Benson CB (2003) Atlas of ultrasound in obstetrics and gynecology: a multimedia reference. Lippincott Williams & Wilkins, Philadelphia

The wall of the ranula will enhance and there should be no enhancing tissue within the cystic part of the abnormality. Initially the ranula is limited by the mylohyoid muscle. Larger lesions can herniate beyond the posterior edge of the muscle or through the muscle into the submandibular space. The term "plunging" has been applied to ranulas that reach the submandibular space. Some use the term to indicate that the lesion has extended beyond the normal confines of the cystic cavity. Rarely a ranula can present entirely in the submandibular space arising from a small lobule of the gland that herniates through the mylohyoid muscle.

A ranula can be present at birth. If large, the ranula in the oral cavity can interfere with breathing at birth and thus can be of considerable concern in the delivery room. Routine prenatal ultrasound can identify a cystic hypoechoic lesion in the oral region (Fig. 2.9). The lack of internal echoes differentiates the cyst from macroglossia and from prenatal tumors that can occur in the oral region [5]. A very large cyst can be drained prior to delivery or resection can be planned at delivery prior to clamping of the umbilical cord [9, 14]. Smaller cysts may be treated electively after delivery [6].

Minor Salivary Glands

Minor salivary glands are distributed throughout the mucosa of the oral cavity and pharynx as well other regions of the upper aerodigestive tract. The roof of the mouth close to the junction of the hard and soft palates has a particularly high concentration of minor salivary glands (Fig. 2.8). Both benign and malignant neoplasms can arise from the small glands. Retentions cysts can also occur here.

Of particular note is adenoid cystic carcinoma arising from these glands. When such a malignancy occurs in the region of the posterior hard palate the palatine nerves can carry tumor to the pterygopalatine fossa (Fig. 2.10). From the fossa, this perineural spread can pass through the foramen rotundum to the gasserian ganglion at the margin of the cavernous sinus and Meckel's cave. The canal for the greater palatine nerve may be enlarged as these tumors tend to grow slowly. Obliteration of the fat in the pterygopalatine fossa is indicative of tumor extension into the fossa making the fossa one of the most important findings in head and neck cancer imaging . In the normal case, fat is always seen in this narrow slit between the pterygoid plate and the posterior wall of the maxillary sinus. If tumor reaches the fossa, the foramen rotundum and Vidian's canal should be examined for enhancement or enlargement indicating more central spread.

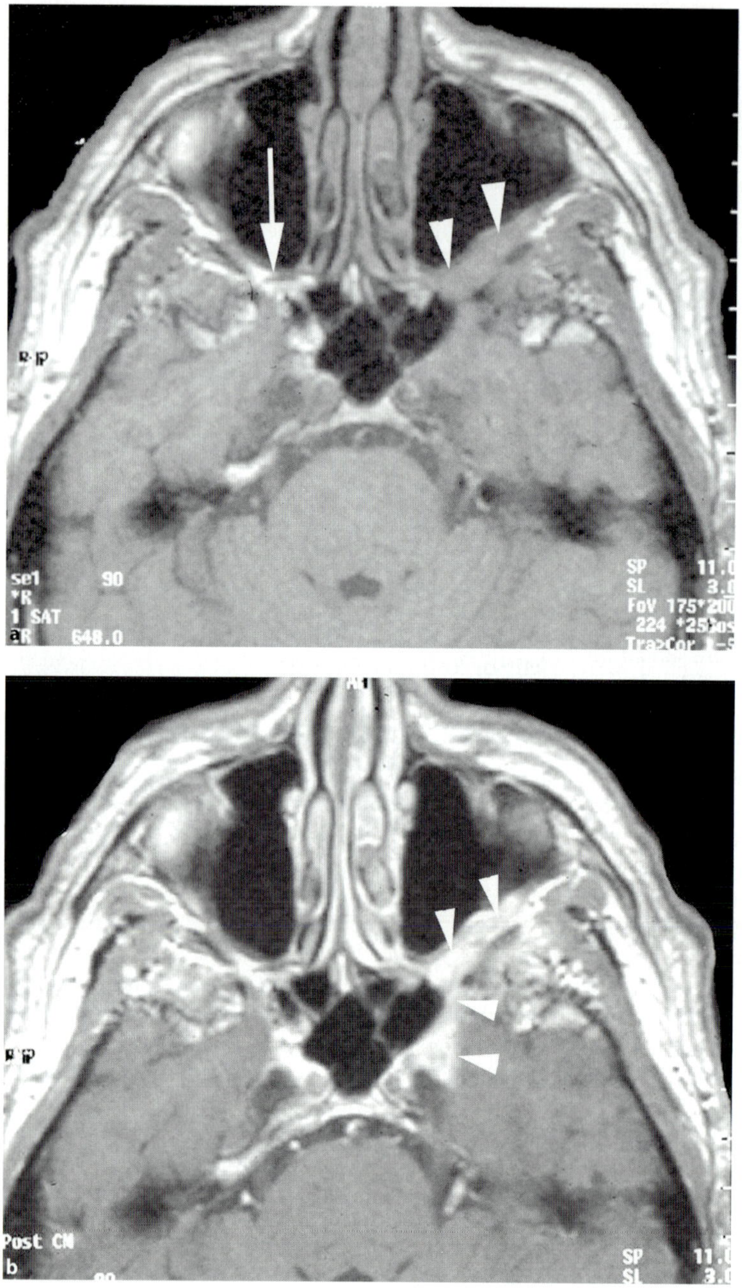

Fig. 2.10: Pterygopalatine fossa obliteration by perineural spread. Adenoid cystic carcinoma of the palate with perineural spread V_2. **a** Axial T1-weighted image precontrast shows tumor (*arrowheads*) filling the pterygopalatine fossa between the maxillary sinus and the pterygoid process of the sphenoid bone. The fat is obliterated. Note the normal fat (*arrow*) in the opposite pterygopalatine fossa. **b** Axial T1-weighted image after contrast at the same level as **a**. The tumor (*arrowheads*) fills the pterygopalatine fossa and follows foramen rotundum to the area of the gasserian ganglion

Inflammation/Obstruction

Obstructed Duct

An obstructed duct usually presents with recurrent swelling and inflammation. This presentation is not usually confused with tumor and is imaged with a different strategy. There are several applicable approaches.

Most calculi in the submandibular duct are dense enough that they can be seen in plain films. However, projecting the course of the submandibular duct away from the bone of the mandible can be very difficult. A specialized projection with the film held between the teeth and the X-ray beam projected upward from below the mandible can be effective. Trying to use plain films to visualize the course of the parotid duct is even more difficult.

Most radiologists consider computed tomography to be more reliable for demonstration of calculi (Fig. 2.11). Axial images done parallel to the occlusal plane will project the entire submandibular duct below dental restorations and the potential artifact that they cause. Similarly this plane of imaging will usually place the entire parotid duct above the dental artifact. The parotid duct can often be followed through the buccal fat, emerging from the buccinator muscle and then curving around the masseter muscle toward the parotid gland.

An obstructing calculus, if radio-opaque, is visualized as a density along the course of the duct. In addition, the dilated duct itself can sometimes be seen extending toward the gland. If there has been recent obstruction, the gland may show increased density that is asymmetric with the opposite normal side. With further inflammation there may be stranding or streaky density in the contiguous fat. The platysma muscle may be thickened if there is inflammation.

Most radiologists do not use contrast if a calculus is suspected. If contrast is injected, a dilated duct may be better seen and the obstructed inflamed gland may enhance more than the opposite side. If there is an abscess suspected then intravenous contrast is very helpful in identifying an enhancing ring.

If a calculus is not dense enough to be radio-opaque, it will not usually be detected on CT. Mucous plugs have been implicated in cases where there is clinical obstruction but no calculus is identified.

Magnetic resonance imaging has been used to assess a potentially obstructed duct. There is no radiation and a dilated duct filled with fluid can be identified on several sequences. Certain sequences or reconstructions

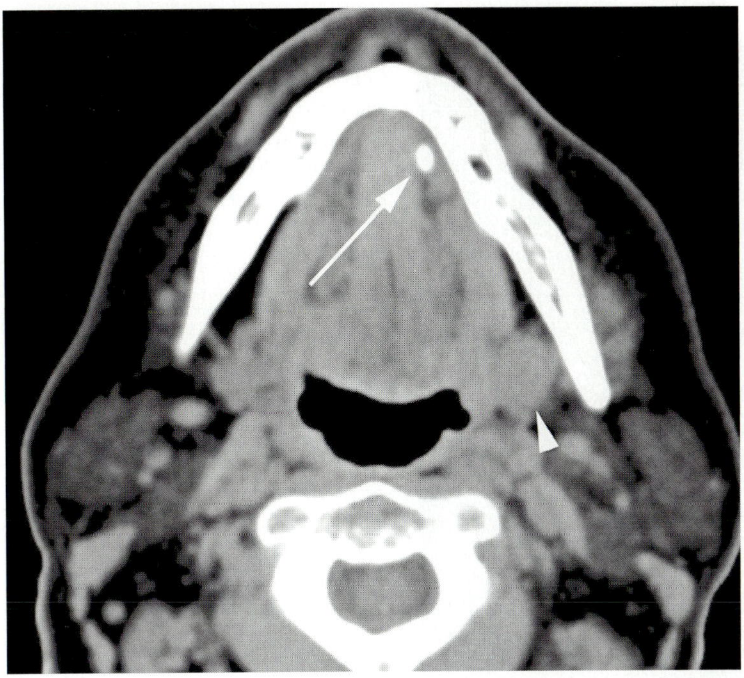

Fig. 2.11: Calculus in the submandibular duct, axial CT scan. There is a calculus (*arrow*) in the anterior sublingual space along the course of the submandibular duct. Note that the submandibular gland (*arrowhead*) is more dense on the abnormal side than on the normal side. This reflects inflammatory obstructive change

can give an image very similar to a sialogram. A filling defect indicates an obstructing calculus or mucous plug. MR sialography is based on detecting the fluid within the obstructed duct. MR gives a good assessment of the gland itself and is very sensitive to minor changes in signal caused by edema or inflammation within the gland. A negative examination with normal signal within the gland and no dilation of the duct is considered to be reliable by some radiologists.

Ultrasound has several definite advantages in assessing obstruction of the duct [20]. There is no radiation and the examination is very fast and inexpensive. One of the major strengths of ultrasound is the ability to define fluid-filled structures. The sound waves reflect from the walls of the structure giving prominent echoes but there are almost no echoes from the fluid. Calcified objects do not transmit sound and so there is acoustic shadowing. An echo-free stripe or band will project away from the calculus on the side opposite to the ultrasound probe. The dilated duct can be followed back into the gland. If a secondary abscess forms, ultrasound will show the fluid-filled space. Ultrasound is operator dependent but where available can be very reliable for this diagnosis.

Injection sialography is a safe but slightly invasive technique that allows excellent demonstration of the ductal anatomy (Fig. 2.12). A small catheter is inserted into the orifice of the duct and iodinated contrast is injected. Contrast passes along the duct into the gland or will opacify to the point of obstruction. Irregularities of the duct indicate prior inflammation with fibrosis. A filling defect indicates a calculus or mucous plug. The examination should not be done if there is acute inflammation present as there is risk of causing further infection within the gland due to retrograde pressure from the injection. Sialography allows visualization of the entire ductal system demonstrating sialectasis confirming the presence of obstructive, inflammatory disease even if a filling defect is not present.

Autoimmune Inflammatory Disease

Recurrent swelling may not be obstructive. Autoimmune sialadenitis or Sjögren's disease also presents with fullness and inflammatory symptoms. On injection sialography there is a very specific appearance at least in relatively early stages. The duct can be normal or even appear to be slightly narrow particularly within the gland. Multiple small collections are seen "budding" off the intraglandular ducts giving the classic "tree in bud" appearance (Fig. 2.12). The small collections tend to be very uniform though can vary with further destruction of the gland.

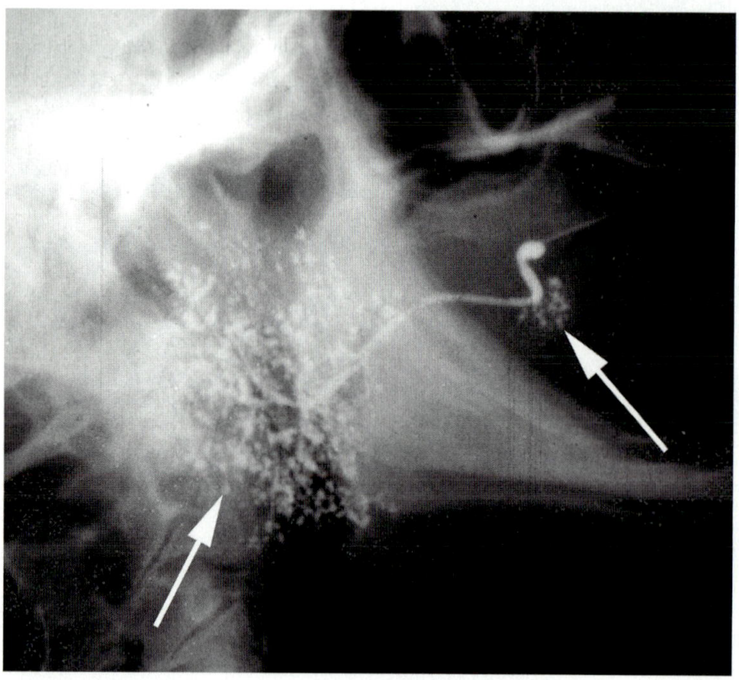

Fig. 2.12: Sjögren's disease, sialogram. Contrast was injected into the parotid duct and shows the "tree in bud" appearance of Sjögren's disease. Note the multiple tiny collections (*arrows*) throughout the gland including the accessory parotid gland

On both CT and MRI, multiple small nodular densities are seen throughout the gland representing the small cystic collections (Fig. 2.13) [11]. The T2-weighted images often show the high signal in the small collections giving an appearance of a multimicrocystic distribution within the gland. In latter stages there can be more confluent fibrotic changes and fatty infiltrations.

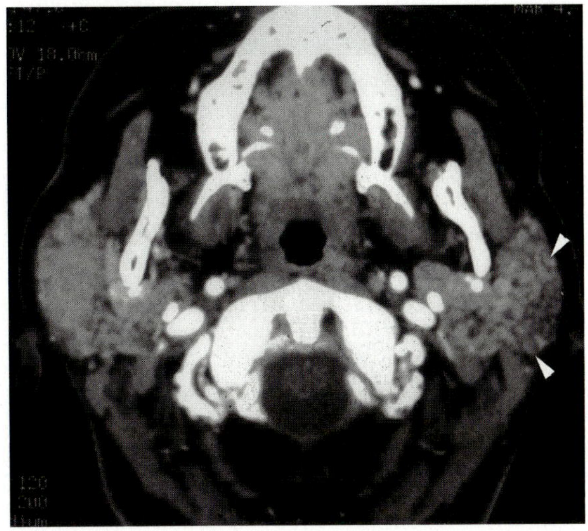

Fig. 2.13: Sjögren's disease, CT. Axial CT after intravenous contrast shows a nodular or granular appearance throughout both parotid glands. Note the multiple small nodular densities (*arrowheads*)

Sialosis

Sialosis or painless, noninflammatory enlargement of the salivary glands gives a variable appearance at imaging depending on the stage. Either MRI or CT will show uniformly large glands. CT can show a dense gland or in more end-stage disease can show enlargement with fatty infiltration. The signal on MRI is relatively uniform throughout a gland but will also vary depending on the stage of the disease. End-stage fat infiltration of the gland shows a very characteristic pattern on T1-weighted sequences. Many times sialosis is seen as an incidental finding. It is important to exclude a mass seen as a more focal abnormality within the gland.

Pitfalls and Common Problems

1. Pleomorphic adenoma may be invisible on initial CT scan if done as the contrast is injected. MRI is considered to be more reliable than CT in finding the margins of the tumor.
2. High enough resolution must be used so that the major neural pathways leading away from a tumor are demonstrated and called negative or positive.
3. Many imaging findings support the preoperative diagnosis of pleomorphic adenoma but no finding is absolutely specific.
4. Complications from imaging are related to contrast allergies. Retrograde sialadenitis can occur if injection sialography is done during acute infection of the gland.

Summary

Imaging of the salivary glands uses many different modalities. There is no established absolute algorithm as to which study should be done in a certain clinical situation. Individual radiologists may prefer one imaging tool over another for evaluation of a particular problem. As always communication between otolaryngologist and radiologist will provide the maximum benefit to the patient.

Take Home Messages

- An irregular margin is the strongest indicator of malignancy but a smooth margin does not necessarily indicate that the tumor is benign.
- The fat pads in the stylomastoid foramen, below the foramen ovale (medial to the lateral pterygoid muscle) and in the pterygopalatine fossa are key check points in the evaluation of perineural spread from salivary malignancy.
- The mylohyoid muscle is a key imaging landmark in sublingual and submandibular disease.
- No imaging modality is perfect for identifying obstructive disease in the salivary glands. The radiologist must know the strengths and weaknesses of each and apply the various studies appropriately.

References

1. Casselman JW, Mancuso AA (1987) Major salivary gland masses: comparison of MR imaging and CT. Radiology 165:183–189
2. Castelijns JA, van den Brekel MWM, Mukherji SK, Lameris JS (2003) Ultrasound of the Neck. In: Som PM, Curtin HD (eds) Head and Neck Imaging. Mosby, St. Louis, Mo., pp 1935–1953
3. Coit WE, Harnsberger HR, Osborn AG, Smoker WR, Stevens MH, Lufkin RB (1987) Ranulas and their mimics: CT evaluation. Radiology 163:211–216
4. Curtin HD (1987) Separation of the masticator space from the parapharyngeal space. Radiology 163:195–204
5. Doubilet PM, Benson CB (2003) Atlas of ultrasound in obstetrics and gynecology: a multimedia reference. Lippincott Williams & Wilkins, Philadelphia
6. Fernandez Moya JM, Cifuentes Sulzberger S, Diaz Recasens J, Ramos C, Sanz R, Perez Tejerizo G (1998) Antenatal diagnosis and management of a ranula. Ultrasound Obstet Gynecol 11:147–148
7. Freling NJ (2000) Imaging of salivary gland disease. Semin Roentgenol 35:12–20
8. Gritzmann N, Rettenbacher T, Hollerweger A, Macheiner P, Hubner E (2003) Sonography of the salivary glands. Eur Radiol 13:964–975
9. Kolker MT, Batti JS, Schoem SR (2004) The ex utero intrapartum treatment procedure for congenital ranula in a Jehovah's Witness. Otolaryngol Head Neck Surg 130:508–510
10. Lev MH, Khanduja K, Morris PP, Curtin HD (1998) Parotid pleomorphic adenomas: delayed CT enhancement. AJNR Am J Neuroradiol 19:1835–1839
11. March DE, Rao VM, Zwillenberg D (1989) Computed tomography of salivary glands in Sjogren's syndrome. Arch Otolaryngol Head Neck Surg 115:105–106
12. Nakamoto Y, Tatsumi M, Hammoud D, Cohade C, Osman MM, Wahl RL (2005) Normal FDG distribution patterns in the head and neck: PET/CT evaluation. Radiology 234:879–885
13. Okamura T, Kawabe J, Koyama K, Ochi H, Yamada R, Sakamoto H, Matsuda M, Ohashi Y, Nakai Y (1998) Fluorine-18 fluorodeoxyglucose positron emission tomography imaging of parotid mass lesions. Acta Otolaryngol Suppl 538:209–213
14. Onderoglu L, Saygan-Karamursel B, Deren O, Bozdag G, Teksam O, Tekinalp G (2003) Prenatal diagnosis of ranula at 21 weeks of gestation. Ultrasound Obstet Gynecol 22:399–401
15. Rabinov JD (2000) Imaging of salivary gland pathology. Radiol Clin North Am 38:1047–1057, x-xi
16. Schlakman BN, Yousem DM (1993) MR of intraparotid masses. AJNR Am J Neuroradiol 14:1173–1180
17. Som PM, Biller HF (1989) High-grade malignancies of the parotid gland: identification with MR imaging. Radiology 173:823–826
18. Som PM, Brandwein MS (2003) Salivary Glands: Anatomy and Pathology. In: Som PM, Curtin HD (eds) Head and Neck Imaging. Mosby, St. Louis, Mo., pp 2005–2133
19. Uchida Y, Minoshima S, Kawata T, Motoori K, Nakano K, Kazama T, Uno T, Okamoto Y, Ito H (2005) Diagnostic value of FDG PET and salivary gland scintigraphy for parotid tumors. Clin Nucl Med 30:170–176
20. Yoshimura Y, Inoue Y, Odagawa T (1989) Sonographic examination of sialolithiasis. J Oral Maxillofac Surg 47:907–912
21. Yousem DM, Kraut MA, Chalian AA (2000) Major salivary gland imaging. Radiology 216:19–29

Chapter 3

Pathology of Salivary Gland Disease

Robert L. Peel and Raja R. Seethala

3

Contents

Core Features

- Salivary gland lesions are rare and can be pathologically challenging due to their wide morphologic spectra.
- Non-neoplastic diseases
  - Acute and chronic non-autoimmune sialadenitis each have fairly characteristic pathologic features though they may have a variety of etiologic factors and pathogenetic mechanisms.
  - Autoimmune sialadenitis is largely comprised of the myoepithelial sialadenitis seen in Sjögren's syndrome, though several autoimmune diseases may manifest in the salivary gland. A complication may be B-cell lymphoproliferative disorders. A subset of chronic sclerosing sialadenitis belongs to this group of diseases.
  - Necrotizing sialometaplasia is a benign self-limited process that may histologically mimic squamous cell carcinoma or mucoepidermoid carcinoma. Subacute necrotizing sialadenitis is a relatively newly described related entity.
  - Sialadenosis is a manifestation of generalized metabolic disturbances while adenomatoid hyperplasia is often an incidental finding.
  - Salivary lymphoepithelial cysts of the salivary gland include salivary type, first branchial cleft cysts, and lymphoepithelial cystic disease of HIV. Dysgenetic polycystic disease is an extremely rare entity.
- Benign tumors
  - Pleomorphic adenomas are the most common benign tumors and have a broad histologic spectrum. These tumors can recur if incompletely excised and may rarely metastasize without having histologic features of malignancy.
  - Basal cell adenomas are benign tumors with specific histologic patterns. The membranous type is associated with cylindromatosis gene (CYLD1) mutations, cutaneous syndromes, and can be multifocal and is more likely to undergo malignant transformation. Canalicular adenomas are minor salivary tumors that are clinicopathologically distinct from basal cell adenomas.
  - Myoepitheliomas also have varied patterns and should show at most a few ducts.
  - Warthin's tumor is linked to smoking and older age and is thus demographically distinct from other cystadenomas. Morphologically it has a characteristic lymphoid stroma resembling a lymph node.
  - Oncocytoma and oncocytosis are benign tumors and tumor-like lesions comprised of solid nests of large polygonal cells with abundant granular eosinophilic cytoplasm that may occasionally mimic metastatic renal cell carcinoma.
  - Sclerosing polycystic adenosis is a rare clonal proliferation that resembles fibrocystic disease of the breast, and though benign, may show changes resembling salivary duct carcinoma.
- Malignant tumors
  - Adenoid cystic carcinoma is a slow growing but relentless malignancy for which stage, histologic grade based on solid component, and p53 expression are important prognosticators. These characteristically overexpress c-kit.
  - Mucoepidermoid carcinoma is the most common salivary malignancy with three cell types (mucous, intermediate, and epidermoid). Most grading systems are three tiered and generally correlate with prognosis; mucoepidermoid carcinomas of the submandibular gland appear more aggressive than those of the parotid gland.

Core Features

- Malignant mixed tumors can be subcategorized into carcinoma ex-pleomorphic adenoma, true malignant mixed tumor (carcinosarcoma), and metastasizing mixed tumor.
- Acinic cell carcinoma is a low-grade tumor that can rarely dedifferentiate into an aggressive high grade tumor.
- Epithelial-myoepithelial carcinoma is a rare biphasic low-grade neoplasm characterized by clear myoepithelial cells and small ducts and may mimic other clear cell lesions of the head and neck.
- Basal cell adenocarcinoma resembles its benign counterpart, basal cell adenoma, and is distinguished mainly by the presence of invasion, though ancillary studies such as immunoperoxidase stains for Ki 67, p53, bcl-2, and epidermal growth factor receptor may help in diagnosis.
- Myoepithelial carcinoma also resembles its benign counterpart and is separated mainly by the presence of invasion, mitoses, and necrosis. Nuclear pleomorphism may be a poor prognostic sign.
- Salivary duct carcinoma is a high grade carcinoma that expresses androgen receptor and her-2-neu. It can be confused with low-grade cribriform cystadenocarcinoma, a recently characterized entity that resembles a low-grade mammary type ductal carcinoma.
- Rare malignant tumors include cystadenocarcinomas, large cell carcinoma, small cell carcinoma, and primary squamous cell carcinomas; all but cystadenocarcinomas behave in an aggressive fashion.

Introduction

The major salivary glands are the paired parotid, submandibular, and sublingual glands. Several hundred smaller minor salivary glands are distributed throughout the mucosa of the oral cavity. Morphologically and functionally similar small aggregates of glands are also present throughout the nasopharynx, sinonasal tract, larynx, trachea, and bronchi. These have also been referred to as minor salivary glands, but are probably more correctly referred to as mucoserous glands. Embryologically they all arise from ingrowths of surface epithelium, are histologically similar, and are affected by the same diseases. The anlage of the parotid can be recognized by the fifth week of embryologic life, the submandibular by the sixth, and the sublingual by the seventh. The parotid is considered to be of ectodermal origin while the submandibular and sublingual glands take origin from endoderm. Origin from surface epithelium is the most likely explanation for the occasional finding of sebaceous glands in the major salivary glands. As the epithelial buds of the future salivary glands enlarge, elongate, and branch they develop lumens and their terminal portions expand into acini lined on the luminal side by a single layer of epithelial cells and on the abluminal side by a single layer of myoepithelial cells. The acini of the parotid gland are lined exclusively by serous cells which are packed with zymogen granules. The acini of the submandibular gland are also mainly serous, but also contain acini lined exclusively by mucous cells and others by serous and mucous cells. The mixed acini are lined by mucous cells with crescentic caps of serous cells known as demilunes of Gianucci. The sublingual gland while composed primarily of mucous acini also contains lesser numbers of serous and mixed acini. Minor salivary glands of the palate, retromolar trigone, and ventral tongue are predominately mucous while those of the lateral tongue, lips, and buccal mucosa are seromucous. Those associated with the circumvallate papillae are referred to as von Ebner's glands and are serous. The acini are drained by a series of ducts the smallest of which are the intralobular intercalated ducts. They are lined by a single layer of cuboidal epithelium and a layer of myoepithelial cells. These in turn drain into the striated ducts so named because of longitudinal infolding of the cell membranes which appears as striations under light microscopy. The striated ducts are also intralobular, but lined by a single layer of epithelium with eosinophilic granular cytoplasm. The intense granular eosinophilia is due to numerous mitochondria. Striated ducts typically lack myoepithelial cells, and are present only in the major salivary glands. Striated ducts drain into the interlobular ducts which are lined by pseudostratified columnar epithelium devoid of a myoepithelial layer. In the major salivary glands these ducts drain into major excretory ducts (Stensen's duct in the parotid gland, Wharton's duct in the submandibular gland, and Bartholin's duct in the sublingual gland) and the epithelium of these ducts changes to squamous as they exit through the oral mucosa. In addition, the sublingual gland also contains several accessory ducts known as Rivinus' ducts. As a result of late encapsulation during embryologic development the parotid gland, unlike the submandibular and sublingual glands, contains intraparenchymal lymph nodes. Late encapsulation is also responsible for the presence of salivary gland structures, usually ducts and less frequency acini, in intra- and periparotid lymph nodes [177, 197, 288, 385, 391, 462].

Lesions of salivary glands are not common but can be pathologically challenging due to their wide range of histologic patterns. Inflammatory and non-neoplastic conditions of salivary glands far outnumber neoplasms which account for less than 3% of all tumors of the head and neck. Approximately one in six parotid tumors, one in three submandibular tumors, and one in two minor salivary gland tumors will be malignant. While tumors of the sublingual gland are extremely uncommon, approximately 80% are malignant [43, 57, 184, 198, 539].

Non-neoplastic Diseases

Acute Sialadenitis

Clinical Features

Acute sialadenitis may involve any salivary gland, though the major salivary glands, particularly the parotid, are most commonly affected [399, 462]. Causes may be bacterial or viral. This entity typically presents unilaterally with localized erythema, swelling, and tenderness in the affected region. Purulent exudate can often be expressed from the excretory duct orifices. Acute viral sialadenitis, in contrast, is preceded by prodromal symptoms including fever, myalgia, and headache and is typically bilateral [399, 462].

Pathology

Grossly, for both acute bacterial and viral sialadenitis, the lobular architecture of the salivary gland is maintained, though the lobules may be expanded and friable with the color ranging from red to yellow. Areas of liquefaction indicative of abscess formation may be present. Cytomegalovirus (CMV) sialadenitis may show no gross abnormalities.

Microscopically, acute bacterial sialadenitis is characterized by acinar destruction with interstitial infiltrates comprised mainly of neutrophils. Multiple small abscesses with necrosis are common. Occasionally, the bacteria can be seen with special stains such as gram stain and acid fast stain, particularly in cases where antibiotics have not yet been administered. Acute viral sialadenitis is rarely examined histopathologically, but consists of a lymphocytic and monocytic infiltrate in the interstitium with vacuolar change in the acini. CMV sialadenitis shows minimal inflammation, but instead may show viral inclusions in both the acini and ducts [195].

Pathogenesis

Bacterial sialadenitis typically occurs as the result of salivary stasis and subsequent retrograde contamination of the salivary ducto-acinar units by oral flora [399, 515]. The parotid is thought to be more prone to bacterial infection since its secretions are predominantly serous and thus lack the protective constituents (IgA, sialic acid, lysozomes) seen in mucinous secretions of the other salivary glands [555, 556]. Causes of salivary stasis include post-surgical setting, dehydration, medical illness, advanced age, radiation, medications, neonatal setting, sialectasia, and sialolithiasis [394, 399, 473]. Bacterial sialadenitis is often polymicrobial. The most common bacterial isolate in acute sialadenitis is *Staphylococcus aureus*. Streptococcal species, most notably the Viridans streptococcal organisms, are also common, and more recently, the contributing role of anaerobic bacteria such as Bacteriodes, peptostreptococcal, and fusobacterial species has been recognized. Rarely, mycobacterial infection may present as an acute sialadenitis rather than a chronic granulomatous sialadenitis (see below) [91, 399, 462, 473, 515].

Viral sialadenitis is typically systemic and can be most commonly attributed to the mumps paramyxovirus. Additional viral isolates include influenza, parainfluenza, Coxsackie A and B, Epstein-Barr, echovirus, and lymphocytic choriomeningitis virus [399, 462]. In the setting of human immunodeficiency virus (HIV), CMV and adenovirus have also rarely been implicated in acute viral parotitis [399].

Prognosis

The prognosis is largely dependent on the patient's underlying disease and its successful treatment. For instance, the reported high mortality (20–50%) reflects the generally poor health status in patients with acute bacterial sialadenitis. A small number will progress to a chronic sialadenitis after resolution of the acute sialadenitis [399].

Chronic Non-autoimmune Sialadenitis

Clinical Features

Chronic non-autoimmune sialadenitis is clinically characterized by a variety of symptoms ranging from a long-standing swelling or mass to xerostomia and superinfection. It may be a result of sialolithiasis which most commonly occurs in the submandibular gland [399, 462]. Chronic sialadenitis, often resulting in xerostomia, is a common and dreaded complication of radiotherapy for head and neck malignant neoplasms [266, 565].

Chronic non-autoimmune sialadenitis is often attributable to a specific etiologic factor such as recurrent obstruction (i.e., sialolithiasis), irradiation, or granulomatous disease [195, 462]. A subset of cases, referred to as chronic recurrent sialadenitis or parotitis, based on the most common site of occurrence, are marked by recurrent painful episodes of swelling and expression of a gray or whitish flocculent material from the duct. Chronic recurrent sialadenitis typically occurs in children or young adults, and may be unilateral or bilateral [60, 462, 503]. Other rare categories of chronic non-autoimmune sialadenitis include infectious granulomatous disease [91, 195].

Pathology

Chronic sialadenitis on gross examination ranges from unremarkable to a firm tan with expansion or atrophy of the lobular architecture depending on the degree of inflammation and chronicity. With sialolithiasis, stones may be grossly evident with associated obstructive changes of sialectasia and periductal fibrosis (Fig. 3.1a).

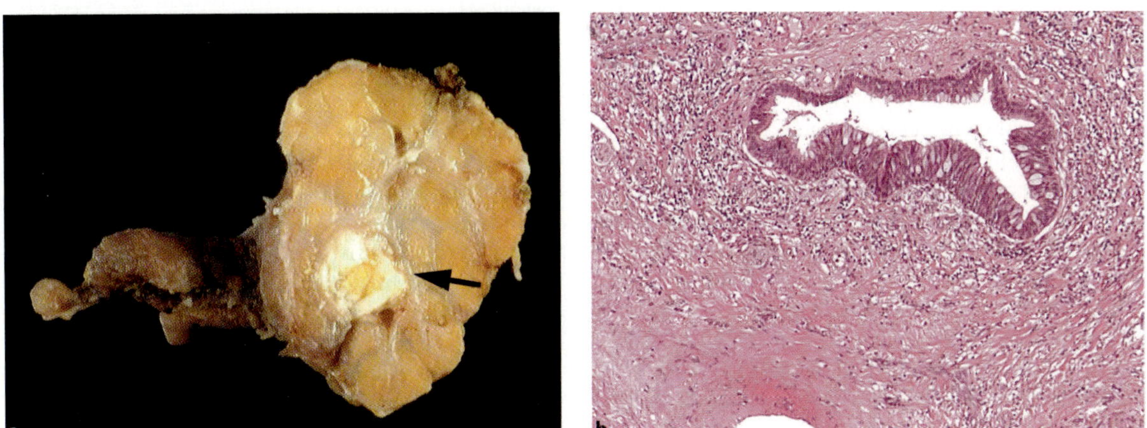

Fig. 3.1: Chronic sialadenitis from sialolithiasis. **a** Submandibular gland with a large sialolith (*arrow*), and mildly ectatic ducts with periductal fibrosis represented by the fibrous white lines radiating from the stone (gross image). **b** Chronic sialadenitis with periductal fibrosis and a mixed chronic inflammatory infiltrate around a large duct that shows mucinous metaplasia (H&E, 100×)

Mucus extravasation may be noted as well [195]. Radiation sialadenitis may show a fibrous white cut surface with involvement of adjacent soft tissue. When the residual lobules are noted, they may be attenuated with interstitial fibrosis.

Microscopically, the classic findings of chronic sialadenitis are a chronic inflammatory infiltrate composed of lymphocytes, plasma cells and macrophages, fibrosis, acinar atrophy, and mucous cell metaplasia of the ductal system (Fig. 3.1b) [462]. A common regenerative phenomenon is the presence of intercalated duct hyperplasia that may be diffuse or nodular. In sialolithiasis, dark calcific stone fragments are noted within the ducts which may have a concomitant squamous metaplasia. Infectious granulomatous sialadenitis ranges from the caseating granulomatosis seen in tuberculosis to foamy histiocytic aggregates seen in atypical mycobacterial infections. Intra- and periparotid lymph node involvement may be seen in the latter [319]. Acid fast stains will highlight the mycobacterial organisms.

Pathogenesis

The predilection of sialoliths to form in the submandibular gland is thought to be a result of the alkaline pH and high mucin content of its secretions. The nidus for stone formation has been postulated to arise as a result of bacteria or organic debris [399, 462]. However, recent scanning electron microscopy and X-ray crystallography studies refuted this as a major cause, finding only hydroxyapatite crystals rich in calcium phosphates [326].

The mechanisms for radiation sialadenitis are not entirely understood, but recent T-cell subset evaluations suggest a possible immune-mediated component of injury [266, 565]. Tuberculous sialadenitis is rare; only 49 cases of tuberculous parotitis have been reported since 1966 [352]. In a review by van der Walt and Leake, tuberculous sialadenitis comprised 8/57 cases of granulomatous sialadenitis [590].

Prognosis

The prognosis depends on the etiologic factor, if identified, and the severity of disease. While surgical treatment of chronic sialadenitis leads to resolution of symptoms of pain and prevention of superinfection with fistula or sinus tract formation [19], xerostomia, often seen in radiation sialadenitis, does not resolve [266, 565].

Autoimmune Sialadenitis

Clinical Features

The majority of autoimmune sialadenitides are in the histopathologic spectrum of myoepithelial sialadenitis (MESA), a term coined as early as 1972 by Donath and Seifert [158], also known as benign lymphoepithelial lesion. The clinical correlates are varied and include terms such as Mikulicz disease, sicca complex, Sjögren's syndrome, and chronic punctate sialadenitis [462].

Other systemic autoimmune diseases that can affect the salivary glands, usually the parotid include Wegener's granulomatosis, sarcoid, and Kimura's disease [383]. Recent evidence indicates that a subset of chronic sclerosing sialadenitides (Kuttner tumor) have an autoimmune etiology [332].

Myoepithelial sialadenitis may present as unilateral or bilateral enlargement of salivary glands, at any age with or without autoimmune disease, but most commonly manifests in females in their fifth to sixth decades as a reflection of the close association with Sjögren's syndrome. Sialograms show sialectasia which ranges from punctate to cavitary [462].

Sjögren's syndrome is an autoimmune exocrinopathy characterized by keratoconjunctivitis, xerostomia, and often other extrasalivary manifestations. It can exist as a primary disease or as a secondary disease associated with other systemic autoimmune diseases, typically rheumatoid arthritis and occasionally progressive systemic sclerosis [224].

Salivary gland involvement in Wegener's granulomatosis, characterized by upper and lower respiratory tract and renal disease, is rare with the parotid being most commonly affected [383]. Fauci et al. [206] report an incidence of less than 1% (n=158) in their experience. In contrast, salivary gland involvement in sarcoidosis is not infrequent ranging from 4% to 30%. A rare syndromic variant of sarcoidosis known as Heerfordt syndrome is characterized by uveitis, bilateral parotitis, and facial nerve palsy [383].

Kimura's disease occurs typically in young Asian males and is characterized clinically by painless lymphadenopathy of the head and neck region, including periparotid and intraparotid lymph nodes [383, 536]. Chronic sclerosing sialadenitis presents as a firm localized swelling of the salivary gland mimicking a neoplasm, most commonly involving the submandibular gland [462]. While originally categorized as a non-specific localized chronic sialadenitis, when excluding cases that are attributable to sialolithiasis or other localized obstruction, at least a subset present with autoimmune extrasalivary disease such as primary sclerosing cholangitis, idiopathic retroperitoneal fibrosis, and lymphoplasmacytic sclerosing pancreatitis warranting placement in the autoimmune sialadenitis category [323, 332].

Pathology

The gross manifestations of myoepithelial sialadenitis are similar to chronic non-immune sialadenitis, ranging from a diffuse to a multinodular expansion. In some cases, the gross cut surface is a tan-pink reminiscent of a lymph node, however, the lobular architecture is maintained distinguishing this from lymphoma. Wegener's granulomatosis may show areas of liquefaction necrosis as a result of vasculitis. Sarcoidosis and Kimura's disease may show preferential enlargement of the intra/periparotid lymph nodes. Chronic sclerosing sialadenitis on gross examination resembles a salivary gland neoplasm and with a well-circumscribed tan-white appearance.

The histologic hallmark of MESA is the presence of epithelial-myoepithelial islands infiltrated by lymphocytes (Fig. 3.2). However, the process begins as a collection of lymphocytes centered on an intralobular duct. This lymphoid infiltrate, when a cluster of at least 50 lymphocytes per 4 mm^2 defines a lymphoid focus, is the basis for grading of labial minor salivary gland biopsies for the diagnosis of Sjögren's syndrome [139, 458]. As these lymphoid infiltrates progress, germinal centers may form, and acinar atrophy ensues. A proliferation of ductal epithelium-myoepithelium arises, obliterating duct lumina and eventually giving rise to classic epithelial-myoepithelial islands. A few studies suggest that these islands may not contain a myoepithelial component, but are composed of metaplastic intercalated ducts with an altered immunophenotype [309, 333].

Salivary glands in the setting of secondary Sjögren's syndrome due to progressive systemic sclerosis may show periglandular fibrosis without inflammation in addition to MESA [458]. Wegener's granulomatosis manifests as a classic triad of vasculitis, necrosis, and granulomatous inflammation, however, only 16% of cases with parotid involvement have the complete triad [383]. Sarcoid is characterized by tight epithelioid granulomas and a lymphoid infiltrate. Biopsies of salivary glands in the lip for the diagnosis of sarcoid show granulomas in 53% of cases [442].

Chronic sclerosing sialadenitis bears a remarkable similarity to lymphoplasmacytic sclerosing pancreatitis [323]. It is characterized by periductal fibrosis with a dense lymphoplasmacytic infiltrate with lymphoid follicles. Eosinophils are variably present. Kitagawa et al. demonstrated the presence of obliterative phlebitis in all cases as demonstrated by elastic stain [332].

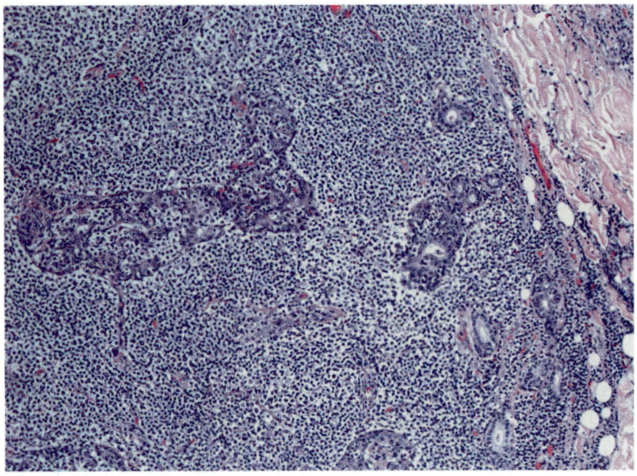

Fig. 3.2: Myoepithelial sialadenitis (MESA) with a florid lymphoid infiltrate and prominent epithelial myoepithelial islands permeated by lymphocytes (H&E, 100×)

Pathogenesis

While Sjögren's syndrome often has a characteristic serology, including anti SS-A, anti SS-B, and occasionally ANA and rheumatoid factor, the pathogenesis of the disease is not entirely clear and is multifactorial as with most autoimmune diseases [224]. In addition to HLA-DR associations, recent studies suggest that polymorphisms in genes, such as minor histocompatibility antigen HA-1, and TNF may play a role in the disease process. Humoral dysregulation and B-cell hyperactivity is thought to be another pathogenic mechanism for Sjögren's syndrome [224, 277].

Similarly, though the serologic manifestations are well known, the pathogenesis of Wegener's granulomatosis, sarcoidosis, Kimura's disease, and chronic sclerosing sialadenitis are not well understood. The classic serologic manifestation of Wegener's granulomatosis is a positive C-ANCA. Sarcoidosis often manifests with hypergammaglobulinemia as well as non-serologic laboratory abnormalities such as hypercalcemia, elevated alkaline phosphatase, and angiotensin-converting enzyme levels. Kimura's disease is characterized by elevated IgE levels and eosinophilia, while the association of chronic sclerosing sialadenitis with elevated IgG4 levels has been noted recently [323, 332, 383].

Prognosis

As with most sialadenitides, the prognosis is related to the severity and treatment of the underlying disorder [75]. Severe recurrent parotitis is amenable to surgical treatment [19]. Of note, patients with Sjögren's syndrome have a forty-fold increased risk for development of small B-cell lymphomas of mucosa-associated lymphoid tissue (MALT) type [224].

Special Considerations

Myoepithelial Sialadenitis and Mucosa-associated Lymphoid Tissue (MALT) Lymphomas

The majority of salivary gland lymphomas are of the MALT type and arise in the setting of MESA. This association was noted as early as 1971 by Azzopardi and Evans [31]. The transition from MESA to MALT lymphoma is postulated to occur as a result of antigenic stimulation, though unlike gastric MALT lymphoma, the etiologic agent (*H. pylori* in gastric MALT lymphoma) has not been identified [32].

Histologic distinction of MESA from early MALT lymphoma is obfuscated by the detection of clonal proliferations in otherwise typical appearing MESA [214, 337]. These MESA clones have a limited VH repertoire even among different patients, suggesting antigenic stimulation from a common epitope [32]. While these clones may eventually give rise to MALT lymphoma, clonality in the setting of typical or even atypical MESA without a significant mass lesion does not indicate lymphoma. The earliest histologic changes of MALT lymphoma are the presence of "halos" of monocytoid or centrocyte-like B cells that are slightly paler on low power magnification [301]. These coalesce into sheets and eventually form mass lesions. Involvement of intra- and periparotid lymph nodes is often seen.

Immunohistochemical and flow cytometric analysis show a population of B cells that are CD19 positive, CD20 positive, CD5 negative, CD10 negative, and CD23 negative. CD43, typically seen on T cells may be aberrantly expressed. MALT lymphomas will often but not always show light chain restriction [1].

Mucosa-associated lymphoid tissue lymphomas have several associated characteristic translocations and trisomies though the frequencies of these vary by site. In the salivary gland, the most common translocation is t(14;18)(q32;q21) which is the fusion of IGH/MALT1, while trisomy 3 was the most common alteration overall. The significance of these alterations is unclear at this point [552].

Myoepithelial Sialadenitis and Carcinoma

In rare instances, MESA can have malignant transformation of the epithelial component. Carcinomas arising in MESA are typically lymphoepithelial carcinomas resembling undifferentiated non-keratinizing nasopharyngeal carcinoma, though keratinizing squamous cell carcinomas have been described [44, 89, 428]. Lymphoepithelial carcinomas of the parotid, akin to their nasopharyngeal counterparts, are often associated with Epstein-Barr virus (EBV) infection. Wu et al. demonstrated the presence of EBV small RNA-1 (EBER-1) in MESA with carcinomatous transformation in both the benign and malignant areas, while typical MESA was negative for EBER [620].

Necrotizing Sialometaplasia

Clinical Features

Necrotizing sialometaplasia (NSM), originally described by Abrams et al. in 1973 [3] is a benign self-healing salivary gland lesion that can mimic malignancy. NSM typically occurs in the fourth decade (mean age 45.9 years) with a male predilection (male:female ratio 1.9:1) [85, 222, 311, 462]. Although the palate is the most frequently involved site, NSM has been described in mucoserous glands throughout the upper and lower respiratory tract [85, 380, 484, 630]. The usual presentation is that of a single unilateral ulcer at the junction of the hard and soft palate [85, 222, 462]. Roughly 10% are bilateral, and 15% are asymptomatic [85].

Pathology

Grossly, NSM is typically a well-demarcated, raised, erythematous ulcer. The underlying salivary tissue is a soft friable gray tan [195, 462]. In a review of 184 cases, the mean size was 1.9 cm (range 0.7–5.0 cm) [85]. The defining microscopic features are: ulceration with pseudoepitheliomatous hyperplasia of the adjacent mucosa, infarction of the salivary lobule, with mucus extravasation, varying degrees of fibrosis, and squamous metaplasia of the ductoacinar units (Fig. 3.3a, b). The latter may be prominent and thus misread as mucoepidermoid carcinoma or squamous cell carcinoma. However, the key distinguishing feature of NSM from the malignant lesions that it may mimic is the maintenance of the lobular architecture despite the often extensive squamous metaplasia. On small biopsy specimens, this may be difficult to assess. Though a high index of suspicion of this lesion is the main requirement for its diagnosis in such a situation, a recent study suggests that NSM in contrast to squamous cell carcinoma does not show evidence of immunohistochemical staining for p53, Ki-67, and bcl-2 and thus may be a useful adjunct for distinguishing between these lesions [418]. It is very important to have an accurate diagnosis of NSM to avoid unnecessary surgery.

Pathogenesis

The classic NSM is thought to be the result of spontaneous infarction of mucoserous glands. However, a clinically and histologically identical picture is seen as a result of surgery, radiation, trauma, or vasculitis among other distortive injuries [26, 487]. The self-limiting nature and histologic features suggest vascular compromise with ischemic injury and subsequent regeneration as the main pathogenic mechanism [85, 462]. The occasional association with repeated emesis seen in bulimia and other disorders raises the possibility of chemical injury as a contributing factor [4, 496].

Prognosis

Prognosis is excellent. NSM is a self-limiting lesion lasting from a few days to a few months and does not recur [85].

Subacute Necrotizing Sialadenitis

Clinical Features

Subacute necrotizing sialadenitis (SANS) is a recently described idiopathic reactive process of minor salivary glands with only 26 cases reported in the literature [106, 222, 371, 588, 612]. SANS shares several clinical and pathologic features with NSM.

In contrast to NSM, SANS occurs typically in the second decade. However, similar to NSM, SANS typically occurs as a painful mass of the palate, though they are non-ulcerated in contrast to NSM. The male predominance is more pronounced (approximately 3:1) though

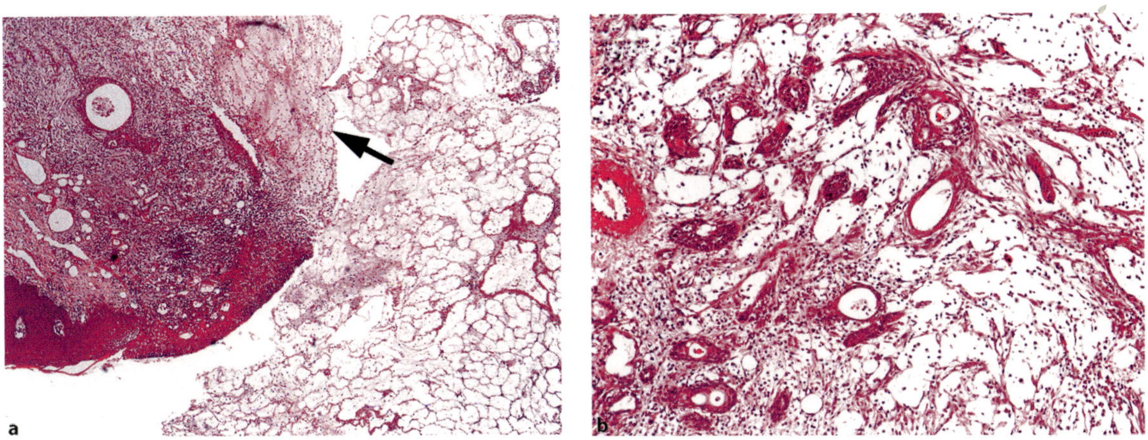

Fig. 3.3: Necrotizing sialometaplasia. **a** Palate with ulcerated squamous mucosa (*left*) and necrotic mucous acini (*right*) showing loss of cellular detail and focal extravasation of mucin (*arrow*) (H&E, 20×). **b** Squamous metaplasia or "sialometaplasia" is noted in the ducts (H&E, 100×)

this may reflect sampling bias, as many of these cases were obtained from a military population [222, 612].

Pathology

Grossly, these are non-ulcerated submucosal masses ranging from 0.3 to 2.5 cm. The histologic criteria put forth by Werning et al. [612] are: acinar cell necrosis and loss, and a mixed inflammatory infiltrate comprised of neutrophils, eosinophils (occasionally prominent), and plasma cells. In contrast to NSM, SANS does not show squamous metaplasia or fibrosis. Ultrastructurally, dense particles have been identified in the acini that either represent viral particles or lysosomes [222, 612].

Pathogenesis

The etiology of SANS is unclear. Because of similar clinical and pathologic characteristics, SANS is viewed by some as a variant of NSM [371]. However, the association in a significant number of patients with upper respiratory tract infections, close living quarters, and a winter month predilection raises the possibility of a viral etiology. Further in support of this is the presence of dense viral-like particles ultrastructurally in the acini in several cases [222].

Prognosis

As in NSM, prognosis is excellent. SANS is also a self-limiting disease with an even more rapid course than NSM; all cases reported resolved within 4 weeks [222, 371, 588].

Sialadenosis

Clinical Features

Sialadenosis is a diffuse enlargement of salivary glands described in several conditions. Sialadenosis usually involves the parotid glands, and less commonly the submandibular glands [121, 157, 462]. Minor salivary gland involvement has also been reported [408]. It is frequently bilateral and has an equal sex distribution. It is typically painless and the enlargement may impart a striking facial appearance. Causes can be categorized as: nutritional (alcoholism, cirrhosis, eating disorders, kwashiorkor, and pellagra), endocrine (diabetes mellitus, thyroid disease, gonadal dysfunction), and neurochemical (vegetative state, lead, mercury, iodine, thiouracil, isoproterenol) [157, 462].

Pathology

Grossly, the salivary glands are unremarkable except for enlargement. Histologically, sialadenosis is a mixture of acinar hypertrophy and fatty infiltration. Morphometric studies have shown an increase in mean acinar cell diameter (approximately 75 microns) as compared to normal (approximately 50 microns) [267]. Additionally zymogen granules are increased in number and size by light and electron microscopy [160]. Most importantly, no inflammation or fibrosis is identified, distinguishing sialadenosis from the sialadenitides. While amyloidosis may present with diffuse enlargement of the salivary glands, histologically, there will be interstitial fibrosis with the characteristic pale amyloid deposition that can be demonstrated with a Congo red stain [195].

Pathogenesis

Despite the variety of predisposing conditions, sialadenosis is thought to be a neurosecretory disorder. Ultrastructural and animal experimental studies point to a disturbance in the autonomic innervation of the salivary glands as the initiating factor for sialadenosis [121, 123, 157, 160, 161].

Prognosis

The persistence of sialadenosis is dependent on the severity and duration of the underlying disease. However, there is usually little morbidity associated with the condition itself; most surgical treatment is performed for cosmetic purposes.

Adenomatoid Hyperplasia

Clinical Features

Adenomatoid hyperplasia is a proliferation of the mucous acini of minor salivary glands. The incidence of this lesion is likely higher than reported in the literature [16, 39, 86, 95, 462]. Adenomatoid hyperplasia typically presents as a painless mass located on the hard and soft palate in up to 95% of cases [39]. Rarely, adenomatoid hyperplasia is located on the retromolar trigone [86, 116]. While it can present at any age it is more common in the fourth decade with a slight male predominance. The typical clinical concern is that of a benign salivary gland tumor [462]. We have occasionally noted these lesions in uvulopalatopharyngoplasty specimens suggesting their role in some cases of obstructive sleep apnea.

Pathology

Grossly, these lesions range from 0.5 to 3 cm [462]. They are usually non-ulcerated well-circumscribed masses. Histologically, the lesion is comprised of expanded lobules of mucous acini. Occasionally, there is mucus extravasation, but without an inflammatory reaction. The overlying mucosa is unremarkable.

Pathogenesis

The pathogenesis is unclear. While Arafat et al. [16] raise the possibility of a hamartomatous origin to this lesion, Barrett and Speight [39] report 14 of 20 (70%) cases to be associated with dentures and/or tobacco suggesting a localized response to trauma. But this apparent association may be the result of sampling bias since the most common clinical setting for the detection of adenomatous hyperplasia is during dental examination [462].

Prognosis

Prognosis is excellent. Recurrences are not seen after excision.

Salivary Duct Cysts

Clinical Features

Salivary duct cysts are also known as sialocysts, simple cysts, and retention cysts. Unlike mucus extravasation phenomenon, salivary duct cysts are true cysts with an epithelial lining [56]. Salivary duct cysts are the most common salivary cysts, comprising about 1.5% of all salivary gland disease in one study [507].

Pathology

These cysts are unilocular and may grossly contain tan serous to gray mucoid material. Long-standing cysts can develop sialoliths. Histologically, these cysts are lined by a cuboidal, columnar, or squamous epithelium. Oncocytic metaplasia may be seen in older individuals. However, these cysts are not associated with lymphoid elements [462].

Pathogenesis

Sialocysts usually occur secondary to obstruction from various causes [56, 195, 462].

Prognosis

Prognosis is excellent. Rare complications include superimposed infections. Recurrences are rare and result from incomplete excision [462].

Lymphoepithelial Cysts

Clinical Features

Lymphoepithelial cysts refer to a group of lesions that include true first branchial cleft cysts, salivary-type lymphoepithelial cysts, and HIV-associated sialadenitis, which may also have overlap with MESA.

True branchial cleft cysts typically present shortly after birth or in childhood though they may not be symptomatic until adulthood. They usually present as a painless unilateral mass near or occasionally in the parotid gland, often with associated sinus tracts and fistulae. Superinfection may cause pain [454, 462, 575].

Salivary duct derived lymphoepithelial cysts rarely present at birth and are not associated with sinus tracts or fistulae. HIV-associated lymphoepithelial cysts have become increasingly common, comprising up to 60% of parotid lymphoepithelial cysts [564]. These tend to be bilateral and associated with lymphadenopathy. The incidence of parotid gland involvement in HIV is about

3–5% [307]. Occasionally these may be the presenting symptom of HIV infection [390]. While the parotid gland is the most frequent site for HIV-associated lymphoepithelial cysts, cysts in the submandibular glands have also been described [262].

Pathology

True first branchial cleft cysts of the parotid region can be divided into type I and type II. Type I anomalies are considered reduplication of the ectodermal component of the ear canal while type II anomalies also include mesodermal components as well [18, 212, 454]. The type II anomalies are more closely associated with the parotid parenchyma [454, 462]. Grossly, these cysts are adjacent to or in the parotid gland and contain cloudy to cheesy material representing keratinaceous debris. In type II anomalies, the cyst wall may grossly contain cartilage. Histologically, branchial cleft cysts will contain a combination of squamous and ciliated respiratory type epithelium. Type II lesions will also contain skin adnexal structures and cartilage. Both types may have lymphoid tissue with germinal centers in the periphery.

Lymphoepithelial cysts may have a nodular inner lining that grossly represents lymphoid tissue. Salivary type lymphoepithelial cysts are lined by a thin squamous or columnar epithelium, and are surrounded by a prominent lymphoid infiltrate with all the architectural features of a lymph node including sinusoidal spaces and primary and secondary germinal centers [56, 467]. Lymphoepithelial cysts in HIV often contain epithelial-myoepithelial islands seen in MESA, and an additional finding is that of multinucleated giant cells [169, 595]. Immunohistochemical detection has identified p24 antigen in the macrophages and giant cells seen in HIV-associated lymphoepithelial cysts [93, 347, 386, 583, 595]. The lymphoid infiltrate differs from that in non-HIV-associated lymphoepithelial cysts and MESA in that it is comprised largely of $CD8^+$ lymphocytes [118, 382].

Pathogenesis

True branchial cleft cysts in the parotid region are derived from the first branchial pouch and are duplication defects. While, initially, the term branchial cleft cyst was used interchangeably for all parotid lymphoepithelial cysts [551, 608], this term has now been reserved only for those cysts that have clinical or histologic features of first branchial pouch derivatives, e.g., early age of onset, presence of sinuses or fistulae, ciliated respiratory epithelium, and the presence of mesodermal elements in type II anomalies. The presence of salivary inclusions within the lymphoid stroma of some lymphoepithelial cysts, as well the documentation of a high amylase content in cyst fluid suggest that most lesions called lymphoepithelial cysts are of the salivary type [230, 467]. These cysts are thus thought to represent cystic dilation of salivary inclusions of the intra- and periparotid lymph nodes.

Human immunodeficiency virus-associated lymphoepithelial cysts are also thought to arise from cystification of salivary elements. However, the histologic spectrum along with three-dimensional reconstruction of 100 parotid lesions [308] suggest that these cysts are cystic dilation of the native ductal system of the salivary gland in the setting of MESA-type lesion akin to that seen in autoimmune disease rather than dilatation of salivary gland inclusions within a lymph node [307, 308].

Prognosis

The recurrence rate for all types of lymphoepithelial cysts is low to absent, however, branchial cleft cysts are more likely to recur than the others, and must be completely excised [18, 212].

Dysgenetic Polycystic Disease

Clinical Features

Dysgenetic polycystic disease is an extremely rare salivary gland disease with only 15 cases reported in the literature [45, 156, 211, 235, 396, 456, 511].

Dysgenetic polycystic disease occurs almost exclusively in the parotid glands of women with an age range of 6–65 years [235]. Only one case has been documented in the submandibular gland of a man [456, 511]. Usually this disease is bilateral, but unilateral disease has been documented [45, 156, 211, 235, 396, 456, 511]. The typical presentation is that of a non-tender mass [211, 511, 534].

Pathology

Grossly, these lesions present as spongy masses of the involved salivary gland. Histologically, there is variable replacement of the parenchyma by cysts of various size and shape. The epithelium is attenuated and cuboidal, and the cyst wall is delicate with minimal fibrosis or inflammation. Occasional invaginations and tufting of epithelium may be seen. The lumina may contain concentric eosinophilic secretions [534].

Pathogenesis

Dysgenetic polycystic disease is thought to be a result of some type of embryologic insult. Though it bears similarities to polycystic disease of other organ sites, such as kidney and liver, this entity has not been associated with extraparotid manifestations. At least three cases have a familial association, though the responsible genetic alteration has not yet been identified [198, 201, 492, 539].

Prognosis

This entity is sufficiently rare as to preclude definitive prediction of behavior. To date, recurrence has been described only occasionally [198, 539].

Benign Tumors

Pleomorphic Adenoma

Clinical Features

Pleomorphic adenoma, also known as benign mixed tumor, is the most common tumor of salivary gland origin, accounting for about 60% of all salivary tumors in large series [298]. Up to 80% occur in the parotid gland, 10% in the submandibular glands, and the rest in the minor salivary glands, throughout the upper and lower aerodigestive tract [449, 508, 624]. While most occur in the lower pole of the superficial lobe, the deep lobe can be involved. Extensions of deep lobe pleomorphic adenomas are the most common tumors of the parapharyngeal space constituting 40% of tumors in this region [198, 201]. Bilateral occurrences of pleomorphic adenoma are rare [201, 462].

Pleomorphic adenomas can occur in any decade, but the mean age is 46 years with a slight female predilection [96, 291, 329]. The typical presentation is that of a painless, slowly growing mass.

Pathology

Grossly, pleomorphic adenomas are typically well-circumscribed ovoid masses. They usually range from 2 to 5 cm in greatest dimension [559], though tumors as large as 50 cm in diameter, weighing over 6 kg have been reported [354, 509, 527]. Larger tumors often have a bosselated surface and may distend overlying skin and cause erosion of bone and remodeling deep to the tumor. In the major glands, they usually have a complete capsule, while in the minor glands they may not. Pleomorphic adenomas usually show a lobulated glistening gray tan cut surface representative of the chondromyxoid stroma characteristic of this tumor (Fig. 3.4a). Areas with less chondroid appear as a homogeneous white tan color. Larger tumors may have areas of calcification/ossification, hemorrhage, and necrosis. Such areas of heterogeneity should be sampled to exclude malignant degeneration. Satellite nodules in primary tumors are rare, but are typical of recurrent tumors.

Histologically, pleomorphic adenoma, as with many salivary tumors, is a biphasic tumor comprised of epithelial (ductal) and myoepithelial cells. It is named for its various histologic patterns or "pleomorphism," rather than actual cellular atypia. The myoepithelial component often predominates with spindled to ovoid cells with wispy pink cytoplasm embedded in a pale chondromyxoid blue gray stroma. These myoepithelial cells are often seen streaming off the ductal component blending into the stroma (Fig. 3.4b). A unique pattern within areas of myoepithelial predominance is a palisaded growth resembling that seen in schwannoma [111]. Cartilaginous differentiation is often seen. Occasionally, osseous metaplasia and even lipomatous metaplasia may be present [201]. Tyrosine-rich crystals are occasionally seen within the chondroid stroma [145, 201].

The tumors can show various epithelial differentiation such as oncocytic, squamous, mucinous, and sebaceous metaplasia, and can be mistaken for squamous cell carcinoma or mucoepidermoid carcinoma, if the overall architecture and configuration is not taken into consideration [445]. The proportions of epithelial and myoepithelial

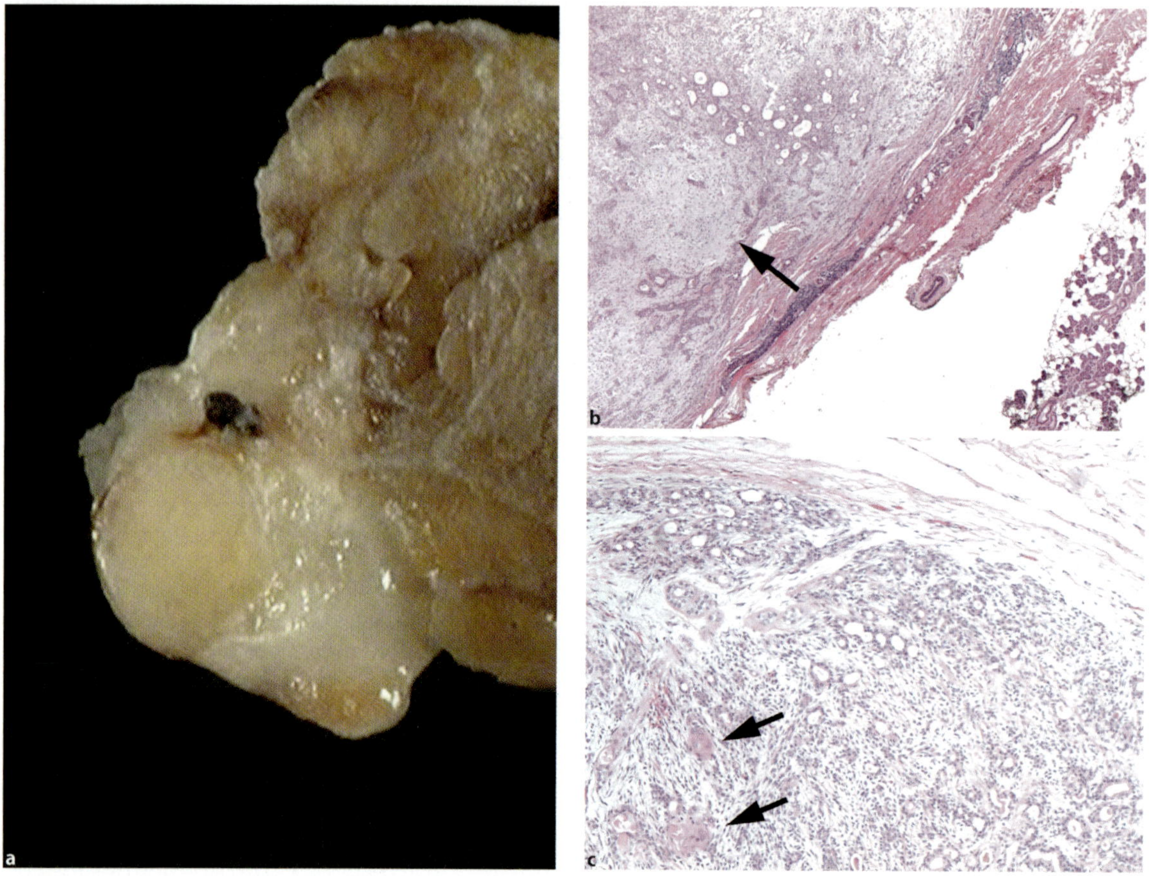

Fig. 3.4: Pleomorphic adenoma. **a** A small well-circumscribed tumor of the tail of the parotid showing a homogeneous glistening gray-tan cut surface (gross image). **b** An encapsulated pleomorphic adenoma with ducts (*top*) and nodular areas of chondroid differentiation (*arrow*) (H&E, 40×). **c** Cellular pleomorphic adenoma with back-to-back ducts lined by myoepithelial cells almost resembling epithelial-myoepithelial carcinoma. Focal squamous metaplasia is present (*small arrows*) (H&E, 100×)

cells vary greatly. Myoepithelial-rich pleomorphic adenomas may be indistinguishable from myoepithelioma if the ductal component is not found. At the other end of the spectrum, cellular pleomorphic adenomas, which contain tubulotrabecular proliferations of ducts and myoepithelial cells with minimal stroma can be mistaken for malignant tumors such as epithelial-myoepithelial carcinoma and adenoid cystic carcinoma if only limited biopsy material is available (Fig. 3.4c).

Immunohistochemically, the ductal components are positive for various cytokeratins: 7, 8, 14, and 19, typically of low molecular weight. The myoepithelial cells are positive for p63, smooth muscle actin, calponin, vimentin, muscle-specific actin, and variably for S-100 protein and glial fibrillary acidic protein (GFAP) [629]. GFAP, though not a sensitive myoepithelial marker, has the benefit of highlighting areas of chondroid stroma, which can distinguish pleomorphic adenoma from other similar histologic types [297]. Similarly, bone morphogenic proteins and type II collagen are expressed in these areas as well [97, 388]. While immunostaining for S-100 also highlights the stromal component, it may also stain some ductal areas [97].

Pathogenesis

Roughly 70% of pleomorphic adenomas have cytogenetic alterations that likely play a central role in tumorigenesis, and can be stratified into four groups: those with 8q12 rearrangements, those with 12q13-15 rearrangements, those with miscellaneous clonal changes, and those that are karyotypically normal [325, 598]. Bullerdiek et al. [597] note that the karyotypically normal individuals are usually a decade older than those with 8q12 rearrangements.

The 8q12 abnormalities are typically translocations involving the PLAG1 gene, juxtaposing this zinc finger gene with a ubiquitously expressed translocation partner gene. The two most common translocations, t(3;8) (p21;q12) and t(5;8) (p13;q12), result in CTTNB1-PLAG1 and LIFR1-PLAG1 fusions, respectively [240, 241]. PLAG1 alterations result in increased IgF2 expression, which is likely contributory to the development of pleomorphic adenoma [5]. The 12q13-15 abnormalities are also usually translocations, involving the HMGA2 (HMGIC) gene that encodes a transcription factor involved in the modulation of DNA structural conformation. The most common alterations are ins(9;12) and t(3;12), which result in HMGA2-NFIB and HMGA2-FHIT fusions, respectively [189].

Interestingly, a t(3;12) was reported in two cases (siblings) of familial pleomorphic adenomas [28, 242, 289, 356, 479]. The aforementioned translocations are also implicated in radiation-associated pleomorphic adenomas [242].

Prognosis

While pleomorphic adenoma is a benign tumor, it has the capacity to recur and to undergo malignant transformation. Recurrence rates range from 0.8% to 6.8% in large series with long-term follow-up [287]. While complete excision is required to ensure a favorable outcome, preservation of anatomic structures is also a major concern. Ghosh et al. [102, 477] argue that the recurrence rate is low (1.8%) even with tumor less than 1 mm from the margin. Capsular rupture and subsequent tumor spillage may play a role in the recurrence of pleomorphic adenoma, however, Henriksson et al. [78, 247, 610] report that the presence of pseudopodia or capsular infiltration was a more significant predictor of recurrence. Recurrent pleomorphic adenomas have a higher likelihood for second recurrence of about 6–15%. Uninodular recurrences have a better outcome than multinodular recurrences [78, 247, 610].

Rarely, a histologically benign pleomorphic adenoma can metastasize and behave like a low-grade malignancy, however, there are no features that can predict this rare occurrence. However, many of these tumors metastasized after at least one initial local recurrence, suggesting the possibility that altered anatomy secondary to surgery gave access to vascular and lymphatic channels [24]. As many as 40% of patients with metastasizing pleomorphic adenomas die with disease [133, 429, 626]. True malignant transformation is rare as well. Clinical features predictive of malignant transformation are age, tumor size, and a long history of a mass in the parotid gland and submandibular location. The presence of hyalinized stroma is the most predictive histologic parameter for malignant transformation [462, 626].

Basal Cell Adenoma

Clinical Features

Basal cell adenomas tend to occur over the age of 50 years with a slight female predilection of 2:1 [199]. They usually occur in the parotid (75%) or submandibular gland (approximately 5%) [626]. These lesions are quite rare in the minor salivary glands when excluding canalicular adenomas which were previously categorized with basal cell adenoma [623, 625]. They typically present as a slowly growing solitary painless mass [462]. A special variant of basal cell adenoma, the membranous type (dermal analog tumor) can be associated with multiple trichoepitheliomas and cylindromas (Brooke-Spiegler syndrome) [429].

Pathology

Grossly, these tumors are a well-circumscribed, solid homogeneous gray-white to tan-brown occasionally mimicking an enlarged lymph node. Rarely, cystic change may be seen grossly [625]. Most tumors are less than 2 cm in diameter [142]. Membranous type basal cell adenomas can be multifocal [429].

Despite the archaic term for these tumors, "monomorphic adenomas," basal cell adenomas can show a variety of histologic patterns: tubular, trabecular, cribriform [141], solid, and membranous. Other than the membranous type, these morphologic patterns have no clinical significance. The common feature to all of these tumors is a "basaloid" morphology to the tumor, namely a proliferation of small dark cells that have a peripheral cuboidal to columnar layer with varying degrees of stratification and palisading. These tumors are reminiscent of cutaneous epidermal and adnexal tumors such as basal cell carcinoma, trichoepithelioma, and cylindroma. Microscopic cystic change is fairly common, present in as many as 65% of tumors, predominating in the tubular/trabecular patterns [622, 625]. Within the center of these tumors, various lines of differentiation can be seen ranging from squamous to sebaceous to mucinous. Basal cell adenomas may have a myxoid or hyaline stroma, and rarely a myoepithelial-rich cellular stroma [606]. However, in contrast to pleomorphic adenoma, the stroma, regardless of cellularity, is distinct from the basaloid proliferation, with no intermingling. Mitoses are rare to absent, as is necrosis, and there is no infiltration of surrounding tissue or perineural invasion, which distinguishes basal cell adenomas from their malignant counterparts, basal cell adenocarcinomas.

The tubular pattern is composed of ductal structures surrounded by a cuboidal to palisaded basal layer, while the trabecular pattern consists of ribbons or cords of cells traversing a myxoid or hyaline stroma resembling a canalicular adenoma in areas (Fig. 3.5a). The solid and cribriform variants consist of broader nests or islands of cells

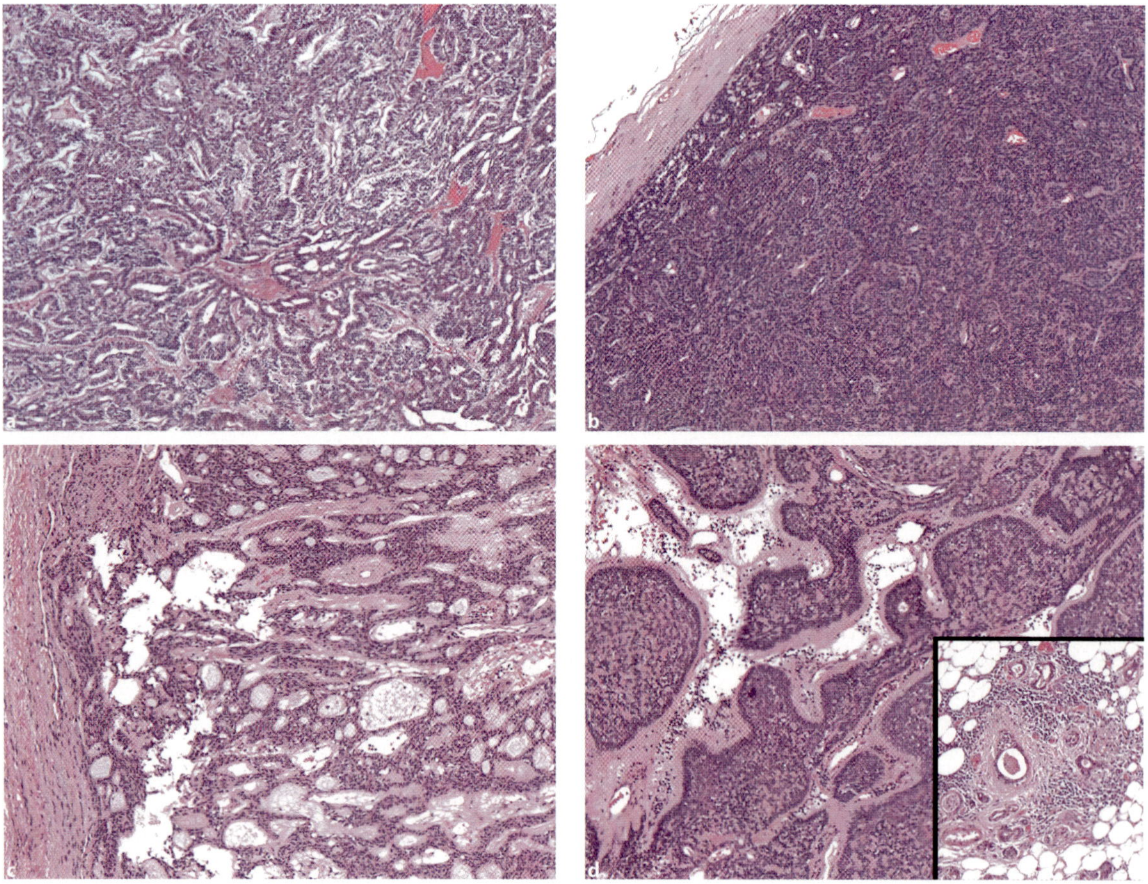

Fig. 3.5: Patterns of basal cell adenoma (all H&E, 100×): **a** tubulotrabecular, **b** solid, **c** cribriform, and **d** membranous or dermal analogue type. *Inset* for **d** a focus of striated duct hyperplasia adjacent to the main tumor

with peripheral palisading, and "cookie cutter" holes in the latter (Fig. 3.5b, c). This latter variant can be confused with adenoid cystic carcinoma. However, the cribriform basal cell adenoma does not infiltrate the surrounding tissue like adenoid cystic carcinoma. Additionally, though often small and dark, the nuclei in this subtype are more vesicular and less angulated than adenoid cystic carcinoma nuclei.

The membranous type of basal cell adenoma consists of nests of cells arranged in a "jigsaw" pattern identical to cutaneous cylindromas. Also similar to cylindroma, is the abundance of hyaline droplets within the nest, occasionally resembling adenoid cystic carcinoma, though the hyaline droplets of membranous basal cell adenomas are smaller, and the nests are more rounded. The surrounding salivary tissue of membranous basal cell adenomas seen in syndromic and multifocal lesions may show areas of striated duct hyperplasia (Fig. 3.5d *inset*) with a focally basaloid appearance representing precursor lesions and explaining the multifocality seen in some of these distinct subtypes of basal cell adenoma [627].

Immunohistochemically, these tumors are strongly and diffusely positive for p63 a progenitor cell marker that is expressed in basal and myoepithelial cells [436]. These tumors may also show varying degrees of true myoepithelial differentiation, staining positively for various smooth muscle markers [296, 519]. Nagao et al. were able to use a combination of a mitotic activity of less that 4 per 10 high power fields along with a low proliferation index by Ki-67 immunostaining, low apoptotic index by TUNEL labeling, and negativity for biomarkers p53, and EGFR to effectively separate basal cell adenomas from basal cell adenocarcinomas [125].

Pathogenesis

For most sporadic basal cell adenomas, the pathogenesis is unclear. Cytogenetic alterations have been only rarely characterized in non-membranous basal cell adenomas, with a trisomy 8 and chromosome 13 alterations being the major abnormalities described [576]. With regards to membranous basal cell adenomas, alterations at the CYLD1 gene locus at chromosome 16q12-13 are seen in both sporadic and familial/syndromic cases, suggesting that this alteration is vital to this subtype's pathogenesis [378]. CYLD1 is a deubiquitinating enzyme whose loss of activity correlates with activation of the NF-kB pathway, hinting at a mechanism of tumorigenesis [375].

Prognosis

Basal cell adenomas have a low rate of recurrence, except for the membranous subtype, which may recur in about 25% of cases. Because of the propensity for multifocality in membranous basal cell adenomas, some of these cases may represent separate tumors rather than true recurrences [179]. Malignant transformation is rare, again favoring the membranous type of basal cell adenoma [137, 179, 210].

Canalicular Adenoma

Clinical Features

Canalicular adenoma, previously categorized with basal cell adenoma, is a rare tumor comprising less than 1% of all salivary tumors [137, 179, 210]. The mean age is 65 years with a female predilection (ratio: 1.8:1) [179, 553]. The anatomic distribution of canalicular adenomas is distinctive, with a marked tendency to involve minor salivary glands of the upper lip in about 80% of cases. The second most common site is the buccal mucosa, where these tumors occur in almost 10% of cases [210]. The remainder of cases occur in the palate [486], and only rarely in the parotid gland [179]. They typically present as painless, slowly growing submucosal nodules. Rarely, multiple/multifocal canalicular adenomas can occur and present clinically with as many as 13 discrete masses, typically occurring in the upper lip and buccal mucosa [462].

Pathology

Grossly tumors are well circumscribed and range from 0.5 to 2.0 cm [209]. They are a homogeneous tan to yellow-tan. Cyst formation is common [627]. Histologically, at low power magnification, these tumors show a characteristic beaded appearance of thin anastomosing cords of cells embedded in a loose paucicellular myxoid stroma with prominent vascularity (Fig. 3.6). On higher magnification, the cords are comprised of two rows of bland monomorphic columnar cells with some stratification. The palisading columnar cells of canalicular adenomas resemble the basal layer of tubular/trabecular basal cell adenomas, however, there are no other cell morphologies as seen in the latter. Additionally the appearance of the tumor cords "floating" in a loose vascular stroma is characteristic and only focally, if ever, seen in basal cell adenoma.

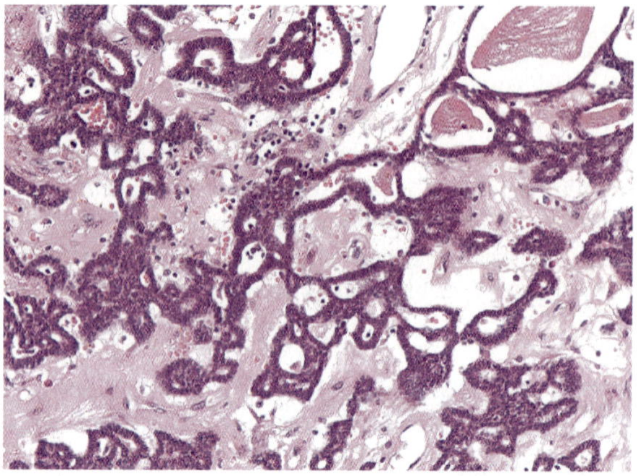

Fig. 3.6: Canalicular adenoma with thin cords of columnar epithelium streaming through a myxohyaline stroma (H&E, 100×)

Immunohistochemically, these tumors are uniformly positive for vimentin, S-100, and cytokeratins and only rarely for GFAP [164]. Muscle markers such as smooth muscle actin, calponin, and smooth muscle myosin heavy chain are uniformly negative suggesting a pure ductal epithelial differentiation [164]. Furthermore, canalicular adenomas are negative for p63, which is a key distinguishing factor immunophenotypically from the strongly p63-positive basal cell adenomas/carcinomas [328].

Polymorphous low-grade adenocarcinoma can be in the differential diagnosis of canalicular adenoma, but as its name suggests, polymorphous low-grade adenocarcinoma has a greater variation in growth pattern and cell type, and will show areas of infiltration and often perineural invasion, though distinction may still be admittedly difficult on small biopsy. Additionally, multifocality of canalicular adenomas may be mistakenly interpreted as infiltration. Both polymorphous low-grade adenocarcinoma and canalicular adenoma are immunophenotypically very similar, though p63 can often be positive in the former [210].

Pathogenesis

The pathogenesis is not well understood, though the presence of multifocality in some cases suggests a field effect [179, 367].

Prognosis

The prognosis is excellent and recurrences are extremely rare. Additionally, some of these recurrences may represent separate tumors [36, 179, 498].

Myoepithelioma

Clinical Features

Myoepitheliomas account for about 1.5% of all salivary tumors. This tumor is primarily one of adults with a peak incidence in the third to fourth decades (range 8–82 years) [62, 63]. The parotid gland is the most common site ranging from 40% to 50%, followed by the minor salivary glands in the palate [462]. Myoepitheliomas of the sinonasal mucoserous glands are rare [101, 143]. Myoepitheliomas usually present as slow-growing painless masses.

Pathology

Grossly, these tumors are a well-circumscribed uniform gray tan. In the parotid gland they usually have a thin fibrous capsule, but in the palate, they may not [143]. The majority measure less than 3 cm [143, 462]. Microscopically, myoepitheliomas have a varied morphology.

In a review of 40 cases, Dardick et al. [524] delineated different cell types: spindled (32.5%), epithelioid (45.0%), hyaline (7.5%), clear (2.5%), and mixed (12.5%). The spindle cell type consists of bland sheets of cells with ovoid nuclei and delicate amphophilic to eosinophilic cytoplasm arranged in interlacing fascicles (Fig. 3.7a). There may be loose myxoid change, occasionally imparting a reticulated or net-like arrangement, but there is never chondroid metaplasia as seen in pleomorphic adenomas [558]. The epithelioid cell type (Fig. 3.7b) consists of cords or solid sheets of polygonal round cells with amphophilic to eosinophilic cytoplasm occasionally arranged in pseudoglandular spaces. Occasionally the cytoplasm is granular and oncocytic with accumulation of mitochondria as seen in oncocytic epithelial lesions [50, 143]. The hyaline or plasmacytoid cell type (Fig. 3.7c) consists of sheets of cells with eccentrically located nuclei and a droplet of prominent dense hyaline eosinophilic cytoplasm. The ultrastructural correlate to these droplets are accumulations of intermediate filaments that in immunoelectron

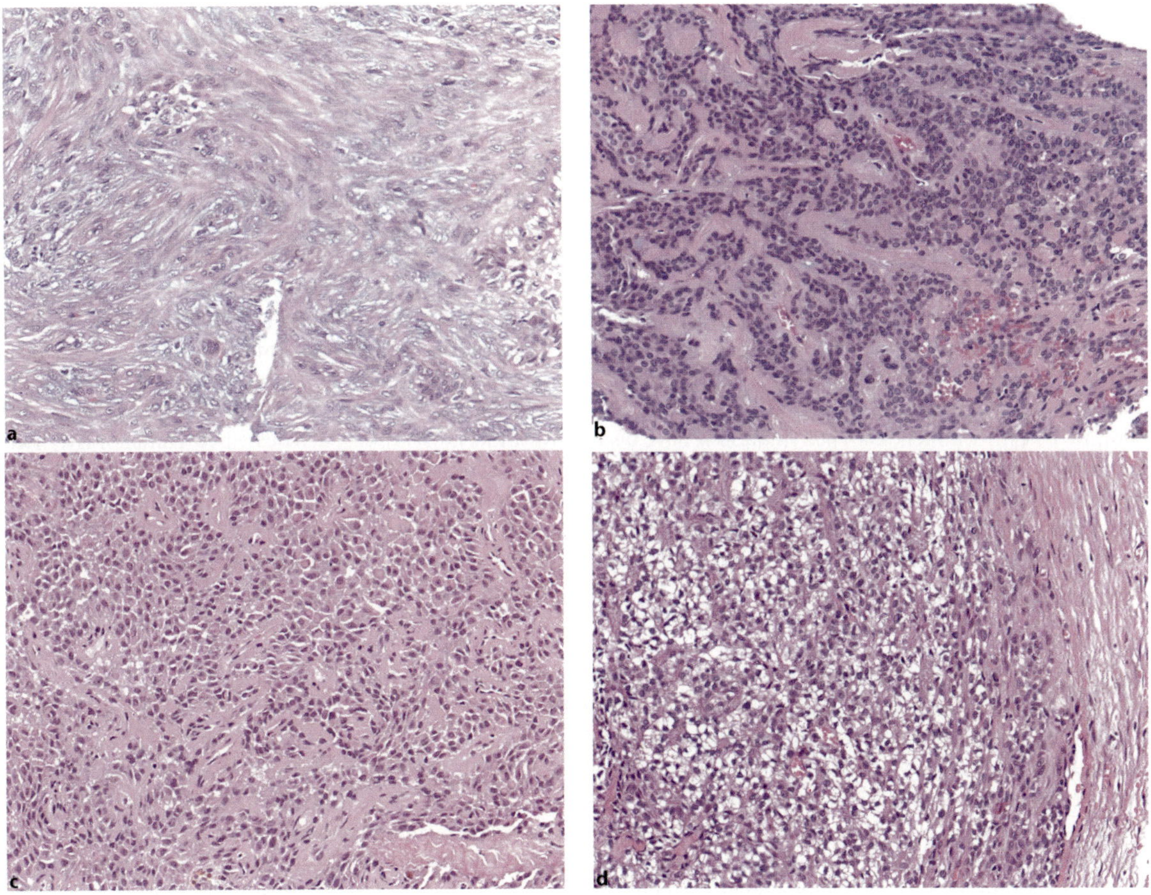

Fig. 3.7: Variants of myoepithelioma (all H&E, 200×): **a** spindled, **b** epithelioid, **c** plasmacytoid, and **d** clear cell type

microscopy show staining for muscle-specific actin [101, 364]. The clear cell type (Fig. 3.7d) most closely resembles the epithelioid cell type but instead shows clear cytoplasm indicative of glycogen accumulation [524]. Additionally, squamous metaplasia can be seen in all subtypes of myoepithelioma, particularly after fine-needle aspiration [101]. Within the oncocytic myoepitheliomas, sebaceous differentiation has rarely been described [495].

The number of true ducts that are allowed in myoepithelioma is debatable and arbitrary, but if there are more than scattered ducts present within a myoepithelial tumor, perhaps a better designation would be a myoepithelial-rich pleomorphic adenoma, or possibly even an epithelial-myoepithelial carcinoma, particularly when the myoepithelial component is of the clear cell subtype [495]. Myoepitheliomas are distinguished from their malignant counterparts by the absence of infiltration [10, 557]. Other useful morphologic features include a low mitotic count, absence of necrosis, and perineural and angiolymphatic invasion [10, 557].

Immunohistochemically, myoepitheliomas will stain with both actins and cytokeratins as well as GFAP and S-100 to varying degrees [231]. These markers are less likely to be expressed in the plasmacytoid and clear cell types, though vimentin, which is rarely expressed in non-neoplastic myoepithelial cells, is strongly and uniformly positive in all cell types in myoepithelioma [476, 500, 606]. The second generation muscle marker calponin shows promising results, staining myoepithelial cells more consistently than smooth muscle actin [167]. Additionally, p63, a basaloid/myoepithelial stem cell marker is also strongly and consistently expressed in myoepithelioma [300] serving as a useful adjunct using the traditional myoepithelial markers.

Pathogenesis

As with many rare salivary gland tumors, the pathogenesis of myoepithelioma is poorly understood. In one myoepithelioma, a t(1:12)(q25;q12) along with deletions of parts of chromosomes 3 and 9 has been described [606]. By comparative genomic hybridization, gross cytogenetic alterations were only present in 25% (3/12) of cases [220, 606]. In 3/12 myoepitheliomas, p53 mutations have been identified [498]. Additionally, p53 homologues p63 and p73 have a unique isoform expression profile in myoepitheliomas as compared to normal salivary tissue, namely the truncated transcriptionally inactive forms (ΔN isoforms) increased in myoepitheliomas [10, 73].

Prognosis

Prognosis is generally favorable; recurrences are relatively rare and are usually related to incomplete excision [495]. Malignant transformation is uncommon [485]. In one series, myoepithelial carcinomas had an antecedent myoepithelioma in only 8% (2/25) of cases [179, 217]. Some authors regard all clear cell myoepitheliomas as tumors of uncertain malignant potential even if they are histologically benign [604]. However, this may stem from the past usage of the term clear cell myoepithelioma interchangeably with epithelial-myoepithelial carcinoma [517].

Warthin's Tumor

Clinical Features

Warthin's tumor, which Warthin himself [420] called *papillary cystadenoma lymphomatosum*, is morphologically similar to other cystadenomas, but the demographic, pathologic, and morphologic features of this lesion are sufficiently distinct to separate it from these other cystadenomas. Warthin's tumor is the second most common salivary tumor overall, comprising 3% of all salivary tumors in the United States [179], though the incidence may be as high as 30% in smaller regions such as central Pennsylvania [517]. The mean age at diagnosis is 62 years, rarely occurring before the age of 40 years [341, 468]. This tumor more commonly occurs in males, though the male to female ratio has decreased dramatically within the past 50 years to about 2:1 [179, 517]. These trends in sex incidence as well as the aforementioned regional variation are likely attributable to the strong link between Warthin's tumor and smoking. Warthin's tumor has an eight times higher incidence in smokers than in non-smokers [535].

Warthin's tumor is essentially restricted to the parotid gland and its lymph nodes, with the tail of the parotid being the most common site of involvement. It is also the salivary gland tumor which occurs most commonly bilateral/multifocal (up to 20%) [587]. Rarely extraparotid Warthin's tumors have been described, comprising as high as 8% of all Warthin's tumors, essentially all occurring in the cervical lymph nodes [517]. Rare examples have been described in the other glands [462], but on close scrutiny these are either from the anterior tail of the parotid or adjacent lymph nodes. Most patients present with a painless mass that may fluctuate in size in as many as 40% of patients. Rarely, infarcted Warthin's tumors (see below) may cause pain [517].

Pathology

Grossly these tumors range from 1 to 10 cm (mean 3.5 cm) [504]. They are typically well circumscribed and often cystic to varying degrees. The cyst lining is often a nodular tan-white with papillary excresence s and the fluid contents are characteristically a granular brown reminiscent of "motor oil." The actual parenchyma is a nodular tan to dark brown (Fig. 3.8a). Microscopically, Warthin's tumor is comprised of a papillary proliferation lined by a double layer composed of surface columnar oncocytic epithelium (Fig. 3.8b) and a smaller basal layer of small cuboidal cells with myoepithelial characteristics. Mucinous, sebaceous, and squamous metaplasia have been seen in Warthin's tumor [200]. The surrounding stroma contains a highly ordered lymphoid architecture similar to an actual lymph node, with germinal centers often found in cores of the epithelial papillae. When Warthin's tumor arises in a lymph node, it may be mistaken for metastatic carcinoma, particularly papillary thyroid carcinoma. However, papillary thyroid carcinoma does not form a two cell layer proliferation, and will have characteristic nuclear features (clearing, overlap, grooves, elongation, and pseudoinclusions) which are absent in Warthin's tumor.

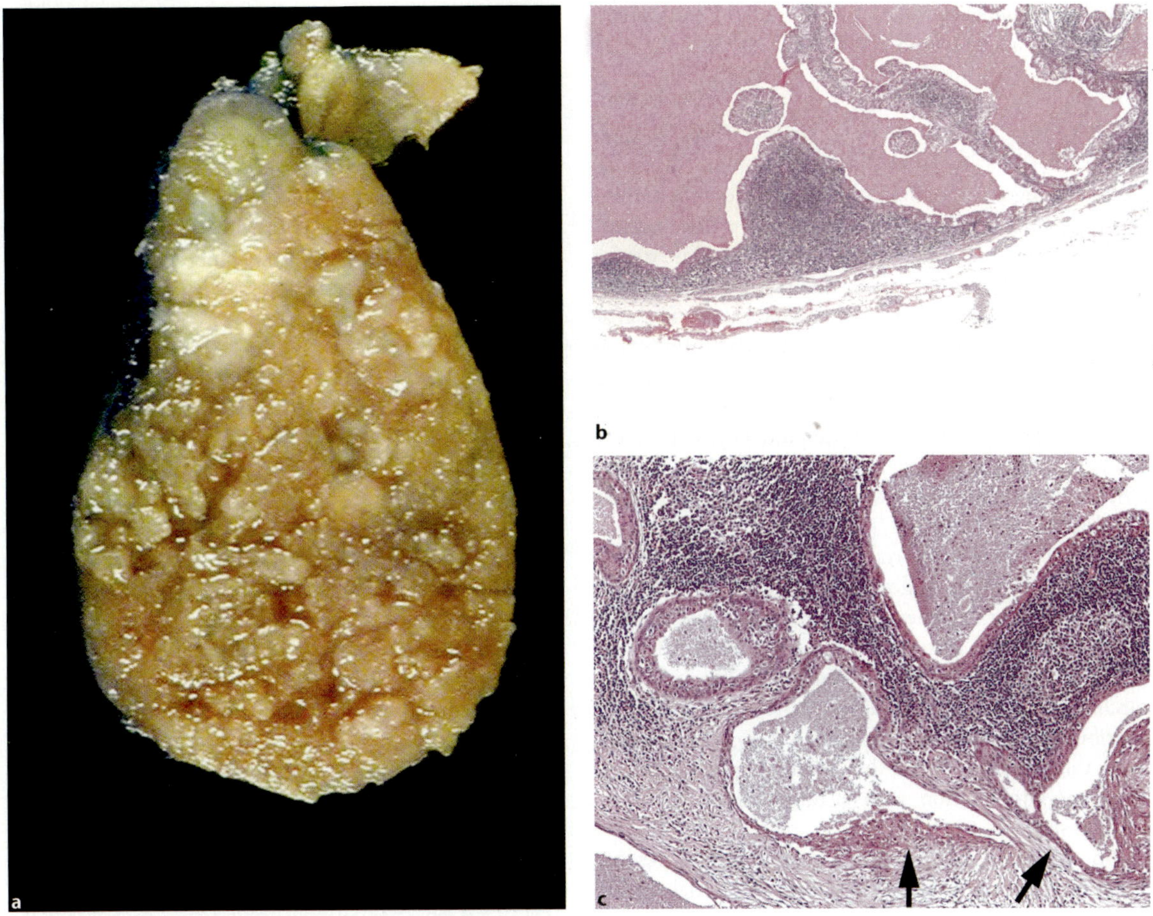

Fig. 3.8: Warthin's tumor. **a** A solid tan-brown tumor of the parotid with central papillary architecture (gross image). **b** A papillary cystic tumor lined by columnar oncocytic cells with a prominent lymphoid stroma including a capsule resembling that of a lymph node (H&E, 20×). **c** "Infarcted" Warthin's tumor with a transition to squamous metaplasia with surrounding fibrosis (*arrows*) (H&E, 100×)

The degree of epithelial proliferation varies greatly, and Seifert et al. classified Warthin's tumor into four histologic subtypes based largely on this epithelial to stromal ratio [153]. Their "type 4" Warthin tumor is of diagnostic interest as this represents Warthin's tumor with extensive squamous metaplasia. This so-called metaplastic or infarcted Warthin's tumor often shows extensive squamous metaplasia (Fig. 3.8c), necrosis, fibrosis, and histiocytic infiltrates, thought to be a result of mechanical or vascular induced changes [462]. In at least some cases, this is secondary to fine-needle aspiration [517]. This variant can be mistaken for a mucoepidermoid carcinoma or a metastatic squamous cell carcinoma. However, infarcted Warthin's tumor will still have a papillary configuration similar to typical Warthin's tumor. Additionally many infarcted Warthin's tumors will on careful examination still show areas of oncocytic columnar epithelium.

Immunohistochemical stains are not usually used for diagnostic purposes, but as with most oncocytic lesions, the epithelial cells of Warthin's tumor are ultrastructurally composed of mitochondria, which can also be stained by for phosphotungstic acid–hematoxylin (PTAH) or immunohistochemically with antibodies to mitochondrial components such as cytochrome c [566, 568]. The immunohistochemical profile of the lymphoid component is that of a reactive lymph node [22].

Pathogenesis

Despite being a fairly common and well-described identity, the pathogenesis of Warthin's tumor is not well understood and is still debated. The prevailing theory for its initial development is that Warthin's tumor is a proliferation of the intercalated and striated ducts of heterotopic salivary inclusions in intra- and periparotid lymph nodes rather than a tumor with a prominent lymphoid response. Since the parotid does not have a complete capsule, the lymph nodes and parotid parenchyma have the ability to intermingle embryologically [506]. While many other salivary gland neoplasms may have a prominent lymphoid stroma [392, 447], the fact that Warthin's tumor almost exclusively occurs in the parotid gland and its associated lymph nodes, and the presence of lymph node architectural elements, occasionally including capsular sinuses, give credence to this hypothesis. Also the involvement of the lymphoid component by metastatic carcinoma, granulomatous disease, and lymphomas in a distribution similar to that in lymph nodes further supports this belief [17, 290]; this is not simply a papillary oncocytic proliferation with a tumor-associated lymphoid response.

Another point of contention is whether this represents a true neoplasm or a reactive proliferation. Initial studies demonstrated cytogenetic alterations in some Warthin's tumors such as loss of the Y chromosome, 6p abnormalities, and t(11;19) which is interestingly also seen in mucoepidermoid carcinomas. However, loss of the Y chromosome is a senescent change that can be seen normal tissues, and many of the cytogenetic alterations seen in these series are usually only minority cell components in an otherwise normal stemline [362, 363]. More recently, Warthin's tumor has not been shown to have monoclonality, either by X chromosome-linked human androgen receptor analysis or by loss of heterozygosity profiling [233, 493, 628].

Regardless of origin and clonality, smoking likely contributes significantly to the pathogenesis of the tumor. One mechanism includes mitochondrial DNA damage resulting in mutations [517]. Possible contributing mechanisms other than smoking include autoimmunity and EBV infection [504, 617].

Prognosis

Prognosis with surgical excision alone is excellent with a recurrence rate of 2–5% [617]. Even these may represent separate tumors, since Warthin's tumor is often multifocal. Malignant transformation is extremely rare with an estimated occurrence of 0.1–2% [523]. Interestingly mucoepidermoid carcinoma is the most common histology, though squamous cell carcinoma and oncocytic carcinomas have been described [179].

Cystadenomas

Clinical Features

Cystadenomas are rare benign cystic salivary tumors that resembles Warthin's tumor, though the clinicopathologic features of this tumor are different. In contrast to Warthin's tumor, there is actually a slight female predilection, and there is no association with smoking [179, 600]. The mean age at presentation is 57 years [80]. The major site of involvement is the parotid gland (45%), though unlike Warthin's tumor, other cystadenomas can be in sites such as the lip and buccal mucosa [523]. Rarely these tumors have been described in the supraglottic larynx as well [243, 522].

Pathology

Cystadenomas range from unicystic (approximately 20%) to multicystic. The multicystic lesions may often have a larger central cyst. These cysts may be filled with a serous or mucinous fluid, and papillary excrescences may be evident within the cysts though these are far less prominent than in cystadenocarcinomas. The histology recapitulates the gross appearance, and the cysts are lined by one to two cell layers comprised of a mixture of oncocytic, mucinous, and focally sebaceous, or squamous epithelium. Papillary oncocytic cystadenomas and mucinous cystadenomas are the most common subtypes. The papillae of the former have a simple architecture with no ramification and minimal multilayering of cells [397]. Luminal tyrosine crystals are occasionally seen [248].

Lymphoid stroma is sparse to absent in contrast to Warthin's tumor. Cystadenocarcinomas and cystic salivary duct carcinomas tend to have more architectural complexity with solid areas and angulated cystic spaces rather than the round contours seen in cystadenomas. Additionally, they will have more cytologic atypia and mitotic activity than cystadenomas. Cystadenomas may resemble low-grade mucoepidermoid carcinomas, but the former, even when they are mucinous, will be lined mostly by columnar epithelium and will not have the three cell populations seen in mucoepidermoid carcinoma. Acinic cell carcinomas may mimic cystadenomas, however, the acinar cell lining in the cysts can be highlighted by a periodic acid-Schiff (PAS) reaction after diastase stain.

Pathogenesis

The pathogenesis is not well understood. While these tumors bear a superficial resemblance to Warthin's tumor, demographics, the lack of a defined risk factor, and the site distribution suggest that these arise through distinct mechanisms.

Prognosis

The prognosis for this benign tumor is excellent; complete excision should be curative. One case of a carcinoma arising in a cystadenoma has been described.

Lymphadenomas

Clinical Features

Lymphadenomas consist of both sebaceous and non-sebaceous tumors. They are rare tumors that also bear resemblance to Warthin's tumor because of their prominent lymphoid stroma, though their epithelial constituents are different.

Sebaceous lymphadenomas, described as early as 1960 [20, 34, 146, 151, 213, 215, 344, 397, 594, 605, 621] are far more common than non-sebaceous lymphadenomas [74, 110, 345, 379]. They tend to occur in the elderly, beyond the sixth decade, and are almost always seen in the parotid gland [403, 461]. All reported non-sebaceous lymphadenomas to date have been described in males (age 13–79 years), exclusively in the parotid gland [379].

The typical presentation is that of a painless mass, mimicking a pleomorphic adenoma. Sebaceous lymphadenomas may occasionally be cystic, clinically resembling Warthin's tumor [379].

Pathology

Sebaceous and non-sebaceous lymphadenomas are grossly solid or cystic well-circumscribed tan masses. Histologically, sebaceous lymphadenomas will have solid to cystic nests of sebaceous cells, foamy polygonal epithelial cells with a slight basaloid appearance on the periphery of the nests embedded within a lymphoid stroma reminiscent of a lymph node (Fig. 3.9a, b). While some reports of non-sebaceous lymphadenomas show a cystic, albeit non-papillary, bilayered oncocytic proliferation within a lymphoid stroma, such tumors may be better classified as variants of Warthin's tumor [248]. The term non-sebaceous lymphadenoma should be reserved for solid basaloid or tubular benign neoplasms with a prominent lymphoid stroma.

These lymphadenomas may mimic MESA, lymphoma, or lymphoepithelial carcinoma. However, the circumscription, lobular nested appearance, and bland cytology of lymphadenomas separate it from lymphoepithelial carcinoma. Unlike MESA, lymphadenomas should only have a localized lymphoid stromal component without significant sialadenitis outside the lesion. Lymphomas should have effacement of lymphoid architecture characterized by abnormal non-polarized follicles or an absence altogether [162]. Sebaceous lymphadenocarcinoma is among the rarest of salivary tumors and can be separated from lymphadenomas by its infiltrative pattern and other features of malignancy such as perineural and angiolymphatic invasion.

Pathogenesis

Lymphadenomas are thought to have an origin from epithelial rests within lymph nodes, similar to Warthin's tumor [385]. In support of this theory is the occasional coexistence of mixed sebaceous lymphadenoma-Warthin's tumors [578]. Sebaceous components are thought to be ectodermally derived and formed embryologically along lines of closure [29, 109]. Ultrastructurally and chemically, the constituents of sebaceous glands in the parotid gland and sebaceous glands of the skin are identical [82].

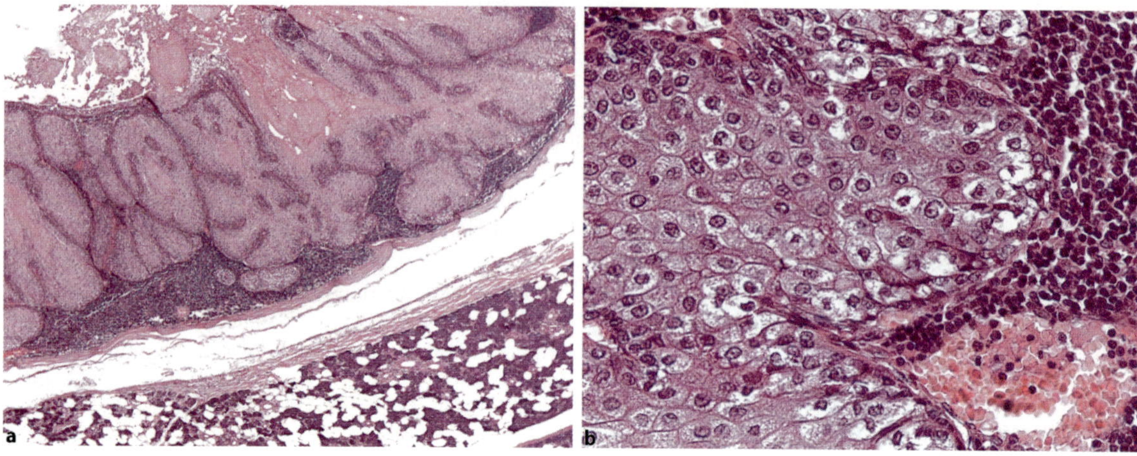

Fig. 3.9: Sebaceous lymphadenoma. **a** A solid and cystic proliferation with a lymphoid stroma reminiscent of a lymph node (H&E, 40×). **b** The proliferation is comprised of foamy polygonal cells defining the sebaceous cell type (H&E, 400×)

Prognosis

Prognosis is excellent; resection is curative.

Oncocytoma and Oncocytosis

Clinical Features

The distinction between oncocytoma and oncocytosis is often arbitrary. Oncocytoma is a rare monomorphic salivary tumor that resembles oncocytosis, which is a diffuse or multifocal proliferation of oncocytes. Oncocytoma is the preferred terminology if an oncocytic lesion is solitary or dominant and/or encapsulated. Hence, by this definition an oncocytoma can arise in the setting of oncocytosis.

It accounts for 1% of salivary tumors. Both oncocytoma and oncocytosis occur usually in the sixth decade, mirroring the increase in the number of oncocytes in salivary glands that is seen with increasing age [324]. About 20% of patients with oncocytoma have an antecedent history of radiation exposure [82]. They may be solitary, bilateral (7%), or arise in the setting of multinodular oncocytic hyperplasia. The parotid gland is the most common (84%) site while the remainder arise almost exclusively in the submandibular gland [381]. Rarely oncocytomas of the minor salivary glands have been described [82].

Clinically oncocytosis presents as unilateral or bilateral salivary gland enlargement, typically of the parotid gland [82, 459]. Multifocal nodular oncocytic hyperplasia is far more common than diffuse oncocytosis.

Pathology

Grossly, oncocytoma is a solid well-circumscribed mass measuring 3–4 cm. Diffuse oncocytosis presents as a diffuse enlargement while multifocal nodular oncocytic hyperplasia has at least two nodules within the salivary parenchyma. As with oncocytic lesions at other sites, oncocytosis and oncocytoma are a tan brown to dark mahogany brown. Oncocytosis can be divided into two main pathologic categories of conditions that clinically and histologically mimic neoplasia: multifocal nodular oncocytic hyperplasia and diffuse oncocytosis.

Microscopically, diffuse oncocytosis involves the entire gland with minimal if any residual normal salivary tissue. In contrast, oncocytoma and multifocal nodular oncocytic hyperplasia consist of solid/trabecular, well-demarcated proliferations of oncocytes, cells with abundant granular pink cytoplasm and round nuclei, embedded in otherwise normal-appearing salivary tissue. Oncocytomas may have capsules, particularly in the parotid gland (Fig. 3.10a). The ultrastructural correlate of the granular cytoplasm of oncocytes is the abundance of mitochondria. Clear cell change can be seen in these lesions and reflects the accumulation of glycogen (Fig. 3.10b) [462, 524].

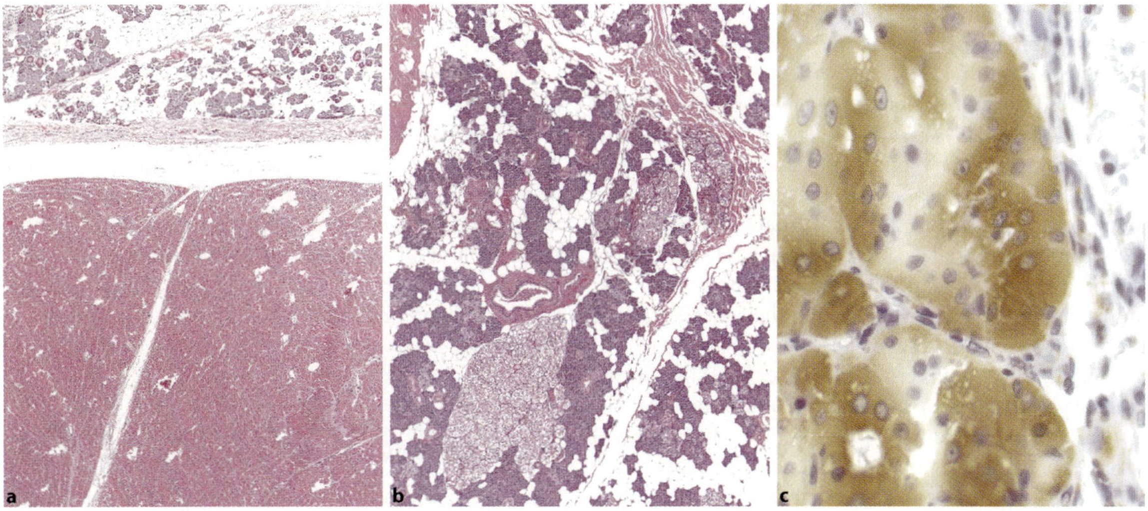

Fig. 3.10: Oncocytoma and oncocytosis. **a** An encapsulated parotid tumor comprised of solid "pink" or oncocytic cells (H&E, 40×). **b** Clear cell oncocytosis of the parotid (H&E, 100×). **c** Immunohistochemical stain for cytochrome c showing positivity in an oncocytoma (DAB chromogen, 400×)

In contrast, oncocytic carcinomas are characterized by necrosis and perineural and vascular invasion. Metastatic carcinomas, particularly renal cell carcinoma and Hürthle cell thyroid carcinoma can mimic oncocytosis or oncocytoma, however, immunohistochemical stains are helpful in ruling out these metastatic tumors [29, 109]. Other considerations include acinic cell carcinoma, oncocytic mucoepidermoid carcinoma, and oncocytic myoepitheliomas. A battery of histochemical stains, PAS with diastase treatment for acinic cell carcinoma, mucicarmine for mucoepidermoid carcinoma, and myoepithelial markers such as smooth muscle actin and vimentin for myoepithelioma, can help to exclude these entities. Additionally oncocytomas, because of their mitochondria, will be positive by phosphotungstic acid–hematoxylin stain or by immunohistochemistry toward mitochondrial cytochromes (Fig. 3.10c) [100].

Pathogenesis

The pathogenesis of oncocytosis and oncocytoma is unclear, but is likely a progression from the age-related precursor of oncocytic metaplasia [381]. While mitochondrial abnormalities are a plausible pathogenic mechanism, mitochondrial DNA C-tract mutations are noted to be rare in these lesions [82].

Prognosis

The prognosis is excellent for lesions classified both as oncocytoma and oncocytosis [87, 178]. Recurrence rates for oncocytomas are roughly 10% in oncocytoma, and may be a result of multifocality rather than incomplete excision. Recurrent cases also tend to have marked clear cell change [8, 90, 279, 537].

Miscellaneous Rare Benign Tumors and Tumor-like Lesions

Ductal Papillomas

Clinical Features

Ductal papillomas are a rare group of benign papillary neoplasms of the large excretory duct. There are three major subtypes of ductal papillomas of salivary gland origin that are about equally rare: intraductal papilloma, inverted ductal papilloma, and sialadenoma papilliferum.

Intraductal papillomas are rare with only 40 cases reported using strict criteria [87]. They are typically a tumor of minor salivary duct origin, though tumors in the parotid, submandibular, and sublingual glands have been described [87, 99, 127, 148, 236, 271, 283, 321, 342, 614,

618]. They typically occur in the fifth or sixth decade as a painless submucosal mass (range 29–77 years) without a gender predilection [236].

Inverted ductal papillomas are also rare with only 35 cases reported [401]. Inverted ductal papilloma is a tumor of minor salivary origin (lip and buccal mucosa) with the only tumor reported in the major salivary gland being debatable [87, 178, 257, 582]. There is no sex predilection and the mean age of occurrence is 53 years. These tumors typically present as a painless submucosal mass with a central dilated pore reflecting their localization to the salivary excretory duct orifice.

Sialadenoma papilliferum resembles its skin adnexal counterparts syringocystadenoma papilliferum and hidradenoma papillferum [87] and is rare with under 50 cases reported, and estimated incidence of approximately 0.2% [87]. These tumors also typically occur in the fifth to sixth decade and they are most frequent on the palate, but unlike other ductal papillomas, they present as granular papillary masses reflecting their often extensive surface component.

Pathology

Grossly, inverted ductal and intraductal papillomas are well-circumscribed masses, the latter more cystic, that are typically less than 3.0 cm. Sialadenoma papilliferum is a granular tan mass that involves the surface mucosa [489]. Microscopically, inverted ductal papilloma has an endophytic growth of transitional/basaloid cells with microcysts reminiscent of its Schneiderian counterpart inverted papilloma. The nests of basaloid cells have central cleft-like spaces that are lined by columnar excretory duct-type mucinous cells. Intraductal papilloma is histologically composed of a cystic dilation of the excretory duct with a papillary arborizing proliferation of a mixture of oncocytic or mucinous cells. Histologically sialadenoma papilliferum shows surface papillary projections of oncocytic columnar cells intermingling with the surface squamous epithelium with a well-demarcated submucosal component that is comprised of large-caliber ducts with uniform "saw tooth" like papillary luminal invaginations.

All ductal papillomas may be mistaken for other papillary salivary gland tumors, particularly cystadenomas and cystadenocarcinomas. Cystadenomas and cystadenocarcinomas are deeper within the salivary gland parenchyma and can be multicystic unlike ductal papillomas [342]. Nonetheless, this distinction in some cases is not well defined. In the pancreas, intraductal papillary mucinous neoplasms and mucinous cystic neoplasms are separated by the fact that the former maintains its connection to the ductal system [401]. In contrast, the understanding of cystadenomas and cystadenocarcinomas of the salivary gland from this standpoint is rudimentary if at all existent; and the possibility that many of these cystadenomas may actually be intraductal papillomas or "papillomatosis" has not been examined in the literature.

Pathogenesis

Other than the presumed excretory ductal origin, not much is know about the pathogenesis of ductal papillomas. Of note, inverted ductal papillomas, unlike Schneiderian papillomas, have no known human papilloma virus association [87]. Also, unlike its cutaneous counterpart syringocystadenoma papilliferum, sialadenoma papilliferum is not a part of the nevus sebaceous complex [439, 514].

Prognosis

Prognosis is generally thought to be excellent, though most series have little or no follow-up [6, 138, 190, 208, 248, 306, 313, 322, 368, 455]. Rare cases of malignant intraductal papillomas and transformation of sialadenoma papilliferum are described [313], but as a rule, excision is thought to be curative.

Sebaceous Adenoma

Clinical Features

While sebaceous differentiation can be seen in a variety of salivary tumors, purely sebaceous adenoma without a lymphoid component is extremely rare with less than 25 cases reported [173]. The mean age is roughly 62 years with a slight male predominance. Sites that are usually involved are the parotid gland and the oral cavity closely mirroring the distribution of Fordyce granules and ectopic sebaceous rests [208].

Pathology

These tumors are well circumscribed and composed of sheets or lobules of sebaceous cells. These must be distinguished from other clear cell neoplasms such as mucoepidermoid carcinoma, acinic cell carcinoma, and clear cell oncocytoma among others [613]. The oil red O stain on frozen sections and electron microscopy remain the two main supportive studies to prove sebaceous differentiation: the presence of intracellular lipids within the foamy cells.

Pathogenesis

Unlike cutaneous sebaceous adenomas there is no described association with Muir-Torre syndrome, a hereditary non-polyposis colorectal carcinoma syndromic variant, suggesting a different pathogenesis [248, 313]. While non-neoplastic ectopic sebaceous rests express androgen receptor just as in their cutaneous counterparts [67, 246, 254, 310, 525, 532], it is not clear whether sebaceous adenomas express this marker.

Prognosis

The prognosis is excellent; none of the cases reported have recurred after excision [254].

Sclerosing Polycystic Adenosis

Clinical Features

Sclerosing polycystic adenosis is an extremely rare cystic lesion resembling fibrocystic disease of the breast with only 37 cases described in the literature [254]. The mean age of occurrence is 44.5 years with no sex predilection [246, 525]. The typical presentation is that of a slow-growing usually painless mass, usually in the parotid.

Pathology

These tumors range from 0.3 to 6.0 cm and are grossly comprised of homogeneous tan masses with a microcystic cut surface. Microscopically, they are well circumscribed with cystic spaces lined by varying proportions of ductal and acinar cells. A spectrum of changes that can be seen in fibrocystic disease of the breast can also be seen in sclerosing polycystic adenosis including sclerosing adenosis, apocrine metaplasia, and atypical ductal hyperplasia [520]. Changes of salivary ductal carcinoma in situ have rarely been identified [77, 538, 546]. There is an outer myoepithelial layer to the ducts and tubules seen in sclerosing polycystic adenosis, distinguishing these lesions from an invasive salivary duct carcinoma.

Pathogenesis

While traditionally considered a non-neoplastic lesion, recent studies of X chromosome-linked human androgen receptor suggest a clonal and thus neoplastic origin to this lesion [77, 295, 481].

Prognosis

The prognosis is fairly good, even in cases with changes of salivary duct carcinoma in situ, with a local recurrence rate of 19%. No metastases or mortality have been reported with this disease.

Malignant Tumors

Adenoid Cystic Carcinoma

Clinical Features

The term adenoid cystic carcinoma was coined by Spies in 1930 [68, 349, 560]. Robin, Lorain and Laboulbene are credited with the first microscopic description which appeared in a paper they published in 1853 [77, 168, 226, 268, 599]. In 1859 Billroth suggested the term cylindroma and over the years numerous other terms have been proposed for this tumor including tubular carcinoma, tubular sarcoma, endothelioma hyalinum, adenocystic basaloid carcinoma, adenocystic carcinoma, adenoepithelioma, basaloma, and basal cell tumor to name just a few [168, 226, 599]. The preferred term is adenoid cystic carcinoma. It has the advantage of identifying the lesion as a carcinoma while avoiding confusion with the benign cutaneous appendage tumor known as cylindroma. The term adenoid cystic carcinoma is still somewhat misleading however since the tumor is not cystic!

Although the majority arise from the major and minor salivary glands, identical tumors can arise from seromucous glands throughout the upper and lower respiratory tract and from the esophagus, lacrimal glands, ceruminous glands, Bartholin's glands, Cowper's glands, breast, uterine cervix, vulva, and rarely the ovary. Adenoid cystic carcinoma accounts for 10% of all salivary gland neoplasms and 30% of all minor salivary gland tumors [351]. It also accounts for 20% of all malignant salivary gland tumors making it the second most common salivary gland malignancy. It is the most common carcinoma of minor salivary glands where the most frequent location is the palate [114]. Adenoid cystic carcinoma makes up 12–15% of parotid gland carcinomas, 30–60% of submandibular gland carcinomas, and 35–55% of minor salivary gland carcinomas [168, 338, 474, 546]. Approximately 25% arise in the major salivary glands and 75% in the minor salivary glands [30, 114, 117].

Adenoid cystic carcinoma is most frequently encountered in individuals between 40 and 60 years of age. It rarely afflicts those younger than 20 years of age. Although some series have a slight female predominance others show either no sex predilection or a male predominance [30]. The most common symptom is a slow-growing frequently painless mass, a feature which may lull both patient and physician into a false sense of security. More ominous signs and symptoms include fixation to adjacent tissues and paraesthesia or paralysis due to the affinity of this tumor for perineural invasion. Ulceration may occur with intraoral tumors and obstruction and epistaxis with those arising from seromucous glands in the sinonasal tract.

Pathologic Features

Adenoid cystic carcinoma, despite its name, is grossly solid rather than cystic and firm. The tumor may be well or poorly circumscribed. The cut surface is pink tan and non-hemorrhagic. Close inspection of those that appear well circumscribed usually reveals areas of infiltration.

Microscopically the tumor is composed of ductal and myoepithelial cells. The predominant cell type consists of cells with dense angular nuclei and scant frequently clear cytoplasm. The cells are considered to be of myoepithelial origin. A second and much less frequent cell type has a nucleus with a more open chromatin pattern and contains more abundant pink cytoplasm. This second cell type is considered to be of ductal origin [30, 103, 114, 164, 182].

Three characteristic growth patterns have been described, namely tubular or trabecular, cribriform, and solid. While all three histologic patterns are often encountered in a single tumor, frequently one pattern predominates. The cribriform pattern is the most common and also most easily recognizable. Proliferation of myoepithelial-type tumor cells form nests in which the cells surround spaces or pseudolumens producing a classic sieve or Swiss cheese pattern (Fig. 3.11a, b). The pseudolumens are filled with dense eosinophilic basement membrane material produced by the myoepithelial cells or basophilic mucinous material [353]. This basement membrane material also surrounds nests of tumor cells. When this material is extensive it can result in disruption of the cribriform pattern in which case thin strands of tumor cells stream through this material. True lumens lined by ductal-type epithelium are rare and smaller than the pseudolumens. They may contain mucicarmine and PAS-positive diastase-resistant mucin. The stroma is commonly dense and hyalinized but may also be myxoid. There is a very strong predilection for perineural invasion.

The tubular growth pattern features ducts and tubules lined by an inner layer of epithelial cells and an outer type of myoepithelial cells. Tubular structures containing eosinophilic hyalinized or basophilic material are also present.

In the solid pattern of adenoid cystic carcinoma, rounded and lobulated solid nests and islands of tumor cells predominate containing few if any pseudolumens or true lumens. While cells similar to those seen in the tubular and cribriform growth patterns may be present, over all the cells in the solid pattern tend to be larger and the nuclei larger and less angular. Cellular pleomorphism and comedonecrosis can also be seen, features not typical of the tubular and cribriform growth patterns. Mitoses are often present and may reach counts as high as 5 or more per 10 high power fields. This is in contrast to the tubular and cribriform growth patterns where mitotic figures are infrequently encountered.

Immunohistochemical stains confirm the presence of both myoepithelial and epithelial cells in adenoid cystic carcinoma. The myoepithelial cells are positive for muscle-specific actin and usually stain for S-100 protein as well as vimentin, p63, and cytokeratin. The epithelial cells stain for cytokeratin, carcinoembryonic antigen, and

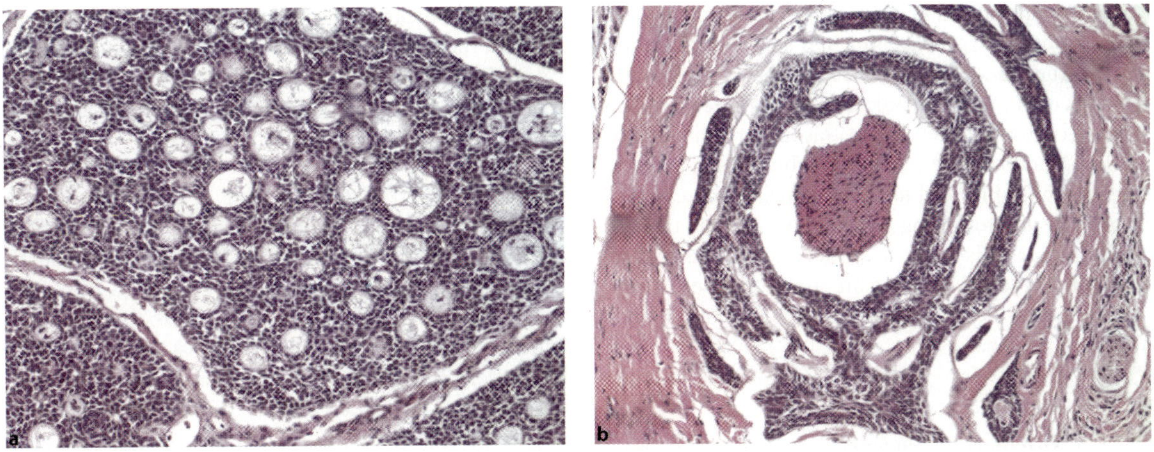

Fig. 3.11: Adenoid cystic carcinoma. **a** Cribriform growth pattern. Cells with dense angular nuclei and scant clear cytoplasm surround spaces producing a classic Swiss cheese pattern (H&E, 200×). **b** Perineural invasion (H&E, 200×)

epithelial membrane antigen and are negative for muscle-specific actin and vimentin. They may or may not express S-100 protein [469]. Recently adenoid cystic carcinomas have been shown to be positive for MUC3 [14, 204, 229, 406]. They may also be estrogen and progesterone receptor positive although not in all cases [182]. Approximately 90% are c-kit (CD117) positive [142].

Differential Diagnosis

Included in the differential diagnosis of adenoid cystic carcinoma are basaloid squamous cell carcinoma, basal cell adenocarcinoma, basal cell adenoma, cellular pleomorphic adenoma, polymorphous low-grade adenocarcinoma, and the basal cell and plexiform subtypes of ameloblastoma. The staining pattern with p63 is useful in distinguishing basaloid squamous cell carcinoma from adenoid cystic carcinoma. Basaloid squamous cell carcinomas consistently display diffuse staining of nearly 100% of the tumor cells with p63. Adenoid cystic carcinomas, on the other hand, show staining of a single peripheral layer of cells or compartmentalized staining with surrounding or interspersed p63 negative cells [463].

Basal cell adenomas, unlike adenoid cystic carcinomas, are characterized by peripheral palisading, a delicate fibrovascular stroma, a circumscribed rather than infiltrating growth pattern and lack of perineural invasion. Rarely, however, they may show trabecular and solid cribriform growth patterns reminiscent of adenoid cystic carcinoma [250]. Basal cell adenocarcinomas show areas of invasive growth and perineural invasion, features in common with adenoid cystic carcinoma, but otherwise resemble basal cell adenomas.

Cellular pleomorphic adenomas can resemble adenoid cystic carcinomas, however, careful examination of the junction of the cellular elements with the stroma aids in the distinction. In pleomorphic adenomas the myoepithelial cells spin off the epithelial elements and blend into the stroma. By contrast, there is a sharp demarcation between the cellular components of adenoid cystic carcinomas and the surrounding, often hyalinized, stroma. In addition, perineural invasion is not present in pleomorphic adenomas. Pleomorphic adenomas are also GFAP positive and adenoid cystic carcinomas are GFAP negative.

Perineural invasion occurs as often in polymorphous low-grade adenocarcinoma (PLGA) as in adenoid cystic carcinoma. However, the cells in PLGA are cuboidal to columnar with eosinophilic or clear cytoplasm and vesicular nuclei. The classic hyperchromatic angulated nucleus of adenoid cystic carcinoma is not present. Expression of c-kit may also be helpful as it is positive in virtually 100% of adenoid cystic carcinomas and in only approximately 50–60% of PLGA [268, 474, 546]. In addition, it has also been reported that where as 90% of tumor cells in PLGA are positive for epithelial membrane antigen, only the epithelial cells lining true lumens stain in adenoid cystic carcinoma [474].

Peripheral palisading is inconspicuous in the basal cell subtype of ameloblastoma and stellate reticulum is absent. The tumor is composed of islands and anastomosing cords of small basaloid cells. These features may lead to confusion in separating this tumor from adenoid cystic carcinoma. The plexiform subtype also lacks peripheral palisading and has a scant stellate reticulum. It consists of anastomosing cords of low columnar to cuboidal tumor cells. Lack of myoepithelial cells and absence of perineural invasion are useful features in separating these subtypes of ameloblastoma from adenoid cystic carcinoma.

Treatment and Prognosis

Surgical resection is the primary treatment for adenoid cystic carcinoma. Lymph node metastases are uncommon and, although controversial, neck dissection may be reserved for patients with clinically positive lymph nodes [94, 104, 268, 338, 351, 407, 474]. Distant metastases, on the other hand, develop in 20–60% of cases and most commonly involve the lung, liver, bone, and brain [77]. Radiation as the sole treatment has proven ineffective since the tumor is radiosensitive but not radiocurable. Postoperative radiotherapy, however, has proven effective in improving local control of the tumor [7, 204, 294, 450]. The best results appear to be obtained by using a combination of radical surgery and postoperative radiation therapy [122, 128, 338, 349, 393, 407, 499, 542, 586]. The usefulness of chemotherapy remains to be proven. Since adenoid cystic carcinomas are usually c-kit positive, clinical trials have been undertaken using Imatinib. These have yielded conflicting results [135].

Data from a combined series of over 800 cases of adenoid cystic carcinoma from all sites shows the following survival rates: 75% at 5 years, 40% at 10 years, 25% at 15 years, and 20% at 20 years [54, 264, 554]. In a series of 129 cases, univariate analysis showed that age over 45 years, paresthesia, advanced clinical stage, solid histological growth pattern, and increased expression of p53 correlated with a poor prognosis. Advanced clinical stage, solid histological growth pattern, and increased expression of p53 were found to be independent significant prognostic factors of a poor prognosis in multivariate analysis of this series [165, 183, 225, 226, 275, 376, 581, 586, 589, 599]. Studies looking only at the histologic growth pattern have shown that grade I tumors (predominately tubular with no solid component), grade II tumors (predominately cribriform with no more than 30% solid component), and grade III tumors (solid component greater than 30%) have cumulative 15-year survival rates of 39%, 26%, and 5%, respectively [71, 259, 339]. The prognostic significance of perineural invasion and DNA ploidy remain controversial [550].

Mucoepidermoid Carcinoma

Clinical Features

Mucoepidermoid carcinoma is the most common cancer of the salivary glands. Although it accounts for 30% of all cancer of the salivary glands, it forms only 10% of all salivary gland tumors and less than 5% of head and neck cancers [219]. Stewart et al. first reported this tumor in the United States in 1945 [83]. They coined the term mucoepidermoid tumor and suggested that it occurred in both a benign and malignant form. Foote and Frazell were the first to point out that all mucoepidermoid tumors are carcinomas albeit those which histologically appear low grade very rarely metastasize [71, 270, 343, 373].

Slightly more than 50–60% arise in the major salivary glands and of these, greater than 80% occur in the parotid, 8–13% in the submandibular gland, and 2–4% in the sublingual gland. Most of the remainder arise from minor salivary glands, usually in the palate. Seromucous glands at other sites such as the sinonasal tract, larynx, and trachea may also be the site of mucoepidermoid carcinomas on rare occasions [83, 258, 259].

Mucoepidermoid carcinoma most commonly occurs in adults (mean age 49 years), although no age group is excluded and indeed it is the most common salivary gland cancer in the pediatric age group [92, 601]. In some series it is more common in women by a ratio of 3:2 while in others there is no sex predominance [71]. The rare intraosseous (central) mucoepidermoid carcinomas, however, have an established female predominance [51, 71, 187].

The most common presenting symptom is a slowly enlarging painless mass of several years duration clinically mimicking a pleomorphic adenoma or other benign neoplasm. Pain and tenderness along with rapid enlargement may be seen with high-grade lesions [452, 563].

Pathologic Features

The gross appearance varies with the grade of the tumor. Low-grade mucoepidermoid tumors produce well-circumscribed though unencapsulated ovoid masses usually

2–4 cm in diameter. Solid gray-white or gray-pink areas are mixed with mucus-filled macrocysts while intermediate grade neoplasms are grossly similar but lack macrocysts. High-grade tumors may be similar in size but grossly are not well circumscribed and gross infiltration is often evident. They do not contain macrocysts although hemorrhage and necrosis, which are not infrequent, may lead to areas of cystic degeneration.

By definition, mucoepidermoid carcinomas are composed of three types of cells, namely mucous cells, epidermoid cells, and intermediate cells. Mucous cells are filled with mucin (mucicarmine and PAS-diastase positive) which compresses the small dark nucleus peripherally. Epidermoid (squamous) cells are polygonal with vesicular nuclei and abundant eosinophilic cytoplasm. Keratinization is rare and never extensive. Intercellular bridges are also not frequently encountered. The third type of cell is the intermediate cell, thought by some to be able to differentiate into mucous and epidermoid cells [88, 273, 315]. Intermediate cells are smaller than either mucous or epidermoid cells and do not stain with either PAS or mucicarmine stains. Intermediate cells range from small basaloid cells to cells just smaller than epidermoid cells and when numerous grow in syncytia. They are also negative with PAS and mucicarmine stains. Less frequently clear cells, oncocytes, spindle cells, and sebaceous cells may predominate. The clear cell variant of mucoepidermoid carcinoma is composed primarily of clear cells with well-defined cell borders and clear cytoplasm due to the presence of glycogen [107, 203, 282, 305, 372, 424, 584]. Oncocytic mucoepidermoid carcinomas show extensive oncocytic change [431]. Other variants include the spindle cell, sebaceous cell, and sclerosing variants [259]. The sclerosing type is characterized by dense central sclerosis with a prominent peripheral inflammatory response composed of lymphocytes, plasma cells, and frequently eosinophils. Possible etiologies of the sclerosis include a reaction to extravasated mucin and/or infarction. In addition there is at least one report of dedifferentiation in a low-grade mucoepidermoid carcinoma [83].

Three histologic grades of mucoepidermoid carcinoma have been described. Low-grade tumors contain numerous cysts of varying size including macrocysts. These cysts are lined predominately by well differentiated mucin containing goblet cells. The cysts are filled with mucus which may extravasate producing an extensive inflammatory reaction in the surrounding stroma. Solid nests of intermediate and epidermoid cells are infrequent and there is essentially no cellular pleomorphism. Mitoses are very infrequent and there is no perineural invasion. Low-grade tumors are well circumscribed both grossly and microscopically (Fig. 3.12a, b). Intermediate-grade tumors have fewer and smaller cysts and fewer cysts lined exclusively by goblet cells. Intermediate cells tend to predominate and they, along with epidermoid cells, produce large cellular sheets. Pleomorphism is absent or minimal, mitoses are infrequent, and perineural invasion is very uncommon. Grossly intermediate-grade tumors are usually circumscribed but microscopically infiltration of the adjacent salivary gland tissue is present. High-grade

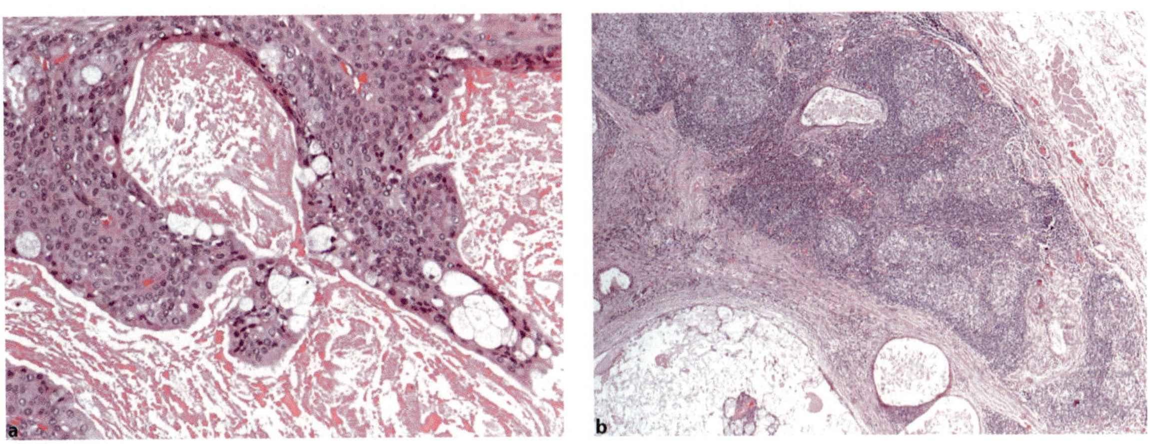

Fig. 3.12: Mucoepidermoid carcinoma. **a** Low-grade mucoepidermoid carcinoma. Tumor is cystic and contains cytologically bland mucous, epidermoid, and intermediate cells (H&E, 200×). **b** Low-grade mucoepidermoid carcinoma with prominent peripheral lymphoid inflammatory response (H&E, 200×)

tumors are characterized by a solid growth pattern composed of various mixtures of intermediate, epidermoid, and squamous cells. Cystic structures are infrequent and small. Mucous cells form less than 10% of the cellular component and indeed may be difficult to recognize unless the tissue is stained with mucicarmine or PAS-diastase. Cytologic and nuclear pleomorphism are present and mitoses are easily found. Perineural invasion may also be present. Grossly the high-grade tumors are not well circumscribed and microscopically tissue infiltration is seen. In an attempt to make grading more objective two numerical scoring systems have been proposed, one by Goode et al. [591] and the other by Brandwein et al. [276, 353, 607]. In one study 89% of high-grade mucoepidermoid carcinomas were aneuploid while 88% of low and intermediate tumors were diploid [11, 276, 607].

Mucoepidermoid carcinomas stain for cytokeratins and may focally stain for vimentin. Negative staining for GFAP and usually for muscle-specific actin and S-100 protein are consistent with an epithelial origin with no significant myoepithelial component. Mucoepidermoid carcinomas also express MUC1, MUC4, and MUC5AC [276]. MUC1 expression increases with tumor grade while staining for MUC4 decreases with grade [444, 591]. Positive staining for MUC5AC may be helpful in separating high-grade mucoepidermoid carcinoma from squamous cell carcinoma [469]. High-grade tumors are typically positive for HER2/neu and typically show greater than 20% nuclear staining for Ki-67, while low-grade tumors are negative for HER2/neu and show less than 20% nuclear staining for Ki-67 [601]. Mucoepidermoid carcinomas do not stain for estrogen receptor [574, 601].

Differential Diagnosis

High-grade mucoepidermoid carcinomas contain few mucin cells and frequently extensive areas of squamous differentiation making distinction from a squamous cell carcinoma difficult. In these cases use of mucin stains to identify the rare mucin-containing cells, positive staining for MUC5AC, and lack of extensive keratinization are useful in recognizing the tumor as a mucoepidermoid carcinoma.

Adenosquamous carcinoma of salivary glands is rare and usually arises in minor rather than major salivary glands. By definition it contains separate distinct foci of adenocarcinoma and squamous cell carcinoma unlike mucoepidermoid carcinoma where both cell types are intimately admixed.

The clear cell variant of mucoepidermoid carcinoma may mimic other primary and non-primary clear cell carcinomas. Proper classification usually comes down to identifying at least some areas containing mucous cells and intermediate and or epidermoid cells.

Cystadenomas and cystadenoma carcinomas tend to have less stroma than mucoepidermoid carcinomas. They also lack the solid proliferations of intermediate and epidermoid cells and typically show a papillary component.

Central mucoepidermoid carcinoma is usually low grade and must be distinguished from glandular odontogenic cysts. According to Waldron and Koh, some areas of glandular odontogenic cysts can be histologically identical to low-grade central mucoepidermoid carcinomas [339, 470]. The epithelial lining of glandular odontogenic cysts, however, is uniformly thin and lacks the more solid areas of epithelial proliferation seen in mucoepidermoid carcinomas [470].

Treatment and Prognosis

The treatment of mucoepidermoid carcinomas is surgical resection. Low-grade tumors are usually treated with wide local excision without neck dissection. Neck dissection in intermediate-grade tumors is probably only indicated if lymph nodes are clinically suspicious. High-grade cancer is treated with neck dissection. Prognosis is influenced by the grade and stage of the tumor, and patient age and sex [470]. Histologic grade is considered one of the most important factors in prognosis. Overall 5-year survival rates range from 92% to 100% for low-grade tumors, 62% to 92% for intermediate-grade tumors, and 0% to 43% for high-grade tumors [531]. Age over 40 years is also associated with a poor prognosis but it should be noted that most cancers in the first and second decades of life are histologically low-grade tumors [470]. Tumors of the submandibular gland have a worse prognosis than tumors of the parotid gland [202, 255, 350, 440, 475, 601, 619]. While all mucoepidermoid carcinomas are capable of metastasizing, metastases most often occur in high-grade lesions. In addition to lymph nodes, the usual sites of metastases are the lungs and bone [601].

Central (Intraosseous) Mucoepidermoid Carcinoma

Central mucoepidermoid carcinomas are rare with less than 100 cases having been reported [202, 440, 601]. They are, however, the most common intraosseous salivary gland tumor [601]. They occur three times more often in the mandible (usually in the region of the third molar) than the maxilla and are twice as common in women. Although they have been reported in both the young and the very old, the mean age at diagnosis is 51 years [40, 72, 186, 194, 245, 360, 370, 415, 453, 567]. Usually low grade, they are thought to arise from the lining of odontogenic cysts or from entrapped salivary gland tissue [567].

Malignant Mixed Tumors

The term malignant mixed tumor is an all inclusive term encompassing three clinically and histologically distinct tumors. They are: (1) carcinoma ex-pleomorphic adenoma, (2) malignant mixed tumor (carcinosarcoma), and (3) metastasizing mixed tumor.

Carcinoma Ex-pleomorphic Adenoma

Clinical Features

Carcinoma ex-pleomorphic adenoma (CEPA) is by definition a carcinoma arising in a pleomorphic adenoma. While it makes up only 5–15% of all salivary gland carcinomas, it accounts for 99% of all malignant mixed tumors [245]. Thackray and Lucas have estimated that left unresected, approximately 25% of pleomorphic adenomas would eventually undergo carcinomatous change [239, 370, 410]. Approximately 80% arise in the major salivary glands and 20% in the minor salivary glands. Among the major salivary glands the parotid gland is the primary site in 81.7% of cases, the submandibular gland in 18%, and the sublingual gland is 0.3% [94, 219, 370, 540]. Origin in minor salivary glands occurs in approximately 20% of cases with the palate being the most frequent intraoral site [61, 186, 453].

Most series show a female to male ratio of 1.2 to 3:1 [61, 186, 194, 239, 245, 370, 540, 567]. In at least three series, however, men outnumbered women by a ratio of 2:1 [21, 41, 61, 130, 194, 245, 370, 540, 567]. The average age at diagnosis is 50–60 years which is approximately 10 years older than most individuals with pleomorphic adenoma. While cases have been reported in patients from the first to the ninth decade, CEPA is extremely uncommon in individuals below the age of 20 years [41, 239, 245, 490].

Reflecting its origin in a pleomorphic adenoma, the most common clinical presentation is sudden rapid enlargement of a long-standing (average 20 years) previously non or slowly enlarging painless mass. In 12–55% of cases this rapid enlargement will be painful and often associated with facial nerve palsy and fixation to the surrounding soft tissues [188]. A minority of patients present with a rapidly enlarging mass and no prior symptoms [41].

Scientific support for the origin of CEPA from pleomorphic adenomas was provided by Eneroth and Zetterberg. They undertook a microspectrophotometric DNA analysis of pleomorphic adenomas and demonstrated a difference in the DNA content between morphologically benign pleomorphic adenomas of short duration and those of long duration [21, 41, 61, 245, 369, 415, 453, 567, 569]. This finding supports the hypothesis that the risk of carcinomatous transformation in a pleomorphic adenoma increases with the age of the tumor. Origin in a small previously undetected pleomorphic adenoma could explain those cases of CEPA presenting without a history of a previous long-standing slowly enlarging mass.

Pathologic Features

Gross features suggestive of CEPA include foci of capsular invasion, hemorrhage, and necrosis in a tumor which in other areas shows classic features of a pleomorphic adenoma. In one series of 47 cases these tumors averaged 4.4 cm in greatest diameter in the parotid gland, 5.0 cm in the submandibular gland, and 2.2 cm in the minor salivary glands [61, 130, 219, 453, 490].

The carcinoma is usually a high-grade adenocarcinoma or an undifferentiated carcinoma although numerous other types including squamous cell carcinoma, mucoepidermoid carcinoma, adenoid cystic carcinoma, myoepithelial carcinoma, clear cell carcinoma, papillary carcinoma, and terminal duct carcinoma have been reported (Fig. 3.13a, b) [453]. Thus when making the diagnosis of CEPA it is important to state the histologic subtype and degree of differentiation of the carcinomatous component. The ratio of pleomorphic adenoma to carcinoma in CEPA is highly variable. Hyalinization is frequently seen in the benign component of the tumor and indeed the presence of hyalinization in an otherwise classic pleomorphic adenoma is reason for additional sampling to avoid missing a small focus of CEPA [370, 453, 540]. On the other hand, residual pleomorphic adenoma may be reduced to a few microscopic foci. In one series residual foci of pleomorphic adenoma were 5 mm in 9% of cases [569].

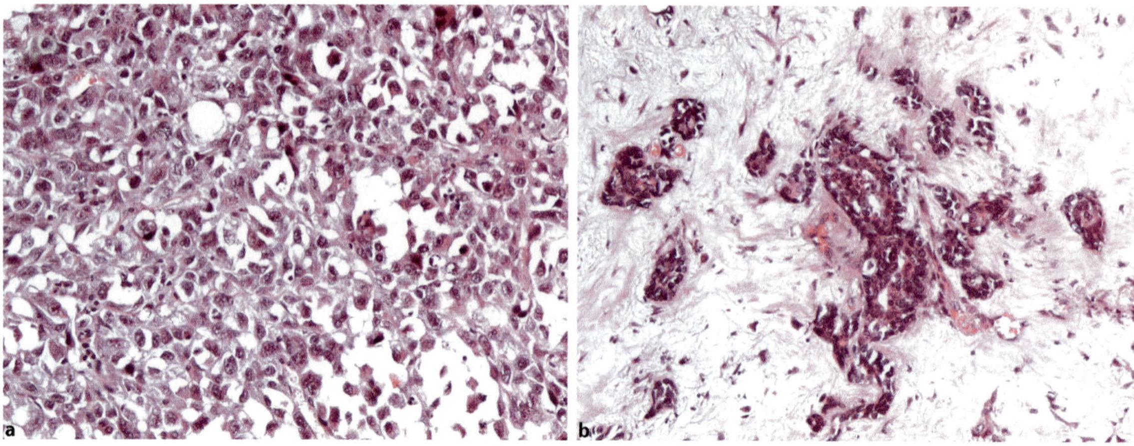

Fig. 3.13: Carcinoma ex-pleomorphic adenoma. **a** Area showing undifferentiated carcinoma (H&E, 200×). **b** Adjacent area of same specimen showing residual pleomorphic adenoma (H&E, 200×)

Treatment and Prognosis

The treatment of CEPA is wide surgical resection usually with a neck dissection. Features associated with an unfavorable prognosis include high tumor grade, large size, soft tissue invasion, perineural invasion, and lymph node metastases [81, 453]. Tortoledo correlated survival with the histologic subtype of the carcinoma and reported 5-year survival rates of 96% for terminal duct carcinoma, 62% for ductal carcinoma, 50% for myoepithelial carcinoma, and 30% for undifferentiated carcinoma [41, 130, 245, 370, 567]. He also found no deaths when the tumor invaded less than 6 mm. Brandwein reported no recurrences in patients with less than 1.5 mm of invasion and Olsen found that patients with less than 5 mm of invasion did not suffer recurrence [81, 154, 207].

Carcinoma ex-pleomorphic adenoma metastasizes exclusively as a carcinoma. Metastases develop in 30–70% of cases and distant metastases occur more frequently than regional metastases. These metastases seem to show a particular affinity for lungs and bone especially the vertebral column [81, 154, 370, 415].

In recent years much has been written about non-invasive (in situ or intracapsular) CEPA [207]. These are carcinomas which arise within a pleomorphic adenoma but have not penetrated the capsule of the pleomorphic adenoma. It has been stated that this finding has no adverse effect and the standard resection for a pleomorphic adenoma is curative [330, 331]. There is, however, at least one well-documented report in which a non-invasive CEPA metastasized to a lymph node [245, 261].

True Malignant Mixed Tumor

Clinical Features

True malignant mixed tumors (TMMT) may be regarded as carcinosarcomas since both the epithelial and stromal components are histologically malignant. Kirklin is credited with the first description of these tumors in 1951 and King was the first to refer to them as carcinosarcomas in 1967 [12, 234, 570].

As of 2000, 60 cases have been reported in the literature, the largest series having been reported by Gnepp in 1998 [66, 346]. TMMT comprise only 0.16–1.0% of all malignant tumors of salivary glands [245, 346]. Although most appear to arise de novo, approximately 33% of patients have either a clinical history or histologic confirmation of a coexisting pleomorphic adenoma [12, 223, 346]. The most common location is the parotid gland. Patients have ranged in age from 14 to 87 years and there is no sex predilection [12, 70, 223, 245, 261, 346, 547, 548, 570]. Signs and symptoms are similar to those of CEPA. Both carcinoma and sarcoma are seen in the metastases of TMMT.

Pathologic Features

The carcinomatous component is most often an adenocarcinoma, a squamous cell carcinoma, or an undifferentiated carcinoma [223]. The sarcomatous element is usually a chondrosarcoma, however, other types of sarcoma have also been reported including spindle cell sarcoma not otherwise specified, osteosarcoma, fibrosarcoma, malignant fibrous histiocytoma, leiomyosarcoma, and rarely liposarcoma and rhabdomyosarcoma [66].

Fowler et al. studied the loss of heterozygosity in tumor suppressor genes in TMMTs and CEPAs. They found that the carcinomatous and sarcomatous components of TMMTs are closely related. These findings also suggested a common clonal origin for the benign and carcinomatous components of CEPA [219].

Treatment and Prognosis

The treatment is radical surgical resection which should be combined with radiation and chemotherapy. Even with such radical treatment most patients die within 5 years [245]. TMMTs metastasize more commonly via a hematogenous rather than lymphatic route with lung and bone being the most frequent sites of metastases.

Metastasizing Mixed Tumor

Clinical Features

Metastasizing mixed tumor is a pleomorphic adenoma, which despite its benign histology, metastasizes. Histologically it is identical to a pleomorphic adenoma and can only be recognized as malignant once it has metastasized. Lung and bone are the most frequent sites of metastatic disease.

Foot and Frazell are credited with the first report of this tumor in 1953 [292]. Gnepp was able to find only 32 reported cases in his 1993 literature search [228, 245, 611]. By 1997 the number had increased to 40 [76, 113, 260, 387]. Approximately 65% occur in the parotid gland and the mean age at presentation is 32 years [245, 610]. Initial signs and symptoms are consistent with those of a pleomorphic adenoma. In almost all cases metastases have been preceded by at least one and frequently numerous local recurrences of a pleomorphic adenoma [610]. The time from initial resection of the pleomorphic adenoma to the appearance of metastatic disease can be as short as 1 year or as long as 20 years.

Pathologic Features

Histologically metastasizing mixed tumors are essentially identical to pleomorphic adenomas and lack any characteristics of malignancy [387]. Flow cytometry has not been helpful in identifying these tumors [387]. A recent analysis of p53, bcl-2, M1B1, CD105, p27, and p21 expression also proved unrewarding in identifying differences between metastasizing and non-metastasizing pleomorphic adenomas [387, 419].

Treatment and Prognosis

Surgical excision is also the treatment of choice for the primary tumor, recurrences, and metastases [610].

Metastases may be related to implantation of tumor cells into blood vessels and lymphatics at the time of surgery [245]. In Wenig's review of 32 patients, 25 (78%) were alive with or without tumor or died of unrelated causes [441]. Gnepp reported follow-up on 20 patients, seven of whom (37%) had died of their disease [98].

Acinic Cell Carcinoma

Clinical Features

The first description of acinic cell carcinoma was published by Nasse in 1892 [361, 539]. Acinic cell tumor, the old name for this neoplasm, reflects the fact that its malignant behavior was not recognized until Buxton's publication in 1953 [539].

Acinic cell carcinoma is a rare low-grade carcinoma accounting for only 2–4% of salivary gland neoplasms [47, 98, 126, 361, 400, 465]. The parotid gland is the most common site (80%) followed by the minor salivary glands (16%) and the submandibular gland (4%). While 80% occur in the parotid gland, acinic cell carcinoma accounts for only 4% of all parotid tumors [47, 269, 357, 400]. Although some series have shown a male predominance and at least one no sexual preference, most report a female to male ratio of approximately 2:1 [47, 172, 400, 457,

494, 579]. The rate of bilateral involvement of the parotid gland is 3%. While this is low, the incidence of bilateral involvement by acinic cell carcinoma is second only to Warthin's tumor which has a 5–10% incidence of bilaterality [166, 409].

The tumor is most frequent in individuals between 40 and 50 years of age but may occur at any age. Although less than 4% of patients are younger than 20 years, it is second only to mucoepidermoid carcinoma among salivary gland carcinomas occurring in the pediatric population [172, 361].

Patients typically present with a history of a slowly enlarging painless mass that is not fixed to the surrounding soft tissue or skin. Pain is a symptom in approximately 22% of patients and facial nerve paresis or paralysis is encountered in approximately 3–8% [278, 361]. The median duration of symptoms prior to treatment is 2 years but may be as long as several decades [191].

Pathologic Features

Grossly the tumors are solitary, firm or rubbery, and well circumscribed ranging in size from 0.5 to 13 cm (median 2.5 cm). Recurrent tumors are frequently multiple and may be poorly demarcated. The cut surface varies from tan to gray and is occasionally cystic [22, 404]. Microscopically multiple growth patterns occur, often within the same tumor. These have been categorized as solid, microcystic, papillary-cystic, and follicular with the solid and microcystic patterns being the most common (Fig. 3.14a–c). In the solid growth pattern the tumor cells grow in large sheets. The microcystic pattern is characterized by interspersed spaces of varying sizes. The microcyst formation may result from accumulation of secretions due to a lack of ducts or may possibly be an artifact of fixation [263, 465]. The papillary-cystic pattern has large cystic spaces containing branching projections of epithelium. In the follicular pattern cystic spaces are distended with a homogeneous proteinaceous material resulting in a pattern mimicking thyroid follicles.

The prototypical cell type is round to polyhedral with a uniform round eccentric nucleus and basophilic granular cytoplasm. These cells very closely resemble normal serous acinar cells and indeed the diagnosis of acinic cell carcinoma is predicated on identifying this cell type. Other cell types include those resembling intercalated duct epithelial cells, vacuolated cells, clear cells, and non-specific glandular cells. Intercalated duct type cells are cuboidal with eosinophilic cytoplasm and centrally placed hyperchromatic nuclei. Vacuolated cells are similar in size to acinar type cells but have vacuolated acidophilic cyto-

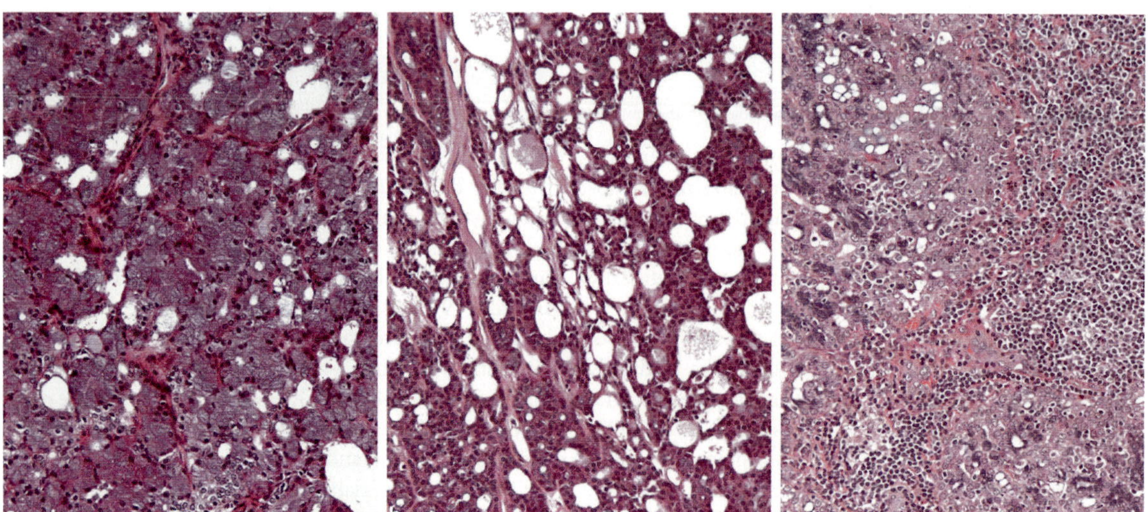

Fig. 3.14: Acinic cell carcinoma. **a** Neoplastic acinic cells with basophilic granular cytoplasm and growing in a predominately solid pattern (H&E, 200×). **b** Microcystic growth pattern (H&E, 200×). **c** Acinic cell carcinoma composed of granular acinic cells (dark granular cells) and non-specific glandular cells. Note presence of abundant lymphoid tissue (H&E, 200×)

plasm and a more open chromatin pattern. Their nuclei may exhibit slight pleomorphism. Although vacuolated, the cells do not contain lipid, glycogen, or epithelial mucin. Clear cells have pale or non-staining cytoplasm but otherwise resemble acinar or non-specific glandular cells. Non-specific glandular cells have eosinophilic cytoplasm, indistinct cell borders, and nuclei which are larger, more vesicular and more pleomorphic than those of the other cell types. Any one tumor may be composed primarily or exclusively of diagnostic acinar type cells or may contain a mixture of cell types. Mitotic figures are rare. Tumors composed primarily of acinar-type cells closely resemble normal serous salivary glands except for the lack of striated ducts. The stroma is typically scant and composed of thin delicate strands of fibrovascular tissue although some tumors may have a dense hyalinized stroma. A relatively frequent finding in the stroma is the presence of abundant lymphoid tissue complete with germinal center formation. This occurs in upward of 30% of acinic cell carcinomas [172, 175, 176].

Like normal acinar cells, the acinar cells of acinic cell carcinoma contain PAS-positive diastase-resistant zymogen granules. The cytoplasm does not stain with mucicarmine or alcian blue stains although, in some cases, intercellular cystic areas may contain material that is weakly mucicarminophilic [145, 172, 176]. Well-differentiated acinar cells are also positive for lactoferrin, amylase, alpha-1-antitrypsin, alpha-1-antichymotrypsin, carcinoembryonic antigen, Leu M-1, and vasoactive intestinal polypeptide [318, 448]. Acinic cell carcinomas are also immunoreactive for cytokeratin and approximately 10% are S-100 positive [353]. They are negative for c-kit and p53 overexpression is low [46, 47, 58, 180, 404, 443]. Acinic cell carcinomas have also been found to be MUC3 positive, MUC5AC negative, and MUC6 negative [361, 443].

Differential Diagnosis

The lack of both ducts and a normal lobular architecture aid in distinguishing acinic cell carcinoma from normal salivary gland parenchyma. Absence of mucous and epidermoid cells permits distinction of the microcystic form of acinic cell carcinoma from mucoepidermoid carcinoma. Identification of zymogen-containing acinar cells separates the papillary-cystic form of acinic cell carcinoma from cystadenocarcinoma. Lack of staining for thyroglobulin and thyroid transcription factor distinguishes the follicular variant of acinic cell carcinoma from metastatic thyroid carcinoma.

Pathogenesis

The name acinic cell carcinoma and the presence of acinar-type cells in the tumor would suggest origin from acinar cells. Most investigators, however, indicate an origin from the stem or reserve cells of the intercalated ducts [443].

Treatment and Prognosis

The treatment of acinic cell carcinoma is complete surgical resection. Neck dissection is usually not recommended because of a relatively low incidence of metastases to regional lymph nodes [361]. There have been only a few reported instances of a favorable response to radiation treatment, most tumors having been radio resistant. Radiation is usually reserved for tumors which cannot be completely resected or for those uncommon cases which have extensive perineural or lymphatic invasion [126, 361, 443].

Acinic cell carcinoma is a low-grade malignancy and there is no correlation between cell type or growth pattern and prognosis [180, 361, 443, 465, 541]. The recurrence rate averages 10–35% and the distant metastatic rate 13–16% [361, 409]. The lungs and bone are the most common sites of distant metastases. Survival rates range from 78 to 90%, 63 to 83%, and 44 to 67% at 5, 10, and 20 years, respectively [166, 521]. The clinical course may be protracted and cases of recurrence have been reported after a disease-free interval of 30 years [284, 521].

Most tumors are diploid and as a result DNA studies are usually not helpful in predicting outcome. El-Nagger, however, reported that in a study of 15 patients, none with diploid tumors developed metastases or died of disease while five of eight with aneuploid tumors developed metastases and four succumbed to their disease [521].

MIB-1 appears to be an independent prognostic factor. Patients with MIB-1-negative tumors have been shown to have significantly better survival than those with MIB-1-positive tumors [545]. In a study by Skalova, five of seven patients with MIB-1 values higher than 10% had unfavorable outcomes while none of the 17 patients with values lower than 5% suffered recurrences during follow-up periods as long as 30 years [286, 545].

3

Dedifferentiated Acinic Cell Carcinoma

A highly aggressive form of acinic cell carcinoma was reported by Stanley in 1988 [152, 166, 497]. He called these tumors dedifferentiated acinic cell carcinomas. In addition to well-differentiated classic acinic cell carcinoma each contained discrete areas of poorly differentiated adenocarcinoma or undifferentiated carcinoma. Transitional areas between the classic acinic cell carcinoma and the high-grade component are not seen.

Unlike classic acinic cell carcinomas, these tumors are highly malignant and metastasize early. It is therefore recommended that these cancers be treated by radical resection and neck dissection [286]. The dedifferentiated component is usually aneuploid [55, 105, 192, 227]. Henley reported a case in which p53 was negative immunohistochemically in both the low- and high-grade components. In addition, polymerase chain reaction and non-isotopic single-stranded conformational polymorphism analysis showed a germ line configuration of the p53 gene, exons five through eight, in both low- and high-grade components of the tumor [249, 562].

Polymorphous Low-grade Adenocarcinoma

Clinical Features

Polymorphous low-grade adenocarcinoma of salivary gland origin (PLGA) was previously known as terminal duct carcinoma and lobular carcinoma because of its histologic resemblance to these forms of breast carcinoma [2, 9, 48, 193, 327, 374, 596]. It is a rare neoplasm with distinctive clinical and morphologic features.

Most of these cancers arise from intraoral minor salivary glands where it accounts for approximately 10% of all intraoral minor salivary gland tumors and 25% of the malignant ones [512, 609]. Sixty to seventy percent involve the palate [238, 327, 402, 411, 471, 480]. Origin from minor salivary glands in the nose and nasopharynx and from the lacrimal glands has also been reported [105]. Origin in major salivary glands is very uncommon and, when it does occur, usually involves the parotid gland [577].

The tumors grow slowly producing a non-ulcerated painless mass ranging in size from 0.4 to 6 cm [105, 193]. Most patients are between 40 and 60 years of age although some patients have been in their early twenties and at least one was diagnosed in a 12-year-old child [105, 134, 252, 464, 571, 609]. PLGA is more common in women than men by a ratio of 2:1 [64, 163, 413, 463].

Pathologic Features

The name PLGA is appropriate because it reflects the main features of this neoplasm. The tumor is polymorphous in its histologic growth patterns but cytologically bland. It is its infiltrating growth pattern, tendency for recurrence, perineural invasion, and ability to metastasize that attest to its malignancy.

Grossly PLGAs are solid and well circumscribed but not encapsulated. The cut surface is homogeneous and tan to tan-yellow. Histologically any combination of six growth patterns, namely solid, tubular, fascicular, cribriform, linear single cell, and papillary/papillary cystic may be observed. Concentric growth around blood vessels and nerves is also characteristic. The tumor cells are cytologically bland and vary from cuboidal to columnar with eosinophilic or clear cytoplasm. Nuclei are round to oval with vesicular chromatin and small nucleoli. Mitotic activity and necrosis are usually not present. The tumor is supported by a stroma which may be scant or abundant and can vary from mucinous to hyalinized. Invasion of soft tissue may be local and easily overlooked. Perineural invasion is typical of PLGA and is seen as often or more often than in adenoid cystic carcinoma (Fig. 3.15a–c).

Polymorphous low-grade adenocarcinomas are positive for cytokeratin and vimentin. They are also strongly positive for S-100. Approximately 10–50% have been reported to be positive for GFAP, muscle-specific actin, and epithelial membrane antigen [105, 526]. Reported results of c-kit expression have been inconsistent [134, 252]. Proliferative activity as measured by Ki-67 is low ranging from 0.2 to 6.4 with a mean of 2.4% [64, 144, 232, 526].

Differential Diagnosis

Included in the differential diagnosis are pleomorphic adenoma, adenoid cystic carcinoma, and acinic cell carcinoma. Pleomorphic and monomorphic adenomas of minor salivary glands do not have a capsule, however, they have a pushing rather than infiltrating destructive margin and lack neurotropism. Adenoid cystic carcinomas infiltrate and have a marked predilection for perineural invasion, however, the prototypical cell of these tumors has an

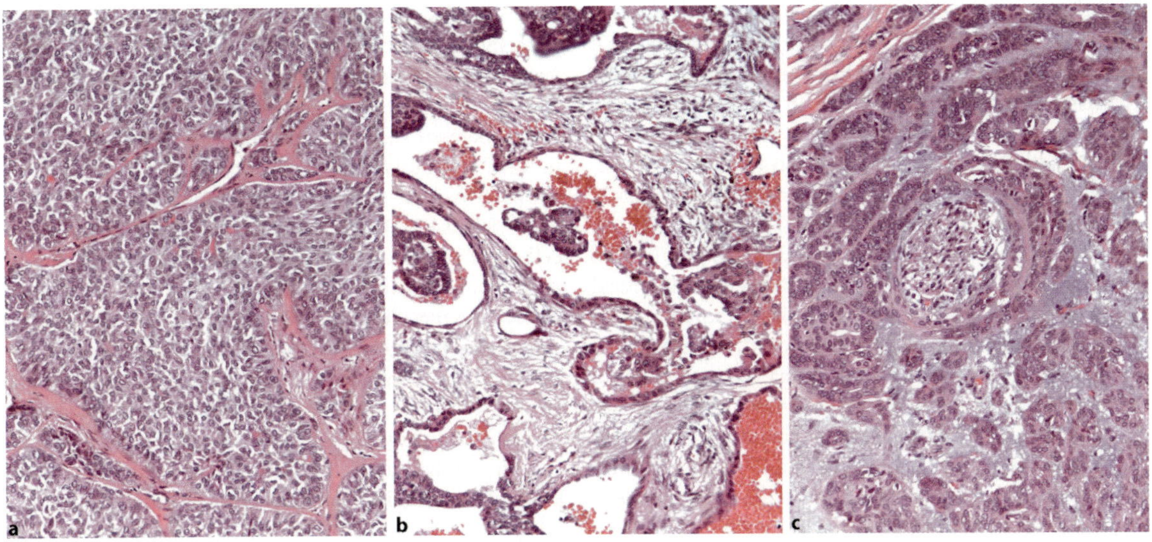

Fig. 3.15: Polymorphous low-grade adenocarcinoma. **a** Cytologically bland tumor cells with eosinophilic to clear cytoplasm. The tumor cells are growing in a solid pattern (H&E, 200×). **b** Papillary cystic growth pattern (H&E, 200×). **c** Tubular growth pattern with perineural invasion (H&E, 200×)

angulated hyperchromatic nucleus and scant cytoplasm. This is in contrast to the typical cell of PLGA which has a vesicular nucleus and more cytoplasm. Acinic cell carcinomas are rare in minor salivary glands and infrequently show perineural invasion. Although there is overlap in the immunohistochemical staining, PLGAs are less frequently and less diffusely positive for GFAP than pleomorphic adenomas. In addition it is the epithelial component that stains in PLGA in contrast to pleomorphic adenomas where the staining is in the stromal component [64, 163, 413, 463]. Positivity for vimentin and a much lower proliferative activity measured by Ki-67 can be helpful in separating PLGA from adenoid cystic carcinoma which shows just the opposite staining results [48, 105, 327, 414]. Some have found c-kit expression helpful in distinguishing between PLGA and adenoid cystic carcinoma while other have not [105].

Treatment and Prognosis

Treatment is complete surgical resection. PLGA is a low-grade indolent tumor with a tendency for local recurrence. In the past it has been associated with a recurrence rate of 20% although a more recent study by Castle et al. reports a recurrence rate of 9.1% [48, 327, 414]. The average time from initial surgery to recurrence is 7 years [193]. In 6–7% of cases there is metastasis to regional lymph nodes [48, 193, 530]. Tumors with a predominately papillary growth pattern have been associated with a higher incidence of cervical lymph node metastases [105, 193]. Postoperative radiation therapy is considered unnecessary due to the low-grade nature of this tumor. Distant metastases have occurred but are very uncommon [159]. Deaths due to tumor are infrequent and usually occur after a prolonged course [25, 217, 312, 572, 573].

Epithelial-myoepithelial Carcinoma

Clinical Features

Epithelial-myoepithelial carcinoma of salivary glands (EMC) is a rare but histologically distinctive low-grade carcinoma. The name was proposed in 1972 by Donath et al. who were the first to appreciate that the tumor is a carcinoma [416, 417, 544]. Prior names applied to this neoplasm include adenomyoepithelioma, clear cell adenoma, and glycogen-rich adenoma and reflect the misconception that it is a benign tumor.

Epithelial-myoepithelial carcinoma accounts for approximately 0.5–1% of all salivary gland neoplasms and favors women by a ratio of 2:1 [446, 466]. The vast majority arise in the major as opposed to the minor salivary glands. The parotid gland is the site of approximately 75% with an additional 10–12% arising in the submandibular gland. Origin from minor salivary glands primarily occurs in the palate [505, 561]. EMC has also arisen in extraoral mucoserous glands in the nasopharynx, larynx, and bronchi [572]. Interestingly a histologically identical tumor occurs in the breast where it is still known as an adenomyoepithelioma [129, 132, 256, 417, 491].

Epithelial-myoepithelial carcinoma is essentially a tumor of older adults (mean age 60 years) although rare cases have been reported in the pediatric age group and we have seen one unreported case in a 6½-year-old child [124, 159]. Patients usually present with an asymptomatic mass. Much less frequently signs and symptoms of a malignant neoplasm, such as facial paralysis and pain, are present. In some instances a mass has been present for several years prior to the patient seeking medical treatment [218].

Pathologic Features

Grossly these tumors are firm, solid, and frequently lobulated. The margins may be sharply circumscribed or infiltrative. The cut surface ranges from yellow to gray-white and cystic spaces are sometimes present. Those involving the palate frequently ulcerate. EMC have ranged in size from 1 to 8 cm.

Histologically four growth patterns have been described namely tubular, cribriform, solid, and papillary [573]. The tubular is the prototypical and most common growth pattern. The tubules are composed of duct-like structures having an inner (luminal) single cell layer of cytologically bland cuboidal epithelial cells with dense granular eosinophilic cytoplasm and an outer (abluminal) single or multiple cell layer of ovoid to polygonal myoepithelial cells with clear cytoplasm and eccentric vesicular nuclei. The epithelial cells are strongly positive with cytokeratin stains and negative for myoepithelial markers. The myoepithelial cells are usually only weakly positive for cytokeratin but stain strongly with myoepithelial markers (S-100, smooth muscle actin, p63, HHF35, and calponin). Their clear cytoplasm is due to the presence of glycogen. Pleomorphism and mitotic activity are absent or minimal although rarely tumors may show pleomorphism and increased mitotic activity. Histologic evidence of malignancy is reflected in areas showing an infiltrative growth pattern and perineural invasion. Prominent collars of PAS-positive diastase-resistant basement membrane material surrounds the duct-like structures which in turn form nests of tumor separated by fibrous bands of connective tissue. This results in a multilobulated appearance (Fig. 3.16). In the cribriform growth pattern two cell populations are still discernable and, while the cribriform pattern can mimic an adenoid cystic carcinoma, no hyaline material is present in the round spaces. The solid growth pattern consists of sheets of myoepithelial cells which, in some areas, may have a spindled shape. Ductal structures are scarce and may be difficult to find. The papillary growth pattern is encountered in cystic areas. The epithelium lining the cystic spaces and papillary structures maintains a biphasic pattern with luminal ductal epithelial cells and abluminal clear myoepithelial cells. In all growth patterns the myoepithelial cells predominate, however, occasionally areas may be present in which apparent atrophy of the clear cells has produced "naked ducts" lined only by a single layer of epithelial cells.

Differential Diagnosis

The differential diagnosis of EMC includes other salivary gland tumors containing clear cells, such as clear cell myoepithelioma, acinic cell carcinoma, and mucoepidermoid carcinoma, and metastatic tumors which may contain clear cells, in particular those from the kidney and thyroid. The clear cells of EMC are myoepithelial cells which contain glycogen and are PAS positive diastase sensitive and mucicarmine negative. The clear cells of clear cell myoepithelioma are also glycogen-containing myoepithelial cells with the same staining characteristics as those in EMC. Clear cell myoepitheliomas, however, lack ducts and may contain foci of other types of myoepithelial cells such as the plasmacytoid, hyaline, and epithelioid forms. Acinic cell carcinoma contains cells with PAS-positive diastase-resistant granules not seen in EMC. Mucoepidermoid carcinoma contains intracytoplasmic droplets of mucin which is PAS positive diastase resistant and mucicarmine positive. The clear cells in renal cell carcinoma contain both glycogen and lipid and will be PAS positive diastase sensitive and will also stain with lipid stains. Clear cell carcinoma of the thyroid is negative for both glycogen and lipid but will stain for thyroglobulin and thyroid transcription factor.

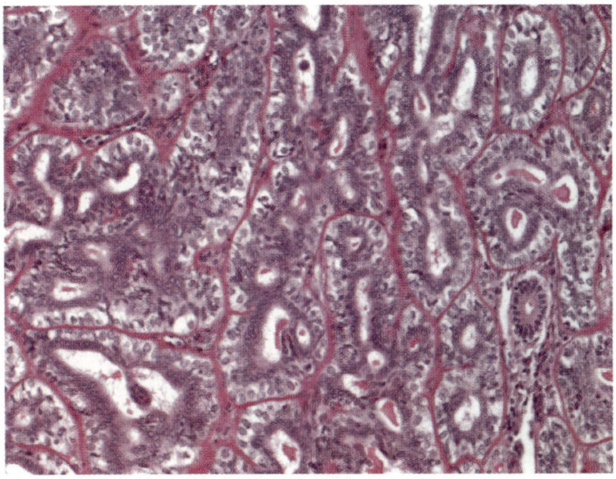

Fig. 3.16: Epithelial-myoepithelial carcinoma. The tumor forms tubules lined by a luminal layer of epithelial cells and an ablumi-nal single or multiple cell layer of myoepithelial cells with clear cytoplasm. Prominent collars of basement membrane material surround the structures. Pleomorphism is absent or minimal (H&E, 200×)

Treatment and Prognosis

The treatment is complete surgical resection. Fonseca et al. found higher values of proliferative cell nuclear antigen in the myoepithelial cells as opposed to the epithelial cells and a higher recurrence rate in those tumors with a predominately solid myoepithelial growth pattern [124, 274]. A study by Tralongo et al. also found that higher proliferative activity occurred in tumors with a more aggressive clinical course [49, 274]. Other studies, however, failed to demonstrate a correlation between proliferative activity or histologic growth pattern and prognosis [124]. The majority of the tumors are diploid [49, 124, 129, 377, 516]. Some studies have found that those which were aneuploid pursued a more aggressive clinical course, however, 60% of those that were diploid also recurred or metastasized [49, 124, 129, 377, 516]. Local recurrence rates for EMC range from 30% to 50% [335, 395]. Regional lymph node metastases occur in 18% of patients and distant metastases in 7–25% [265, 317, 472]. The overall 5-year survival rate is 80%. This drops off to approximately 70% at 10 years.

Basal Cell Adenocarcinoma

Clinical Features

Basal cell adenocarcinoma is the malignant counterpart of basal cell adenoma. It is an uncommon low-grade malignancy first recognized by Klima et al. in 1978 [147, 317, 423]. It accounts for 1.6% of all salivary gland neoplasms and 2.9% of all salivary gland malignancies [423].

Most patients are in their sixth or seventh decade (mean age 60 years) although cases have been reported in individuals as young as 2 months and as old as 92 years [265, 317, 423, 436, 603]. Basal cell adenocarcinoma occurs with equal frequency in men and women [265]. Most of these tumors arise de novo. Origin in a pre-existing basal cell adenoma is uncommon and when it does occur it usually involves the membranous type of basal cell adenoma [15, 147, 265, 317]. Approximately 90% of the tumors arise in the major salivary glands with the vast majority involving the parotid gland [181]. Origin in minor salivary glands is uncommon [52, 423]. Patients usually present with an asymptomatic swelling which may be of weeks to years in duration. Pain and tenderness are uncommon [502]. In approximately 10–15% of cases basal cell adenocarcinoma of salivary glands occurs in conjunction with dermal cylindromas and trichoepitheliomas. This association, while significant, is lower than the 40% association of basal cell adenomas with these dermal tumors [603].

Pathologic Features

Basal cell adenocarcinomas are solid tan to gray tumors up to 7 cm in diameter. Infiltration into adjacent salivary gland parenchyma and soft tissue may be readily apparent or very subtle.

Microscopically there is a striking resemblance to basal cell adenomas both in growth pattern and cytology. Four growth patterns, identical to those in basal cell adenoma, occur. The tubular pattern is characterized by multiple small ductal structures, the trabecular by anastomosing cords of cells, the solid by rounded nests or large sheets of cells, and the membranous by overproduction of basement membrane material which accumulates both around cell nests and intercellularly. While any combination of growth patterns may be seen in a single tumor, one usually predominates. Of the four patterns, the solid is the most common.

Cytologically two cell types similar to those in basal cell adenomas are present. One is a small round cell with a round dark staining nucleus and scant cytoplasm and the other a larger cell with a lighter staining nucleus and amphophilic cytoplasm. In most tumors the smaller cells are arranged peripherally and perpendicular alignment of their nuclei produces a palisading effect, which may, however, not be as conspicuous as in basal cell adenomas. Centrally located larger cells may produce swirls and squamous eddies.

Cellular and nuclear pleomorphism are minimal and necrosis, if present, is focal and not extensive. Mitoses are not frequent averaging two or less per 10 high power fields. Careful examination, however, will reveal invasive growth. In addition there is a 25–35% incidence of perineural and intravascular invasion [65, 265, 502, 616].

Immunohistochemically basal cell adenocarcinoma does not differ from basal cell adenoma [502]. Staining results support both epithelial and myoepithelial differentiation in both the small and large cells. While all tumors stain for cytokeratin, the majority are also at least focally positive for S-100, smooth muscle actin, vimentin, carcinoembryonic antigen, and epithelial membrane antigen [115, 181, 375].

Pleuro-potential ductal reserve cells are thought to give rise to this tumor [436]. The membranous variant of basal cell adenoma is the most common variant to give rise to basal cell adenocarcinoma, however, this is uncommon, most basal cell adenocarcinomas apparently arising de novo [423].

Differential Diagnosis

Included in the differential diagnosis of basal cell adenocarcinoma are basal cell adenoma, adenoid cystic carcinoma, cutaneous basal cell carcinoma, and small cell carcinoma. In some instances basal cell adenocarcinoma may only be differentiated from basal cell adenoma by identifying an infiltrative growth pattern and/or perineural and intravascular invasion. Some have found staining for Ki-67, p53, bcl-2, and epidermal growth factor receptor helpful in making this distinction [336, 580]. The membranous variant of basal cell adenoma is typically multifocal and care must be taken not to mistake multifocality for invasion.

Basal cell adenocarcinoma and adenoid cystic carcinoma both show perineural invasion and both produce hyalinized basement membrane material. Intercellular deposits of basement membrane material, squamous eddies, and peripheral palisading, however, are features associated with basal cell adenocarcinoma and not adenoid cystic carcinoma. A dual population of small and large cells is also characteristic of basal cell adenocarcinoma and not adenoid cystic carcinoma.

Perineural invasion and immunohistochemical evidence of myoepithelial differentiation would aid in distinguishing basal cell adenocarcinoma from cutaneous basal cell carcinoma. Clinical information as to the location of the tumor would also be invaluable.

Basal cell adenocarcinoma lacks the nuclear molding, brisk mitotic activity, and prominent necrosis of small cell carcinomas. Unlike small cell carcinoma, it is negative for synaptophysin and chromogranin.

Treatment and Prognosis

Treatment is complete surgical excision. Since it is a low-grade carcinoma, neck dissection is usually reserved for patients with clinically positive lymph nodes. In a recent review of a large series of basal cell adenocarcinomas Muller and Barnes found a local recurrence rate of 37%. Cervical lymph node metastases were present in 8% and distant metastases in 4%. There was a mean follow-up of 54 months on 45 patients. Of these patients, 37 were alive without disease, 4 were alive with disease, 1 died of disease, and 3 died of other causes [10, 35, 120, 437, 488, 495].

Myoepithelial Carcinoma

Clinical Features

Myoepithelial carcinoma (malignant myoepithelioma) is the malignant counterpart of myoepithelioma. By definition it is composed exclusively or almost exclusively of myoepithelial cells with an infiltrative growth pattern.

Myoepithelial carcinomas account for only 0.2% of all epithelial salivary gland tumors and 10% of all myoepithelial salivary gland tumors [437, 495]. Approximately 84 cases have been reported to date [580]. Seventy-five percent occur in the parotid gland [10, 120, 336, 437, 488, 495, 580, 593]. When minor salivary glands are involved there is a distinct predilection for those in the palate [495]. The tumors are most common in the sixth and seventh decades (range 24–81 years) and occur with equal frequency in men and women [495]. A painless mass is usually the only clinical complaint. Approximately 50% of cases have arisen in a pre-existing benign tumor, usually a pleomorphic adenoma or a myoepithelioma.

Pathologic Features

Grossly myoepithelial carcinomas are unencapsulated soft to firm and often nodular. They vary in size from 2 to 10 cm. The cut surface is tan to gray-white and may show areas of necrosis and cystic degeneration. Glassy gelatinous areas may also be observed [303, 405, 495].

Microscopically there is infiltrative destructive growth into the adjacent salivary gland or soft tissues. These tumors frequently have a multinodular growth pattern. The nodules of tumor cells are separated by fibrous stroma and often have myxoid or necrotic centers. As in myoepitheliomas any of four cell types may be present and in any proportion. These cell types are: (1) epithelioid, (2) plasmacytoid (or hyaline), (3) spindle, and (4) clear cell. The epithelioid cells have a moderate amount of eosinophilic cytoplasm. The plasmacytoid or hyaline cells have eccentrically placed nuclei reminiscent of plasma cells and a glassy eosinophilic cytoplasm. They tend to be particularly numerous in palatal tumors. The spindle cells are elongated and resemble plump fibroblasts. The clear cells have clear cytoplasm due to the presence of glycogen. In some myoepithelial carcinomas the cytologic atypia is obvious whereas in others cytologic features of malignancy are very subtle and indeed the diagnosis of malignancy may rest solely on identifying areas of invasive destructive growth. In the 25 cases reported by Savera et al. 40% were classified as high grade and 60% as low grade [171, 174, 221].

The stromal component of these tumors is characterized by the presence of amphophilic to blue-gray myxoid material and or eosinophilic hyalinized material. The myxoid material is particularly characteristic and often accumulates around nests of plasmacytoid cells.

Results of immunoperoxidase stains are essentially the same as obtained with myoepitheliomas. Myoepithelial carcinomas are positive for AE1/3, vimentin, and S-100 in virtually all cases. Vimentin and S-100 are infrequently present in normal myoepithelial cells but are sensitive (although non-specific) markers of neoplastic myoepithelial cells. Reactivity for other myoepithelial cell markers such as muscle specific actin, GFAP, smooth muscle actin, and calponin is variable.

Differential Diagnosis

The differential diagnosis is lengthy and includes a number of other salivary gland tumors such as: polymorphous low-grade adenocarcinoma, epithelial-myoepithelial carcinoma, oncocytoma and hyalinizing clear cell carcinoma, benign and malignant spindle cell tumors, plasmacytomas, and metastatic renal cell carcinoma. Documentation of exclusive myoepithelial differentiation by immunohistochemistry will usually permit distinction of myoepithelial carcinomas from other neoplasms.

Treatment and Prognosis

The treatment is complete surgical excision. The clinical behavior of myoepithelial carcinomas is unpredictable. Although tumors showing cytologic pleomorphism, numerous mitoses and necrosis are usually associated with an adverse outcome, some with aggressive histologic features have been clinically indolent. In addition there have been reports of histologically low-grade tumors that have metastasized and resulted in death [221].

Cystadenocarcinoma

Clinical Features

Cystadenocarcinomas of the salivary glands are low-grade cystic neoplasms which have been reported in the past under a variety of names including malignant papillary cystadenoma, mucus-producing adenopapillary carcinoma, low-grade papillary adenocarcinoma, papillary adenocarcinoma, adenopapillary carcinoma, papillary cystadenocarcinoma, and papillary cystic adenocarcinoma [9, 27, 69, 112, 140, 171, 174, 185, 221, 320, 412, 422, 501, 510, 529, 543, 544, 615].

The tumor is twice as common in the major salivary glands as opposed to the minor salivary glands and most frequently occurs in the parotid [221]. Cystadenocarcinomas have been reported over an age range of 20–86 years, however, 75% of patients are over the age of 50 years (mean age 58.8 years) [334].

Microscopically there are haphazardly arranged cystic spaces that vary in size and shape. Mucin released from ruptured cysts can produce an inflammatory response. The cystic spaces are separated by scant to abundant stroma. Solid cellular areas and ducts may be present between the cysts and at the periphery of tumor but they never comprise the major portion of the neoplasm. The cysts and ducts are lined by small and large cuboidal and columnar cells with eosinophilic, clear, or mucinous cytoplasm. In some tumors the columnar cells impart a decidedly enteric appearance. The epithelium lining the cystic spaces may form a single layer to multiple layers. In over three fourths of cases there is a prominent intracystic papillary growth. This may range from small collections of cells lacking a fibrovascular core to large elongated and branching structures supported by fibrovascular cores. A cribriform growth pattern may also be seen. Nuclei are typically bland and mitoses are infrequent. Although some tumors may show a moderate degree of nuclear pleomorphism this has not been predictive of a more aggressive course. In contrast, tumors composed predominately of columnar cells may prove to be more aggressive [314, 585].

Recognizing these tumors as carcinomas is predicated upon finding areas of infiltrative growth. Tumors arising in minor salivary glands infiltrate adjacent soft tissue and skeletal muscle and may even infiltrate bone. In major salivary glands the infiltrative growth may be limited to the gland parenchyma making it more difficult to appreciate. Perineural invasion is not a feature of this neoplasm.

Differential Diagnosis

Included in the differential diagnosis are cystadenomas and all other salivary gland neoplasms that may have a cystic component. Cystadenomas are the benign counterpart of cystadenocarcinomas and do not have the infiltrative growth pattern of the latter.

Low-grade mucoepidermoid carcinomas are predominately cystic and often papillary cystic but unlike cystadenocarcinomas contain a mixture of mucous, epidermoid, and intermediate cells. Epidermoid differentiation is uncommon in cystadenocarcinomas. Also the solid proliferative component is usually larger in mucoepidermoid carcinomas than in cystadenocarcinomas.

The cystic and papillary areas of polymorphous low-grade adenocarcinoma can also be confused with cystadenocarcinoma. Features of polymorphous low-grade adenocarcinoma which can aid in the distinction from cystadenocarcinoma include a more variable growth pattern, mucinous and hyalinized stroma, and perineural invasion.

The papillary cystic form of acinic cell carcinoma is distinguished from cystadenocarcinoma by its microcystic growth pattern and tumor cells with basophilic, PAS-positive diastase-resistant zymogen granules.

Treatment and Prognosis

Cystadenocarcinomas are low-grade tumors and complete surgical excision is usually curative.

These tumors are uncommon and the series by Foss et al. remains the largest to date [293]. They had follow-up on 40 of their 57 patients. Local recurrence occurred in three patients and four had regional lymph node metastasis, three at the time of diagnosis and one 4.5 years following initial surgery. Three patients developed local recurrences which were successfully treated. Of the 40 patients, 36 were alive and 4 died of other causes after a mean postsurgical interval of 59 months.

Salivary Duct Carcinoma

Clinical Features

First described by Kleinsasser et al. in 1968, salivary duct carcinoma is a rare high-grade tumor thought to arise from the large excretory ducts [314]. The name is somewhat misleading since essentially all salivary gland carcinomas are believed to arise from reserve cells of the ductal system.

The peak incidence of this tumor occurs in the sixth and seventh decades. It is more common in men than women by a ratio of 2.5:1. It occurs most commonly in the parotid gland (78%) followed by the submandibular gland (12%) and the minor salivary glands (10%) [293]. Salivary duct carcinoma comprises approximately 6–10% of all carcinomas of the parotid [13]. Many patients present with signs and symptoms reflecting the aggressive behavior of this tumor including a rapidly enlarging painful mass and facial nerve paresis or paralysis. In the series by Jaehne et al., approximately two thirds of the patients presented with T3 or T4 tumors [293]. Hosal et al. reported the presence of calcifications seen on CT scans in 5 of their 15 patients [84, 150, 272, 358, 425, 451, 533].

Pathologic Features

Grossly salivary duct carcinomas are firm and gray white. Tumor margins may be obviously infiltrating or, less frequently, may appear deceptively discrete. Central comedo-type necrosis may be apparent on cross-section.

Microscopically the tumor is very reminiscent of ductal carcinoma of the breast. An intraductal component is characterized by solid, papillary, cribriform, and comedo growth patterns similar to intraductal carcinoma of the breast. All four growth patterns may be present in the same tumor. The invasive component typically grows as ribbons and small clusters of cells in a desmoplastic often hyalinized stroma reminiscent of invasive ductal carcinoma of the breast. It should also be stressed that invasive disease may also produce growth patterns similar to intraductal disease. In these instances invasion is recognized by a lack of a smooth round contour to the nests of tumor cells and also by a lack of a peripheral layer of myoepithelial cells [136, 205, 244, 314, 358, 451, 528]. The tumor cells are moderately large with an increased nuclear cytoplasmic ratio, abundant eosinophilic cytoplasm, hyperchromatic pleomorphic nuclei with prominent nucleoli, and frequent and abnormal mitotic figures (Fig. 3.17a, b). Perineural invasion is present in approximately 80% of cases [37, 155, 358, 398, 451]. The tumor cells are typically positive for cytokeratin and epithelial membrane antigen. Immunoreactivity for CEA has varied from 0% to 72% while staining for S-100 has varied from 0% to 41% depending on the series [285, 433, 434, 460, 518]. Salivary duct carcinomas are also frequently positive for gross cystic disease fluid protein, androgen receptor, and HER2/neu [304, 433, 460]. They are seldom positive for estrogen and progesterone receptors [433, 460]. Proliferative activity as measured by Ki-67 is usually high.

Histologic variants of salivary duct carcinoma include sarcomatoid, micropapillary, and mucin-rich [434]. The sarcomatoid variant is biphasic consisting of both carcinomatous and sarcomatous areas histologically. The sarcomatous change is considered to be a dedifferentiated phenomenon and has also been seen in mucoepidermoid, acinic cell, adenoid cystic, squamous cell, and epithelial-myoepithelial salivary gland carcinomas [285, 518]. The sarcomatous component expresses cytokeratin and epithelial membrane antigen in addition to being positive for vimentin [316, 592]. The micropapillary variant has foci where the tumor produces morula-like papillary cell clusters which lack fibrovascular cores and are surrounded by clear spaces [13, 119]. Mucin-rich sal-

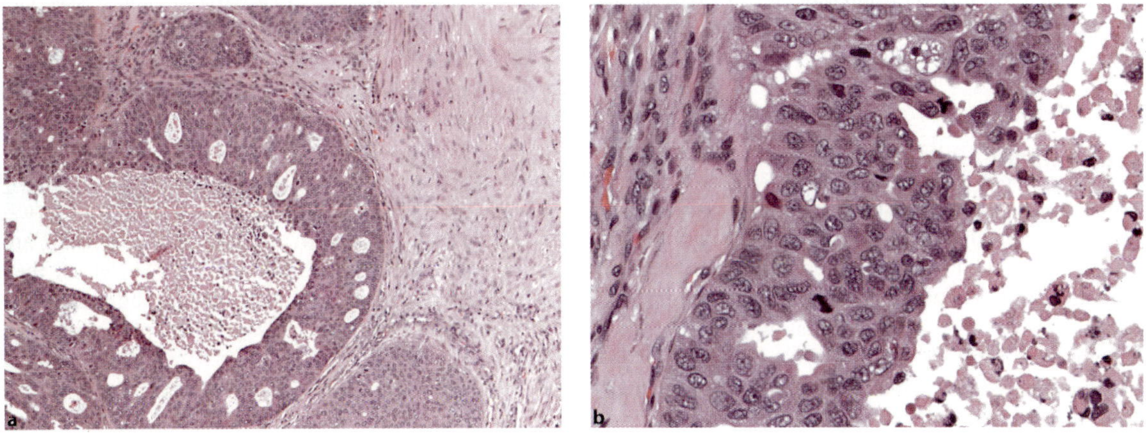

Fig. 3.17: Salivary duct carcinoma. **a** Cribriform and comedo growth patterns (H&E, 100×). **b** Higher magnification to show marked pleomorphism of tumor cells and abnormal mitotic figures (H&E, 400×)

ivary duct carcinoma is characterized by islands of tumor cells surrounded by pools of mucus which in turn are separated into compartments by bands of fibrous tissue [293].

Differential Diagnosis

The differential diagnosis includes metastatic adenocarcinoma from the prostate and metastatic ductal carcinoma of the breast. Immunoperoxidase staining for prostate-specific antigen aids in ruling out metastatic prostate carcinoma [38]. It is more difficult to exclude metastatic ductal carcinoma of the breast since, in rare instances, salivary duct carcinoma is positive for estrogen and progesterone receptors. Identifying areas of intraductal (in situ) tumor would serve to distinguish salivary duct carcinoma from both metastatic prostate and breast carcinoma [293]. Less frequently other primary salivary gland cancers, namely mucoepidermoid carcinoma and low-grade papillary adenocarcinoma, enter into the differential diagnosis. Mucoepidermoid carcinomas, unlike salivary duct carcinomas, are not characterized by papillary, cribriform, and comedo growth patterns. Moreover mucoepidermoid carcinomas have a more heterogeneous cell population consisting of intermediate, epidermoid, and mucin cells. This is in contradistinction to the single, albeit pleomorphic, cell type that comprises salivary duct carcinoma. Papillary growth in a low-grade adenocarcinoma should not cause confusion with salivary duct carcinoma since this is cytologically a low-grade tumor. In addition it is primarily a cancer of minor rather than major salivary glands.

Treatment and Prognosis

Because of its aggressive clinical behavior, salivary duct carcinoma is treated by complete surgical excision of the primary combined with neck dissection and adjuvant radiotherapy. Cervical lymph node metastases are present in 60–80% of cases. Hosal et al. found that 50% of patients with clinically negative (N0) lymph nodes had histologically positive lymph nodes [149]. The incidence of distant metastases ranges from 33% to 66%. Two thirds of patients die of their disease usually within 4 years of treatment [79, 149]. Death is usually from distant metastases which occur most commonly to the lungs and bone [79, 149].

Low-grade Cribriform Cystadenocarcinoma

Clinical Features

This tumor was first described by Delgado et al. in 1996 [79, 149]. The authors proposed the term low-grade salivary duct carcinoma. Currently the preferred term is low-grade cribriform cystadenocarcinoma (LGCC) which avoids confusion with conventional salivary duct carcinoma which is a high-grade tumor with a poor prognosis.

This is an uncommon tumor, less than 30 cases having been reported [221]. Patients have a median age of 64 years and the tumor occurs with equal frequency in men and women. In a combined series of 26 cases, 25 arose in the parotid gland and one in the submandibular gland [79, 149]. Most patients seek treatment because of the presence of an asymptomatic mass.

Pathologic Features

Tumors range in size from 0.7 to 4 cm. Grossly they are well circumscribed and typically have a cystic component which may be either focal or extensive.

Microscopically LGCC resembles atypical ductal hyperplasia of the breast or micropapillary/cribriform in situ ductal carcinoma of the breast. Single or multiple cystically dilated ducts and smaller ducts are filled by cells forming cribriform, micropapillary, and filigree papillary patterns. Areas showing a solid growth pattern may also be present. The tumor cells are cytologically bland ductal cells (Fig. 3.18a, b). Some may contain a golden brown lipofuscin-like pigment in the cytoplasm imparting an apocrine-like appearance to the cells. Immunoperoxidase stains for myoepithelial cells demonstrate that most of the tumors are in situ although some will show foci of microinvasion or small focal areas of limited invasive disease.

Low-grade cribriform cystadenocarcinomas are strongly and diffusely positive for S-100, however, they do not show evidence of myoepithelial differentiation. Stains for HER-2/neu and androgen are typically negative [170, 196, 299].

Differential Diagnosis

The differential diagnosis of LGCC centers around cystadenocarcinoma and the papillary cystic variant of acinic

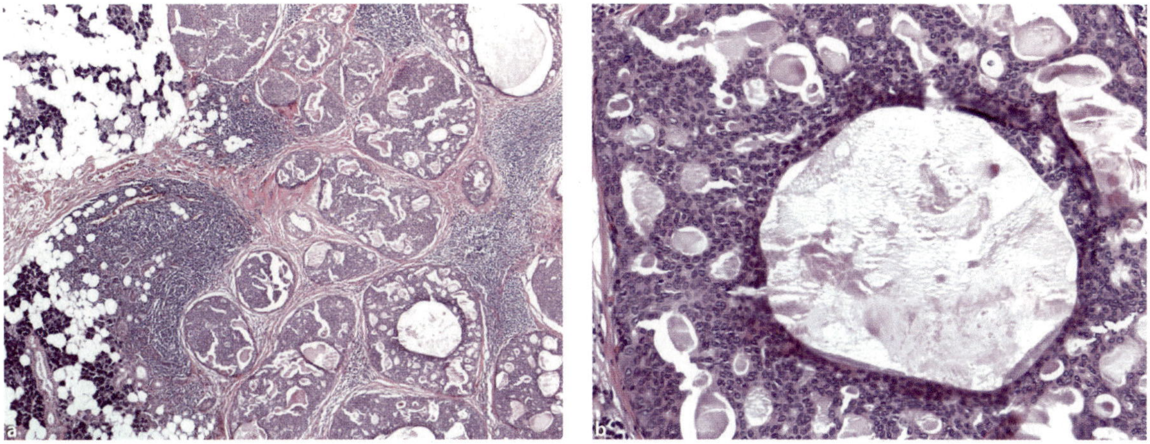

Fig. 3.18: Low-grade cribriform cystadenocarcinoma. **a** Infiltrating tumor with cribriform/micropapillary growth pattern (H&E, 40×). **b** Higher magnification to show that the tumor cells are cytologically bland. This is in marked contrast to the pleomorphism seen in salivary duct carcinomas (H&E, 200×)

cell carcinoma. Although cystadenocarcinomas often have a papillary component they lack the resemblance to atypical ductal hyperplasia and ductal carcinoma in situ of the breast which is so characteristic of LGCC. In addition cystadenocarcinomas tend to have a more obvious invasive component, while LGCCs are frequently entirely in situ carcinomas or only minimally invasive [299, 421, 430, 602].

The papillary cystic variant of acinic cell carcinoma will contain acinar cells with basophilic zymogen granules which are PAS positive diastase resistant. These are not present in LGCC. LGCC may, however, contain intracytoplasmic golden yellow granules of lipofuschin-like material.

Low-grade cribriform cystadenocarcinoma is strongly and diffusely positive for S-100 and negative for androgen receptor and HER-2/neu. This is exactly opposite to the staining pattern of salivary duct carcinoma and argues against LGCC being a low- grade form of salivary duct carcinoma.

Treatment and Prognosis

The treatment is complete surgical resection. Follow-up is limited because of the small number of reported cases, however, to date none have recurred [170, 196, 421, 602].

Large Cell Carcinoma

Clinical Features

Large cell carcinoma of the salivary glands is a rare high-grade neoplasm composed of large undifferentiated cells lacking any features of squamous cell carcinoma or adenocarcinoma. In some series it is two to three times less common than small cell carcinoma of salivary glands, however, in at least one series it was more common than small cell carcinoma of salivary glands [33, 280, 421].

These tumors are more common in the major than the minor salivary glands and most frequently occur in the parotid gland [348, 438]. They are rapidly growing and patients often present with involvement of adjacent soft tissue and skin. Cervical metastasis is also frequently present. Most patients are in their seventh decade when diagnosed and there is no sex bias with regard to incidence [53, 299].

Pathologic Features

Grossly the tumors tend to be large, averaging 3 cm at the time of surgery. Large cell carcinomas are poorly circumscribed firm gray-white tumors which may be solid and partially cystic. The cut surface frequently has areas of hemorrhage and necrosis. Infiltration into the salivary gland parenchyma and frequently the surrounding soft tissues is obvious grossly in most cases.

Microscopically the tumor is composed of sheets, nests, and trabeculae of large undifferentiated cells which may be strikingly pleomorphic or relatively uniform (Fig. 3.19). The individual tumor cells are two to three times larger than those of small cell carcinoma and have abundant eosinophilic to amphophilic cytoplasm. Some cells may have clear cytoplasm due to the presence of glycogen. Mucin, however, is not present. Nuclei are large and pleomorphic with prominent single or multiple nucleoli. Some cells may be elongated and spindle shaped. A few large cell carcinomas have contained numerous osteoclast-like giant cells [59, 170, 253, 281, 302, 340, 426, 478, 482]. Mitotic figures are abundant and foci of necrosis are common as are perineural and angiolymphatic invasion. Some tumors may be positive for neuroendocrine markers such as synaptophysin and chromogranin A [170, 196, 251].

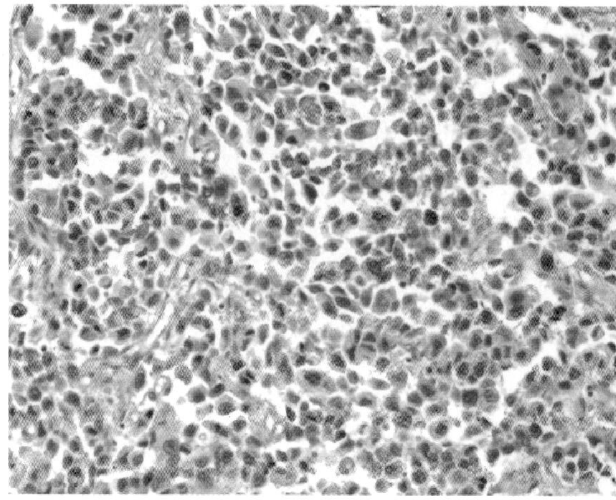

Fig. 3.19: Large cell carcinoma. The tumor is composed of sheets and nests of large pleomorphic cells. There is no evidence of squamous or glandular differentiation (H&E, 200×)

Differential Diagnosis

Metastatic undifferentiated or poorly differentiated carcinomas, large cell and anaplastic lymphomas, and metastatic melanomas must be considered in the differential diagnosis. A thorough history and physical examination are critical in excluding the possibility of a metastatic poorly differentiated or undifferentiated carcinoma.

Large cell carcinomas have a tendency to grow in a dyscohesive cell pattern which can closely mimic large cell and anaplastic lymphomas. Unlike large cell carcinomas, lymphomas will be negative for cytokeratin and positive for lymphoid markers with immunohistochemistry techniques.

Immunohistochemistry is also invaluable in separating amelanotic melanomas from large cell carcinomas. The melanomas will be negative for cytokeratin but positive for markers such as S-100, HMB45, and Melan A.

Treatment and Prognosis

Large cell carcinoma is a highly malignant tumor which requires aggressive treatment. This frequently entails radical surgery combined with radiation and chemotherapy. With undifferentiated carcinomas, cell size (large cell carcinoma versus small cell carcinoma) does not appear to alter the prognosis [170, 251, 427].

Small Cell Carcinoma

Clinical Features

Although most common in the lung, approximately 4% of small cell carcinomas arise from a variety of extrapulmonary sites including the head and neck where they have been reported in the larynx, pharynx, cervical esophagus, nose and paranasal sinuses, oral cavity, and salivary glands [281, 340, 366, 482]. The most common site in the head and neck is the larynx.

Small cell carcinoma accounts for less than 2% of salivary gland malignancies and less than 1% of all salivary gland neoplasms [170, 196, 482]. Over 80% arise in the parotid gland [170, 196, 251, 482]. Less frequently they arise in the submandibular gland or the minor salivary glands [427]. Approximately 60% occur in men although in some series the male to female ratio may be as high as 6:1 [251]. Patients are usually over the age of 50 years (mean 54 years) although rarely these cancers have been reported in children [483]. Most patients complain of a rapidly enlarging mass which may or may not be painful. Unlike pulmonary small cell carcinoma, there is no association between smoking and small cell carcinoma of the salivary gland [108, 432].

Pathologic Features

The tumors are gray to gray-white and firm. Infiltrative growth is usually obvious grossly.

Microscopically small cell carcinoma forms infiltrative sheets, nests, and trabeculae of cells supported by a fibrovascular stroma. Focal rosette-like formations, peripheral palisading, and ductal differentiation may be present [108]. Individual tumor cells are 1.5 to 2 times the diameter of a lymphocyte. They have round to fusiform hyperchromatic nuclei, small inconspicuous nucleoli, and scant cytoplasm. Nuclear molding and crush artifact are common. Mitoses are frequent and foci of tumor necrosis are commonly seen.

Some tumors are composed of cells which are slightly larger and have more cytoplasm corresponding to the intermediate type of small cell carcinoma of the lung. Foci of squamous differentiation may occasionally be seen [432].

Small cell carcinomas of salivary glands are typically positive for the cytokeratin stains AE1/3, CK20, and CAM5.2 frequently in a perinuclear dot-like pattern. CK7 is positive in addition to CK20 in approximately one third of cases [432]. These tumors are also positive for neuroendocrine markers, most commonly neuron-specific enolase, chromogranin, and synaptophysin.

Differential Diagnosis

Most frequently entertained in the differential diagnosis are metastatic small cell carcinoma of the lung, metastatic Merkel cell carcinoma of the skin, malignant lymphoma, and the solid variant of adenoid cystic carcinoma.

Small cell carcinoma of the lung and small cell carcinoma of the salivary gland are histologically identical. Knowledge of the clinical history and physical examination along with the results of special stains will usually lead to the correct diagnosis. Small cell carcinomas of the lung are positive for CK7 and negative for CK20. In addition the perinuclear dot-like staining pattern is not seen [251, 253]. They are also positive for thyroid transcription factor while small cell carcinomas of salivary glands are usually negative, although in one series of 15 cases of small cell carcinoma of salivary glands three were positive for thyroid transcription factor [432].

Merkel cell carcinoma and small cell carcinoma of salivary gland origin have an identical immunohistochemical staining pattern including a characteristic perinuclear dot-like pattern with cytokeratin stains. A detailed history and physical examination is critical in excluding a diagnosis of Merkel cell carcinoma.

Malignant lymphomas are negative for cytokeratin and neuroendocrine markers and positive for lymphocyte markers such as leukocyte common antigen. The exact opposite is true for small cell carcinomas.

Rarely the solid variant of adenoid cystic carcinoma may mimic small cell carcinoma on routine hematoxylin and eosin stained sections. Unlike small cell carcinoma, however, it does not show a perinuclear dot-like staining pattern with cytokeratin stains and neuroendocrine stains are negative.

Treatment and Prognosis

Although not as aggressive as small cell carcinoma of the lung or larynx, small cell carcinoma of the salivary glands is a high-grade malignancy and is treated aggressively. This frequently involves a combination of surgery, radiation, and chemotherapy [216, 513, 549]. Gnepp et al. reported 2- and 5-year survival rates of 70% and 46% for small cell carcinoma of salivary glands compared to 16% and 5% for those of the larynx [539]. Another series by Nagao et al. reported 2- and 5-year survival rates of 38% and 13% for small cell carcinoma of salivary glands [237, 513].

Primary Squamous Cell Carcinoma

Clinical Features

Primary squamous cell carcinomas of the salivary glands (PSSC) are rare, extremely aggressive neoplasms, the majority of patients presenting with advanced disease [384, 513]. In Spiro's review of 2,807 salivary gland tumors, PSSC accounted for only 1.9% [23, 513]. Nine percent of patients have a history of prior radiation exposure [23, 131, 237, 355, 389, 513].

In over two thirds of cases the cancer arises in the parotid gland and most of the remaining cases originate in the submandibular gland [513]. Rare cases probably arise in minor salivary glands although these may be difficult or impossible to distinguish from mucosal squamous cell carcinomas with extension into underlying minor salivary glands. PSSC is twice as common in men as women [365]. Although it has been reported in all decades of life, it is most common in the seventh decade. It is extremely uncommon in individuals below the age of 20 years [435]. Signs and symptoms include a painful rapidly enlarging mass and facial nerve palsy, although up to 50% may present with an asymptomatic mass [42, 237, 355, 389, 513].

Pathologic Features

Primary squamous cell carcinomas are gray-white, firm, usually grossly infiltrative, and average 3 cm in diameter. The cut surface may show focal areas of necrosis.

Histologically the tumors are usually moderately differentiated squamous cell carcinomas. Keratin production, often with keratin pearl formation, and intercellular bridge formation are easily identified (Fig. 3.20). Less frequently the tumors are high grade. Perineural invasion is frequently present. The stroma typically show a desmoplastic response.

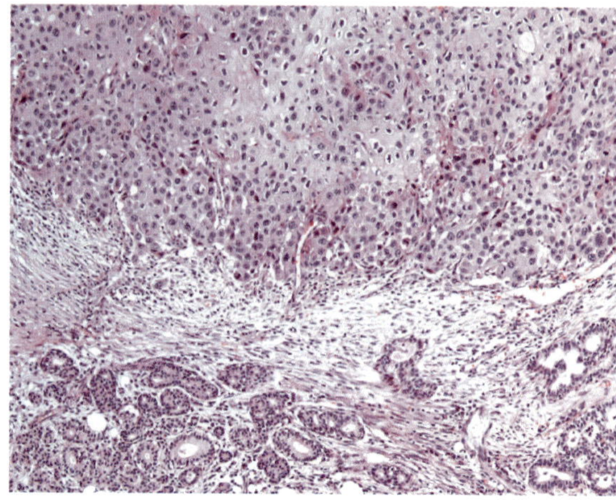

Fig. 3.20: Primary squamous cell carcinoma. Glassy cytoplasm and intercellular bridges identify this tumor as a squamous cell carcinoma (top half of figure). Residual salivary gland is present in the lower half of figure (H&E, 100×)

Differential Diagnosis

Squamous metaplasia, necrotizing sialometaplasia, keratocystoma, high-grade mucoepidermoid carcinoma, and metastatic squamous cell carcinoma all enter into the differential diagnosis.

Squamous metaplasia may occur in other neoplasms in response to inflammation and leakage of cyst contents such as may occur for example in Warthin's tumor. Prior fine-needle aspiration of benign tumors may also induce squamous metaplasia [216, 237, 355].

Preservation of normal lobular architecture and lack of invasion best serve to distinguish necrotizing sialometaplasia from PSSC. These features may, however, be difficult to appreciate in a small biopsy.

Keratocystoma is a benign cystic neoplasm in which cystic spaces are filled with keratin and lined by regularly oriented bland squamous cells. Although some solid squamous islands may be present there is no evidence of invasive, destructive growth [23, 216, 237, 355].

Mucoepidermoid carcinomas must, by definition, contain mucous cells. Mucous cells, however, are not numerous in high-grade tumors and indeed may not be recognized in some cases, unless the sections are stained with PAS-diastase or mucicarmine stains. While composed primarily of squamous (epidermoid cells), high-grade mucoepidermoid carcinomas do not show the extensive intracellular keratinization, keratin pearl formation, and intercellular bridge formation characteristic of PSSC.

Metastatic squamous cell carcinoma to salivary glands is more common than PSSC. This is particularly true in the parotid with its rich supply of both peri- and intraglandular lymph nodes [359]. The presence of a focus of squamous cell carcinoma in situ would serve to distinguish PSSC from metastatic squamous cell carcinoma. Such foci are seldom seen however because most PSSCs present at an advanced stage with obliteration of any foci of in situ disease. The clinical history and physical examination may provide valuable information. Squamous cell carcinoma metastatic to the parotid usually originates from skin lesions of the head and neck. The skin of the frontal and temporal areas, the periorbital region, the cheek, the pinna, the external ear canal, and the pre- and postauricular areas are favored sites. Tumors at these sites are usually clinically obvious long before metastases to the parotid.

Treatment and Prognosis

This is an aggressive tumor and radical resection with neck dissection is usually indicated. The facial nerve may be spared if not directly infiltrated by tumor. Up to 75% of patients have histologically positive cervical lymph nodes. There is a significant incidence of local-regional recurrence which has led to the use of postoperative radiation therapy in may instances. Distant metastases occur in 20–30% of patients. The 5-year survival rate is 25%.

Take Home Messages

- Salivary gland pathologic entities have a wide morphologic spectrum, and there may be considerable overlap between non-neoplastic, benign, and malignant entities.
- Non-neoplastic disease is often a manifestation of an underlying systemic disease. Necrotizing sialometaplasia is important to consider as it may histologically mimic malignancy. Marginal zone B-cell lymphoma may be a late complication of autoimmune MESA.
- Benign tumors are varied and named for their cell type. They have an appreciable recurrence rate if incompletely excised. Pleomorphic adenomas can behave aggressively after multiple recurrences without having malignant histologic features. Some tumors that are multifocal such as canalicular adenomas and Warthin's tumors, imply a field effect, while membranous type basal cell adenoma is multifocal often as a result of known mutations. Malignant transformation is extremely rare.
- Malignant tumors are as varied as their benign counterparts. Certain tumors are almost always low grade (i.e., polymorphous low-grade adenocarcinoma, acinic cell carcinoma, epithelial-myoepithelial carcinoma), while others are definitionally high grade (i.e., salivary duct carcinoma, large cell carcinoma, and small cell carcinoma). Malignant mixed tumor should be considered a category of disease with several clinicopathologic variants rather than a distinct entity. Histologic grading systems are most important in adenoid cystic carcinoma and mucoepidermoid carcinoma, while understanding of pathologic prognosticators in other malignant tumors is still not well established.

References

1. Abbondanzo SL (2001) *Extranodal marginal-zone B-cell lymphoma of the salivary gland.* Ann Diagn Pathol 5:246–254
2. Aberle AM, Abrams AM, Bowe R, et al. (1985) *Lobular (polymorphous low-grade) carcinoma of minor salivary glands. A clinicopathologic study of twenty cases.* Oral Surg Oral Med Oral Pathol 60:387–395
3. Abrams AM, Melrose RJ, Howell FV (1973) *Necrotizing sialometaplasia. A disease simulating malignancy.* Cancer 32:130–135
4. Aframian D, Milhem II, Kirsch G, et al. (1995) *Necrotizing Sialometaplasia after Silastic Ring Vertical Gastroplasty: Case Report and Review of Literature.* Obes Surg 5:179–182
5. Ahn MS, Hayashi GM, Hilsinger RL Jr., et al. (1999) *Familial mixed tumors of the parotid gland.* Head Neck 21:772–775
6. Albores-Saavedra J, Morris AW (1963) *Sebaceous adenoma of the submaxillary salivary gland. Report of a case.* Arch Otolaryngol 77:500–503
7. Alcedo JC, Fabrega JM, Arosemena JR, et al. (2004) *Imatinib mesylate as treatment for adenoid cystic carcinoma of the salivary glands: report of two successfully treated cases.* Head Neck 26:829–831
8. Alho OP, Kristo A, Luotonen J, et al. (1996) *Intraductal papilloma as a cause of a parotid duct cyst. A case report.* J Laryngol Otol 110:277–278
9. Allen MS Jr., Fitz-Hugh GS, Marsh WL Jr. (1974) *Low-grade papillary adenocarcinoma of the palate.* Cancer 33:153–158
10. Alos L, Cardesa A, Bombi JA, et al. (1996) *Myoepithelial tumors of salivary glands: a clinicopathologic, immunohistochemical, ultrastructural, and flow-cytometric study.* Semin Diagn Pathol 13:138–147
11. Alos L, Lujan B, Castillo M, et al. (2005) *Expression of membrane-bound mucins (MUC1 and MUC4) and secreted mucins (MUC2, MUC5AC, MUC5B, MUC6 and MUC7) in mucoepidermoid carcinomas of salivary glands.* Am J Surg Pathol 29:806–813
12. Alvarez-Canas C, Rodilla IG (1996) *True malignant mixed tumor (carcinosarcoma) of the parotid gland. Report of a case with immunohistochemical study.* Oral Surg Oral Med Oral Pathol Oral Radiol Endod 81:454–458
13. Anderson C, Muller R, Piorkowski R, et al. (1992) *Intraductal carcinoma of major salivary gland.* Cancer 69:609–614
14. Andreadis D, Epivatianos A, Poulopoulos A, et al. (2006) *Detection of C-KIT (CD117) molecule in benign and malignant salivary gland tumours.* Oral Oncol 42:57–65

15. Andreadis D, Nomikos A, Epivatianos A, et al. (2005) *Basaloid squamous cell carcinoma versus basal cell adenocarcinoma of the oral cavity.* Pathology 37:560–563
16. Arafat A, Brannon RB, Ellis GL (1981) *Adenomatoid hyperplasia of mucous salivary glands.* Oral Surg Oral Med Oral Pathol 52:51–55
17. Arida M, Barnes EL, Hunt JL (2005) *Molecular assessment of allelic loss in Warthin tumors.* Mod Pathol 18:964–968
18. Aronsohn RS, Batsakis JG, Rice DH, et al. (1976) *Anomalies of the first branchial cleft.* Arch Otolaryngol 102:737–740
19. Arriaga MA, Myers EN (1990) *The surgical management of chronic parotitis.* Laryngoscope 100:1270–1275
20. Assor D (1970) *Sebaceous lymphadenoma of the parotid gland. A case report.* Am J Clin Pathol 53:100–103
21. Attie JN, Sciubba JJ (1981) *Tumors of major and minor salivary glands: clinical and pathologic features.* Curr Probl Surg 18:130–133
22. Auclair PL (1994) *Tumor-associated lymphoid proliferation in the parotid gland. A potential diagnostic pitfall.* Oral Surg Oral Med Oral Pathol 77:19–26
23. Auclair PL, Ellis GL (1991) *Primary squamous cell carcinoma* Surgical pathology of the salivary glands. Edited by Ellis GL, Auclair PL, Gnepp DR. Philadelphia, WB Saunders Co., pp 369–378
24. Auclair PL, Ellis GL (1996) *Atypical features in salivary gland mixed tumors: their relationship to malignant transformation.* Mod Pathol 9:652–657
25. Avitia S, Hamilton JS, Osborne RF (2005) *Epithelial-myoepithelial carcinoma.* Ear Nose Throat J 84:764, 767
26. Aydin O, Yilmaz T, Ozer F, et al. (2002) *Necrotizing sialometaplasia of parotid gland: a possible vasculitic cause.* Int J Pediatr Otorhinolaryngol 64:171–174
27. Aydm E, Turkoglu S, Ozen O, et al. (2005) *Mucinous cystadenocarcinoma of a minor salivary gland in the upper lip: Case report.* Auris Nasus Larynx 32:301–304
28. Ayoub OM, Bhatia K, Mal RK (2002) *Pleomorphic adenoma of the parotid gland: is long-term follow-up needed?* Auris Nasus Larynx 29:283–285
29. Azevedo LR, Damante JH, Lara VS, et al. (2005) *Age-related changes in human sublingual glands: a post mortem study.* Arch Oral Biol 50:565–574
30. Azumi N, Battifora H (1987) *The cellular composition of adenoid cystic carcinoma. An immunohistochemical study.* Cancer 60:1589–1598
31. Azzopardi JG, Evans DJ (1971) *Malignant lymphoma of parotid associated with Mikulicz disease (benign lymphoepithelial lesion).* J Clin Pathol 24:744–752
32. Bahler DW, Swerdlow SH (1998) *Clonal salivary gland infiltrates associated with myoepithelial sialadenitis (Sjogren's syndrome) begin as nonmalignant antigen-selected expansions.* Blood 91:1864–1872
33. Balogh K, Wolbarsht RL, Federman M, et al. (1985) *Carcinoma of the parotid gland with osteoclastlike giant cells. Immunohistochemical and ultrastructural observations.* Arch Pathol Lab Med 109:756–761
34. Baratz M, Loewenthal M, Rozin M (1976) *Sebaceous lymphadenoma of the parotid gland.* Arch Pathol Lab Med 100:269–270
35. Barnes L, Appel B, Perez H, et al. (1985) *Myoepitheliomas of the head and neck: Case report and review.* J Surg Oncol 28:21–28
36. Barnes L, Appel BN, Perez H, et al. (1985) *Myoepithelioma of the head and neck: case report and review.* J Surg Oncol 28:21–28
37. Barnes L, Rao U, Contis L, et al. (1994) *Salivary duct carcinoma. Part II. Immunohistochemical evaluation of 13 cases for estrogen and progesterone receptors, cathepsin D, and c-erbB-2 protein.* Oral Surg Oral Med Oral Pathol 78:74–80
38. Barnes L, Rao U, Krause J, et al. (1994) *Salivary duct carcinoma. Part I. A clinicopathologic evaluation and DNA image analysis of 13 cases with review of the literature.* Oral Surg Oral Med Oral Pathol 78:64–73
39. Barrett AW, Speight PM (1995) *Adenomatoid hyperplasia of oral minor salivary glands.* Oral Surg Oral Med Oral Pathol Oral Radiol Endod 79:482–487
40. Batsakis J (1979) *Tumors of the Head and Neck.* Clinical and Pathological Considerations, 2nd edition. Baltimore, Williams and Wilkins and Wilkins Co., pp 26–30
41. Batsakis JG (1982) *Malignant mixed tumor.* Ann Otol Rhinol Laryngol 91:342–343
42. Batsakis JG (1983) *Primary squamous cell carcinomas of major salivary glands.* Ann Otol Rhinol Laryngol 92:97–98
43. Batsakis JG (1991) *Sublingual gland.* Ann Otol Rhinol Laryngol 100:521–522
44. Batsakis JG, Bernacki EG, Rice DH, et al. (1975) *Malignancy and the benign lymphoepithelial lesion.* Laryngoscope 85:389–399
45. Batsakis JG, Bruner JM, Luna MA (1988) *Polycystic (dysgenetic) disease of the parotid glands.* Arch Otolaryngol Head Neck Surg 114:1146–1148
46. Batsakis JG, Chinn E, Regezi JA, et al. (1978) *The pathology of head and neck tumors: salivary glands, part 2.* Head Neck Surg 1:167–180
47. Batsakis JG, Chinn EK, Weimert TA, et al. (1979) *Acinic cell carcinoma: a clinicopathologic study of thirty-five cases.* J Laryngol Otol 93:325–340

48. Batsakis JG, el-Naggar AK (1991) *Terminal duct adenocarcinomas of salivary tissues.* Ann Otol Rhinol Laryngol 100:251–253
49. Batsakis JG, el-Naggar AK, Luna MA (1992) *Epithelial-myoepithelial carcinoma of salivary glands.* Ann Otol Rhinol Laryngol 101:540–542
50. Batsakis JG, Kraemer B, Sciubba JJ (1983) *The pathology of head and neck tumors: the myoepithelial cell and its participation in salivary gland neoplasia, Part 17.* Head Neck Surg 5:222–233
51. Batsakis JG, Luna MA (1990) *Histopathologic grading of salivary gland neoplasms: I. Mucoepidermoid carcinomas.* Ann Otol Rhinol Laryngol, 99:835–838
52. Batsakis JG, Luna MA (1991) *Basaloid salivary carcinoma.* Ann Otol Rhinol Laryngol 100:785–787
53. Batsakis JG, Luna MA (1991) *Undifferentiated carcinomas of salivary glands.* Ann Otol Rhinol Laryngol 100:82–84
54. Batsakis JG, Luna MA, el-Naggar A (1990) *Histopathologic grading of salivary gland neoplasms: III. Adenoid cystic carcinomas.* Ann Otol Rhinol Laryngol 99:1007–1009
55. Batsakis JG, Pinkston GR, Luna MA, et al. (1983) *Adenocarcinomas of the oral cavity: a clinicopathologic study of terminal duct carcinomas.* J Laryngol Otol 97:825–835
56. Batsakis JG, Raymond AK (1989) *Sialocysts of the parotid glands.* Ann Otol Rhinol Laryngol 98:487–489
57. Batsakis JG, Regezi JA (1978) *The pathology of head and neck tumors: salivary glands, part 1.* Head Neck Surg 1:59–68
58. Batsakis JG, Wozniak KJ, Regezi JA (1977) *Acinous cell carcinoma: a histogenetic hypothesis.* J Oral Surg 35:904–906
59. Baugh RF, Wolf GT, McClatchey KD (1986) *Small cell carcinoma of the head and neck.* Head Neck Surg 8:343–354
60. Baurmash HD (2004) *Chronic recurrent parotitis: a closer look at its origin, diagnosis, and management.* J Oral Maxillofac Surg 62:1010–1018
61. Beahrs OH, Woolner LB, Kirklin JW, et al. (1957) *Carcinomatous transformation of mixed tumors of the parotid gland.* AMA Arch Surg, 75:605–613; discussion 613–604
62. Begin LR, Black MJ (1993) *Salivary-type myxoid myoepithelioma of the sinonasal tract: a potential diagnostic pitfall.* Histopathology 23:283–285
63. Begin LR, Rochon L, Frenkiel S (1991) *Spindle cell myoepithelioma of the nasal cavity.* Am J Surg Pathol 15:184–190
64. Beltran D, Faquin WC, Gallagher G, et al. (2006) *Selective immunohistochemical comparison of polymorphous low-grade adenocarcinoma and adenoid cystic carcinoma.* J Oral Maxillofac Surg 64:415–423
65. Berean KW, Watts MC, Mills SE (1995) *Basal cell adenocarcinoma of salivary glands.* Lab Invest 72:99A
66. Bhalla RK, Jones TM, Taylor W, et al. (2002) *Carcinosarcoma (malignant mixed tumor) of the submandibular gland: A case report and review of the literature.* J Oral Maxillofac Surg 60:1067–1069
67. Bharadwaj G, Nawroz I, O'Regan B (2007) *Sclerosing polycystic adenosis of the parotid gland.* Br J Oral Maxillofac Surg 45:74–76
68. Billroth T (1859) *Beobachtungen Uber Geschwulste der Speichisdrusen Virch.* Pathol Anat 17:357–375
69. Blanck C, Eneroth CM, Jakobsson PA (1971) *Mucus-producing adenopapillary (non-epidermoid) carcinoma of the parotid gland.* Cancer 28:676–685
70. Bleiweiss IJ, Huvos AG, Lara J, et al. (1992) *Carcinosarcoma of the submandibular salivary gland. Immunohistochemical findings.* Cancer 69:2031–2035
71. Boahene DK, Olsen KD, Lewis JE, et al. (2004) *Mucoepidermoid carcinoma of the parotid gland: the Mayo clinic experience.* Arch Otolaryngol Head Neck Surg 130:849–856
72. Boles R, Johns ME, Batsakis JG (1973) *Carcinoma in pleomorphic adenomas of salivary glands.* Ann Otol Rhinol Laryngol 82:684–690
73. Bombi JA, Alos L, Rey MJ, et al. (1996) *Myoepithelial carcinoma arising in a benign myoepithelioma: immunohistochemical, ultrastructural, and flow-cytometrical study.* Ultrastruct Pathol 20:145–154
74. Bos I, Meyer S, Merz H (2004) *[Lymphadenoma of the parotid gland without sebaceous differentiation. Immunohistochemical investigations].* Pathologe 25:73–78
75. Bowman SJ (2002) *Collaborative research into outcome measures in Sjogren's syndrome. Update on disease assessment.* Scand J Rheumatol Suppl (116):23–27
76. Bradley P (2005) *Metastasizing pleomorphic salivary adenoma should now be considered a low grade malignancy with a lethal potential.* Otolaryngol Head Neck Surg 13:123–126
77. Bradley PJ (2004) *Adenoid cystic carcinoma of the head and neck: a review.* Curr Opin Otolaryngol Head Neck Surg 12:127–132
78. Bradley PJ (2005) *Metastasizing pleomorphic salivary adenoma should now be considered a low-grade malignancy with a lethal potential.* Curr Opin Otolaryngol Head Neck Surg 13:123–126
79. Brandwein-Gensler M, Hille J, Wang BY, et al. (2004) *Low-grade salivary duct carcinoma: description of 16 cases.* Am J Surg Pathol 28:1040–1044
80. Brandwein M, Huvos A (1995) *Laryngeal oncocytic cystadenomas. Eight cases and a literature review.* Arch Otolaryngol Head Neck Surg 121:1302–1305

3

81. Brandwein M, Huvos AG, Dardick I, et al. (1996) *Noninvasive and minimally invasive carcinoma ex mixed tumor: a clinicopathologic and ploidy study of 12 patients with major salivary tumors of low (or no?) malignant potential.* Oral Surg Oral Med Oral Pathol Oral Radiol Endod 81:655–664
82. Brandwein MS, Huvos AG (1991) *Oncocytic tumors of major salivary glands. A study of 68 cases with follow-up of 44 patients.* Am J Surg Pathol 15:514–528
83. Brandwein MS, Ivanov K, Wallace DI, et al. (2001) *Mucoepidermoid carcinoma: a clinicopathologic study of 80 patients with special reference to histological grading.* Am J Surg Pathol 25:835–845
84. Brandwein MS, Jagirdar J, Patil J, et al. (1990) *Salivary duct carcinoma (cribriform salivary carcinoma of excretory ducts). A clinicopathologic and immunohistochemical study of 12 cases.* Cancer 65:2307–2314
85. Brannon RB, Fowler CB, Hartman KS (1991) *Necrotizing sialometaplasia. A clinicopathologic study of sixty-nine cases and review of the literature.* Oral Surg Oral Med Oral Pathol 72:317–325
86. Brannon RB, Houston GD, Meader CL (1985) *Adenomatoid hyperplasia of mucous salivary glands: a case involving the retromolar area.* Oral Surg Oral Med Oral Pathol 60:188–190
87. Brannon RB, Sciubba JJ, Giulani M (2001) *Ductal papillomas of salivary gland origin: A report of 19 cases and a review of the literature.* Oral Surg Oral Med Oral Pathol Oral Radiol Endod 92:68–77
88. Brannon RB, Willard CC (2003) *Oncocytic mucoepidermoid carcinoma of parotid gland origin.* Oral Surg Oral Med Oral Pathol Oral Radiol Endod 96:727–733
89. Brauneis J, Laskawi R, Schroder M, et al. (1990) *[Squamous cell carcinoma in the area of the parotid gland. Metastasis or primary tumor?].* HNO 38:292–294
90. Brehmer D, Hohbach M, Laubert A (1999) *[Intraductal papilloma of the parotid gland].* Laryngorhinootologie 78:332–334
91. Brook I (2003) *Acute bacterial suppurative parotitis: microbiology and management.* J Craniofac Surg 14:37–40
92. Browand BC, Waldron CA (1975) *Central mucoepidermoid tumors of the jaws. Report of nine cases and review of the literature.* Oral Surg Oral Med Oral Pathol 40:631–643
93. Bruner JM, Cleary KR, Smith FB, et al. (1989) *Immunocytochemical identification of HIV (p24) antigen in parotid lymphoid lesions.* J Laryngol Otol 103:1063–1066
94. Buchholz TA, Shimotakahara SG, Weymuller EA Jr., et al. (1993) *Neutron radiotherapy for adenoid cystic carcinoma of the head and neck.* Arch Otolaryngol Head Neck Surg 119:747–752
95. Buchner A, Merrell PW, Carpenter WM, et al. (1991) *Adenomatoid hyperplasia of minor salivary glands.* Oral Surg Oral Med Oral Pathol 71:583–587
96. Buenting JE, Smith TL, Holmes DK (1998) *Giant pleomorphic adenoma of the parotid gland: case report and review of the literature.* Ear Nose Throat J 77:637–640
97. Bullerdiek J, Wobst G, Meyer-Bolte K, et al. (1993) *Cytogenetic subtyping of 220 salivary gland pleomorphic adenomas: correlation to occurrence, histological subtype, and in vitro cellular behavior.* Cancer Genet Cytogenet 65:27–31
98. Buxton RW, Maxwell JH, French AJ (1953) *Surgical treatment of epithelial tumors of the parotid gland.* Surg Gynecol Obstet 97:401–416
99. Cabov T, Macan D, Manojlovic S, et al. (2004) *Oral inverted ductal papilloma.* Br J Oral Maxillofac Surg 42:75–77
100. Capone RB, Ha PK, Westra WH, et al. (2002) *Oncocytic neoplasms of the parotid gland: a 16-year institutional review.* Otolaryngol Head Neck Surg 126:657–662
101. Cardesa A, Alos L (2005) *Myoepithelioma.* Pathology and Classification of Head and Neck Tumours. Edited by Barnes EL, Eveson JW, Reichart P, Sidransky D. Lyon, IARC, pp 259–260
102. Carew JF, Spiro RH, Singh B, et al. (1999) *Treatment of recurrent pleomorphic adenomas of the parotid gland.* Otolaryngol Head Neck Surg 121:539–542
103. Caselitz J, Schulze I, Seifert G (1986) *Adenoid cystic carcinoma of the salivary glands: an immunohistochemical study.* J Oral Pathol 15:308–318
104. Casler JD, Conley JJ (1992) *Surgical management of adenoid cystic carcinoma in the parotid gland.* Otolaryngol Head Neck Surg 106:332–338
105. Castle JT, Thompson LD, Frommelt RA, et al. (1999) *Polymorphous low grade adenocarcinoma: a clinicopathologic study of 164 cases.* Cancer 86:207–219
106. Castro WH, Drummond SN, Gomez RS (2002) *Subacute necrotizing sialadenitis in the buccal mucosa.* J Oral Maxillofac Surg 60:1494–1496
107. Chan JK, Saw D (1987) *Sclerosing mucoepidermoid tumour of the parotid gland: report of a case.* Histopathology 11:203–207
108. Chan JK, Suster S, Wenig BM, et al. (1997) *Cytokeratin 20 immunoreactivity distinguishes Merkel cell (primary cutaneous neuroendocrine) carcinomas and salivary gland small cell carcinomas from small cell carcinomas of various sites.* Am J Surg Pathol 21:226–234
109. Chang A, Harawi SJ (1992) *Oncocytes, oncocytosis, and oncocytic tumors.* Pathol Annu 27 Pt 1:263–304
110. Chang JY, Hsiao CH (2004) *Lymphadenoma lacking sebaceous differentiation in the parotid gland.* J Formos Med Assoc 103:459–462

111. Chaplin AJ, Darke P, Patel S (1983) *Tyrosine-rich crystals in pleomorphic adenomas of parotid glands.* J Oral Pathol 12:342–346
112. Chaudhry AP, Vickers RA, Gorlin RJ (1961) *Intraoral minor salivary gland tumors: An analysis of 1,414 cases.* Oral Surg Oral Med Oral Path 14:1194–1226
113. Chen I, Tu H (2000) *Pleomorphic adenoma of the parotid gland metastasizing to the cervical lymph node.* Otolaryngol Head Neck Surg 122:455–457
114. Chen JC, Gnepp DR, Bedrossian CW (1988) *Adenoid cystic carcinoma of the salivary glands: an immunohistochemical analysis.* Oral Surg Oral Med Oral Pathol 65:316–326
115. Chen KT (1985) *Carcinoma arising in monomorphic adenoma of the salivary gland.* Am J Otolaryngol 6:39–41
116. Chen YK, Lin CC, Lin LM, et al. (1999) *Adenomatoid hyperplasia in the mandibular retromolar area. Case report.* Aust Dent J 44:135–136
117. Cheng J, Saku T, Okabe H, et al. (1992) *Basement membranes in adenoid cystic carcinoma. An immunohistochemical study.* Cancer 69:2631–2640
118. Chetty R (1998) *HIV-associated lymphoepithelial cysts and lesions: morphological and immunohistochemical study of the lymphoid cells.* Histopathology 33:222–229
119. Cheuk W, Miliauskas JR, Chan JKC (2004) *Intraductal carcinoma of the oral cavity: a case report and a reappraisal of the concept of pure ductal carcinoma in situ in salivary duct carcinoma.[see comment].* Am J Surg Pathol 28:266–270
120. Chhieng DC, Paulino AF (2002) *Cytology of myoepithelial carcinoma of the salivary gland.* Cancer 96:32–36
121. Chilla R (1981) *Sialadenosis of the salivary glands of the head. Studies on the physiology and pathophysiology of parotid secretion.* Adv Otorhinolaryngol 26:1–38
122. Chilla R, Schroth R, Eysholdt U, et al. (1980) *Adenoid cystic carcinoma of the head and neck. Controllable and uncontrollable factors in treatment and prognosis.* ORL J Otorhinolaryngol Relat Spec 42:346–367
123. Chilla R, Witzemann V, Opaitz M, et al. (1981) *Possible involvement of parotid beta-adrenergic receptors in the etiology of sialadenosis.* Arch Otorhinolaryngol 230:113–120
124. Cho KJ, el-Naggar AK, Ordonez NG, et al. (1995) *Epithelial-myoepithelial carcinoma of salivary glands. A clinicopathologic, DNA flow cytometric, and immunohistochemical study of Ki-67 and HER-2/neu oncogene.* Am J Clin Pathol 103:432–437
125. Choi HR, Batsakis JG, Callender DL, et al. (2002) *Molecular analysis of chromosome 16q regions in dermal analogue tumors of salivary glands: a genetic link to dermal cylindroma?* Am J Surg Pathol 26:778–783
126. Chong GC, Beahrs OH, Woolner LB (1974) *Surgical management of acinic cell carcinoma of the parotid gland.* Surg Gynecol Obstet 138:65–68
127. Clark DB, Priddy RW, Swanson AE (1990) *Oral inverted ductal papilloma.* Oral Surg Oral Med Oral Pathol 69:487–490
128. Conley J, Dingman DL (1974) *Adenoid cystic carcinoma in the head and neck (cylindroma).* Arch Otolaryngol 100:81–90
129. Corio RL, Sciubba JJ, Brannon RB, et al. (1982) *Epithelial-myoepithelial carcinoma of intercalated duct origin. A clinicopathologic and ultrastructural assessment of sixteen cases.* Oral Surg Oral Med Oral Pathol 53:280–287
130. Cornog J, Gray S (1976) *Surgical and clinical pathology of salivary gland tumors.* Diseases of the Salivary Glands. Edited by Rankow R, Polayes I. Philadelphia, WB Saunders Co., pp 130–142
131. Cornog JL (1970) *Surgical and clinical pathology of salivary gland tumors* Diseases of Salivary Glands Edited by Rankow R, Polayes I. Philadelphia, WB Saunders Co., pp 92–142
132. Corridan M (1956) *Glycogen-rich clear cell adenoma of the parotid.* J Pathol Bacteriol 72:623–627
133. Crumpler C, Scharfenberg JC, Reed RJ (1976) *Monomorphic adenomas of salivary glands. Trabecular-tubular, canalicular, and basaloid variants.* Cancer 38:193–200
134. Curran AE, White DK, Damm DD, et al. (2001) *Polymorphous low-grade adenocarcinoma versus pleomorphic adenoma of minor salivary glands: resolution of a diagnostic dilemma by immunohistochemical analysis with glial fibrillary acidic protein.* Oral Surg Oral Med Oral Pathol Oral Radiol Endod 91:194–199
135. da Cruz Perez DE, de Abreu Alves F, Nobuko Nishimoto I, et al. (2006) *Prognostic factors in head and neck adenoid cystic carcinoma.* Oral Oncol 42:139–146
136. Dagrada GP, Negri T, Tamborini E, et al. (2004) *Expression of HER-2/neu gene and protein in salivary duct carcinomas of parotid gland as revealed by fluorescence in-situ hybridization and immunohistochemistry.[comment].* Histopathology 44:301–302
137. Daley TD, Gardner DG, Smout MS (1984) *Canalicular adenoma: not a basal cell adenoma.* Oral Surg Oral Med Oral Pathol 57:181–188
138. Dalforno S, Donna A (1967) *[Sebaceous adenoma of the salivary gland].* Cancro 20:667–673
139. Daniels TE (1984) *Labial salivary gland biopsy in Sjogren's syndrome. Assessment as a diagnostic criterion in 362 suspected cases.* Arthritis Rheum 27:147–156
140. Dardick I (1996) *Salivary Gland Tumor Pathology.* New York, Igaku-shoin, pp 235–239

141. Dardick I, Daley TD, van Nostrand AW (1986) *Basal cell adenoma with myoepithelial cell-derived stroma: a new major salivary gland tumor entity.* Head Neck Surg 8:257–267
142. Dardick I, Lytwyn A, Bourne AJ, et al. (1992) *Trabecular and solid-cribriform types of basal cell adenoma. A morphologic study of two cases of an unusual variant of monomorphic adenoma.* Oral Surg Oral Med Oral Pathol 73:75–83
143. Dardick I, Thomas MJ, van Nostrand AW (1989) *Myoepithelioma – new concepts of histology and classification: a light and electron microscopic study.* Ultrastruct Pathol 13:187–224
144. Darling MR, Schneider JW, Phillips VM (2002) *Polymorphous low-grade adenocarcinoma and adenoid cystic carcinoma: a review and comparison of immunohistochemical markers.* Oral Oncol 38:641–645
145. de Araujo VC, de Sousa SO, Carvalho YR, et al. (2000) *Application of immunohistochemistry to the diagnosis of salivary gland tumors.* Appl Immunohistochem Mol Morphol 8:195–202
146. De la Maza LM, Schwartz MM, Soto EA (1971) *Sebaceous lymphadenoma of the parotid region.* Arch Pathol 92:294–295
147. de Sousa SO, Schwarzschild M, de Araujo NS, et al. (2000) *Basal cell adenocarcinoma of the palate with squamous metaplasia.* J Clin Pathol 53:153–156
148. de Sousa SO, Sesso A, de Araujo NS, et al. (1995) *Inverted ductal papilloma of minor salivary gland origin: morphological aspects and cytokeratin expression.* Eur Arch Otorhinolaryngol 252:370–373
149. Delgado R, Klimstra D, Albores-Saavedra J (1996) *Low grade salivary duct carcinoma. A distinctive variant with a low grade histology and a predominant intraductal growth pattern.* Cancer 78:958–967
150. Delgado R, Vuitch F, Albores-Saavedra J (1992) *High grade salivary duct carcinoma.* Mod Pathol 5:71A
151. Deysine M, Mann BF Jr. (1969) *Sebaceous lymphadenoma of the parotid gland: associated with a case of bilateral parotid gland tumors.* Ann Surg 169:437–443
152. Di Palma S, Corletto V, Lavarino C, et al. (1999) *Unilateral aneuploid dedifferentiated acinic cell carcinoma associated with bilateral-low grade diploid acinic cell carcinoma of the parotid gland.* Virchows Arch 434:361–365
153. Di Palma S, Simpson RH, Skalova A, et al. (1999) *Metaplastic (infarcted) Warthin's tumour of the parotid gland: a possible consequence of fine needle aspiration biopsy.* Histopathology 35:432–438
154. Di Palma S, Skalova A, Vanieek T, et al. (2005) *Non-invasive (intracapsular) carcinoma ex pleomorphic adenoma: recognition of focal carcinoma by HER-2/neu and MIB1 immunohistochemistry.* Histopathology 46:144–152
155. Dimery IW, Jones LA, Verjan RP, et al. (1987) *Estrogen receptors in normal salivary gland and salivary gland carcinoma.* Arch Otolaryngol Head Neck Surg 113:1082–1085
156. Dobson CM, Ellis HA (1987) *Polycystic disease of the parotid glands: case report of a rare entity and review of the literature.* Histopathology 11:953–961
157. Donath K (1976) *[Sialadenosis of the parotid gland. Ultrastructural, clinical and experimental findings in disturbances of secretion (author's transl)].* Veroff Pathol (103):1–122
158. Donath K, Seifert G (1972) *[Ultrastructure and pathogenesis of myoepithelial sialadenitis. Occurrence of myoepithelial cells in the benign lymphoepithelial lesion (Sjogren's syndrome)].* Virchows Arch A Pathol Anat 356:315–329
159. Donath K, Seifert G (1972) *Zur Diagnose and Ultrastruktur des tubularen Speichelgangcarcinoms. Epithelial-myoepitheliales Schaltstruckcarcinom.* Virchows Arch A Pathol Anat 356:16–31
160. Donath K, Seifert G (1975) *Ultrastructural studies of the parotid glands in sialadenosis.* Virchows Arch A Pathol Anat Histol 365:119–135
161. Donath K, Spillner M, Seifert G (1974) *The influence of the autonomic nervous system on the ultrastructure of the parotid acinar cells. Experimental contribution to the neurohormonal sialadenosis.* Virchows Arch A Pathol Anat Histol 364:15–33
162. Dreyer T, Battmann A, Silberzahn J, et al. (1993) *Unusual differentiation of a combination tumor of the parotid gland. A case report.* Pathol Res Pract 189:577–581; discussion 581–575
163. Edwards PC, Bhuiya T, Kelsch RD (2003) *C-kit expression in the salivary gland neoplasms adenoid cystic carcinoma, polymorphous low-grade adenocarcinoma, and monomorphic adenoma.* Oral Surg Oral Med Oral Pathol Oral Radiol Endod 95:586–593
164. Edwards PC, Bhuiya T, Kelsch RD (2004) *Assessment of p63 expression in the salivary gland neoplasms adenoid cystic carcinoma, polymorphous low-grade adenocarcinoma, and basal cell and canalicular adenomas.* Oral Surg Oral Med Oral Pathol Oral Radiol Endod 97:613–619
165. Eibling DE, Johnson JT, McCoy JP Jr., et al. (1991) *Flow cytometric evaluation of adenoid cystic carcinoma: correlation with histologic subtype and survival.* Am J Surg 162:367–372
166. el-Naggar AK, Batsakis JG, Luna MA, et al. (1990) *DNA flow cytometry of acinic cell carcinomas of major salivary glands.* J Laryngol Otol 104:410–416
167. el-Naggar AK, Lovell M, Callender DL, et al. (1999) *Cytogenetic analysis of a primary salivary gland myoepithelioma.* Cancer Genet Cytogenet 113:49–53

168. el-Naggar AK (2005) *Adenoid cystic carcinomas in Pathology and Genetics Head and Neck Tumors.* Edited by Barnes EL, Eveson JW, Reichart P, Sidransky D. Lyon, IARC Press, pp 221–222
169. Elliott JN, Oertel YC (1990) *Lymphoepithelial cysts of the salivary glands. Histologic and cytologic features.* Am J Clin Pathol 93:39–43
170. Ellis G, Auclair P *(1996) Tumors of the Salivary Glands, Atlas of Tumor Pathology, third series, fascicle 17.* Washington DC, Armed Forces Institute of Pathology, pp 296–369
171. Ellis G, Auclair P *(1996) Tumors of the Salivary Glands, Atlas of Tumor Pathology, third series, fascicle 17.* Washington DC, Armed Forces Institute of Pathology, pp 289–296
172. Ellis G, Simpson R *(2005) Acinic cell carcinoma in Pathology and Genetics Head and Neck Tumours (edited by Barnes L, Eveson J, Reichart P, Sidransky D) WHO, Lyon.* France, IARC Press, pp 216–218
173. Ellis GL (1998) *Clear cell neoplasms in salivary glands: clearly a diagnostic challenge.* Ann Diagn Pathol 2:61–78
174. Ellis GL, Auclair PL, Gnepp DR, et al. (1991) *Other malignant neoplasms in.* Surgical Pathology of the Salivary Glands. Philadelphia, WB Saunders, pp 455–488
175. Ellis GL, Auclair PL *(1991) Acinic cell adenocarcinoma in Surgical Pathology of the Salivary Glands (Ellis GL, Auclair PL, Gnepp DR, editors).* Philadelphia, WB Saunders Co., pp 299–317
176. Ellis GL, Auclair PL *(1996) Acinic cell carcinoma in Tumors of the Salivary Glands, Atlas of Tumor Pathology, third series, fascicle 17.* Washington DC, Armed Forces Institute of Pathology, pp 183–203
177. Ellis GL, Auclair PL *(1996) Tumors of the Salivary Glands, Atlas of Tumor Pathology, third series, fascicle 17.* Washington DC, Armed Forces Institute of Pathology, pp 1–26
178. Ellis GL, Auclair PL (1991) *Ductal Papillomas.* Surgical pathology of the salivary glands. Philadelphia, W.B. Saunders, pp 238–252
179. Ellis GL, Auclair PL (1996) *Tumors of the salivary glands.* Washington D.C., Armed Forces Institute of Pathology, pp 268–281
180. Ellis GL, Corio RL (1983) *Acinic cell adenocarcinoma. A clinicopathologic analysis of 294 cases.* Cancer 52:542–549
181. Ellis GL, Wiscovitch JG (1990) *Basal cell adenocarcinomas of the major salivary glands.* Oral Surg Oral Med Oral Pathol 69:461–469
182. Emanuel P, Wang B, Wu M, et al. (2005) *p63 Immunohistochemistry in the distinction of adenoid cystic carcinoma from basaloid squamous cell carcinoma.* Mod Pathol 18:645–650
183. Enamorado I, Lakhani R, Korkmaz H, et al. (2004) *Correlation of histopathological variants, cellular DNA content, and clinical outcome in adenoid cystic carcinoma of the salivary glands.* Otolaryngol Head Neck Surg 131:646–650
184. Eneroth CM (1970) *Incidence and prognosis of salivary glands tumors at different sites. A study of parotid, submandibular and palatal tumors in 2632 patients.* Acta Otolaryngol Suppl 263:174–178
185. Eneroth CM (1971) *Salivary gland tumors in the parotid gland, submandibular gland, and the palate region.* Cancer 27:1415–1418
186. Eneroth CM, Blanck C, Jakobsson PA (1968) *Carcinoma in pleomorphic adenoma of the parotid gland.* Acta Otolaryngol 66:477–492
187. Eneroth CM, Hjertman L, Moberger G, et al. (1972) *Mucoepidermoid carcinomas of the salivary glands with special reference to the possible existence of a benign variety.* Acta Otolaryngol 73:68–74
188. Eneroth CM, Zetterberg A (1974) *Malignancy in pleomorphic adenoma. A clinical and microspectrophotometric study.* Acta Otolaryngol 77:426–432
189. Enlund F, Nordkvist A, Sahlin P, et al. (2002) *Expression of PLAG1 and HMGIC proteins and fusion transcripts in radiation-associated pleomorphic adenomas.* Int J Oncol 20:713–716
190. Epker BN, Henny FA (1971) *Intra-oral sebaceous gland adenoma.* Cancer 27:987–1000
191. Erlandson RA, Tandler B (1972) *Ultrastructure of acinic cell carcinoma of the parotid gland.* Arch Pathol Lab Med 93:130–140
192. Evans HL, Batsakis JG (1984) *Polymorphous low-grade adenocarcinoma of minor salivary glands. A study of 14 cases of a distinctive neoplasm.* Cancer 53:935–942
193. Evans HL, Luna MA (2000) *Polymorphous low-grade adenocarcinoma: a study of 40 cases with long-term follow up and an evaluation of the importance of papillary areas.* Am J Surg Pathol 24:1319–1328
194. Evans R, Cruickshank A (1970) *Epithelial Tumors of the Salivary Glands.* Philadelphia, W.B. Saunders Co., pp 226–241
195. Eversole L (2001) *Salivary gland pathology.* Head and neck pathology: with clinical correlations. Edited by Fu Y, Wenig BM, Abemayor E, Wenig BL. Philadelphia, Churchill-Livingstone, pp 242–291
196. Eversole LR, Gnepp DR, Eversole GM *(1991) Undifferentiated carcinoma in Surgical Pathology of the Salivary Glands, (Ellis GL, Auclair PL, Gnepp DR, editors)* Philadelphia, WB Saunders Co., pp 422–440

197. Eveson JW, Auclair PL, Gnepp D, et al. (2005) *Tumors of Salivary Glands in Pathology and Genetics Head and Neck Tumors*. Edited by Barnes EL, Eveson JW, Reichart P, Sidransky D. Lyon, IARC Press, pp 212–215
198. Eveson JW, Cawson RA (1985) *Salivary gland tumours. A review of 2410 cases with particular reference to histological types, site, age and sex distribution*. J Pathol 146:51–58
199. Eveson JW, Cawson RA (1985) *Tumours of the minor (oropharyngeal) salivary glands: a demographic study of 336 cases*. J Oral Pathol 14:500–509
200. Eveson JW, Cawson RA (1989) *Infarcted (infected) adenolymphomas. A clinicopathological study of 20 cases*. Clin Otolaryngol 14:205–210
201. Eveson JW, Kusafuka K, Stenman G, et al. (2005) *Pleomorphic adenoma*. Pathology and Classification of Head and Neck Tumours. Edited by Barnes EL, Eveson JW, Reichart P, Sidransky D. Lyon, IARC
202. Ezsias A, Sugar AW, Milling MA, et al. (1994) *Central mucoepidermoid carcinoma in a child*. J Oral Maxillofac Surg 52:512–515
203. Fadare O, Hileeto D, Gruddin YL, et al. (2004) *Sclerosing mucoepidermoid carcinoma of the parotid gland*. Arch Pathol Lab Med 128:1046–1049
204. Faivre S, Raymond E, Casiraghi D, et al. (2005) *Imatinib mesylate can induce objective response in progressing, highly expressing KIT adenoid cystic carcinoma of the salivary glands*. J Clin Oncol 23:6271–6273
205. Fan CY, Melhem MF, Hosal AS, et al. (2001) *Expression of androgen receptor, epidermal growth factor receptor, and transforming growth factor alpha in salivary duct carcinoma*. Arch Otolaryngol Head Neck Surg 127:1075–1079
206. Fauci AS, Haynes BF, Katz P, et al. (1983) *Wegener's granulomatosis: prospective clinical and therapeutic experience with 85 patients for 21 years*. Ann Intern Med 98:76–85
207. Felix A, Rosa-Santos J, Mendonca ME, et al. (2002) *Intracapsular carcinoma ex pleomorphic adenoma. Report of a case with unusual metastatic behaviour*. Oral Oncol 38:107–110
208. Ferguson JW, Geary CP, MacAlister AD (1987) *Sebaceous cell adenoma. Rare intra-oral occurrence of a tumour which is a frequent marker of Torre's syndrome*. Pathology 19:204–208
209. Ferreiro JA (1994) *Immunohistochemical analysis of salivary gland canalicular adenoma*. Oral Surg Oral Med Oral Pathol 78:761–765
210. Ferreiro JA (2005) *Canalicular adenoma*. Pathology and Classification of Head and Neck Tumours. Edited by Barnes EL, Eveson JW, Reichart P, Sidransky D. Lyon, IARC, pp 267
211. Ficarra G, Sapp JP, Christensen RE, et al. (1996) *Dysgenetic polycystic disease of the parotid gland: report of case*. J Oral Maxillofac Surg 54:1246–1249
212. Finn DG, Buchalter IH, Sarti E, et al. (1987) *First branchial cleft cysts: clinical update*. Laryngoscope 97:136–140
213. Firat P, Hosal S, Tutar E, et al. (2000) *Sebaceous lymphadenoma of the parotid gland*. J Otolaryngol 29:114–116
214. Fishleder A, Tubbs R, Hesse B, et al. (1987) *Uniform detection of immunoglobulin-gene rearrangement in benign lymphoepithelial lesions*. N Engl J Med 316:1118–1121
215. Fleming DA, Morrice I (1973) *Sebaceous lymphadenoma of the parotid gland: a report of a case*. J Pathol 110:259–261
216. Flynn MB, Maguire S, Martinez S, et al. (1999) *Primary squamous cell carcinoma of the parotid gland: the importance of correct histological diagnosis*. Ann Surg Oncol 6:768–770
217. Fonseca I, Soares J (1993) *Epithelial-myoepithelial carcinoma of the salivary glands. A study of 22 cases*. Virchows Arch A Pathol Anat Histopathol 422:389–396
218. Fonseca I, Soares J (1993) *Proliferating cell nuclear antigen immunohistochemistry in epithelial-myoepithelial carcinoma of the salivary glands*. Arch Pathol Lab Med 117:993–995
219. Foote FW Jr., Frazell EL (1953) *Tumors of the major salivary glands*. Cancer 6:1065–1133
220. Foschini MP, Gaiba A, Cocchi R, et al. (2005) *p63 expression in salivary gland tumors: role of DeltaNp73L in neoplastic transformation*. Int J Surg Pathol 13:329–335
221. Foss RD, Ellis GL, Auclair PL (1996) *Salivary gland cystadenocarcinomas. A clinicopathologic study of 57 cases*. Am J Surg Pathol 20:1440–1447
222. Fowler CB, Brannon RB (2000) *Subacute necrotizing sialadenitis: report of 7 cases and a review of the literature*. Oral Surg Oral Med Oral Pathol Oral Radiol Endod 89:600–609
223. Fowler MH, Fowler J, Ducatman B, et al. (2006) *Malignant mixed tumors of the salivary gland: a study of loss of heterozygosity in tumor suppressor genes*. Mod Pathol 19:350–355
224. Fox RI (2005) *Sjogren's syndrome*. Lancet 366:321–331
225. Franzen G, Klausen OG, Grenko RT, et al. (1991) *Adenoid cystic carcinoma: DNA as a prognostic indicator*. Laryngoscope 101:669–673
226. Franzen G, Nordgard S, Boysen M, et al. (1995) *DNA content in adenoid cystic carcinomas*. Head Neck 17:49–55
227. Freedman PD, Lumerman H (1983) *Lobular carcinoma of intraoral minor salivary gland origin. Report of twelve cases*. Oral Surg Oral Med Oral Pathol 56:157–166
228. Freeman SB, Kennedy KS, Parker GS, et al. (1990) *Metastasizing pleomorphic adenoma of the nasal septum*. Arch Otolaryngol Head Neck Surg 116:1331–1333

229. Freier K, Flechtenmacher C, Walch A, et al. (2005) *Differential KIT expression in histological subtypes of adenoid cystic carcinoma (ACC) of the salivary gland.* Oral Oncol 41:934–939
230. Fujibayashi T, Itoh H (1981) *Lymphoepithelial (so-called branchial) cyst within the parotid gland. Report of a case and review of the literature.* Int J Oral Surg 10:283–292
231. Furuse C, Sousa SO, Nunes FD, et al. (2005) *Myoepithelial cell markers in salivary gland neoplasms.* Int J Surg Pathol 13:57–65
232. Furuse C, Tucci R, Machado de Sousa SO, et al. (2003) *Comparative immunoprofile of polymorphous low-grade adenocarcinoma and canalicular adenoma.* Ann Diagn Pathol 7:278–280
233. Gallo O, Bocciolini C (1997) *Warthin's tumour associated with autoimmune diseases and tobacco use.* Acta Otolaryngol 117:623–627
234. Gandour-Edwards RF, Donald PJ, Vogt PJ, et al. (1994) *Carcinosarcoma (malignant mixed tumor) of the parotid: report of a case with a pure rhabdomyosarcoma component.* Head Neck 16:379–382
235. Garcia S, Martini F, Caces F, et al. (1998) *[Polycystic disease of the salivary glands: report of an attack of the submaxillary glands].* Ann Pathol 18:58–60
236. Gardiner GW, Briant TD, Sheman L (1984) *Inverted ductal papilloma of the parotid gland.* J Otolaryngol 13:23–26
237. Gaughan RK, Olsen KD, Lewis JE (1992) *Primary squamous cell carcinoma of the parotid gland.* Arch Otolaryngol Head Neck Surg 118:798–801
238. George MK, Mansour P, Pahor AL (1991) *Terminal parotid duct carcinoma.* J Laryngol Otol 105:780–781
239. Gerughty RM, Scofield HH, Brown FM, et al. (1969) *Malignant mixed tumors of salivary gland origin.* Cancer 24:471–486
240. Geurts JM, Schoenmakers EF, Roijer E, et al. (1998) *Identification of NFIB as recurrent translocation partner gene of HMGIC in pleomorphic adenomas.* Oncogene 16:865–872
241. Geurts JM, Schoenmakers EF, Roijer E, et al. (1997) *Expression of reciprocal hybrid transcripts of HMGIC and FHIT in a pleomorphic adenoma of the parotid gland.* Cancer Res 57:13–17
242. Ghosh S, Panarese A, Bull PD, et al. (2003) *Marginally excised parotid pleomorphic salivary adenomas: risk factors for recurrence and management. A 12.5-year mean follow-up study of histologically marginal excisions.* Clin Otolaryngol 28:262–266
243. Gilcrease MZ, Nelson FS, Guzman-Paz M (1998) *Tyrosine-rich crystals associated with oncocytic salivary gland neoplasms.* Arch Pathol Lab Med 122:644–649
244. Glisson B, Colevas AD, Haddad R, et al. (2004) *HER2 expression in salivary gland carcinomas: dependence on histological subtype.* Clin Cancer Res 10:944–946
245. Gnepp DR (1993) *Malignant mixed tumors of the salivary glands: a review.* Pathol Annu 28 Pt 1:279–328
246. Gnepp DR (2003) *Sclerosing polycystic adenosis of the salivary gland: a lesion that may be associated with dysplasia and carcinoma in situ.* Adv Anat Pathol 10:218–222
247. Gnepp DR (2005) *Metastasizing pleomorphic adenoma.* Pathology and Classification of Head and Neck Tumours. Edited by Barnes EL, Eveson JW, Reichart P, Sidransky D. Lyon, IARC, p 245
248. Gnepp DR, Brannon R (1984) *Sebaceous neoplasms of salivary gland origin. Report of 21 cases.* Cancer 53:2155–2170
249. Gnepp DR, Chen JC, Warren C (1988) *Polymorphous low-grade adenocarcinoma of minor salivary gland. An immunohistochemical and clinicopathologic study.* Am J Surg Pathol 12:461–468
250. Gnepp DR, Chen JC, Warren C (1988) *Polymorphous low-grade adenocarcinoma of minor salivary gland. An immunohistochemical and clinicopathologic study.* Am J Surg Pathol 12:461–468
251. Gnepp DR, Corio RL, Brannon RB (1986) *Small cell carcinoma of the major salivary glands.* Cancer 58:705–714
252. Gnepp DR, el-Mofty S (1997) *Polymorphous low-grade adenocarcinoma: glial fibrillary acidic protein staining in the differential diagnosis with cellular mixed tumors.* Oral Surg Oral Med Oral Pathol Oral Radiol Endod 83:691–695
253. Gnepp DR, Ferlito A, Hyams V (1983) *Primary anaplastic small cell (oat cell) carcinoma of the larynx. Review of the literature and report of 18 cases.* Cancer 51:1731–1745
254. Gnepp DR, Wang LJ, Brandwein-Gensler M, et al. (2006) *Sclerosing polycystic adenosis of the salivary gland: a report of 16 cases.* Am J Surg Pathol 30:154–164
255. Goldfarb D, Mikaelian D, Keane WM (1994) *Mucoepidermoid carcinoma of the mandible.* Am J Otolaryngol 15:54–57
256. Goldman RL, Klein HZ (1972) *Glycogen-rich adenoma of the parotid gland. An uncommon benign clear-cell tumor resembling certain clear-cell carcinomas of salivary origin.* Cancer 30:749–754
257. Gomes AP, Sobral AP, Loducca SV, et al. (2004) *Sialadenoma papilliferum: immunohistochemical study.* Int J Oral Maxillofac Surg 33:621–624
258. Goode R, El-Nagger A (2005) *Mucoepidermoid carcinoma.* Pathology and Genetics Head and Neck Tumors. Edited by Barnes L, Eveson J, Reichart P, Sidransky D. Lyon, IARC Press, pp 219–220

259. Goode RK, Auclair PL, Ellis GL (1998) *Mucoepidermoid carcinoma of the major salivary glands: clinical and histopathologic analysis of 234 cases with evaluation of grading criteria.* Cancer 82:1217–1224
260. Goodisson DW, Burr RG, Creedon AJ, et al. (1999) *A case of metastasizing pleomorphic adenoma.* Oral Surg Oral Med Oral Pathol Oral Radiol Endod 87:341–345
261. Gotte K, Riedel F, Coy JF, et al. (2000) *Salivary gland carcinosarcoma: immunohistochemical, molecular genetic and electron microscopic findings.* Oral Oncol 36:360–364
262. Gottesman RI, Som PM, Mester J, et al. (1996) *Observations on two cases of apparent submandibular gland cysts in HIV positive patients: MR and CT findings.* J Comput Assist Tomogr 20:444–447
263. Grage TB, Lober PH, Arhelger SW (1961) *Acinic cell carcinoma of the parotid gland.* Am J Surg 102:765–768
264. Greiner TC, Robinson RA, Maves MD (1989) *Adenoid cystic carcinoma. A clinicopathologic study with flow cytometric analysis.* Am J Clin Pathol 92:711–720
265. Gross M, Maly B, Goldfarb A, et al. (2004) *Basal cell adenocarcinoma in a buccal minor salivary gland.* Acta Otolaryngolog (Stockh) 124:213–216
266. Grotz KA, Wustenberg P, Kohnen R, et al. (2001) *Prophylaxis of radiogenic sialadenitis and mucositis by coumarin/troxerutine in patients with head and neck cancer – a prospective, randomized, placebo-controlled, double-blind study.* Br J Oral Maxillofac Surg 39:34–39
267. Gupta S, Sodhani P (1998) *Sialadenosis of parotid gland: a cytomorphologic and morphometric study of four cases.* Anal Quant Cytol Histol 20:225–228
268. Gurney TA, Eisele DW, Weinberg V, et al. (2005) *Adenoid cystic carcinoma of the major salivary glands treated with surgery and radiation.* Laryngoscope 115:1278–1282
269. Gustafsson H, Carlsoo B (1985) *Multiple acinic cell carcinoma. Some histological and ultrastructural features of a case.* J Laryngol Otol 99:1183–1193
270. Gustafsson H, Dahlqvist A, Anniko M, et al. (1987) *Mucoepidermoid carcinoma in a minor salivary gland in childhood.* J Laryngol Otol 101:1320–1323
271. Haberland-Carrodeguas C, Fornatora ML, Reich RF, et al. (2003) *Detection of human papillomavirus DNA in oral inverted ductal papillomas.* J Clin Pathol 56:910–913
272. Haines K, Murad T (1989) *Infiltrating salivary duct carcinoma of the parotid.* Lab Invest 60:36A
273. Hamed G, Shmookler BM, Ellis GL, et al. (1994) *Oncocytic mucoepidermoid carcinoma of the parotid gland.* Arch Pathol Lab Med 118:313–314
274. Hamper K, Brugmann M, Koppermann R, et al. (1989) *Epithelial-myoepithelial duct carcinoma of salivary glands: a follow-up and cytophotometric study of 21 cases.* J Oral Pathol Med 18:299–304
275. Hamper K, Lazar F, Dietel M, et al. (1990) *Prognostic factors for adenoid cystic carcinoma of the head and neck: a retrospective evaluation of 96 cases.* J Oral Pathol Med 19:101–107
276. Handra-Luca A, Lamas G, Bertrand JC, et al. (2005) *MUC1, MUC2, MUC4, and MUC5AC expression in salivary gland mucoepidermoid carcinoma: diagnostic and prognostic implications.* Am J Surg Pathol 29:881–889
277. Hansen A, Lipsky PE, Dorner T (2005) *Immunopathogenesis of primary Sjogren's syndrome: implications for disease management and therapy.* Curr Opin Rheumatol 17:558–565
278. Hanson TA (1975) *Acinic cell carcinoma of the parotid salivary gland presenting as a cyst. Report of two cases.* Cancer 36:570–575
279. Hara H, Oyama T, Omori K, et al. (1999) *Fine needle aspiration cytology of an intraductal papilloma originating in a sublingual gland. A case report.* Acta Cytol 43:457–463
280. Hayashi Y, Aoki N (1983) *Undifferentiated carcinoma of the parotid gland with bizarre giant cells. Clinicopathologic report with ultrastructural study.* Acta Pathol Jpn 33:169–176
281. Hayashi Y, Nagamine S, Yanagawa T, et al. (1987) *Small cell undifferentiated carcinoma of the minor salivary gland containing exocrine, neuroendocrine, and squamous cells.* Cancer 60:1583–1588
282. Hayes MM, Cameron RD, Jones EA (1993) *Sebaceous variant of mucoepidermoid carcinoma of the salivary gland. A case report with cytohistologic correlation.* Acta Cytol 37:237–241
283. Hegarty DJ, Hopper C, Speight PM (1994) *Inverted ductal papilloma of minor salivary glands.* J Oral Pathol Med 23:334–336
284. Hellquist HB, Sundelin K, Di Bacco A, et al. (1997) *Tumour growth fraction and apoptosis in salivary gland acinic cell carcinomas. Prognostic implications of Ki-67 and bcl-2 expression and of in situ end labelling (TUNEL).* J Pathol 181:323–329
285. Henley J, Summerlin DJ, Potter D, et al. (2005) *Intraoral mucin-rich salivary duct carcinoma.[comment].* Histopathology 47:436–437
286. Henley JD, Geary WA, Jackson CL, et al. (1997) *Dedifferentiated acinic cell carcinoma of the parotid gland: a distinct rarely described entity.* Hum Pathol 28:869–873

287. Henriksson G, Westrin KM, Carlsoo B, et al. (1998) *Recurrent primary pleomorphic adenomas of salivary gland origin: intrasurgical rupture, histopathologic features, and pseudopodia.* Cancer 82:617–620
288. Hiatt JL, Sank JJ (1991) *Embryology and anatomy of salivary glands.* Surgical Pathology of the Salivary Glands. Edited by Ellis GL AP, Gnepp DR. Philadelphia WB Saunders Co., pp 2–9
289. Hickman RE, Cawson RA, Duffy SW (1984) *The prognosis of specific types of salivary gland tumors.* Cancer 54:1620–1624
290. Honda K, Kashima K, Daa T, et al. (2000) *Clonal analysis of the epithelial component of Warthin's tumor.* Hum Pathol 31:1377–1380
291. Honda T, Yamamoto Y, Isago T, et al. (2005) *Giant pleomorphic adenoma of the parotid gland with malignant transformation.* Ann Plast Surg 55:524–527
292. Hoorweg JJ, Hilgers FJ, Keus RB, et al. (1998) *Metastasizing pleomorphic adenoma: a report of three cases.* Eur J Surg Oncol 24:452–455
293. Hosal AS, Fan C, Barnes L, et al. (2003) *Salivary duct carcinoma.* Otolaryngology – Head Neck Surg 129:720–725
294. Hotte SJ, Winquist EW, Lamont E, et al. (2005) *Imatinib mesylate in patients with adenoid cystic cancers of the salivary glands expressing c-kit: a Princess Margaret Hospital phase II consortium study.* J Clin Oncol 23:585–590
295. Howard DJ, Lund VJ (1985) *Reflections on the management of adenoid cystic carcinoma of the nasal cavity and paranasal sinuses.* Otolaryngol Head Neck Surg 93:338–341
296. Hrynchak M, White V, Berean K, et al. (1994) *Cytogenetic findings in seven lacrimal gland neoplasms.* Cancer Genet Cytogenet 75:133–138
297. Huang JW, Ming Z, Shrestha P, et al. (1996) *Immunohistochemical evaluation of the Ca(2+)-binding S-100 proteins S-100A1, S-100A2, S-100A4, S-100A6 and S-100B in salivary gland tumors.* J Oral Pathol Med 25:547–555
298. Hughes KV 3rd, Olsen KD, McCaffrey TV (1995) *Parapharyngeal space neoplasms.* Head Neck 17:124–130
299. Hui KK, Luna MA, Batsakis JG, et al. (1990) *Undifferentiated carcinomas of the major salivary glands.* Oral Surg Oral Med Oral Pathol 69:76–83
300. Hungermann D, Roeser K, Buerger H, et al. (2002) *Relative paucity of gross genetic alterations in myoepitheliomas and myoepithelial carcinomas of salivary glands.* J Pathol 198:487–494
301. Hyjek E, Smith WJ, Isaacson PG (1988) *Primary B-cell lymphoma of salivary glands and its relationship to myoepithelial sialadenitis.* Hum Pathol 19:766–776
302. Ibrahim NB, Briggs JC, Corbishley CM (1984) *Extrapulmonary oat cell carcinoma.* Cancer 54:1645–1661
303. Ibrahim R, Bird DJ, Sieler MW (1991) *Malignant myoepithelioma of the larynx with massive metastatic spread to the liver: an ultrastructural and immunocytochemical study.* Ultrastruct Pathol 15:69–76
304. Ide F, Mishima K, Saito I (2003) *Sarcomatoid salivary duct carcinoma of the oral cavity.* Virchows Archiv 443:686–689
305. Ide F, Obara K, Enatsu K, et al. (2005) *Sclerosing mucoepidermoid carcinoma of the oral cavity.* J Oral Pathol Med 34:187–189
306. Iezzi G, Rubini C, Fioroni M, et al. (2002) *Sebaceous adenoma of the cheek.* Oral Oncol 38:111–113
307. Ihrler S, Steger W, Riederer A, et al. (1996) *[HIV-associated cysts of the parotid glands. An histomorphologic and magnetic resonance tomography study of formal pathogenesis].* Laryngorhinootologie 75:671–676
308. Ihrler S, Zietz C, Riederer A, et al. (1996) *HIV-related parotid lymphoepithelial cysts. Immunohistochemistry and 3-D reconstruction of surgical and autopsy material with special reference to formal pathogenesis.* Virchows Arch 429:139–147
309. Ihrler S, Zietz C, Sendelhofert A, et al. (1999) *Lymphoepithelial duct lesions in Sjogren-type sialadenitis.* Virchows Arch 434:315–323
310. Imamura Y, Morishita T, Kawakami M, et al. (2004) *Sclerosing polycystic adenosis of the left parotid gland: report of a case with fine needle aspiration cytology.* Acta Cytol 48:569–573
311. Imbery TA, Edwards PA (1996) *Necrotizing sialometaplasia: literature review and case reports.* J Am Dent Assoc 127:1087–1092
312. Inoue Y, Nomura J, Hashimoto M, et al. (2001) *Epithelial-myoepithelial carcinoma of the palate: a case report.* J Oral Maxillofac Surg 59:1502–1505
313. Izutsu T, Kumamoto H, Kimizuka S, et al. (2003) *Sebaceous adenoma in the retromolar region: report of a case with a review of the English literature.* Int J Oral Maxillofac Surg 32:423–426
314. Jaehne M, Roeser K, Jaekel T, et al. (2005) *Clinical and immunohistologic typing of salivary duct carcinoma: a report of 50 cases.* Cancer 103:2526–2533
315. Jahan-Parwar B, Huberman RM, Donovan DT, et al. (1999) *Oncocytic mucoepidermoid carcinoma of the salivary glands.* Am J Surg Pathol 23:523–529
316. James GK, Pudek M, Berean KW, et al. (1996) *Salivary duct carcinoma secreting prostate-specific antigen.* Am J Clin Pathol 106:242–247

3

317. Jayakrishnan A, Elmalah I, Hussain K, et al. (2003) *Basal cell adenocarcinoma in minor salivary glands.* Histopathology 42:610–614
318. Jeng YM, Lin CY, Hsu HC (2000) *Expression of the c-kit protein is associated with certain subtypes of salivary gland carcinoma.* Cancer Lett 154:107–111
319. Jervis PN, Lee JA, Bull PD (2001) *Management of non-tuberculous mycobacterial peri-sialadenitis in children: the Sheffield otolaryngology experience.* Clin Otolaryngol 26:243–248
320. Johnston N, Rose D, Lutterloch M (2005) *Cystadenocarcinoma of salivary gland presenting as a cystic lesion in the mandible.* Oral Surg Oral Med Oral Pathol Oral Radiol Endod 101:201–204
321. Jurgens PE (2004) *Inverted ductal papilloma of the lower lip: a case report.* J Oral Maxillofac Surg 62:1158–1161
322. Kaminagakura E, Andrade CR, Rangel AL, et al. (2003) *Sebaceous adenoma of oral cavity: report of case and comparative proliferation study with sebaceous gland hyperplasia and Fordyce's granules.* Oral Dis 9:323–327
323. Kamisawa T, Nakajima H, Egawa N, et al. (2005) *IgG4-Related Sclerosing Disease Incorporating Sclerosing Pancreatitis, Cholangitis, Sialadenitis and Retroperitoneal Fibrosis with Lymphadenopathy.* Pancreatology 6:132–137
324. Kanazawa H, Furuya T, Murano A, et al. (2000) *Oncocytoma of an intraoral minor salivary gland: report of a case and review of literature.* J Oral Maxillofac Surg 58:894–897
325. Kas K, Voz ML, Roijer E, et al. (1997) *Promoter swapping between the genes for a novel zinc finger protein and beta-catenin in pleiomorphic adenomas with t(3;8)(p21;q12) translocations.* Nat Genet 15:170–174
326. Kasaboglu O, Er N, Tumer C, et al. (2004) *Micromorphology of sialoliths in submandibular salivary gland: a scanning electron microscope and X-ray diffraction analysis.* J Oral Maxillofac Surg 62:1253–1258
327. Kemp BL, Batsakis JG, el-Naggar AK, et al. (1995) *Terminal duct adenocarcinomas of the parotid gland.* J Laryngol Otol 109:466–468
328. Khullar SM, Best PV (1992) *Adenomatosis of minor salivary glands. Report of a case.* Oral Surg Oral Med Oral Pathol 74:783–787
329. Kici S, Peytral C (2001) *[Giant pleomorphic adenoma of the parotid gland: a case report and review of the literature].* Ann Otolaryngol Chir Cervicofac 118:330–332
330. King OH Jr. (1967) *Carcinosarcoma of accessory salivary gland. First report of a case.* Oral Surg Oral Med Oral Pathol 23:651–659
331. Kirklin JW, Mc DJ, Harrington SW, et al. (1951) *Parotid tumors; histopathology, clinical behavior, and end results.* Surg Gynecol Obstet 92:721–733
332. Kitagawa S, Zen Y, Harada K, et al. (2005) *Abundant IgG4-positive plasma cell infiltration characterizes chronic sclerosing sialadenitis (Kuttner's tumor).* Am J Surg Pathol 29:783–791
333. Kjorell U, Ostberg Y (1984) *Distribution of intermediate filaments and actin microfilaments in parotid autoimmune sialoadenitis of Sjogren syndrome.* Histopathology 8:991–1011
334. Kleinsasser O, Klein HJ, Hubner G (1968) *Salivary duct carcinoma. A group of salivary gland tumors analogous to mammary duct carcinoma.* Arch Klin Exp Ohren- Nasen-Kehlkopfheilk 192:100–105
335. Klima M, Wolfe K, Johnson PE (1978) *Basal cell tumors of the parotid gland.* Arch Otolaryngol 104:111–116
336. Klumpp TR, Mohr RM, Silverman CL, et al. (1995) *Malignant myoepithelioma of the parotid gland: case report and review of the literature.* J Laryngol Otol 109:995–998
337. Knowles DM, Athan E, Ubriaco A, et al. (1989) *Extranodal noncutaneous lymphoid hyperplasias represent a continuous spectrum of B-cell neoplasia: demonstration by molecular genetic analysis.* Blood 73:1635–1645
338. Koka VN, Tiwari RM, van der Waal I, et al. (1989) *Adenoid cystic carcinoma of the salivary glands: clinicopathological survey of 51 patients.* J Laryngol Otol 103:675–679
339. Kokemueller H, Brueggemann N, Swennen G, et al. (2005) *Mucoepidermoid carcinoma of the salivary glands – clinical review of 42 cases.* Oral Oncol 41:3–10
340. Koss LG, Spiro RH, Hajdu S (1972) *Small cell (oat cell) carcinoma of minor salivary gland origin.* Cancer 30:737–741
341. Kotwall CA (1992) *Smoking as an etiologic factor in the development of Warthin's tumor of the parotid gland.* Am J Surg 164:646–647
342. Koutlas IG, Jessurun J, Iamaroon A (1994) *Immunohistochemical evaluation and in situ hybridization in a case of oral inverted ductal papilloma.* J Oral Maxillofac Surg 52:503–506
343. Krolls SO, Trodahl JN, Boyers RC (1972) *Salivary gland lesions in children. A survey of 430 cases.* Cancer 30:459–469
344. Kunze P (1979) *[Sebaceous lymphadenoma of the parotid gland (author's transl)].* Zentralbl Allg Pathol 123:210–213
345. Kwon GY, Kim EJ, Go JH (2002) *Lymphadenoma arising in the parotid gland: a case report.* Yonsei Med J 43:536–538
346. Kwon MY, Gu M (2001) *True malignant mixed tumor (carcinosarcoma) of parotid gland with unusual mesenchymal component: a case report and review of the literature.* Arch Pathol Lab Med 125:812–815
347. Labouyrie E, Merlio JP, Beylot-Barry M, et al. (1993) *Human immunodeficiency virus type 1 replication within cystic lymphoepithelial lesion of the salivary gland.* Am J Clin Pathol 100:41–46

348. Larsson LG, Donner LR (1999) *Large cell neuroendocrine carcinoma of the parotid gland: fine needle aspiration, and light microscopic and ultrastructural study.* Acta Cytol 43:534–536
349. Leafstedt SW, Gaeta JF, Sako K, et al. (1971) *Adenoid cystic carcinoma of major and minor salivary glands.* Am J Surg 122:756–762
350. Lebsack JP, Marrogi AJ, Martin SA (1990) *Central mucoepidermoid carcinoma of the jaw with distant metastasis: a case report and review of the literature.* J Oral Maxillofac Surg 48:518–522
351. Lee DJ, Smith RR, Spaziani JT, et al. (1985) *Adenoid cystic carcinoma of the nasopharynx. Case reports and literature review.* Ann Otol Rhinol Laryngol 94:269–272
352. Lee IK, Liu JW (2005) *Tuberculous parotitis: case report and literature review.* Ann Otol Rhinol Laryngol 114:547–551
353. Lee JH, Lee JH, Kim A, et al. (2005) *Unique expression of MUC3, MUC5AC and cytokeratins in salivary gland carcinomas.* Pathol Int 55:386–390
354. Lee KC, Chan JK, Chong YW (1992) *Ossifying pleomorphic adenoma of the maxillary antrum.* J Laryngol Otol 106:50–52
355. Lee S, Kim GE, Park CS, et al. (2001) *Primary squamous cell carcinoma of the parotid gland.* Am J Otolaryngol 22:400–406
356. Leverstein H, van der Wal JE, Tiwari RM, et al. (1997) *Surgical management of 246 previously untreated pleomorphic adenomas of the parotid gland.* Br J Surg 84:399–403
357. Levin JM, Robinson DW, Lin F (1975) *Acinic cell carcinoma.* Arch Surg 110:64–68
358. Lewis JE, McKinney BC, Weiland LH, et al. (1996) *Salivary duct carcinoma. Clinicopathologic and immunohistochemical review of 26 cases.* Cancer 77:223–230
359. Lewis JE, Olsen KD (2005) *Tumors of Salivary Glands.* Pathology and Genetics Head and Neck Tumors. Edited by Barnes EL, Eveson J, Reichart P, Sidransky D. Lyon, IARC, pp 245–246
360. Lewis JE, Olsen KD, Sebo TJ (2001) *Carcinoma ex pleomorphic adenoma: pathologic analysis of 73 cases.* Hum Pathol 32:596–604
361. Lewis JE, Olsen KD, Weiland LH (1991) *Acinic cell carcinoma. Clinicopathologic review.* Cancer 67:172–179
362. Lewis PD, Baxter P, Paul Griffiths A, et al. (2000) *Detection of damage to the mitochondrial genome in the oncocytic cells of Warthin's tumour.* J Pathol 191:274–281
363. Lewis PD, Fradley SR, Griffiths AP, et al. (2002) *Mitochondrial DNA mutations in the parotid gland of cigarette smokers and non-smokers.* Mutat Res 518:47–54
364. Li S, Baloch ZW, Tomaszewski JE, et al. (2000) *Worrisome histologic alterations following fine-needle aspiration of benign parotid lesions.* Arch Pathol Lab Med 124:87–91
365. Li S, Baloch ZW, Tomaszewski JE, et al. (2000) *Worrisome histologic alterations following fine-needle aspiration of benign parotid lesions.* Arch Pathol Lab Med 124:87–91
366. Lin Y, Wu H, Tzeng J (2005) *Small-cell undifferentiated carcinoma of the submandibular gland: An extremely rare extrapulmonary site.* Am J Otolaryngol 26:60–63
367. Lins JE, Gnepp DR (1986) *Myoepithelioma of the palate in a child.* Int J Pediatr Otorhinolaryngol 11:5–13
368. Lipani C, Woytash JJ, Greene GW Jr. (1983) *Sebaceous adenoma of the oral cavity.* J Oral Maxillofac Surg 41:56–60
369. Littman CD, Alguacil-Garcia A (1987) *Clear cell carcinoma arising in pleomorphic adenoma of the salivary gland.* Am J Clin Pathol 88:239–243
370. LiVolsi VA, Perzin KH (1977) *Malignant mixed tumors arising in salivary glands. I. Carcinomas arising in benign mixed tumors: a clinicopathologic study.* Cancer 39:2209–2230
371. Lombardi T, Samson J, Kuffer R (2003) *Subacute necrotizing sialadenitis: a form of necrotizing sialometaplasia?* Arch Otolaryngol Head Neck Surg 129:972–975
372. Love GL, Sarma DP (1986) *Spindle cell mucoepidermoid carcinoma of submandibular gland.* J Surg Oncol 31:66–68
373. Loy TS, McLaughlin R, Odom LF, et al. (1989) *Mucoepidermoid carcinoma of the parotid as a second malignant neoplasm in children.* Cancer 64:2174–2177
374. Lucarini JW, Sciubba JJ, Khettry U, et al. (1994) *Terminal duct carcinoma. Recognition of a low-grade salivary adenocarcinoma.[see comment].* Arch Otolaryngol Head Neck Surg 120:1010–1015
375. Luna MA, Batsakis JG, Tortoledo ME, et al. (1989) *Carcinomas ex monomorphic adenoma of salivary glands.* J Laryngol Otol 103:756–759
376. Luna MA, el-Naggar A, Batsakis JG, et al. (1990) *Flow cytometric DNA content of adenoid cystic carcinoma of submandibular gland. Correlation of histologic features and prognosis.* Arch Otolaryngol Head Neck Surg 116:1291–1296
377. Luna MA, Ordonez NG, Mackay B, et al. (1985) *Salivary epithelial-myoepithelial carcinomas of intercalated ducts: a clinical, electron microscopic, and immunocytochemical study.* Oral Surg Oral Med Oral Pathol 59:482–490
378. Luna MA, Tortoledo ME, Allen M (1987) *Salivary dermal analogue tumors arising in lymph nodes.* Cancer 59:1165–1169
379. Ma J, Chan JK, Chow CW, et al. (2002) *Lymphadenoma: a report of three cases of an uncommon salivary gland neoplasm.* Histopathology 41:342–350

380. Maisel RH, Johnston WH, Anderson HA, et al. (1977) *Necrotizing sialometaplasia involving the nasal cavity.* Laryngoscope 87:429–434
381. Mandel L, Carrao V (2005) *Bilateral parotid diffuse hyperplastic oncocytosis: case report.* J Oral Maxillofac Surg 63:560–562
382. Mandel L, Kim D, Uy C (1998) *Parotid gland swelling in HIV diffuse infiltrative CD8 lymphocytosis syndrome.* Oral Surg Oral Med Oral Pathol Oral Radiol Endod 85:565–568
383. Mandel L, Surattanont F (2002) *Bilateral parotid swelling: a review.* Oral Surg Oral Med Oral Pathol Oral Radiol Endod 93:221–237
384. Marciani RD, Trodahl JN, Dauchess VG, et al. (1976) *Squamous cell carcinoma of the submandibular gland.* J Oral Surg 34:646–650
385. Mariappan MR, Fadare O, Jain D (2004) *Sebaceous differentiation in salivary glands.* Arch Pathol Lab Med 128:245–246
386. Marie B, Labouyrie E, Scheid P, et al. (1997) *Human immunodeficiency virus type 1 in an unusual cystic lymphoepithelial lesion of the lung.* Histopathology 31:83–86
387. Marioni G, Marino F, Stramare R, et al. (2003) *Benign metastasizing pleomorphic adenoma of the parotid gland: a clinicopathologic puzzle.* Head Neck 25:1071–1076
388. Mark J, Dahlenfors R, Wedell B (1997) *Impact of the in vitro technique used on the cytogenetic patterns in pleomorphic adenomas.* Cancer Genet Cytogenet 95:9–15
389. Marks MW, Ryan RF, Litwin MS, et al. (1987) *Squamous cell carcinoma of the parotid gland.* Plast Reconstr Surg 79:550–554
390. Marmary Y, Gomori JM, Nitzan DW (1990) *Lymphoepithelial parotid cysts as presenting symptom of immunodeficiency virus infection: clinical, sialographic, and magnetic resonance imaging findings.* J Oral Maxillofac Surg 48:981–984
391. Martinez-Madrigal F, Micheau C (1989) *Histology of the major salivary glands.* Am J Surg Pathol 13:879–899
392. Martins C, Fonseca I, Roque L, et al. (1997) *Cytogenetic characterisation of Warthin's tumour.* Oral Oncol 33:344–347
393. Matsuba HM, Simpson JR, Mauney M, et al. (1986) *Adenoid cystic salivary gland carcinoma: a clinicopathologic correlation.* Head Neck Surg 8:200–204
394. McAdams RM, Mair EA, Rajnik M (2005) *Neonatal suppurative submandibular sialadenitis: case report and literature review.* Int J Pediatr Otorhinolaryngol 69:993–997
395. McCluggage G, Sloan J, Cameron S, et al. (1995) *Basal cell adenocarcinoma of the submandibular gland.* Oral Surg Oral Med Oral Pathol Oral Radiol Endod 79:342–350
396. McFerran DJ, Ingrams DR, Gallimore AP, et al. (1995) *Polycystic disease of salivary glands.* J Laryngol Otol 109:165–167
397. McGavran MH, Bauer WC, Ackerman LV (1960) *Sebaceous lymphadenoma of the parotid salivary gland.* Cancer 13:1185–1187
398. McKinney B, Lewis J, Weiland L, et al. (1994) *Salivary duct carcinoma. Clinicopathologic and immunohistochemical review of 26 cases.* Lab Invest 70:100A
399. McQuone SJ (1999) *Acute viral and bacterial infections of the salivary glands.* Otolaryngol Clin North Am 32:793–811
400. Mehta RP, Faquin WC, Deschler DG (2004) *Pathology quiz case 1. Acinic cell carcinoma of the parotid gland with ductal extension.* Arch Otolaryngol Head Neck Surg 130:790, 792–793
401. Mentzel T (2004) *[Skin adnexal and salivary gland neoplasms. Similarities and differences of selected patients].* Pathologe 25:79–88
402. Merchant WJ, Cook MG, Eveson JW (1996) *Polymorphous low-grade adenocarcinoma of parotid gland.* Br J Oral Maxillofac Surg 34:328–330
403. Merwin WH Jr., Barnes L, Myers EN (1985) *Unilocular cystic sebaceous lymphadenoma of the parotid gland.* Arch Otolaryngol 111:273–275
404. Michal M, Skalova A, Simpson RH, et al. (1997) *Well-differentiated acinic cell carcinoma of salivary glands associated with lymphoid stroma.* Hum Pathol 28:595–600
405. Michal M, Skalova A, Simpson RH, et al. (1996) *Clear cell malignant myoepithelioma of the salivary glands.* Histopathology 28:309–315
406. Miettinen M, Lasota J (2005) *KIT (CD117): a review on expression in normal and neoplastic tissues, and mutations and their clinicopathologic correlation.* Appl Immunohistochem Mol Morphol 13:205–220
407. Miglianico L, Eschwege F, Marandas P, et al. (1987) *Cervico-facial adenoid cystic carcinoma: study of 102 cases. Influence of radiation therapy.* Int J Radiat Oncol Biol Phys 13:673–678
408. Mignogna MD, Fedele S, Lo Russo L (2004) *Anorexia/bulimia-related sialadenosis of palatal minor salivary glands.* J Oral Pathol Med 33:441–442
409. Miki H, Masuda E, Ohata S, et al. (1999) *Late recurrence of acinic cell carcinoma of the parotid gland.* J Med Invest 46:213–216
410. Milford CA, Mugliston TA, O'Flynn P, et al. (1989) *Carcinoma arising in a pleomorphic adenoma of the epiglottis.* J Laryngol Otol 103:324–327
411. Miliauskas JR (1991) *Polymorphous low-grade (terminal duct) adenocarcinoma of the parotid gland.* Histopathology 19:555–557

412. Mills SE, Garland TA, Allen MS Jr. (1984) *Low-grade papillary adenocarcinoma of palatal salivary gland origin.* Am J Surg Pathol 8:367–374
413. Mino M, Pilch BZ, Faquin WC (2003) *Expression of KIT (CD117) in neoplasms of the head and neck: an ancillary marker for adenoid cystic carcinoma.* Mod Pathol 16:1224–1231
414. Mitchell DA, Eveson JW, Ord RA (1989) *Polymorphous low-grade adenocarcinoma of minor salivary glands – a report of three cases.* Br J Oral Maxillofac Surg 27:494–500
415. Moberger JG, Eneroth CM (1968) *Malignant mixed tumors of the major salivary glands. Special reference to the histologic structure in metastases.* Cancer 21:1198–1211
416. Mohamed AH (1976) *Ultrastructure of glycogen-rich clear cell carcinoma of the palate.* J Oral Pathol 5:103–121
417. Mohamed AH, Cherrick HM (1975) *Glycogen-rich adenocarcinoma of minor salivary glands. A light and electron microscopic study.* Cancer 36:1057–1066
418. Mohammed BS, Liu Z, Tang W, et al. (2006) *BCL-2, Ki67 and P53 expression in oral necrotizing sialometaplasia and squamous cell carcinoma.* Mod Pathol 19:105A
419. Molina CP, Chaljub G, Campbell GA (2003) *Pathologic quiz case: a 37-year-old man with spinal cord compression.* Arch Pathol Lab Med 127:887–889
420. Monk JS Jr., Church JS (1992) *Warthin's tumor. A high incidence and no sex predominance in central Pennsylvania.* Arch Otolaryngol Head Neck Surg 118:477–478
421. Moore JG, Bocklage T (1998) *Fine-needle aspiration biopsy of large-cell undifferentiated carcinoma of the salivary glands: presentation of two cases, literature review, and differential cytodiagnosis of high-grade salivary gland malignancies.* Diagn Cytopathol 19:44–50
422. Mostofi R, Wood RS, Christison W, et al. (1992) *Low-grade papillary adenocarcinoma of minor salivary glands. Case report and literature review.* Oral Surg Oral Med Oral Pathol 73:591–595
423. Muller S, Barnes L (1996) *Basal cell adenocarcinoma of the salivary glands. Report of seven cases and review of the literature.* Cancer 78:2471–2477
424. Muller S, Barnes L, Goodurn WJ Jr. (1997) *Sclerosing mucoepidermoid carcinoma of the parotid.* Oral Surg Oral Med Oral Pathol Oral Radiol Endod 83:685–690
425. Murrah VA, Batsakis JG (1994) *Salivary duct carcinoma.* Ann Otol Rhinol Laryngol 103:244–247
426. Myerowitz RL, Barnes EL, Myers E (1978) *Small cell anaplastic (oat cell) carcinoma of the larynx: report of a case and review of the literature.* Laryngoscope 88:1697–1702
427. Nadiminti H, Thomas GR, Regalado J (2004) *Pathology quiz case 1. Small cell carcinoma (SmCC) of the parotid gland.* Arch Otolaryngol Head Neck Surg 130:474–477
428. Nagao K, Matsuzaki O, Saiga H, et al. (1983) *A histopathologic study of benign and malignant lymphoepithelial lesions of the parotid gland.* Cancer 52:1044–1052
429. Nagao K, Matsuzaki O, Saiga H, et al. (1982) *Histopathologic studies of basal cell adenoma of the parotid gland.* Cancer 50:736–745
430. Nagao K, Matsuzaki O, Saiga H, et al. (1982) *Histopathologic studies of undifferentiated carcinoma of the parotid gland.* Cancer 50:1572–1579
431. Nagao T, Gaffey TA, Kay PA, et al. (2003) *Dedifferentiation in low-grade mucoepidermoid carcinoma of the parotid gland.* Hum Pathol 34:1068–1072
432. Nagao T, Gaffey TA, Olsen KD, et al. (2004) *Small cell carcinoma of the major salivary glands: clinicopathologic study with emphasis on cytokeratin 20 immunoreactivity and clinical outcome.* Am J Surg Pathol 28:762–770
433. Nagao T, Gaffey TA, Serizawa H, et al. (2004) *Sarcomatoid variant of salivary duct carcinoma: clinicopathologic and immunohistochemical study of eight cases with review of the literature.* Am J Clin Pathol 122:222–231
434. Nagao T, Gaffey TA, Visscher DW, et al. (2004) *Invasive micropapillary salivary duct carcinoma: a distinct histologic variant with biologic significance.* Am J Surg Pathol 28:319–326
435. Nagao T, Serizawa H, Iwaya K, et al. (2002) *Keratocystoma of the parotid gland: a report of two cases of an unusual pathologic entity.* Mod Pathol 15(9):1005–1010.
436. Nagao T, Sugano I, Ishida Y, et al. (1998) *Basal cell adenocarcinoma of the salivary glands: comparison with basal cell adenoma through assessment of cell proliferation, apoptosis, and expression of p53 and bcl-2.* Cancer 82:439–447
437. Nagao T, Sugano I, Ishida Y, et al. (1998) *Salivary gland malignant myoepithelioma: a clinicopathologic and immunohistochemical study of ten cases.* Cancer 83:1292–1299
438. Nagao T, Sugano I, Ishida Y, et al. (2000) *Primary large-cell neuroendocrine carcinoma of the parotid gland: immunohistochemical and molecular analysis of two cases.* Mod Pathol 13:554–561
439. Nagao T, Sugano I, Matsuzaki O, et al. (2000) *Intraductal papillary tumors of the major salivary glands: case reports of benign and malignant variants.* Arch Pathol Lab Med 124:291–295
440. Namin AK, Moshref M, Shahoon H, et al. (2005) *Intraosseous mucoepidermoid carcinoma of the maxilla in a teenager: a case report and review of literature.* Oral Surg Oral Med Oral Pathol Oral Radiol Endod 100:e93–96
441. Nasse D (1892) *Die Geschwulste der Speicheldrusen und verwandte Tumoren des Kopfes.* Langenbecks Arch Klin Chir 44:233–302

442. Nessan VJ, Jacoway JR (1979) *Biopsy of minor salivary glands in the diagnosis of sarcoidosis.* N Engl J Med 301:922–924
443. Neto AG, Pineda-Daboin K, Spencer ML, et al. (2005) *Sinonasal acinic cell carcinoma: a clinicopathologic study of four cases.* Head Neck 27:603–607
444. Nguyen LH, Black MJ, Hier M, et al. (2003) *HER2/neu and Ki-67 as prognostic indicators in mucoepidermoid carcinoma of salivary glands.* J Otolaryngol 32:328–331
445. Nishimura T, Furukawa M, Kawahara E, et al. (1991) *Differential diagnosis of pleomorphic adenoma by immunohistochemical means.* J Laryngol Otol 105:1057–1060
446. Nistal M, Garcia-Viera M, Martinez-Garcia C, et al. (1994) *Epithelial-myoepithelial tumor of the bronchus.* Am J Surg Pathol 18:421–425
447. Nordkvist A, Mark J, Dahlenfors R, et al. (1994) *Cytogenetic observations in 13 cystadenolymphomas (Warthin's tumors).* Cancer Genet Cytogenet 76:129–135
448. Nordkvist A, Roijer E, Bang G, et al. (2000) *Expression and mutation patterns of p53 in benign and malignant salivary gland tumors.* Int J Oncol 16:477–483
449. Norlin R (1965) *Bilateral mixed tumor of the parotid initially regarded as pharyngeal neoplasm.* Pract Otorhinolaryngol (Basel) 27:298–301
450. Ochel HJ, Gademann G, Rocken C, et al. (2005) *Effects of imatinib mesylate on adenoid cystic carcinomas.* Anticancer Res 25:3659–3664
451. Ockner DM, Mills SE, Swanson PE, et al. (1994) *Salivary duct carcinoma: An immunohistologic comparison with invasive ductal carcinoma of the breast.* Lab Invest 70:100A
452. Ogawa I, Nikai H, Takata T, et al. (1992) *Clear-cell variant of mucoepidermoid carcinoma: report of a case with immunohistochemical and ultrastructural observations.* J Oral Maxillofac Surg 50:906–910
453. Olsen KD, Lewis JE (2001) *Carcinoma ex pleomorphic adenoma: a clinicopathologic review.* Head Neck 23:705–712
454. Olsen KD, Maragos NE, Weiland LH (1980) *First branchial cleft anomalies.* Laryngoscope 90:423–436
455. Orlian AI, Salman L, Reddi T, et al. (1987) *Sebaceous adenoma of the oral mucosa.* J Oral Med 42:38–39
456. Ortiz-Hidalgo C, Cervantes J, de la Vega G (1995) *Unilateral polycystic (dysgenetic) disease of the parotid gland.* South Med J 88:1173–1175
457. Orvidas LJ, Kasperbauer JL, Lewis JE, et al. (2000) *Pediatric parotid masses.* Arch Otolaryngol Head Neck Surg 126:177–184
458. Osial TA Jr., Whiteside TL, Buckingham RB, et al. (1983) *Clinical and serologic study of Sjogren's syndrome in patients with progressive systemic sclerosis.* Arthritis Rheum 26:500–508
459. Ozolek JA, Bastacky SI, Myers EN, et al. (2005) *Immunophenotypic comparison of salivary gland oncocytoma and metastatic renal cell carcinoma.* Laryngoscope 115:1097–1100
460. Padberg B-C, Sasse B, Huber A, et al. (2005) *Sarcomatoid salivary duct carcinoma.* Ann Diagn Pathol 9:86–92
461. Pai RR, Bharathi S, Naik R, et al. (1994) *Unilocular cystic sebaceous lymphadenoma of the parotid gland.* Indian J Pathol Microbiol 37:327–330
462. Peel R (2001) *Diseases of the salivary gland.* Surgical pathology of the head and neck. Edited by Barnes L. New York, Marcel-Dekker, pp 634–690
463. Penner CR, Folpe AL, Budnick SD (2002) *C-kit expression distinguishes salivary gland adenoid cystic carcinoma from polymorphous low-grade adenocarcinoma.* Mod Pathol 15:687–691
464. Perez-Ordonez B, Linkov I, Huvos AG (1998) *Polymorphous low-grade adenocarcinoma of minor salivary glands: a study of 17 cases with emphasis on cell differentiation.* Histopathology 32:521–529
465. Perzin KH, LiVolsi VA (1979) *Acinic cell carcinomas arising in salivary glands: a clinicopathologic study.* Cancer 44:1434–1457
466. Pesavento G, Ferlito A, Recher G (1980) *Primary clear cell carcinoma of the larynx.* J Clin Pathol 33:1160–1164
467. Piattelli A, Tete S (1995) *Lymphoepithelial cyst of the parotid gland.* Acta Stomatol Belg 92:137–138
468. Pinkston JA, Cole P (1996) *Cigarette smoking and Warthin's tumor.* Am J Epidemiol 144:183–187
469. Pires FR, da Cruz Perez DE, de Almeida OP, et al. (2004) *Estrogen receptor expression in salivary gland mucoepidermoid carcinoma and adenoid cystic carcinoma.* Pathol Oncol Res 10:166–168
470. Pires FR, de Almeida OP, de Araujo VC, et al. (2004) *Prognostic factors in head and neck mucoepidermoid carcinoma.* Arch Otolaryngol Head Neck Surg 130:174–180
471. Puxeddu R, Puxeddu P, Parodo G, et al. (1998) *Polymorphous low-grade adenocarcinoma of the parotid gland.* Eur J Morphol 36(suppl):262–266
472. Quddus MR, Henley JD, Affify AM, et al. (1999) *Basal cell adenocarcinoma of the salivary gland: an ultrastructural and immunohistochemical study.* Oral Surg Oral Med Oral Pathol Oral Radiol Endod 87:485–492
473. Raad, II, Sabbagh MF, Caranasos GJ (1990) *Acute bacterial sialadenitis: a study of 29 cases and review.* Rev Infect Dis 12:591–601
474. Rapidis AD, Givalos N, Gakiopoulou H, et al. (2005) *Adenoid cystic carcinoma of the head and neck. Clinicopathological analysis of 23 patients and review of the literature.* Oral Oncol 41:328–335

475. Raslan WF, Sawyer DR, Mercuri LG (1998) *Central mucoepidermoid carcinoma.* J Can Dent Assoc 64:420–424
476. Reis-Filho JS, Schmitt FC (2002) *Taking advantage of basic research: p63 is a reliable myoepithelial and stem cell marker.* Adv Anat Pathol 9:280–289
477. Renehan A, Gleave EN, McGurk M (1996) *An analysis of the treatment of 114 patients with recurrent pleomorphic adenomas of the parotid gland.* Am J Surg 172:710–714
478. Richardson RL, Weiland LH (1982) *Undifferentiated small cell carcinomas in extrapulmonary sites.* Semin Oncol 9:484–496
479. Righi PD, Li YQ, Deutsch M, et al. (1994) *The role of the p53 gene in the malignant transformation of pleomorphic adenomas of the parotid gland.* Anticancer Res 14:2253–2257
480. Ritland F, Lubensky I, LiVolsi VA (1993) *Polymorphous low-grade adenocarcinoma of the parotid salivary gland.* Arch Pathol Lab Med 117:1261–1263
481. Robin C, Laboulbene A (1853) *Memoire sur trois productions morbides non decrites.* C R Soc Biol 5:185–196
482. Rodriguez J, Forcelledo M, Gutierrez L, et al. (2004) *Small cell undifferentiated carcinoma of the submandibular gland with neurosecretory features.* Ann Otol Rhinol Laryngol 113:55–59
483. Rollins CE, Yost BA, Costa MJ, et al. (1995) *Squamous differentiation in small-cell carcinoma of the parotid gland.* Arch Pathol Lab Med 119:183–185
484. Romagosa V, Bella MR, Truchero C, et al. (1992) *Necrotizing sialometaplasia (adenometaplasia) of the trachea.* Histopathology 21:280–282
485. Rosai J (1996) *Major and minor salivary glands.* Ackerman's surgical pathology. Edited by Rosai J. St. Louis, Mosby, pp 834–835
486. Rousseau A, Mock D, Dover DG, et al. (1999) *Multiple canalicular adenomas: a case report and review of the literature.* Oral Surg Oral Med Oral Pathol Oral Radiol Endod 87:346–350
487. Rye LA, Calhoun NR, Redman RS (1980) *Necrotizing sialometaplasia in a patient with Buerger's disease and Raynaud's phenomenon.* Oral Surg Oral Med Oral Pathol 49:233–236
488. Said S, Compana J (2005) *Myoepithelial carcinoma ex-pleomorphic adenoma of salivary glands: A problematic diagnosis.* Oral Surg Oral Med Oral Pathol Oral Radiol Endod 99:196–201
489. Sakorafas GH, Sarr MG, van de Velde CJ, et al. (2005) *Intraductal papillary mucinous neoplasms of the pancreas: A surgical perspective.* Surg Oncol 14:155–178
490. Saksela E, Tarkkanen J, Kohonen A (1970) *The malignancy of mixed tumors of the parotid gland. A clinicopathological analysis of 70 cases.* Acta Otolaryngol 70:62–70
491. Saksela E, Tarkkanen J, Wartiovaara J (1972) *Parotid clear-cell adenoma of possible myoepithelial origin.* Cancer 30:742–748
492. Santucci L, Smorlesi L (1954) *[I tumori misti, benigni e maligni, di tipo salivare, in sede extra-macro-salivare con particolare riguardo alle localizzazioni eccezionali.].* Arch De Vecchi Anat Patol 22:623–692
493. Santucci M, Gallo O, Calzolari A, et al. (1993) *Detection of Epstein-Barr viral genome in tumor cells of Warthin's tumor of parotid gland.* Am J Clin Pathol 100:662–665
494. Sato T, Kamata SE, Kawabata K, et al. (2005) *Acinic cell carcinoma of the parotid gland in a child.* Pediatr Surg Int 21:377–380
495. Savera AT, Sloman A, Huvos AG, et al. (2000) *Myoepithelial carcinoma of the salivary glands: a clinicopathologic study of 25 patients.* Am J Surg Pathol 24:761–774
496. Schoning H, Emshoff R, Kreczy A (1998) *Necrotizing sialometaplasia in two patients with bulimia and chronic vomiting.* Int J Oral Maxillofac Surg 27:463–465
497. Schultz AM, Thomas AB, Henley JD, et al. (2004) *Pathologic quiz case: a 42-year-old man with right facial swelling and weakness. Dedifferentiated acinic cell carcinoma of the parotid gland.* Arch Pathol Lab Med 128:e52–53
498. Sciubba JJ, Brannon RB (1982) *Myoepithelioma of salivary glands: report of 23 cases.* Cancer 49:562–572
499. Seaver PR Jr., Kuehn PG (1979) *Adenoid cystic carcinoma of the salivary glands. A study of ninety-three cases.* Am J Surg 137:449–455
500. Seethala RR, LiVolsi VA, Zhang PJ, et al. (2005) *Comparison of p63 and p73 expression in benign and malignant salivary gland lesions.* Head Neck 27:696–702
501. Seifert G (1991) *Histologic Typing of Salivary Gland Tumors.* Springer, New York p 26
502. Seifert G (1996) *Classification and differential diagnosis of clear and basal cell tumors of the salivary glands.* Semin Diagn Pathol 13:95–103
503. Seifert G (1997) *Aetiological and histological classification of sialadenitis.* Pathologica 89:7–17
504. Seifert G (1997) *[Carcinoma in pre-existing Warthin tumors (cystadenolymphoma) of the parotid gland. Classification, pathogenesis and differential diagnosis].* Pathologe 18:359–367
505. Seifert G (1998) *Are adenomyoepithelioma of the breast and epithelial-myoepithelial carcinoma of the salivary glands identical tumours?* Virchows Arch 433:285–288
506. Seifert G, Bull HG, Donath K (1980) *Histologic subclassification of the cystadenolymphoma of the parotid gland. Analysis of 275 cases.* Virchows Arch A Pathol Anat Histol 388:13–38

3

507. Seifert G, Donath K (1976) *Classification of the pathohistology of diseases of the salivary glands – review of 2,600 cases in the Salivary Gland Register.* Beitr Pathol 159:1–32
508. Seifert G, Donath K (1996) *Multiple tumours of the salivary glands – terminology and nomenclature.* Eur J Cancer B Oral Oncol 32B:3–7
509. Seifert G, Donath K, Schafer R (1999) *Lipomatous pleomorphic adenoma of the parotid gland. Classification of lipomatous tissue in salivary glands.* Pathol Res Pract 195:247–252
510. Seifert G, Miehlke A, Haubrich J, et al. (1986) *Diseases of the Salivary Glands: Diagnosis, Pathology, Treatment, Facial Nerve Surgery,* Stuttgart, Georg Theime Verlag, pp 248–252
511. Seifert G, Thomsen S, Donath K (1981) *Bilateral dysgenetic polycystic parotid glands. Morphological analysis and differential diagnosis of a rare disease of the salivary glands.* Virchows Arch A Pathol Anat Histol 390:273–288
512. Selva D, Davis GJ, Dodd T, et al. (2004) *Polymorphous low-grade adenocarcinoma of the lacrimal gland.* Arch Ophthalmol 122:915–917
513. Shemen LJ, Huvos AG, Spiro RH (1987) *Squamous cell carcinoma of salivary gland origin.* Head Neck Surg 9:235–240
514. Shimoda M, Kameyama K, Morinaga S, et al. (2004) *Malignant transformation of sialadenoma papilliferum of the palate: a case report.* Virchows Arch 445:641–646
515. Silvers AR, Som PM (1998) *Salivary glands.* Radiol Clin North Am 36:941–966, vi
516. Simpson RH, Clarke TJ, Sarsfield PT, et al. (1991) *Epithelial-myoepithelial carcinoma of salivary glands.* J Clin Pathol 44:419–423
517. Simpson RHW, Eveson JW (2005) *Warthin tumor.* Pathology and Classification of Head and Neck Tumours. Edited by Barnes EL, Eveson JW, Sidransky D. Lyons, IARC, pp 263–265
518. Simpson RHW, Prasad AR, Lewis JE, et al. (2003) *Mucin-rich variant of salivary duct carcinoma: a clinicopathologic and immunohistochemical study of four cases.* Am J Surg Pathol 27:1070–1079
519. Sjogren H, Dahlenfors R, Stenman G, et al. (2003) *Observations by G-banding and multicolor spectral karyotyping in a salivary gland basal cell adenoma.* Virchows Arch 442:86–87
520. Skalova A, Gnepp DR, Simpson RH, et al. (2006) *Clonal Nature of Sclerosing Polycystic Adenosis of Salivary Glands Demonstrated by Using the Polymorphism of the Human Androgen Receptor Locus (HUMARA) as a Marker.* Mod Pathol 19:105A
521. Skalova A, Leivo I, Von Boguslawsky K, et al. (1994) *Cell proliferation correlates with prognosis in acinic cell carcinomas of salivary gland origin. Immunohistochemical study of 30 cases using the MIB 1 antibody in formalin-fixed paraffin sections.* J Pathol 173:13–21
522. Skalova A, Leivo I, Wolf H, et al. (2000) *Oncocytic cystadenoma of the parotid gland with tyrosine-rich crystals.* Pathol Res Pract 196:849–851
523. Skalova A, Michal M (2005) *Cystadenoma.* Pathology and Classification of Head and Neck Tumours. Edited by Barnes EL, Eveson JW, Sidransky D. Lyons, IARC, pp 273–274
524. Skalova A, Michal M, Ryska A, et al. (1999) *Oncocytic myoepithelioma and pleomorphic adenoma of the salivary glands.* Virchows Arch 434:537–546
525. Skalova A, Michal M, Simpson RH, et al. (2002) *Sclerosing polycystic adenosis of parotid gland with dysplasia and ductal carcinoma in situ. Report of three cases with immunohistochemical and ultrastructural examination.* Virchows Arch 440:29–35
526. Skalova A, Simpson RH, Lehtonen H, et al. (1997) *Assessment of proliferative activity using the MIB1 antibody help to distinguish polymorphous low grade adenocarcinoma from adenoid cystic carcinoma of salivary glands.* Pathol Res Pract 193:695–703
527. Skalova A, Starek I, Simpson RH, et al. (2001) *Spindle cell myoepithelial tumours of the parotid gland with extensive lipomatous metaplasia. A report of four cases with immunohistochemical and ultrastructural findings.* Virchows Arch 439:762–767
528. Skalova A, Starek I, Vanecek T, et al. (2003) *Expression of HER-2/neu gene and protein in salivary duct carcinomas of parotid gland as revealed by fluorescence in-situ hybridization and immunohistochemistry.[see comment].* Histopathology 42:348–356
529. Slootweg PJ (1993) *Low-grade adenocarcinoma of the oral cavity: polymorphous or papillary?* J Oral Pathol Med 22:327–330
530. Slootweg PJ, Muller H (1987) *Low-grade adenocarcinoma of the oral cavity. A comparison between the terminal duct and the papillary type.* J Craniomaxillofac Surg 15:359–364
531. Smith A, Winkler B, Perzin KH, et al. (1985) *Mucoepidermoid carcinoma arising in an intraparotid lymph node.* Cancer 55:400–403
532. Smith BC, Ellis GL, Slater LJ, et al. (1996) *Sclerosing polycystic adenosis of major salivary glands. A clinicopathologic analysis of nine cases.* Am J Surg Pathol 20:161–170
533. Smith JA, Warhol MJ, Brodsky GL (1983) *An immunohistochemical study of a carcinoma of the parotid gland exhibiting both ductal and acinic cell differentiation.* Oral Surg Oral Med Oral Pathol 55:267–273

534. Smyth AG, Ward-Booth RP, High AS (1993) *Polycystic disease of the parotid glands: two familial cases.* Br J Oral Maxillofac Surg 31:38–40
535. Snyderman C, Johnson JT, Barnes EL (1986) *Extraparotid Warthin's tumor.* Otolaryngol Head Neck Surg 94:169–175
536. Som PM, Biller HF (1992) *Kimura disease involving parotid gland and cervical nodes: CT and MR findings.* J Comput Assist Tomogr 16:320–322
537. Soofer SB, Tabbara S (1999) *Intraductal papilloma of the salivary gland. A report of two cases with diagnosis by fine needle aspiration biopsy.* Acta Cytol 43:1142–1146
538. Spies JW (1930) *Adenoid cystic carcinoma.* Arch Surg 21:365–404
539. Spiro RH (1986) *Salivary neoplasms: overview of a 35-year experience with 2,807 patients.* Head Neck Surg 8:177–184
540. Spiro RH, Huvos AG, Strong EW (1977) *Malignant mixed tumor of salivary origin: a clinicopathologic study of 146 cases.* Cancer 39:388–396
541. Spiro RH, Huvos AG, Strong EW (1978) *Acinic cell carcinoma of salivary origin. A clinicopathologic study of 67 cases.* Cancer 41:924–935
542. Spiro RH, Huvos AG, Strong EW (1979) *Adenoid cystic carcinoma: factors influencing survival.* Am J Surg 138:579–583
543. Spiro RH, Huvos AG, Strong EW (1982) *Adenocarcinoma of salivary origin. Clinicopathologic study of 204 patients.* Am J Surg 144:423–431
544. Spiro RH, Koss LG, Hajdu SI, et al. (1973) *Tumors of minor salivary origin. A clinicopathologic study of 492 cases.* Cancer 31:117–129
545. Stanley RJ, Weiland LH, Olsen KD, et al. (1988) *Dedifferentiated acinic cell (acinous) carcinoma of the parotid gland.* Otolaryngol Head Neck Surg 98:155–161
546. Stell PM (1986) *Adenoid cystic carcinoma.* Clin Otolaryngol 11:267–291
547. Stephen J, Batsakis JG, Luna MA, et al. (1986) *True malignant mixed tumors (carcinosarcoma) of salivary glands.* Oral Surg Oral Med Oral Pathol 61:597–602
548. Stephen J, Luna MA, Batsakis J (1985) *Malignant mixed (heterologous) tumors of salivary glands.* Lab Invest 52:65A
549. Sterman BM, Kraus DH, Sebek BA, et al. (1990) *Primary squamous cell carcinoma of the parotid gland.* Laryngoscope 100:146–148
550. Stewart FW, Foote FW, Becker WF (1945) *Mucoepidermoid tumors of salivary glands.* Ann Surg 122:820–844
551. Stewart S, Levy R, Karpel J, et al. (1974) *Lymphoepithelial (branchial) cyst of the parotid gland.* J Oral Surg 32:100–106
552. Streubel B, Simonitsch-Klupp I, Mullauer L, et al. (2004) *Variable frequencies of MALT lymphoma-associated genetic aberrations in MALT lymphomas of different sites.* Leukemia 18:1722–1726
553. Suarez P, Hammond HL, Luna MA, et al. (1998) *Palatal canalicular adenoma: report of 12 cases and review of the literature.* Ann Diagn Pathol 2:224–228
554. Szanto PA, Luna MA, Tortoledo ME, et al. (1984) *Histologic grading of adenoid cystic carcinoma of the salivary glands.* Cancer 54:1062–1069
555. Tabak LA (1995) *In defense of the oral cavity: structure, biosynthesis, and function of salivary mucins.* Annu Rev Physiol 57:547–564
556. Tabak LA, Levine MJ, Mandel ID, et al. (1982) *Role of salivary mucins in the protection of the oral cavity.* J Oral Pathol 11:1–17
557. Takai Y, Dardick I, Mackay A, et al. (1995) *Diagnostic criteria for neoplastic myoepithelial cells in pleomorphic adenomas and myoepitheliomas. Immunocytochemical detection of muscle-specific actin, cytokeratin 14, vimentin, and glial fibrillary acidic protein.* Oral Surg Oral Med Oral Pathol Oral Radiol Endod 79:330–341
558. Takai Y, Mori M, Dardick I, et al. (1994) *Myofilament localization and immunoelectron microscopic detection of muscle-specific actin in neoplastic myoepithelial cells in pleomorphic adenomas and myoepitheliomas.* Ultrastruct Pathol 18:575–591
559. Takeda Y, Shimono M (1999) *Pleomorphic adenoma with nuclear palisading arrangement of modified myoepithelial cells: histopathologic and immunohistochemical study.* Bull Tokyo Dent Coll 40:27–34
560. Tauxe WN, Mc DJ, Devine KD (1962) *A century of cylindromas. Short review and report of 27 adenoid cystic carcinomas arising in the upper respiratory passages.* Arch Otolaryngol 75:364–376
561. Tavassoli FA (1991) *Myoepithelial lesions of the breast. Myoepitheliosis, adenomyoepithelioma, and myoepithelial carcinoma.* Am J Surg Pathol 15:554–568
562. Tay HL, Reilly PG, Akosa AB (1992) *Salivary terminal duct carcinoma.* J Laryngol Otol 106:649–651
563. Terada T, Ikeuchi S, Inomoto C, et al. (2004) *Mucoepidermoid carcinoma of the palate composed exclusively of clear cells (clear cell variant).* Virchows Arch 445:541–543
564. Terry JH, Loree TR, Thomas MD, et al. (1991) *Major salivary gland lymphoepithelial lesions and the acquired immunodeficiency syndrome.* Am J Surg 162:324–329
565. Teymoortash A, Simolka N, Schrader C, et al. (2005) *Lymphocyte subsets in irradiation-induced sialadenitis of the submandibular gland.* Histopathology 47:493–500

566. Teymoortash A, Werner JA (2005) *Tissue that has lost its track: Warthin's tumour*. Virchows Arch 446:585–588
567. Thackray A, Lucas R (1974) *Tumors of the Major Salivary Glands*. Atlas of Tumor Pathology, Series 2, Fascicle 10. Washington, DC, Armed Forces Institute of Pathology, pp 107–117
568. Thompson AS, Bryant HC Jr. (1950) *Histogenesis of papillary cystadenoma lymphomatosum (Warthin's tumor) of the parotid salivary gland*. Am J Pathol 26:807–849
569. Tortoledo ME, Luna MA, Batsakis JG (1984) *Carcinomas ex pleomorphic adenoma and malignant mixed tumors. Histomorphologic indexes*. Arch Otolaryngol 110:172–176
570. Toynton S, Wilkins M, Cook H, et al. (1994) *True malignant mixed tumor of a minor salivary gland*. J Laryngol Otol 108:76–79
571. Tralongo V, Becchina G, Genovese F, et al. (2002) *Polymorphous low-grade adenocarcinoma of the salivary glands: clinicopathological and immunohistochemical study of a case*. Anticancer Res 22:1347–1352
572. Tralongo V, Daniele E (1998) *Epithelial-myoepithelial carcinoma of the salivary glands: a review of literature*. Anticancer Res 18:603–608
573. Tralongo V, Rodolico V, Nagar C, et al. (1997) *Epithelial-myoepithelial carcinoma of the salivary glands: a clinicopathologic, immunohistochemical and DNA flow cytometric study of three cases*. Anticancer Res 17:761–768
574. Tran PT, Cunningham CJ, Baughman RA (2004) *Glandular odontogenic cyst*. J Endod 30:182–184
575. Triglia JM, Nicollas R, Ducroz V, et al. (1998) *First branchial cleft anomalies: a study of 39 cases and a review of the literature*. Arch Otolaryngol Head Neck Surg 124:291–295
576. Trompouki E, Hatzivassiliou E, Tsichritzis T, et al. (2003) *CYLD is a deubiquitinating enzyme that negatively regulates NF-kappaB activation by TNFR family members*. Nature 424:793–796
577. Tsang YW, Tung Y, Chan JK (1991) *Polymorphous low grade adenocarcinoma of the palate in a child*. J Laryngol Otol 105:309–311
578. Tschen JA, McGavran MH (1979) *Sebaceous lymphadenoma: ultrastructural observations and lipid analysis*. Cancer 44:1388–1392
579. Tucci FM, Bianchi PM, Bottero S, et al. (1993) *Acinic cell carcinoma of the parotid gland in childhood*. Int J Pediatr Otorhinolaryngol 27:187–191
580. Tuncel U, Ergul G, Ozlugedik S, et al. (2004) *Myoepithelial carcinoma in the nasopharynx: an unusual localization*. Yonsei Med J 45:161–165
581. Tytor M, Gemryd P, Grenko R, et al. (1995) *Adenoid cystic carcinoma: significance of DNA ploidy*. Head Neck 17:319–327
582. Ubaidat MA, Robinson RA, Belding PJ, et al. (2001) *Sialadenoma papilliferum of the hard palate: report of 2 cases and immunohistochemical evaluation*. Arch Pathol Lab Med 125:1595–1597
583. Uccini S, Riva E, Antonelli G, et al. (1999) *The benign cystic lymphoepithelial lesion of the parotid gland is a viral reservoir in HIV type 1-infected patients*. AIDS Res Hum Retroviruses 15:1339–1344
584. Urano M, Abe M, Horibe Y, et al. (2002) *Sclerosing mucoepidermoid carcinoma with eosinophilia of the salivary glands*. Pathol Res Pract 198:305–310
585. Urban SD, Hall JM, Bentkover SH, et al. (2002) *Salivary duct carcinoma of minor salivary gland origin: report of a case involving the cavernous sinus*. J Oral Maxillofac Surg 60:958–962
586. van der Schans EJ, Knegt P, de Jong PC, et al. (1985) *Adenoid cystic carcinoma of the upper digestive and respiratory tracts. A retrospective study of 59 cases*. Clin Otolaryngol 10:63–67
587. van der Wal JE, Davids JJ, van der Waal I (1993) *Extraparotid Warthin's tumours – report of 10 cases*. Br J Oral Maxillofac Surg 31:43–44
588. van der Wal JE, Kraaijenhagen HA, van der Waal I (1995) *Subacute necrotising sialadenitis: a new entity?* Br J Oral Maxillofac Surg 33:302–303
589. van der Wal JE, Snow GB, van der Waal I (1990) *Intraoral adenoid cystic carcinoma. The presence of perineural spread in relation to site, size, local extension, and metastatic spread in 22 cases*. Cancer 66:2031–2033
590. van der Walt JD, Leake J (1987) *Granulomatous sialadenitis of the major salivary glands. A clinicopathological study of 57 cases*. Histopathology 11:131–144
591. Van Heerden WF, Raubenheimer EJ, Dreyer L (2005) *The role of DNA ploidy and Ki-67 in the grading of mucoepidermoid carcinomas*. Anticancer Res 25:2589–2592
592. Van Krieken JH (1993) *Prostate marker immunoreactivity in salivary gland neoplasms. A rare pitfall in immunohistochemistry.[see comment]*. Am J Surg Pathol 17:410–414
593. Van Roggen G, Baatenburg-De J, Verschuur B, et al. (1998) *Myoepithelial carcinoma (malignant myoepithelioma): First report of an occurrence in the maxillary sinus*. Histopathology 32:239–241
594. Verghese S, Lalitha MK (1975) *Sebaceous lymphadenoma of the parotid region report of a case*. Indian J Pathol Bacteriol 18:46–48
595. Vicandi B, Jimenez-Heffernan JA, Lopez-Ferrer P, et al. (1999) *HIV-1 (p24)-positive multinucleated giant cells in HIV-associated lymphoepithelial lesion of the parotid gland. A report of two cases*. Acta Cytol 43:247–251

596. Vincent SD, Hammond HL, Finkelstein MW (1994) *Clinical and therapeutic features of polymorphous low-grade adenocarcinoma*. Oral Surg Oral Med Oral Pathol 77:41–47
597. Voz ML, Agten NS, Van de Ven WJ, et al. (2000) *PLAG1, the main translocation target in pleomorphic adenoma of the salivary glands, is a positive regulator of IGF-II*. Cancer Res 60:106–113
598. Voz ML, Astrom AK, Kas K, et al. (1998) *The recurrent translocation t(5;8)(p13;q12) in pleomorphic adenomas results in upregulation of PLAG1 gene expression under control of the LIFR promoter*. Oncogene 16:1409–1416
599. Vrielinck LJ, Ostyn F, van Damme B, et al. (1988) *The significance of perineural spread in adenoid cystic carcinoma of the major and minor salivary glands*. Int J Oral Maxillofac Surg 17:190–193
600. Waldron CA, el-Mofty SK, Gnepp DR (1988) *Tumors of the intraoral minor salivary glands: a demographic and histologic study of 426 cases*. Oral Surg Oral Med Oral Pathol 66:323–333
601. Waldron CA, Koh ML (1990) *Central mucoepidermoid carcinoma of the jaws: report of four cases with analysis of the literature and discussion of the relationship to mucoepidermoid, sialodontogenic, and glandular odontogenic cysts*. J Oral Maxillofac Surg 48:871–877
602. Wang C-P, Chang Y-L, Ko J-Y, et al. (2004) *Lymphoepithelial carcinoma versus large cell undifferentiated carcinoma of the major salivary glands*. Cancer 101:2020–2027
603. Warrick PD, Irish JC, Mancer K, et al. (2000) *Basal cell adenocarcinoma: a rare malignancy of the salivary glands*. J Otolaryngol 29:102–109
604. Warthin AS (1929) *Papillary cystadenoma lymphomatosum. A rare teratoid of the parotid*. J Cancer Res 13:116–125
605. Wasan SM (1971) *Sebaceous lymphadenoma of the parotid gland*. Cancer 28:1019–1022
606. Weber A, Langhanki L, Schutz A, et al. (2002) *Expression profiles of p53, p63, and p73 in benign salivary gland tumors*. Virchows Arch 441:428–436
607. Weed D, Gomez-Fernancez C, Pacheo J, et al. (2004) *MUC4 and ERBB2 expression in major and minor salivary gland mucoepidermoid carcinoma*. Head Neck 26:353–364
608. Weitzner S (1973) *Lymphoepithelial (branchial) cyst of parotid gland*. Oral Surg Oral Med Oral Pathol 35:85–88
609. Wenig BM, Harpaz N, DelBridge C (1989) *Polymorphous low-grade adenocarcinoma of seromucous glands of the nasopharynx. A report of a case and a discussion of the morphologic and immunohistochemical features*. Am J Clin Pathol 92:104–109
610. Wenig BM, Hitchcock CL, Ellis GL, et al. (1992) *Metastasizing mixed tumor of salivary glands. A clinicopathologic and flow cytometric analysis*. Am J Surg Pathol 16:845–858
611. Wermuth DJ, Mann CH, Odere F (1988) *Metastasizing pleomorphic adenoma arising in the soft palate*. Otolaryngol Head Neck Surg 99:505–508
612. Werning JT, Waterhouse JP, Mooney JW (1990) *Subacute necrotizing sialadenitis*. Oral Surg Oral Med Oral Pathol 70:756–759
613. Whitaker SB, Vigneswaran N, Singh BB (1997) *Androgen receptor status of the oral sebaceous glands*. Am J Dermatopathol 19:415–418
614. White DK, Miller AS, McDaniel RK, et al. (1982) *Inverted ductal papilloma: a distinctive lesion of minor salivary gland*. Cancer 49:519–524
615. Whittaker JS, Turner EP (1976) *Papillary tumours of the minor salivary glands*. J Clin Pathol 29:795–805
616. Williams SB, Ellis GL, Auclair PL (1993) *Immunohistochemical analysis of basal cell adenocarcinoma*. Oral Surg Oral Med Oral Pathol 75:64–69
617. Williamson JD, Simmons BH, el-Naggar A, et al. (2000) *Mucoepidermoid carcinoma involving Warthin tumor. A report of five cases and review of the literature*. Am J Clin Pathol 114:564–570
618. Wilson DF, Robinson BW (1984) *Oral inverted ductal papilloma*. Oral Surg Oral Med Oral Pathol 57:520–523
619. Winkle MR, Harrington PC, Maronian N (1999) *Central mucoepidermoid carcinoma of the mandible*. Am J Otolaryngol 20:169–171
620. Wu LY, Cheng J, Lu Y, et al. (2004) *[Epstein-Barr virus infection in benign lymphoepithelial lesions with malignant transformation of salivary glands]*. Zhonghua Kou Qiang Yi Xue Za Zhi 39:291–293
621. Wuketich S, Kittinger G (1966) *[Sebaceous lymphadenoma of the parotid]*. Arch Klin Exp Ohren Nasen Kehlkopfheilkd 187:836 844
622. Yu G, Ussmueller J, Donath K (2000) *[A clinicopathologic study on membranous basal cell adenoma]*. Zhonghua Kou Qiang Yi Xue Za Zhi 35:88–90
623. Yu G, Ussmueller J, Donath K (2000) *[Histogenesis and development of membranous basal cell adenoma of the salivary gland]*. Zhonghua Kou Qiang Yi Xue Za Zhi 35:31–33
624. Yu GY, Ma DQ, Zhang Y, et al. (2004) *Multiple primary tumours of the parotid gland*. Int J Oral Maxillofac Surg 33:531–534
625. Yu GY, Ubmuller J, Donath K (1998) *Membranous basal cell adenoma of the salivary gland: a clinicopathologic study of 12 cases*. Acta Otolaryngol 118:588–593

626. Zarbo RJ (2002) *Salivary gland neoplasia: a review for the practicing pathologist.* Mod Pathol 15:298–323
627. Zarbo RJ, Prasad AR, Regezi JA, et al. (2000) *Salivary gland basal cell and canalicular adenomas: immunohistochemical demonstration of myoepithelial cell participation and morphogenetic considerations.* Arch Pathol Lab Med 124:401–405
628. Zarbo RJ, Regezi JA, Lloyd RV, et al. (1987) *HLA-DR antigens in normal, inflammatory, and neoplastic salivary glands.* Oral Surg Oral Med Oral Pathol 64:577–584
629. Zhao M, Takata T, Ogawa I, et al. (1998) *Immunohistochemical demonstration of bone morphogenetic protein-2 and type II collagen in pleomorphic adenoma of salivary glands.* J Oral Pathol Med 27:293–296
630. Zschoch H (1992) *[Mucus gland infarct with squamous epithelial metaplasia in the lung. A rare site of so-called necrotizing sialometaplasia].* Pathologe 13:45–48

Chapter 4

Biopsy of Minor Salivary Glands of the Lip

William L. Chung

4

Contents

Core Features

- Discussion of common systemic conditions affecting minor salivary glands.
- Armamentarium and technique for biopsy procedure.
- Complications related to biopsy.

Complications to Avoid
- Hemorrhage
- Recurrence of minor salivary gland lesion
- Sensory disturbance

Introduction

Surgery for minor salivary gland pathology requires a high degree of individualization due to the wide range of presenting symptoms. The size and location of the lesion also determines the planned treatment. A number of diagnostic tests can be ordered when minor salivary gland dysfunction is suspected, but a definitive diagnosis of minor salivary gland disease requires histopathologic confirmation. We will review the basic development, anatomy, and function of minor salivary glands in addition to discussing the more common systemic conditions and tumors which affect the minor salivary glands. Additionally the chapter focuses on the armamentarium and technique associated with the biopsy of minor salivary glands.

Development and Anatomy of Minor Salivary Glands and Associated Structures of the Oral Cavity

The salivary glands are divided into two groups: major and minor glands. Three pairs of major salivary glands exist (parotid, submandibular, and sublingual). In adults a variable number of minor salivary glands ranging in the hundreds are located just beneath the epithelium throughout the oral cavity and under the mucosal surface of the lips. Specifically, minor glands are found labially, bucally, lingually, palatally, and glossopalatally.

The developing salivary glands appear as a bud that forms terminal bulbs. These bulbs undergo branching and ultimately form a lumen. Minor salivary glands begin to develop between six and seven weeks in utero. Minor glands are well developed in the newborn infant. The primary function of minor salivary glands is not to produce saliva to mix with foods. Rather, the minor salivary glands secrete minor amounts of saliva to keep the mucosal lining of the oral cavity moist. Approximately 10% of the total saliva comes from the minor salivary glands. The majority of minor salivary glands are mucous, while some are purely serous and others are mixed glands. Minor salivary glands have a structure and histology similar to major glands, but minor glands are significantly smaller and have far less branching than major glands. They do not have any distinct capsule. Each minor gland consists of several small secretory units and it has its own short duct that opens directly into the oral cavity.

The oral cavity is lined by various types of mucosa. The mucosa lining the lips varies in structure and function from other types of mucosa located in the oral cavity. The submucosa consists of connective tissue located just beneath the mucosa. The submucosa contains the blood vessels and nerves. Its presence helps determine the degree of mobility of the mucosal layer depending on the length of the connective tissue ridges and pegs. The arterial supply to the lips arises from the superior and inferior labial branches of the facial artery, while the venous supply occurs through the superior and inferior labial veins. The upper lip is innervated by superior labial branches of the infraorbital nerve and the lower lip is innervated by the mental branch of the inferior alveolar (mandibular) nerve.

Most Common Benign Disorders of Minor Salivary Glands

Mucus extravasation cysts are the most common form of mucoceles of minor salivary glands. Mucus extravasation cysts most frequently occur in the lower lip in a paramedian location, but can also occur in the buccal mucosa or floor of mouth. They are soft, dome-shaped, fluid-filled vesicles that take on a bluish appearance as a result of the mucin (Fig. 4.1). Mucus extravasation cysts often result from trauma to the lip that causes tearing of a duct with extravasation of the mucus into the surrounding connective tissue. They are rarely painful and are usually no greater than a centimeter in diameter. These lesions are typically seen in children and young adults with a peak incidence in the second and third decades. Treatment consists of complete excision with any associated underlying minor salivary glands.

Mucus retention cysts are far less common but clinically indistinguishable from mucus extravasation cysts and are treated in an identical fashion. Mucus retention cysts also have a blue appearance and the onset of these lesions may be uncertain. Other lesions that have a similar color, such as a venous varix, hemangioma, lymphangioma, and a low-grade mucoepidermoid carcinoma, should be considered carefully in the differential diagnosis.

Systemic Disorders Affecting Minor Salivary Glands

Several systemic conditions have been shown to affect minor salivary gland structure and function. These disorders range from an autoimmune, genetic, or noninfectious inflammatory origin to a late complication from bone marrow transplantation. The most significant autoimmune disorder affecting minor salivary glands is *Sjögren's syndrome*. Sjögren's syndrome is characterized by dry eyes (keratoconjunctivitis sicca) and dry mouth (xerostomia). The condition is a result of immune-mediated destruction of the lacrimal and salivary glands. When Sjögren's syndrome occurs as an isolated condition, it is referred to as primary Sjögren's syndrome. When it is associated with another autoimmune disorder, most often rheumatoid arthritis, it is termed secondary Sjögren's syndrome. Sjögren's syndrome predominantly affects women (9:1) over the age of 40 years.

Multiple autoantibody formation is characteristic of Sjögren's syndrome. Approximately 70% of patients with primary Sjögren's syndrome have autoantibodies to two nuclear antigens (SS-A and SS-B). Both SS-A and rheumatoid factor are detectable in nearly 75% of secondary Sjögren's syndrome patients. Several human lymphocyte-associated (HLA) antigens are also commonly linked to Sjögren's syndrome. HLA-B8 and HLA-DR3 are found in primary Sjögren's syndrome, while HLA-DR4 is associated with secondary Sjögren's syndrome. Rheumatoid factor is often positive even in the absence of any clinical manifestations.

The primary histologic feature is progressive periductal lymphocytic infiltration with scattered plasma cells [1, 2]. It is believed that B cells destroy the glandular acinar cells due to a surface antigenicity. Proliferation of ductal epithelium with resultant epimyoepithelial island formation, another characteristic of Sjögren's syndrome, occurs because the myoepithelium and ductal elements lack the antigenicity of the acinar cells. The epimyoepithelial islands commonly occur in major salivary glands but are usually absent in the minor glands.

Numerous studies ranging from advanced imaging techniques and sialography to serology and ophthalmologic studies (Schirmer's test) all help to establish a di-

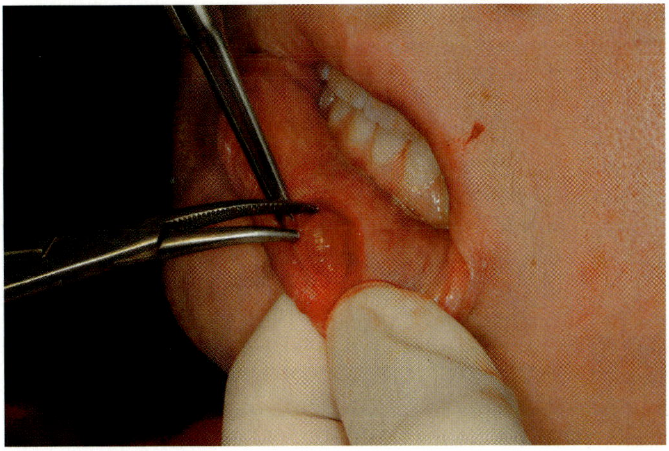

Fig. 4.1: Mucus extravasation cyst. Lower lip everted and mosquito hemostat used to dissect around the cyst

agnosis of Sjögren's syndrome. However, confirmation of Sjögren's syndrome requires a histopathologic diagnosis. Biopsy of labial salivary glands is not preferred over that of parotid glands because the parotid gland is usually more severely affected than minor salivary glands. Nonetheless, biopsy of minor salivary glands in the lips is carried out with far greater ease compared to parotid biopsy. A minimum of five to seven minor glands should be harvested from beneath normal mucosa. One looks for a large (greater than 50) number of lymphocytic foci next to normal acini. More than five foci of lymphocytes per 4 mm^2 is highly consistent with a diagnosis of Sjögren's syndrome.

Cystic fibrosis is the most common fatal genetic disease affecting Caucasian children. Cystic fibrosis has an incidence of 1 in 2,000 live births and is transmitted as an autosomal recessive trait. It affects the secretory process of all exocrine glands, which includes the minor salivary glands. The primary functional abnormality arises when viscous mucous secretions block the respiratory tree and pancreatic ducts, causing the most common and significant clinical manifestations of recurrent and chronic respiratory infections and pancreatic insufficiency. Although the clinical manifestations on the salivary glands are far less profound than those for the other exocrine glands, salivary gland function and salivary composition are altered nonetheless. The structural integrity of the minor salivary glands is only minimally altered by this disorder [3]. However, its function can be significantly compromised, as reported by Mandel [4].

Mandel's studies noted elevated levels of salivary calcium and proteins, particularly in the submandibular and sublingual glands as well as the minor salivary glands [4]. These increases in calcium and protein likely form precipitates that may explain the turbidity in the fluid excreted from the affected glands. Mandel further proposes that these complexes create blockage of the normally narrow, small minor salivary gland ducts. The resultant decrease in salivary excretory rates from the minor glands can be significant. Capillary tubes can be used to measure the flow from the labial glands as a diagnostic test to determine cystic fibrosis. The histology of these labial glands will reveal dilated acini and ducts that are filled with inspissated mucus or plugs.

Granulomatous diseases can affect minor salivary glands. One specific granulomatous, inflammatory condition is *granulomatous cheilitis*. Granulomatous cheilitis has a predilection for the minor glands in the lower lip and causes them to become thickened. The condition is occasionally a manifestation of Melkersson-Rosenthal syndrome, which consists of facial paralysis, labial edema, particularly of the upper lip, and fissured tongue [5, 6]. Granulomatous cheilitis can also be associated with leprosy and Crohn's disease. Another rare granulomatous disorder is *cheilitis glandularis*. The etiology of this condition is unknown, but smoking and prolonged sun exposure have been implicated. The lower lip becomes edematous and fistulous tracts can occur in the most severe forms. The underlying minor glands become inflamed and nodular. Histologically bacterial infiltration with glandular hyperplasia and ductal dilatation can be noted.

Chronic graft-versus-host disease is a late complication of bone marrow transplantation and a major cause of morbidity and mortality. Several studies have reported decreased salivary flow rates ranging from 55% to 90% in patients with this condition [7, 8]. The glandular dysfunction associated with chronic graft-versus-host disease is secondary to chronic sialoadenitis [9, 10]. Alborghetti et al [11] report that the xerostomia ensuing chronic graft-versus-host disease treatment is a result of a persistent lymphocytic infiltrate and the subsequent lack of minor salivary gland secretory unit recovery.

Common Minor Salivary Gland Tumors

Minor salivary gland tumors are usually slow-growing and asymptomatic. The overlying mucosa is typically intact unless occlusal trauma has occurred. Most studies report the majority of minor salivary gland tumors as malignant and major salivary gland tumors as benign. Two studies have reported a higher incidence of minor salivary gland tumors as being malignant [12, 13]. When these tumors occur in older patients, they are more often malignant than when they present in younger patients who are more likely to have benign tumors.

Minor salivary gland tumors are located throughout the oral cavity with the hard palate being the most frequently reported site. Malignant labial minor salivary gland tumors are more commonly located in the lower lip, whereas benign labial minor salivary gland tumors are more often found in the upper lip [12, 13]. Although it is not the intended purpose of this chapter to discuss salivary gland tumors, one particular tumor, the polymorphous low-grade tumor, occurs only in minor salivary glands and has been reported with some frequency in the lips. Thus it will be briefly reviewed so as to coincide with the primary topic of this chapter – biopsy of labial minor salivary glands.

Polymorphous Low-Grade Adenocarcinoma

The *polymorphous low-grade adenocarcinoma* is a slow-growing tumor that does not occur in any of the major salivary glands. It is small, rarely exceeding 4 cm, and typically presents as a firm painless swelling in the palate. This tumor also has been reported in the buccal mucosa, upper lip, and floor of mouth. The polymorphous low-grade adenocarcinoma has a 3:1 predilection for females, with one study even reporting exclusivity to females [14]. Because this tumor has been reported to develop in the tongue base, adenoid cystic carcinoma must also be considered in the differential diagnosis. Both tumors can display perineural invasion, but the polymorphous low-grade adenocarcinoma usually does not spread through the nerves to other structures or invade bone. Histologically the polymorphous low-grade adenocarcinoma consists of cytologically uniform cells with rare mitotic figures. However, the tumor exhibits a significant amount of invasion and infiltration at its margins.

Armamentarium and Technique for Biopsy

The following materials and instruments are helpful when performing an office biopsy of minor salivary glands in the lip: 4×4 gauze pads, no. 15 blade, tissue forceps (Adson's with teeth), mosquito hemostat, tissue scissors, needle driver, and suture scissor. A local anesthetic with epinephrine (1% or 2% lidocaine with 1:100,000 epinephrine) provides improved hemostasis versus a similar anesthetic without a vasoconstrictor. A 4×4 gauze pad is preferred over mechanical suction for keeping the surgical field dry to avoid minor salivary glands or specimens from being accidentally lost to the suction device. The gauze pad is also useful as it allows the clinician to firmly hold the everted lip while absorbing any saliva, so as not to lose handle of the lip.

The lips are the most readily assessable location in the oral cavity to visualize the minor salivary glands. After the lower lip has been firmly grasped and everted, the mucosa is dried with a gauze sponge. Small drops of saliva may become apparent on the mucosal surface, indicating the location of the minor salivary gland ducts. As with any other office-based procedure, biopsy of minor salivary glands of the lip requires the surgeon to adhere to universal precautions to avoid an occupational exposure with the patient's blood or saliva. After obtaining consent from the patient for the biopsy, a local anesthetic with vasoconstrictor is administered in an area of normal overlying mucosa. The no. 15 blade is used to make an 8- to 10-mm incision through the mucosa in the anterior portion of the lip posterior to the vermillion border and wet-dry line. A mosquito hemostat is then used to bluntly dissect through the submucosal layer while the lower lip is tightly and firmly everted. The numerous minor salivary glands will become readily visible as they begin to extrude through the submucosal layer (Fig. 4.2).

The glands can be grasped with tissue forceps and cut at their base with tissue scissors then placed in a bottle of 10% formalin for submission to a pathologist (Figs. 4.3, 4.4). After obtaining the necessary gland, the incision is closed with resorbable suture such as 4-0 chromic in an interrupted fashion.

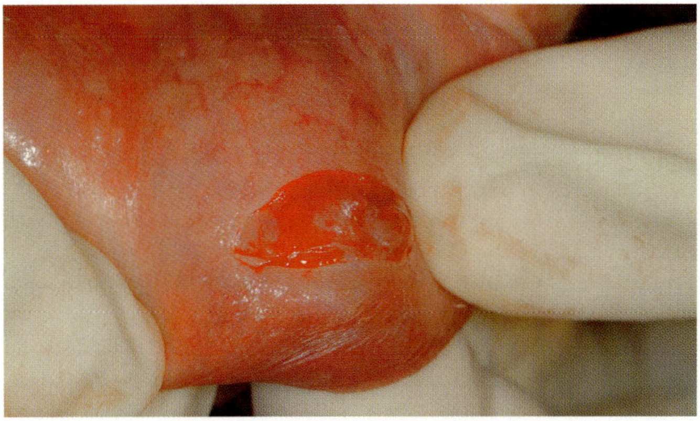

Fig. 4.2: Numerous minor salivary glands visible immediately beneath mucosal incision

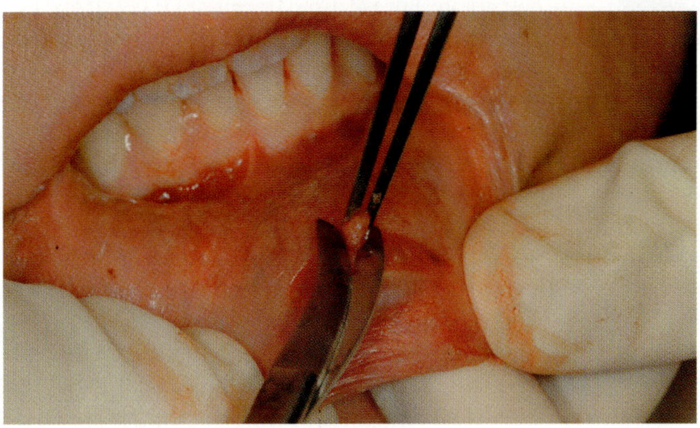

Fig. 4.3: Minor salivary gland held in tissue forceps with scissors used to cut gland at base

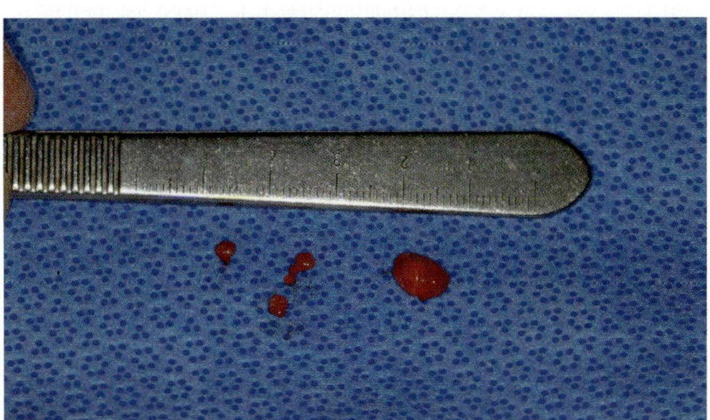

Fig. 4.4: Minor salivary glands along with excised mucocele

4

Complications with Biopsy of Minor Salivary Glands of the Lip

The most common complication associated with biopsy of labial minor salivary glands is hemorrhage. Most hemorrhage can be controlled with direct pressure followed by cauterization of bleeding tissue and/or vessel. Injecting a local anesthetic with a vasoconstrictor into the bleeding tissue also helps to provide hemostasis. If a mucocele or any of its related lesions is incompletely excised or removed without any accessory minor glands deep to the lesion, the lesion may recur. Caution should be exercised when performing a biopsy of the lower lip in a paramedian location. If the incision is carried too deep through the mucosa in an area overlying a terminal branch of the mental nerve, a resultant sensory deficit is possible.

Summary

Treatment for minor salivary gland disease is highly individualized and variable. When definitive diagnosis of certain systemic conditions that affect minor salivary glands is required, histopathologic confirmation can be achieved by a biopsy of the lip. This biopsy is readily performed in the office under local anesthesia. Hemorrhage is the main complication that occurs with biopsy of labial salivary glands. The lower lip is typically chosen for its accessibility.

Take Home Messages

- Lower lip is easiest location for a biopsy of minor salivary glands.
- Local anesthetic with a vasoconstrictor provides better hemostasis for biopsy.
- Biopsy to confirm Sjögren's syndrome requires at least five to seven minor salivary glands.
- When excising a mucus extravasation cyst, remove several minor salivary glands beneath the cyst.

References

1. Tarpley TM, Andersen LG, White CL (1974) Minor salivary gland involvement in Sjogren's syndrome. Oral Surg 37: 64–74
2. Friedman H, Kilmar V, Galletta VP, Cossermelli W (1979) Lip biopsy in connective tissue diseases. Oral Surg 47: 256–262
3. Doggett RG, Belitinck B, Harrison GM (1971) Structure and ultrastructure of the labial salivary glands in patient with cystic fibrosis. J Clin Pathol 24: 270–282
4. Mandel ID (1990) The diagnostic uses of saliva. Oral Med 19:119–125
5. Seifert G, Mielke A, Haubrich J, Chilla R (1986) Diseases of the salivary glands. Thieme, New York
6. Cawson RA, Gleeson MJ, Eveson JW (1997) Pathology and Surgery of the Salivary Glands Isis Medical Media, Oxford
7. Nagler R, Marmary Y, Chisin R, et al. (1996) Major salivary gland dysfunction in human acute and chronic graft versus host disease. Bone Marrow Transplant 17: 219–224
8. Nagler RM, Laufer D, Nagler A (1996) Parotid gland dysfunction in an animal model of chronic graft versus host disease. Arch Otolaryngol Head Neck Surg 122: 1057–1060
9. Schubert MM, Sullivan KM, Morton TH, et al. (1984) Oral manifestations of chronic graft vs. host disease. Arch Intern Med 144: 1591–1595
10. Sale GE, Shulman HM, Schubert MM, et al. (1981) Oral and ophthalmic pathology of graft versus host disease in man: predictive value of the lip biopsy. Hum Pathol 12: 1022–1030
11. Alborghetti MR, Correa MEP, Adam RL, et al. (2005) Late effect of chronic graft-vs.-host disease in minor salivary glands. J Oral Pathol Med 34: 486–493
12. Yih WY, Kratochuil FJ, Stewart JC (2005) Intraoral minor salivary gland neoplasms: review of 212 cases. J Oral Maxillofac Surg 63: 805–810
13. Jansisyanont P, Blanchaert RH Jr, Ord RA (2002) Intraoral minor salivary gland neoplasm: a single institution experience of 80 cases. Int J Oral Maxillofac Surg 31: 257–261
14. Freedman PD, Lumerman H (1983) Lobular carcinoma of intraoral minor salivary gland origin: Report of twelve cases. Oral Surg Oral Med Oral Pathol 56: 157–165

Chapter 5

Treatment of Frey's Syndrome

Pavel Dulguerov

5

Contents

Core features

- Understand the anatomy of the autonomic innervation of the parotid gland and facial skin.
- Frey's syndrome is secondary to the sympathetic denervation of sweat glands – the reinnervation through the auriculotemporal nerve is a secondary event.
- The aberrant regeneration theory explains the physiopathology of Frey's syndrome; other described variants do not represent true Frey's syndrome cases.
- A topographic and quantitative testing for Frey's is required prior to its treatment – the ISPH test described has the majority of desired features.
- Frey's syndrome incidence after parotidectomy, without prevention techniques, is 40–80% by clinical questioning and 80–100% by objective testing.
- Intradermic botulinum toxin injection is a well-tolerated and efficient treatment. The recommended dilution is 50 IU/1 ml, inter-injection distance is 1 cm, and injection volume is 0.1 ml.

Complications to Avoid

- Facial muscle paralysis (rare and reversible complication): inject only intradermally and avoid injecting toward the midline
- Pain during injection: if bothersome could be decreased by the prior application of topical anesthetic cream

Introduction

Frey's syndrome or gustatory sweating and flushing is characterized by sweating and flushing of the facial skin during meals [44]. The area involved is on the lateral aspect of the face and upper neck, usually around the parotid region. There is no direct relation with chewing [44]. Once present, the gustatory sweating and flushing remain unchanged, i.e., there is no spontaneous resolution, even after numerous years [76].

Frey's syndrome is named after Dr. Lucia Frey, a neurologist at the University of Warsaw, who published a landmark paper on the "syndrome du nerf auriculotemporal" in 1923 [44], despite the fact that similar cases were already reported in the nineteenth century [33].

Anatomy and Physiology

During eating, a reflex arc is stimulated leading to increased salivary secretion of minor and major salivary glands, including the parotid gland. The origin of the afferent limb is at the level of the gustatory papillae of the oral cavity and oropharynx. The afferent neurons terminate in the nucleus solitarius and project to the inferior salivary nucleus.

Preganglionic parasympathetic efferent fibers leave the inferior salivary nucleus and the brain stem with the glossopharyngeal nerve. After passing through the jugular foramen and the superior and inferior glossopharyngeal ganglions, the parasympathetic fibers follow the tympanic (Jacobson's) nerve. Jacobse's nerve enters the temporal bone on its inferior aspect and travels in the inferior tympanic canaliculus toward the middle ear cavity. A plexus is formed on the promontory, but the parasympathetic fibers not supplying the middle ear unite to form the lesser superficial petrosal nerve. This nerve exits the temporal bone and travels on the floor of the middle cranial fossa. The fibers then exit the skull through the foramen ovale and reach the otic ganglion where they synapse with postganglionic parasympathetic fibers. These postganglionic parasympathetic fibers then join the auriculotemporal nerve and reach the parotid gland through its medial aspect in the parapharyngeal space. Like all postganglionic parasympathetic neurons, the neurotransmitter of these fibers is acetylcholine. The muscarinic receptors of the parotid gland are of the M3 subtype [21].

The secretion of the parotid gland is controlled predominantly by the parasympathetic system. In cats, stimulation of the parasympathetic fibers produces an important increase of salivary output, while sympathetic stimulation results only in a discrete increase [111]. In human volunteers undergoing stapedectomy for otosclerosis, electric stimulation of the tympanic plexus resulted in an increase of parotid salivary output proportional to the intensity of the applied current [113].

The sympathetic fibers for the cutaneous vessels and sweat glands follow the cervical sympathetic chain and a synaptic relay is found in the sympathetic cervical ganglions. The fibers then follow the periarterial plexuses of the internal and external carotid arteries and their branches before joining and following the branches of the trigeminal nerve supplying the cutaneous sensation of the skin [89, 93]. Thus, for the preauricular skin, these sympathetic fibers also travel within the auriculotemporal nerve. While the overall organization is described in anatomic textbooks, the exact pathway is still debatable [143] and it remains unclear at what exact level of the lower face, a switch from sympathetic fibers traveling along the internal carotid artery to sympathetic fibers traveling with the external carotid artery takes place [32, 93, 143]. It is also possible that at midface there is some overlap, with double sympathetic innervation coursing along the trigeminal nerve and along the external carotid artery [32, 121].

The result of sympathetic activation is increased secretion from sweat glands [116] and vasoconstriction [93]. A vasodilatation role of the parasympathetic facial system [17] has been demonstrated [12] and found to follow the facial nerve and then the greater superficial petrosal branch [82]. Fibers probably synapse in the sphenopalatine ganglion before joining the corresponding branches of the trigeminal nerve [82], in our case the auriculotemporal nerve.

In contradistinction to other postganglionic sympathetic fibers, which are adrenergic, sweat glands have acetylcholine as the main neurotransmitter [42, 86]. The cholinergic receptors on sweat glands are muscarinic, predominantly of the M3 subtype [140] similar to that of parasympathetic salivary gland nerves.

Pathogenesis of Frey's Syndrome

André Thomas [135] and later Ford and Woodhall [41] postulated that the severed parasympathetic fibers to the parotid gland regenerate along the wrong neurilemmal sheaths of the sectioned cutaneous sympathetic fibers, the so-called aberrant regeneration theory. Several experimental and clinical observations support the aberrant regeneration theory: (1) auriculotemporal nerve block by local anesthetics induces a local anesthesia and an abolishment of gustatory sweating of similar cutaneous distribution [41, 48]; (2) stimulation of the tympanic plexus results in sweating in the involved skin area [113]; (3) symptoms are unaffected by anesthesia of the stellate ganglion, despite the appearance of a temporary Horner syndrome [30, 41, 48]; (4) in the involved area, there is an impairment of the normal sympathetic function, such as reduced thermoregulatory sweating [29, 41, 48, 58, 89] and absence of emotional flushing [29, 41, 58, 89]; (5) a latent period (minimum 1–2 months [77]) is present between the initial injury and the appearance of gustatory flushing and sweating [48, 58, 88, 89, 145]; (6) if patients are followed sequentially with an appropriate sweat test, the positivity of the test increases and the involved area progressively increases in size [77, 88]; (7) the symptoms can be abolished by the local injection of anticholinergic substances such as atropine [41, 48], as well as botulinum toxin (see below); (8) a localized hypersensitivity to cholinergic drugs is described with mecholine [145], acetylcholine [41, 48], and pilocarpine [48, 145]; and (9) the syndrome appears after various lesions or resections of the homolateral cervical sympathetic chain [29, 58, 89, 102, 145].

The postulated etiology is an aberrant regeneration of the sectioned parasympathetic fibers normally innervating the parotid gland (Fig. 5.1). The traumatized fibers lose their parotid targets and regenerate to innervate the vessels and sweat glands of the overlying skin. In order for this aberrant regeneration to occur, the sympathetic fibers to these vessels and sweat glands have to be damaged, a frequent event in either parotid surgery or penetrating parotid trauma. The regular function of the parotid parasympathetic fibers is to increase salivary secretion during eating. The activation following aberrant regeneration produces an activation of the new targets during meals, resulting in a local vasodilatation ("gustatory flushing") and localized sweating ("gustatory sweating"). Despite all these convincing arguments, the aberrant regeneration remains a hypothesis until the demonstration of parasympathetic neurons on reinnervated sweat glands.

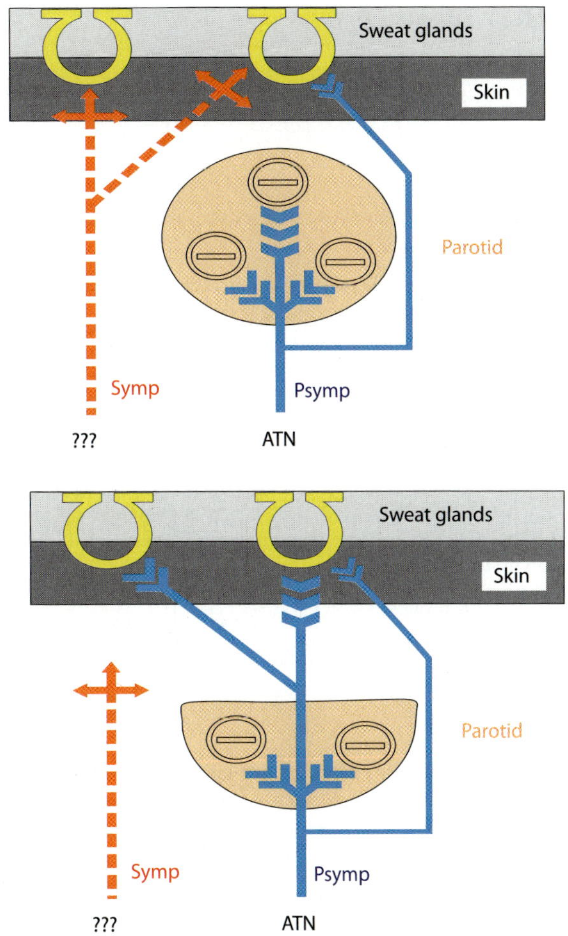

Fig. 5.1: Schematic representation of the aberrant regeneration theory. *Top* Normal situation. *Bottom* Situation after superficial parotidectomy. *Symp* Sympathetic innervation of sweat glands, *Psymp* parasympathetic innervation of the parotid and facial skin, *ATN* auriculotemporal nerve, *???* sympathetic nerve, the exact pathway of which is still unclear (auriculotemporal nerve, great auricular nerve, perivascular plexuses)

Etiology

Since Frey, emphasis has been placed on the auriculotemporal nerve [113] and the regeneration of the parasympathetic fibers it contains [41, 135] to explain gustatory sweating and flushing. Although parotidectomy is the most frequent etiology [35], the syndrome has been described with other surgical procedures in the parotid region such as mandibular surgery [54, 72, 138], drainage of parotid or other local abscesses [6, 50, 98, 103, 107, 144] and neck dissection [56, 84, 99, 133]; with regional trauma such as mandibular fractures [47, 52, 85, 148] or penetrating wounds [5, 37]; and with surgery or lesions of the cervical sympathetic chain [20, 58, 83, 89, 102, 105, 145] (Table 5.1).

5

Table 5.1. Etiology of Frey's syndrome

Typical Frey's syndrome etiologies:
1. Trauma in the parotid region • Parotidectomy • Other surgical procedures in the parotid region (mandibular surgery, drainage of parotid abscess, neck dissection) • Penetrating trauma parotid region • Closed mandibular fractures
2. Trauma to the cervical sympathetic chain
3. Other aberrant regeneration locations • Cerebellopontine angle • Middle ear • Otic ganglion
4. Autonomic neuropathies • Diabetic neuropathy
Atypical variants of gustatory sweating:
1. Physiologic
2. Pediatric gustatory flushing
3. Gustatory neuralgia

The development of gustatory sweating after cervical sympathectomy can only be explained if one is to admit that the primary event of gustatory sweating is a degeneration of the cervical sympathetic neurons. The initial event is the loss of postganglionic sympathetic neurons and the resulting denervation of the corresponding facial sweat glands. Regeneration of parasympathetic fibers, within the degenerating sympathetic neurilemmal sheets, is a secondary event although it accounts for the observed symptoms. If sympathetic degeneration is the primary event then Frey's syndrome could occur in any location where close contact between parasympathetic sialogogue fibers and sympathetic sudomotor efferents is present. This perspective allows the explanation of the location of Frey's syndrome outside the auriculotemporal nerve territory [84], the presence of gustatory sweating away from the flap elevation area [84], as well as such etiologies as cervical sympathectomy, diabetic and possibly other autonomic neuropathy [91].

Often in the preantibiotic literature, gustatory sweating is described as following "parotitis." A closer look at most of these publications shows that most of the cases described had had drainage of a parotid abscess, although in these publications various etiologies were proposed. The cause of Frey's syndrome is not the infection but the surgical drainage. No recent case of gustatory sweating resulting from parotid infection has been reported.

More bizarre etiologies for facial gustatory sweating, in single case reports, include herpes simplex of the mandibular division of the trigeminal nerve [31], a case of a large cerebellopontine angle tumor [123], and "gustatory otorrhea" [115]. These cases could also be explained by the aberrant regeneration theory, with the locus of cross-fiber regeneration being at the level of the maxillary division of the trigeminal nerve [123], at the level of the middle ear [115], or in the deep portion of the auriculotemporal nerve instead of the parotid space portion of the auriculotemporal nerve [31]. A similar explanation, i.e., peripheral parasympathetic sprouting to degenerated sympathetic fibers, has been offered for the observed facial, and often neck and upper chest, gustatory sweating seen in patients with severe diabetic neuropathy [13, 15, 43, 59, 65, 134, 139, 142].

A certain amount of "physiologic" gustatory sweating and flushing can be induced by certain spicy foods such as chilies in normal subjects [86]. A variation of the threshold of individual cutaneous regions appears to be present, since only certain head and neck areas are found to respond in a given individual [86]. In contradistinction to Frey's syndrome, this "physiologic" gustatory sweating and flushing is bilateral and usually symmetrical [86], similar to physiologic thermal sweating [109]. In fact the cutaneous distribution of this physiologic gustatory sweating was found to be similar to that of hyperthermic head and neck sweating and flushing [86].

The few cases of gustatory sweating in the pediatric age group that have been described [7, 8, 22, 40, 68, 70, 130, 147] merit careful review because they possibly represent the only etiology, not easily explained by the aberrant regeneration theory. The majority of the cases described are normal children with unilateral [7, 8, 22, 40, 70, 130, 147] or bilateral gustatory facial flushing [22, 68], without any sweating. The absence of facial sweating, a hallmark of Frey's syndrome, in these cases tends to make us consider them as variations of normal. Maybe the term "gustatory flushing syndrome," as proposed by Kozma and Gabriel [70], might be more appropriate. Another argument against accepting these few cases as Frey's syndrome is that, with a follow-up of several years, a gradual resolution of the symptoms occur [22, 70, 95], in contradistinction to typical gustatory sweating. A final consideration is the possible role of traumatic forceps delivery, pointed out by Balfour and Bloom [7] because about half of the pediatric "gustatory flushing" cases follow a forceps delivery [7, 8, 22, 68, 130].

In addition, a "gustatory otorrhea" in a two patients without any previous pathology has been reported [110, 131].

Recently several cases of facial pain in the territory of the auriculotemporal nerve have been described [24, 124, 127, 136] and the name "gustatory neuralgia" proposed [124]. Other specific characteristics of gustatory neuralgia include an electric, burning (neuralgic) pain, pain distribution in the territory of the auriculotemporal nerve, triggering of the pain by eating, numbness in the auriculotemporal territory because of surgery, and lack of response to anticonvulsant medication [124]. Gustatory neuralgia should be differentiated from classical Frey's syndrome because of the absence of sweating and flushing and because pain is not a symptom in patients with Frey's syndrome [30, 38]. The authors describing this "gustatory neuralgia" refer to the 1979 paper of Hanowell et al. [56] as a justification for the presence of pain in Frey's syndrome patients, however Hanowell's patients had composite resections and neck dissections which was probably responsible for the observed pain.

Investigation of Gustatory Sweating

Since the most troublesome symptom of Frey's syndrome is sweating, testing for Frey's syndrome has in general been limited to the evaluation of sweating. Only Laage-Hellmann investigated flushing, and this was done by simple direct observation and without any quantification [74, 77]. We attempted to study skin color changes, without being convincingly able to demonstrate them in patients with Frey's syndrome (Dulguerov, unpublished). Temperature skin changes were demonstrated in four patients in one study [64] and another used lactate content in an attempt to quantify the amount of sweat [79].

Testing for gustatory sweating is, therefore, assessing the function of eccrine sweat glands. The major function of sweat glands in humans is thermoregulation [118]. About 2–4 million sweat glands are distributed over the entire human body with a density varying from 60 glands/cm^2 on the back to 600 glands/cm^2 on the palms and soles [117]. The maximal sweat rate is about 2–20 nl/min per gland [118]. The face has about 250 glands/cm^2 and thus the maximal facial sweat rate should be about 0.5–5 µl/min per cm^2 or 5–50 ml/min per m^2. Sweat is a hypotonic solution that contains mainly sodium chloride, potassium, and bicarbonate, as well as certain inorganic compounds such as lactate, urea, and ammonia [116, 118].

Tests of autonomic thermoregulatory function are complex [90] and the measure of sweat output is just one of the aspects assessed. Tests of sweat output function measure the production of sweat by a group of sweat glands and these tests could be classified as: (1) topographic, where a chemical reaction provides a view of the anatomic location of sweat secretion; (2) electric, where a change of skin impedance by the humidity of sweat is measured; and (3) thermodynamic, where the skin humidity is evaporated and a "sudometer" measures the thermal mass of the air stream [90]. Advantages of the electric and thermodynamic tests include the possibility of repeated and dynamic measures, while topographic tests give a better representation of surface and anatomic distribution.

The ideal test method for gustatory sweating should provide topographic information and quantification of the amount of sweating. While dynamic measures might be interesting in investigational studies, their use in clinical practice is of limited value. Further characteristics of the test should include: (1) simplicity (one-step); (2) sensitivity; (3) reliability; (4) adequate dynamic range, so that different sweating rates could be appreciated; (5) absence of toxicity and allergenicity of the agents used; (6)

easy removal from the skin of the applied agents; and (7) low cost [36, 117].

The most frequently used method of sweat secretion assessment for gustatory sweating was originally described by Victor Minor, a Russian neurologist [96]. The original solution described contains 1.5 g iodine, 10 g castor oil, and 88.5 g of absolute alcohol and is painted on the skin to be tested. Actually, any colored iodine solution used for disinfections, such as Betadine, will work [49]. After drying, the areas are powdered with starch (regular baking corn starch works fine). The water in the sweat produces blue coloring by a reduction reaction of the iodine-starch mixture. With limited sweat production, the apertures of individual sweat glands are marked as small blue dots, while with larger amounts of sweat secretion the blue dots are larger and eventually become confluent. Therefore, the Minor test is seen as a topographic method allowing accurate mapping of the involved surface.

Disadvantages of the Minor test include the necessary application of several layers of reagents, the difficulty of removing the iodine paint, the possible allergy to iodine [119], and the difficulty of using the method with heavy perspiration, since the sweat tends to drip down, obscuring the assessment of the more dependently located skin [36]. While it could be seen as objective, it is not a quantitative test and therefore might not be suited for the comparison of two treatments [34, 35]. In addition the topographic information provided by the Minor test is cumbersome to use with the newer treatments involving local intradermal injections, because the applied reagents should be removed and the skin disinfected prior to injection while maintaining the topographic mapping.

Several modifications of the Minor test have been proposed but all of these share the inconveniences of the original test [1, 36]. Randall [109], noting that some papers have starch coatings, modified the method by using paper instead of starch, but continued to paint the skin with the iodine-based mixture. Dole and Thaysen [26] further simplified the process by the use of paper that was coated with iodine. Unfortunately this method seems to have been forgotten until recently [36].

We recently applied two techniques for the evaluation of gustatory sweating [36]. The blotting paper method simply uses the difference in weight of a piece of blotting paper before and after gustatory stimulation. In the iodine-sublimated paper histogram (ISPH) method, regular office paper is sublimated with iodine and acquires the property of changing color when wetted. The paper is than digitized and a histogram algorithm applied to measure the area of color change [36]. A calibration of these tests with known and appropriate quantities of saline was performed and an excellent correlation found.

These tests (blotting paper and ISPH) satisfy most of the requirements of an ideal sweat test: quantitative test, simplicity, sensitivity, reliability, adequate dynamic range, absence of toxicity and allergenicity, easy removal from the skin of the applied agents, and low cost. In addition, these two tests give complementary data. While the quantitative data obtained with the blotting paper method is excellent, the topographic information is suboptimal. The topographic data of ISPH technique is excellent, providing a mirror image of the facial sweating area.

Incidence

The reported incidence of gustatory sweating after parotidectomy is highly variable and "depends on the diligence with which it is sought and the time-interval from surgery" [132]. The publications of Laage-Hellmann [74–77] in the late 1950s constitute the first serious attempt to study this problem. A group of 123 patients who underwent a parotidectomy was evaluated retrospectively with a questionnaire and clinical testing. On questioning, 62% of the patients complained of problems during eating: 22% had both sweating and flushing, 26% had sweating only, and 14% had only flushing. When a gustatory stimulus was used, flushing was observed in 92% of patients, and 98% of patients exhibited a positive Minor test. Laage-Hellmann [74–77] concluded that gustatory sweating is an unavoidable sequel of parotidectomy that is not overtly symptomatic in all patients. The incidence of clinical and objective gustatory sweating following parotidectomy in publications using an objective evaluation technique is summarized in Table 5.2.

The severity of the gustatory sweating was judged moderate by 58% of patients, important by 15%, and embarrassing by 27% [74]. Lower percentage of important and embarrassing symptoms have been found in other studies [88]. The correlation between the severity of sweating and intensity of the Minor test was not good [39, 74].

More recently, the clinical severity has been correlated to the surface involved [79, 88] and to the extent of parotid surgery (superficial versus total) [46, 53, 79]. There has been an ongoing debate on the role of the thickness of the flap raised prior to the actual parotidectomy, as originally suggested by Singleton and Cassisi [129]. Others have not substantiated this point of view [88].

Table 5.2. Incidence of Frey's syndrome

Author	Year	Number of patients	Incidence of clinical Frey's syndrome (%)	Incidence of objective Frey's syndrome (%)
Laage-Hellman [74]	1958	123	62	98
Kornblut et al. [69]	1974	35	43	97
Gordon and Fiddian [53]	1976	50	34	100
Farrell and Kalnins [39][a]	1991	21	14	43
Yu and Hamilton [146]	1992	35	6	14
Allison and Rappaport [2]	1993	35	83	87
Linder et al. [88]	1997	26	43	96
Nosan et al. [104]	1991	23	44	70
Dulguerov et al. [35]	1999	24	53	76
Laskawi et al. [84]	1998	81	63	100
Cavalot [16]	2000	86	47	86

Incidence of Frey's syndrome in the literature using questioning (clinical) and objective testing. No Frey's syndrome prevention techniques were used in these patient cohorts

[a]Farrell and Kalnins [39] used a modified Minor test with Betadine and four of their patients underwent postoperative radiation therapy. Modified from Dulguerov et al. [35]

The delay between parotidectomy and the appearance of gustatory sweating was examined by sequential Minor tests by Laage-Hellman [77]. The minimal delay was 5 weeks and the median delay for a positive Minor test was approximately 8 weeks. The test was positive before patients started to complain about gustatory sweating. In some patients, the test became positive at 9 months and in less then 1% of patients did gustatory sweating appear after 1 year. While most other authors [84, 88] have confirmed this timeframe, clinical manifestation of gustatory sweating have been reported to appear up to 8.5 years after parotidectomy [60].

Available Treatments

The treatment modalities proposed for gustatory sweating can be classified in five main groups: (1) external radiotherapy; (2) local or systemic application of anticholinergic drugs; (3) section of some portion of the efferent neural arc; (4) interposition of a subcutaneous barrier, as used for Frey's syndrome prevention; and (5) injection of botulinum toxin in the involved skin. Considering that the symptoms are not always very troublesome, it is important that the treatment itself does not result in more serious side effects.

Radiotherapy

Radiotherapy was first attempted by Needles [101]. In Laage-Hellman's studies irradiated patients had a lower incidence of gustatory sweating [74], with the involved surface often outside the radiotherapy fields. Similar hints can be drawn from other publications [4, 23, 88], indicating that should radiotherapy be indicated, the expected incidence and severity of gustatory sweating will be low.

Anticholinergic Medication

The attempts to treat gustatory sweating with systemic anticholinergic medications [101] were put to rest by the study of Shelley and Horvath who showed that none of the substances available could be used in accepted doses to reduce the sweating produced by 0.1 cc intradermal injection of pilocarpine [128]. In addition, these authors showed that local iontophoresis or application of anticholinergic drugs such as scopolamine could be used to reduce sweating [128]. Laage-Hellman was the first to apply scopolamine (3% cream) for the treatment of gustatory sweating [77], with symptom reduction in male and abolition in female patients. The difference was tentatively explained by a thinner female skin. Double-blind studies, have shown topical glycopyrrolate [60, 61, 94], aluminum chloride [11, 63, 122], and diphemanil methylsulfate [80] to be superior to placebo. Few patients experienced minor side effects such as dry mouth. However, the population in each of these studies was small, and only one publication is available on patients treated with these drugs for longer periods [61]. Despite the effectiveness of these preparations, patients seem, in the long run [88], to abandon the cumbersome daily application requiring skin drying with a hairdryer and avoiding shaving for 12 h [132]. In addition, skin wounds or infection, as well as application to the mucosa of the eyes, mouth, and nose result in an enhanced absorption and side effects [60].

Interruption of the Efferent Pathway

Section of the auriculotemporal nerve was originally described by Leriche for the treatment of traumatic parotid fistula [87]. Coldwater [19] and more recently Debets and Munting [25] attempted auriculotemporal nerve section, with only partial and temporary decrease of the symptoms [57]. Also, the access to this deeply located region is complex and carries the risk of injuring several important structures, including the facial nerve. At the other end of the efferent pathway, a division of the intracranial portion of the glossopharyngeal nerve was done by Gardner and McCubbin [45], with a good result lasting 5 years in one patient and a short period of relief in a second one. Because of the extensive surgery, this therapy has not been pursued.

Hemenway [62] in 1960 suggested interrupting the efferent neuronal pathway at the level of the middle ear, by sectioning the tympanic nerve of Jacobson. The first such procedure for gustatory sweating was carried out by Golding-Wood, who named it "tympanic neurectomy" [51], in three patients with apparently excellent results. Other authors' experience [57, 60, 106, 113] has been less enthusiastic: all patients were initially improved, but a longer follow-up was associated with recurrence of symptoms in most cases. While tympanic neurectomy appears to be based on solid physiopathologic grounds, does not seem too risky, and can be done under local anesthesia, the paucity of recent reports probably attests its lack of effectiveness.

Surgical Interposition

Sessions et al. [125] pioneered the use of a barrier between the facial skin and the parotid bed in the treatment of established Frey's syndrome. They used the surgical interposition of a fascia lata graft in four patients with excellent results. This technique appeared to be effective in the small group of patients reported [125, 141]. Probably a major deterrent of its use is the risk of facial nerve paralysis during reoperation, since the nerve lies just under the skin after superficial or total parotidectomy. A variation of this technique with the use of a pedicled temporal fascia has been reported [114] in a case without prior facial nerve dissection.

Botulinum Toxin

The injection of botulinum A toxin in the skin involved by gustatory sweating was recently proposed by Drobik and Laskawi [28]. Following their case report, the technique has been progressively adopted [3, 9, 10, 16, 28, 34, 38, 55, 73, 78, 81, 84, 100, 108, 137]. Numerous advantages can be cited for the use of botulinum toxin in the treatment of Frey's syndrome. The substance is relatively well known and has been used for a variety of pathologies in the last 25 years with few side effects [66]. Its use is rather simple in the office setting, and avoids complex procedures in the operating room. The only disadvantages are the pain associated with the needle sticking and the secondary reluctance of some patients to be stuck, especially on the face.

Mechanism of Botulinum Toxin Action

Eight serotypes (A, B, Cα, Cβ, D, E, F, and G) of botulinum toxins are produced by different strains of the anaerobic bacteria *Clostridium botulinum* of which only four (A, B, E, and F) are toxic to humans [71]. Although these serotypes are structurally (dimers of a large 150-kD and light

50-kD chains) and functionally (acetylcholine release inhibition) similar, they represent different pharmacologic entities because of the differences in membrane receptor binding sites and intracellular targets.

The action of botulinum toxins is that of highly specific endopeptidases that cleave cytosol proteins involved in the fusion of exocytosis vesicles with the cell membrane [97], with type A toxin acting on synaptosome-associated protein (SNAP)-25 [14] and type B toxin acting on vesicle-associated membrane protein (VAMP) [120]. This action is highly specific for cholinergic synapses because the specific membrane proteins required for the internalization of botulinum toxins are found only in the presynaptic endings of cholinergic synapses [18]. By blocking the exocytosis mechanism of the presynaptic terminal, the release of acetylcholine is inhibited. The synapse remains intact but is non-functional and for neuromuscular junctions results in muscle paralysis. The recovery of function is due to collateral sprouting from the same or other axons and the formation of new synapses.

Practical Aspects

Botulinum toxin A has been approved by the Food and Drug Administration (FDA) since 1989 and is commercially available as Botox (Allergan, Irvine, CA) and Dysport (Speywood Pharmaceuticals, Maidenhead, UK). In the USA only Botox is available and FDA approved for muscular dystonia, blepharospasm, and glabellar rhytids. Type B toxin has more recently become available as Myobloc in the USA and Neurobloc in Europe (Elan Pharmaceuticals, San Francisco, CA) and is approved by the FDA for cervical muscular dystonia [27].

A Botox vial contains 100 IU of botulinum toxin A, 0.5 mg of human albumin, and 0.9 mg of NaCl as a sterile powder that can remain in a refrigerator for at least 24 months. A Dysport vial contains 500 IU of type A toxin–hemagglutinin complex, 125 g of albumin solution, and 2.5 mg of lactose in a sterile powder form. Botox is diluted with 2–5 ml of 0.9% saline solution, while 1 ml is typically used for Dysport [27]. The solution should also remain refrigerated and is said to lose potency after a few hours. Lowe demonstrated that 1 IU of Botox was approximately equivalent in potency to 4 m.u. of Dysport for the treatment of hyperfunctional upper facial expression lines [92], however more recent data seem to indicate a factor of 3 [112].

The practical considerations for botulinum toxin treatment in Frey's syndrome include:

Mapping of the facial surface to be treated by a technique described earlier; we use the ISPH method because it gives excellent topographic information without dripping and staining [34]. With any technique the contour of the area to be injected is drawn on the patient's face.

A grid of 1 cm squares is drawn either physically on the face or an "imaginary" one is created by the physician. We prefer the latter approach and use the minute bleeding from the needle puncture sites as guides.

If anesthetic is to be used it should be applied at this time. Local anesthetic cream (EMLA, Astra, Sweden) is what we have used occasionally.

The delimited area is injected at sites 1 cm apart which are infiltrated with 0.1 ml (5 IU) of a solution containing botulinum toxin at a concentration of 5 IU/0.1 ml (2 cc per bottle of Botox powder) [34]. The injection should be strictly intradermal, rising tiny wheals at each injection site. A light massage of the area is used for local diffusion.

While a consensus on the exact botulinum toxin injection modalities for gustatory sweating treatment is lacking, experimental data favor the 10-mm inter-injection distance and an injection dose of 0.1 ml (Table 5.3). The 10-mm inter-injection distance is supported by the data of Shaari and Sanders for neuromuscular junctions [126]: injections 10 mm away from the motor end plate band of rat tibialis anterior muscle are ineffective in inducing paralysis. In the same experimental system, increasing the dose and volume of botulinum toxin resulted in increased paralysis. A 20-fold increase in dose doubled the paralysis; however, little gain was achieved with injection doses above 5 IU [126]. As far as volume is concerned, a 100-fold increase in volume was necessary to double the paralysis [126].

Studies on human sweat glands partially support these data [71]. Small volumes of concentrated botulinum toxin have the advantage of minimizing the diffusion and possible side effects. However, if side effects do occur they would be more disabling because of the higher concentration [126]. We [34] and others [55] used a concentration of 50 IU/ml, with the idea that a smaller volume of injection will produce less discomfort and be more efficacious. This is probably necessary in zones with intense facial gustatory sweating. Others [10, 78, 81, 84, 100] have

5

Table 5.3. Botulinum toxin treatment of Frey's syndrome

Study	Year	Patients	Botox dilution (U/ml)	Inter-injection distance (cm)	Dose per injection	Dose per patient (U)	Maximal dose used
Bjerkhoel [10]	1997	14	25	1	0.1 ml	38±12	62.5
Naumann [100]	1997	45	20	1.5	0.05–0.1 ml	21±14	72
Laccourreye [81]	1998	12	25	1	0.1 ml	65	88
Laskawi [84]	1998	19	25	2	0.1 ml	31	100
Cavalot [16]	2000	40	25	1	0.1 ml	?	200
Dulguerov [34]	2000	16	50	1	0.1 ml	41±22	75
Guntinas-Lichius [55][a]	2002	20	25	1	0.1 ml	37±9	?
		20	50	1	0.1 ml	62±20	?
Beerens [9][a]	2002	13	20	2	0.1 ml	25	38
Tugnoli [137][a]	2002	17	20	1.5	0.1 ml	25–55	55
Eckardt [38]	2003	33	?	1.5	1 IU	16–80	80

Principal characteristics of botulinum toxin injections used for the treatment of Frey's syndrome. Only publications with more than 10 patients were included. Data from Kuttner et al. [73] were not tabulated because several of the selected parameters could not be extracted

[a]The botulinum toxin preparation used was Dysport and the Botox equivalents are approximate, with a presumed equivalence of 1 IU Botox = 4 m.u. Dysport [92]. Modified from Dulguerov [35]

obtained good results with a lower dilution (25 IU/ml), and this dosage might be advantageous in patients who have a large surface of gustatory sweating. Guntinas-Lichius compared two concentrations of botulinum toxin and found that the higher concentration is associated with longer recurrence-free intervals [55]. However, a total dose per patient should remain limited to less than 100 IU per session.

Side Effects

We did not experience any facial paralysis side effects of the botulinum toxin injection, as reported by others [9, 10, 81]. It is difficult to understand how a strictly intradermal injection can result in paralysis of facial nerve branches, because the membrane receptors responsible for the cholinergic specificity of botulinum toxins are located only in the presynaptic terminals and not in nerve fiber trunks. Therefore, the most plausible explanation of this rare and partial temporary paresis [9] is an injection deep to the dermis and/or diffusion to facial motor end plates.

The pain associated with the needle injection was evaluated by our patients to be minimal (2/10 on an analog visual pain scale) [34], a result found also in other studies [10, 81]. The use of local anesthetic cream (EMLA, Astra, Sweden) might be tried in the few patients reluctant to undergo this procedure [10].

Since the various botulinum toxins are foreign proteins it is surprising that the incidence of antibodies and allergic reaction is low. The development of antibodies seems related to the amount of protein load injected and the shortness of the interval between injections [27]. The incidence was about 5–10% with the original Allergan batch (#79-11) but has decreases to less than 1% with current Botox preparations [27, 67]. There is no overt hypersensitivity reaction but the blocking antibodies result in decreased effectiveness of the botulinum toxin preparation. These patients could benefit from botulinum toxin B or F preparations.

Therapeutic Results

In our and most published series, all patients treated have a complete resolution of their clinical symptoms. Lower total doses per patient were used by Arad-Cohen and Blitzer resulting in the necessity to repeat the injections several times prior to obtaining a complete response [3]. In our study, objective testing demonstrated a decrease of the surface involved from 29±22 cm^2, before treatment, to 0.6±0.4 cm^2, after treatment [34].

The duration of the effect of botulinum toxin on gustatory sweating is rather long lasting, with an average of 15 months [9, 78, 84]. An actuarial estimate puts the clinical gustatory sweating recurrence at 1, 2, and 3 years at 27%, 63%, and 92%, respectively [78]. The severity of the recurrent Frey's syndrome was found to be reduced when compared to that of the initial episode and retreatment with botulinum toxin was still effective [78]. A clear explanation for this longer timeframe relative to neuromuscular indications is lacking, but different possibilities have been suggested [84], such as an atrophy of the sweat glands, poor sprouting of autonomic fibers, and increased scarring impeding regenerating axons.

Take Home Messages

- Frey's syndrome is an almost unavoidable complication of parotidectomy, if no preventive techniques are employed.
- Frey's syndrome occurs months to years after surgery and is explained by aberrant regeneration of parasympathetic sialogogue fibers to cutaneous sweat glands.
- The treatment of Frey's syndrome with botulinum toxin is effective and is, in experienced hands, almost free of complications.

References

1. Adie R (1968) Gustatory sweating. Aust N Z J Surg 38:98–103
2. Allison GR, Rappaport I (1993) Prevention of Frey's syndrome with superficial musculoaponeurotic system interposition. Am J Surg 166:407–410
3. Arad-Cohen A, Blitzer A (2000) Botulinum toxin treatment for symptomatic Frey's syndrome. Otolaryngol Head Neck Surg 122:237–240
4. Armitstead PR, Smiddy FG, Frank HG (1979) Simple enucleation and radiotherapy in the treatment of the pleomorphic salivary adenoma of the parotid gland. Br J Surg 66:716–717
5. Baddour HM, Ripley JF, Cortez EA, et al. (1980) Treatment of Frey's syndrome by an interpositional fascia graft: report of case. J Oral Surg 38:778–781
6. Baillarger M (1853) Mémoire sur l'oblitération du canal de Sténon. Gaz Med Paris 23:194–197
7. Balfour HH Jr., Bloom JE (1970) The auriculotemporal syndrome beginning in infancy. J Pediatr 77:872–874
8. Beck SA, Burks AW, Woody RC (1989) Auriculotemporal syndrome seen clinically as food allergy. Pediatrics 83:601–603
9. Beerens AJ, Snow GB (2002) Botulinum toxin A in the treatment of patients with Frey syndrome. Br J Surg 89:116–119
10. Bjerkhoel A, Trobbe O (1997) Frey's syndrome: treatment with botulinum toxin. J Laryngol Otol 111:839–844
11. Black MJ, Gunn A (1990) The management of Frey's syndrome with aluminium chloride hexahydrate antiperspirant. Ann R Coll Surg Engl 72:49–52
12. Blair DA, Glover WE, Roddie JC (1961) Cutaneous vasomotor nerves to the head and trunk. J Appl Physiol 16:119–122
13. Blair DI, Sagel J, Taylor I (2002) Diabetic gustatory sweating. South Med J 95:360–362
14. Blasi J, Chapman ER, Link E, et al. (1993) Botulinum neurotoxin A selectively cleaves the synaptic protein SNAP-25. Nature 365:160–163
15. Bronshvag MM (1978) Spectrum of gustatory sweating, with especial reference to its presence in diabetics with autonomic neuropathy. Am J Clin Nutr 31:307–309
16. Cavalot AL, Palonta F, Preti G, et al. (2000) Post-parotidectomy Frey's syndrome. Treatment with botulinum toxin type A. Acta Otorhinolaryngol Ital 20:187–191
17. Chorobski J, Penfield W (1932) Cerebral vasodilatator nerves and their pathway from the medulla oblongata, with observation on the pial and intracerebral vascular plexus. Arch Neurol Psychiatr 28:1257–1289
18. Coffield JA, Considine RV, Simpson LL (1994) The site and mechanism of action of botulinum neurotoxin. In: Jankovic J, Hallett M, editors. (1994) The site and mechanism of action of botulinum neurotoxin. ed. New York: Marcel Drekker Inc
19. Coldwater KB (1954) Surgical treatment of the auriculotemporal syndrome. AMA Arch Surg 69:54–57
20. Cunliffe WJ, Johnson CE (1967) Gustatory hyperhidrosis. A complication of thyroidectomy. Br J Dermatol 79:519–526

5

21. Dai YS, Ambudkar IS, Horn VJ, et al. (1991) Evidence that M3 muscarinic receptors in rat parotid gland couple to two second messenger systems. Am J Physiol 261:C1063–1073
22. Davis RS, Strunk RC (1981) Auriculotemporal syndrome in childhood. Am J Dis Child 135:832–833
23. Dawson AK, Orr JA (1985) Long-term results of local excision and radiotherapy in pleomorphic adenoma of the parotid. Int J Radiat Oncol Biol Phys 11:451–455
24. De Benedittis G (1990) Auriculotemporal syndrome (Frey's syndrome) presenting as tic douloureux. Report of two cases. J Neurosurg 72:955–958
25. Debets JM, Munting JD (1992) Parotidectomy for parotid tumours: 19-year experience from The Netherlands. Br J Surg 79:1159–1161
26. Dole VP, Thaysen JH (1953) Variation in the functional power of human sweat glands. J Exp Med 98:129–144
27. Dressler D, Hallett M (2006) Immunological aspects of Botox, Dysport and Myobloc/NeuroBloc. Eur J Neurol 13(suppl 1):11–15
28. Drobik C, Laskawi R (1995) Frey's syndrome: treatment with botulinum toxin. Acta Otolaryngol 115:459–461
29. Drummond PD (1994) Sweating and vascular responses in the face: normal regulation and dysfunction in migraine, cluster headache and harlequin syndrome. Clin Auton Res 4:273–285
30. Drummond PD (1995) Mechanisms of physiological gustatory sweating and flushing in the face. J Auton Nerv Syst 52:117–124
31. Drummond PD, Boyce GM, Lance JW (1987) Postherpetic gustatory flushing and sweating. Ann Neurol 21:559–563
32. Drummond PD, Lance JW (1987) Facial flushing and sweating mediated by the sympathetic nervous system. Brain 110 793–803
33. Dulguerov P, Marchal F, Gysin C (1999) Frey syndrome before Frey: the correct history. Laryngoscope 109:1471–1473
34. Dulguerov P, Quinodoz D, Cosendai G, et al. (2000) Frey syndrome treatment with botulinum toxin. Otolaryngol Head Neck Surg 122:821–827
35. Dulguerov P, Quinodoz D, Cosendai G, et al. (1999) Prevention of Frey syndrome during parotidectomy. Arch Otolaryngol Head Neck Surg 125:833–839
36. Dulguerov P, Quinodoz D, Vaezi A, et al. (1999) New objective and quantitative tests for gustatory sweating. Acta Otolaryngol 119:599–603
37. Duphenix M (1757) Observations sur les fistules du canal salivaire de Stenon. Sur une playe compliquée à la joue ou le canal salivaire fut déchiré. Mem Acad R Chir 3:431–439
38. Eckardt A, Kuettner C (2003) Treatment of gustatory sweating (Frey's syndrome) with botulinum toxin A. Head Neck 25:624–628
39. Farrell ML, Kalnins IK (1991) Frey's syndrome following parotid surgery. Aust N Z J Surg 61:295–301
40. Feiwel M (1959) Auriculotemporal syndrome. Proc R Soc Med 52:191
41. Ford FR, Woodhall B (1938) Phenomena due to misdirection of regenerating fibers of cranial, spinal, and autonomic nerves: Clinical observations. Arch Surg 36:480–496
42. Fox RH, Goldsmith R, Kidd DJ (1962) Cutaneous vasomotor control in the human head, neck and upper chest. J Physiol 161:298–312
43. Freedman A (1973) Facial sweating after food in diabetes. Br Med J 3:291
44. Frey L (1923) Le syndrome du nerf auriculo-temporal. Rev Neurol 2:92–104
45. Gardner WJ, McCubbin JW (1956) Auriculotemporal syndrome; gustatory sweating due to misdirection of regenerated nerve fibers. J Am Med Assoc 160:272–277
46. Gavric M (1991) Aurikulotemporalni sindrom kao posledica parotidektomija. Stomatol Glas Srb 37:385–391
47. Gerbino G, Roccia F, Grosso M, et al. (1997) Pseudoaneurysm of the internal maxillary artery and Frey's syndrome after blunt facial trauma. J Oral Maxillofac Surg 55:1485–1490
48. Glaister DH, Hearnshaw JR, Heffron PF, et al. (1958) The mechanism of post-parotidectomy gustatory sweating (the auriculo-temporal syndrome). Br Med J:942–946
49. Glogau RG (2004) Hyperhidrosis and botulinum toxin A: patient selection and techniques. Clin Dermatol 22:45–52
50. Goatcher PD (1954) The auriculo-temporal syndrome. Br Med J 4873:1233–1234
51. Golding-Wood PH (1962) Tympanic neurectomy. J Laryngol Otol 76:683–693
52. Goodman RS (1986) Frey's syndrome: secondary to condylar fracture. Laryngoscope 96:1397–1398
53. Gordon AB, Fiddian RV (1976) Frey's syndrome after parotid surgery. Am J Surg 132:54–58
54. Guerrissi J, Stoyanoff J (1998) Atypical Frey syndrome as a complication of Obwegeser osteotomy. J Craniofac Surg 9:543–547
55. Guntinas-Lichius O (2002) Increased botulinum toxin type A dosage is more effective in patients with Frey's syndrome. Laryngoscope 112:746–749
56. Hanowell S, Lees DE, MacNamara T (1979) Auriculotemporal syndrome after combined modality therapy for cancer. South Med J 72:1116–1117

57. Harrison K, Donaldson I (1979) Frey's syndrome. J R Soc Med 72:503–508
58. Haxton HA (1948) Gustatory sweating. Brain 71:16–25
59. Hayes PC, Tulloch JA (1982) An unusual case of gustatory sweating. Postgrad Med J 58:656–657
60. Hays LL (1978) The Frey syndrome: a review and double blind evaluation of the topical use of a new anticholinergic agent. Laryngoscope 88:1796–1824
61. Hays LL, Novack AJ, Worsham JC (1982) The Frey syndrome: a simple, effective treatment. Otolaryngol Head Neck Surg 90:419–425
62. Hemenway WG (1960) Gustatory sweating and flushing. The auriculo-temporal syndrome – Frey's syndrome. Laryngoscope 70:84–90
63. Huttenbrink KB (1986) Die Therapie des gustatorischen Schwitzens nach Parotidektomie. Freysches Syndrom. Laryngol Rhinol Otol (Stuttg) 65:135–137
64. Isogai N, Kamiishi H (1997) Application of medical thermography to the diagnosis of Frey's syndrome. Head Neck 19:143–147
65. Janka HU, Standl E, Mehnert H (1979) Clonidine effect on diabetic gustatory sweating. Ann Intern Med 91:130
66. Jankovic J, Hallet M (1994) Therapy with botulinum toxin. New York: Marcel Dekker Inc
67. Jankovic J, Vuong KD, Ahsan J (2003) Comparison of efficacy and immunogenicity of original versus current botulinum toxin in cervical dystonia. Neurology 60:1186–1188
68. Johnson IJ, Birchall JP (1995) Bilatral auriculotemporal syndrome in childhood. Int J Pediatr Otorhinolaryngol 32:83–86
69. Kornblut AD, Westphal P, Miehlke A (1974) The effectiveness of a sternomastoid muscle flap in preventing post-parotidectomy occurrence of the Frey syndrome. Acta Otolaryngol 77:368–373
70. Kozma C, Gabriel S (1993) Gustatory flushing syndrome. A pediatric case report and review of the literature. Clin Pediatr (Phila) 32:629–631
71. Kreyden OP, Scheidegger EP (2004) Anatomy of the sweat glands, pharmacology of botulinum toxin, and distinctive syndromes associated with hyperhidrosis. Clin Dermatol 22:40–44
72. Kryshtalskyj B, Weinberg S (1989) An assessment for auriculotemporal syndrome following temporomandibular joint surgery through the preauricular approach. J Oral Maxillofac Surg 47:3–6
73. Kuttner C, Troger M, Dempf R, et al. (2001) Effektivität von Botulinum-toxin A in der Behandlung des gustatorischen Schwitzens. Nervenarzt 72:787–790
74. Laage-Hellman JE (1957) Gustatory sweating and flushing after conservative parotidectomy. Acta Otolaryngol 48:234–252
75. Laage-Hellman JE (1958) Gustatory sweating and flushing: aetiological implications of response of separate sweat glands to various stimult. Acta Otolaryngol 49:363–374
76. Laage-Hellman JE (1958) Gustatory sweating and flushing; aetiological implications of latent period and mode of development after parotidectomy. Acta Otolaryngol 49:306–314
77. Laage-Hellman JE (1958) Treatment of gustatory sweating and flushing. Acta Otolaryngol 49:132–143
78. Laccourreye O, Akl E, Gutierrez-Fonseca R, et al. (1999) Recurrent gustatory sweating (Frey syndrome) after intracutaneous injection of botulinum toxin type A: incidence, management, and outcome. Arch Otolaryngol Head Neck Surg 125:283–286
79. Laccourreye O, Bernard D, de Lacharriere O, et al. (1993) Frey's syndrome analysis with biosensor. A preliminary study. Arch Otolaryngol Head Neck Surg 119:940–944
80. Laccourreye O, Bonan B, Brasnu D, et al. (1990) Treatment of Frey's syndrome with topical 2% diphemanil methylsulfate (Prantal): a double-blind evaluation of 15 patients. Laryngoscope 100:651–653
81. Laccourreye O, Muscatelo L, Naude C, et al. (1998) Botulinum toxin type A for Frey's syndrome: a preliminary prospective study. Ann Otol Rhinol Laryngol 107:52–55
82. Lambert GA, Bogduk N, Goadsby PJ, et al. (1984) Decreased carotid arterial resistance in cats in response to trigeminal stimulation. J Neurosurg 61:307–315
83. Lance JW, Drummond PD, Gandevia SC, et al. (1988) Harlequin syndrome: the sudden onset of unilateral flushing and sweating. J Neurol Neurosurg Psychiatry 51:635–642
84. Laskawi R, Drobik C, Schonebeck C (1998) Up-to-date report of botulinum toxin type A treatment in patients with gustatory sweating (Frey's syndrome). Laryngoscope 108:381–384
85. Laws IM (1967) Two unusual complications of fractured condyles. Br J Oral Surg 5:51–59
86. Lee TS (1954) Physiological gustatory sweating in a warm climate. J Physiol 124:528–542
87. Leriche R (1914) Behandlung der permanenten parotis Fisteln durch die Entnervung der Speicheldrüse Ausreissen des N. auriculotemporalis. Zentralblatt Chir 41:754–755
88. Linder TE, Huber A, Schmid S (1997) Frey's syndrome after parotidectomy: a retrospective and prospective analysis. Laryngoscope 107:1496–1501

89. List CF, Peet MM (1938) Sweat secretion in man: IV. Sweat secretion of the face and its disturbance. Arch Neurol Psychol 40:443–470
90. Low PA (2003) Testing the autonomic nervous system. Semin Neurol 23:407–421
91. Low PA, Vernino S, Suarez G (2003) Autonomic dysfunction in peripheral nerve disease. Muscle Nerve 27:646–661
92. Lowe NJ (1998) Botulinum toxin type A for facial rejuvenation. United States and United Kingdom perspectives. Dermatol Surg 24:1216–1218
93. Matthews B, Robinson PP (1980) The course of post-ganglionic sympathetic fibres distributed with the trigeminal nerve in the cat. J Physiol 303:391–401
94. May JS, McGuirt WF (1989) Frey's syndrome: treatment with topical glycopyrrolate. Head Neck 11:85–89
95. Mellinkoff SM, Mellinkoff J (1950) Gustatory hyperhidrosis of the left knee. J Am Med Assoc 142:901
96. Minor V (1927) Ein neues Verfahren zu der klinischen Untersuchung der Schweissabsonderung. Dtsch Z Nervenheilkd 101:302–308
97. Montecucco C, Schiavo G, Tugnoli V, et al. (1996) Botulinum neurotoxins: mechanism of action and therapeutic applications. Mol Med Today 2:418–424
98. Morfit HM, Kramish D (1961) Auriculotemporal syndrome (Frey's syndrome) following surgery of parotid tumors. Am J Surg 102:777–780
99. Myers EN, Conley J (1970) Gustatory sweating after radical neck dissection. Arch Otolaryngol 91:534–542
100. Naumann M, Zellner M, Toyka KV, et al. (1997) Treatment of gustatory sweating with botulinum toxin. Ann Neurol 42:973–975
101. Needles W (1936) The auriculotemporal syndrome. With a suggestion regarding therapy. Arch Neurol Psychiatr 35:357–360
102. Nesathurai S, Harvey DT, Schatz SW (1995) Gustatory facial sweating subsequent to upper thoracic sympathectomy. Arch Phys Med Rehabil 76:104–107
103. New GB, Bozer HE (1922) Hyperhydrosis of the cheek associated with the parotid region. Minn Med 5:652–657
104. Nosan DK, Ochi JW, Davidson TM (1991) Preservation of facial contour during parotidectomy. Otolaryngol Head Neck Surg 104:293–298
105. Ottomo M, Heimburger RF (1980) Alternating Horner's syndrome and hyperhidrosis due to dural adhesions following cervical spinal cord injury: case report. J Neurosurg 53:97–100
106. Parisier SC, Binder WJ, Blitzer A, et al. (1978) Evaluation of tympanic neurectomy and chorda tympanectomy for gustatory sweating and benign salivary gland disease. Ear Nose Throat J 57:213–223
107. Payne RT (1940) Pneumococcal parotiditis and antecedent auriculotemporal syndrome. Lancet i:634–636
108. Quinodoz D, Dulguerov P, Cosenday G, et al. (1997) Traitement du syndrome de Frey avec la toxine botulinique. Med Hyg 55:2070–2073
109. Randall WC, (1946) Sweat gland activity and changing patterns of sweat secretion on the skin surface. Am J Physiol 147:391–398
110. Redleaf MI, McCabe BF (1993) Gustatory otorrhea: Frey's syndrome of the external auditory canal. Ann Otol Rhinol Laryngol 102:438–440
111. Richins CA, Kuntz A (1953) Role of sympathetic nerves in the regulation of salivary secretions. Brain Res 173:471–473
112. Rosales RL, Bigalke H, Dressler D (2006) Pharmacology of botulinum toxin: differences between type A preparations. Eur J Neurol 13(suppl 1):2–10
113. Ross JA (1970) The function of the tympanic plexus as related to Frey's syndrome. Laryngoscope 80:1816–1833
114. Rubinstein RY, Rosen A, Leeman D (1999) Frey syndrome: treatment with temporoparietal fascia flap interposition. Arch Otolaryngol Head Neck Surg 125:808–811
115. Saito H (1999) Gustatory otalgia and wet ear syndrome: a possible cross-innervation after ear surgery. Laryngoscope 109:569–572
116. Sato K (1977) The physiology, pharmacology, and biochemistry of the eccrine sweat gland. Rev Physiol Biochem Pharmacol 79:51–131
117. Sato K, Kang WH, Saga K, et al. (1989) Biology of sweat glands and their disorders. I. Normal sweat gland function. J Am Acad Dermatol 20:537–563
118. Sato K, Kang WH, Saga K, et al. (1989) Biology of sweat glands and their disorders. II. Disorders of sweat gland function. J Am Acad Dermatol 20:713–726
119. Sato KT, Richardson A, Timm DE, et al. (1988) One-step iodine starch method for direct visualization of sweating. Am J Med Sci 295:528–531
120. Schiavo G, Benfenati F, Poulain B, et al. (1992) Tetanus and botulinum-B neurotoxins block neurotransmitter release by proteolytic cleavage of synaptobrevin. Nature 359:832–835
121. Schliack H, Schiffter R, Goebel HH, et al. (1972) Untersuchungen zur Frage der Schweissdrusseninnervation im Bereich des Gesichts. Acta Anat (Basel) 81:421–438
122. Schmelzer A, Rosin V, Steinbach E (1992) Zur Therapie des Freyschen Syndroms durch ein Anhidrotisches Gel. Laryngorhinootologie 71:59–63
123. Schnarch A, Markitziu A (1990) Dysgeusia, gustatory sweating, and crocodile tears syndrome induced by a cerebellopontine angle meningioma. Oral Surg Oral Med Oral Pathol 70:711–714

124. Scrivani SJ, Keith DA, Kulich R, et al. (1998) Posttraumatic gustatory neuralgia: a clinical model of trigeminal neuropathic pain. J Orofac Pain 12:287–292
125. Sessions RB, Roark DT, Alford BR (1976) Frey's syndrome – a technical remedy. Ann Otol 85:734–739
126. Shaari C, Sanders I (1994) Assessment of the biological activity of botulinum toxin. In: Jankovic J, Hallett M, editors. (1994) Assessment of the biological activity of botulinum toxin. ed. New York: Marcel Drekker Inc
127. Sharav Y, Benoliel R, Schnarch A, et al. (1991) Idiopathic trigeminal pain associated with gustatory stimuli. Pain 44:171–174
128. Shelley WB, Horvath PN (1951) Comparative study on the effect of anticholinergic compounds on sweating. J Invest Dermatol 16:267–274
129. Singleton GT, Cassisi NJ (1980) Frey's syndrome: incidence related to skin flap thickness in parotidectomy. Laryngoscope 90:1636–1639
130. Sly RM (1981) Auriculotemporal syndrome. Cutis 28:423, 5
131. Sonsale A, Sharp JF, Johnson IJ (1999) Gustatory sweating of the external auditory canal. J Laryngol Otol 113:1000–1001
132. Sood S, Quraishi MS, Bradley PJ (1998) Frey's syndrome and parotid surgery. Clin Otolaryngol 23:291–301
133. Spiro RH, Martin H (1967) Gustatory sweating following parotid surgery and radical neck dissection. Ann Surg 165:118–127
134. Stuart DD (1978) Diabetic gustatory sweating. Ann Intern Med 89:223–224
135. Thomas A (1927) Le double réflexe vaso-dilatateur et sudoral de la face consécutif aux blessures de la loge parotidienne. Rev Neurol (Paris) 1:447–460
136. Truax BT (1989) Gustatory pain: a complication of carotid endarterectomy. Neurology 39:1258–1260
137. Tugnoli V, Ragona RM, Eleopra R, et al. (2002) The role of gustatory flushing in Frey's syndrome and its treatment with botulinum toxin type A. Clin Auton Res 12:174–178
138. Tuinzing DB, van der Kwast WA (1982) Frey's syndrome. A complication after sagittal splitting of the mandibular ramus. Int J Oral Surg 11:197–200
139. van der Linden J, Sinnige HA, van den Dorpel MA (2000) Gustatory sweating and diabetes. Neth J Med 56:159–162
140. Vilches JJ, Navarro X, Verdu E (1995) Functional sudomotor responses to cholinergic agonists and antagonists in the mouse. J Auton Nerv Syst 55:105–111
141. Wallis KA, Gibson T (1978) Gustatory sweating following parotidectomy: correction by a fascia lata graft. Br J Plast Surg 31:68–71
142. Watkins PJ (1973) Facial sweating after food: a new sign of diabetic autonomic neuropathy. Br Med J 1:583–587
143. Watson C, Vijayan N (1995) The sympathetic innervation of the eyes and face: a clinicoanatomic review. Clin Anat 8:262–272
144. Weber FP (1897) Clinical cases V: a case of localized sweating and blushing on eating, possibly due to temporary compression of vasomotor fibers. Trans Clin Soc Lond 31:277–280
145. Wilson WC (1936) Observations relating to the innervation of the sweat glands of the face. Clin Sci 2:273–286
146. Yu LT, Hamilton R (1992) Frey's syndrome: prevention with conservative parotidectomy and superficial musculoaponeurotic system preservation. Ann Plast Surg 29:217–222
147. Zalzal GH (1991) Congenital gustatory facial flushing. Otolaryngol Head Neck Surg 104:878–880
148. Zoller J, Herrmann A, Maier H (1993) Frey's syndrome secondary to a subcondylar fracture. Otolaryngol Head Neck Surg 108:751–753

Chapter 6

Sialendoscopy

6

Francis Marchal

Contents

6

Core features

- Sialendoscopy can be either a diagnostic or an interventional procedure.
- Diagnostic sialendoscopy is an evaluation procedure that aims to replace most of the radiological investigations of the salivary ductal system.
- Interventional sialendoscopy, alone or combined with external surgery, is an operation for obstructive salivary ductal pathology.

Complications to Avoid

- The diameter of Wharton's duct is 2–3 mm in the normal gland, and Stensen's duct is less than 2 mm, so endoscopes of smaller diameter than these measurements must be used.
- Avoid sialendoscopy during an acute inflammatory process because of the increased fragility of the ductal system.

Introduction

Salivary gland pathologies are traditionally divided into neoplastic and non-neoplastic, the latter being further subdivided into inflammatory and non-inflammatory [48, 49]. The advent of new endoscopic techniques [31, 33] allows a complete exploration of the salivary ductal system and a precise evaluation of its pathologies. This new approach helps to support the division of non-neoplastic salivary gland diseases into: (1) parenchymal, which require traditional treatments, or (2) ductal, which can, in the majority of cases, be handled endoscopically.

Sialendoscopy [31, 35, 42] aims to visualize the lumen of the salivary ducts, as well as to diagnose and treat ductal diseases. Because of the required equipment, the complexity, the duration, and the potential complications of the procedure, it appears important to distinguish two different procedures: diagnostic sialendoscopy and interventional sialendoscopy [34]. Diagnostic sialendoscopy is an evaluation procedure that aims to replace most of the radiological investigations of the ductal system. Interventional sialendoscopy, alone or combined with external surgery (see Chapter 7, Removal of Calculi or Strictures in Salivary Ducts that Cannot be Removed by Sialendoscopy), must be considered as an operation on the obstructive ductal pathology, avoiding almost totally the removal of the salivary gland.

Anatomical Considerations

The papilla of Wharton's duct is extremely thin and difficult to catheterize. By entering Wharton's duct, the bifurcation toward the sublingual gland appears immediately, followed by a relatively long main duct that divides within the gland. A sphincter mechanism has been discussed in the literature, but so far no convincing demonstration has been published. The diameter of Wharton's duct is approximately 2–3 mm in the normal gland, and it is possible to explore the second, third, and occasionally the fourth generation branches (Figs. 6.1, 6.2). In the parotid gland, the papilla has a wider opening, allowing easier catheterization. The overall diameter of the duct is about 1 mm smaller than the submandibular duct, but its endoscopic appearance is similar (see Fig. 6.1).

As the diameter of Stensen's is often less than 2 mm, it is impossible to explore it with a large endoscope without producing local trauma to the duct. After having passed the masseter muscle angle, the parotid ductal divisions occur earlier than those in the submandibular duct. As the gland extends into wider and broader territory, it is possible to explore the second, third, fourth, fifth, and even more branches (Fig. 6.2). Both glands can be explored, almost to the end of the anatomical limits of the gland, as the ductal size does not decrease rapidly (Fig. 6.3).

Sialolithiasis

Sialolithiasis results in a mechanical obstruction of the salivary duct, causing repetitive swelling during meals, which can remain transitory or can be complicated by bacterial infections [7, 28]. Traditionally, recurrent episodes of infection lead to open surgery and sialolithiasis still represents the most frequent indication for excision of the submandibular gland [5, 15].

Epidemiology

Sialolithiasis is the main cause of unilateral diffuse parotid or submandibular gland swellings. Its incidence has been poorly studied, but seems to be much higher than the classic Rauch data of 1/300,000. In a study based

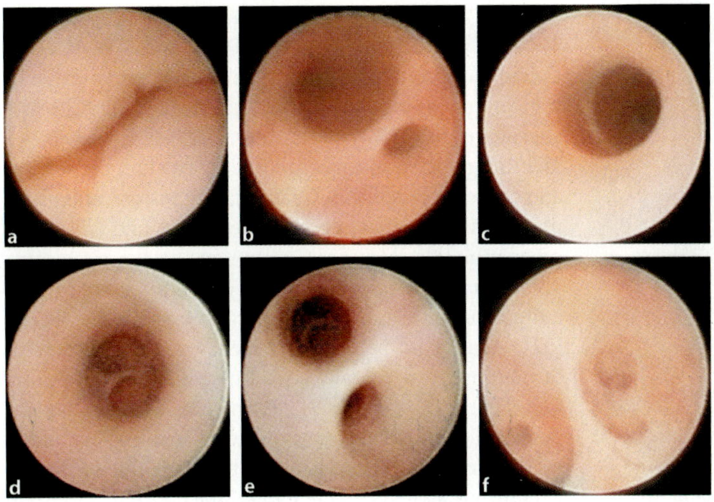

Fig. 6.1: Wharton's duct. **a** First few centimeters of Wharton's duct. **b** Junction of the sublingual duct. **c** Main duct. **d** First generation branches. **e** Second generation branches. **f** Third generation branches

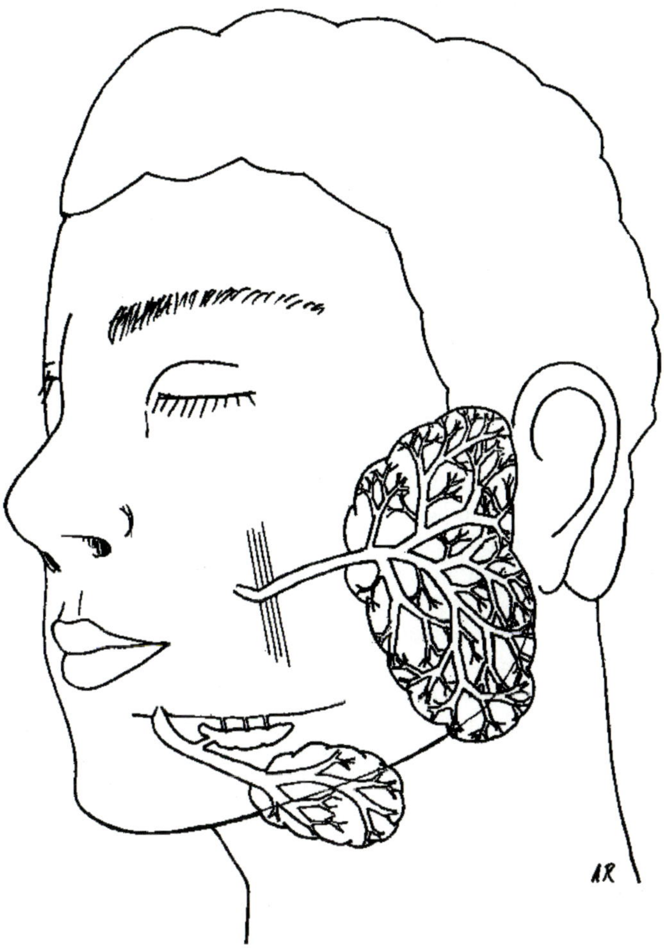

Fig. 6.2: View of both ductal systems. Parotid ducts are smaller in diameter, with more branching than submandibular ducts

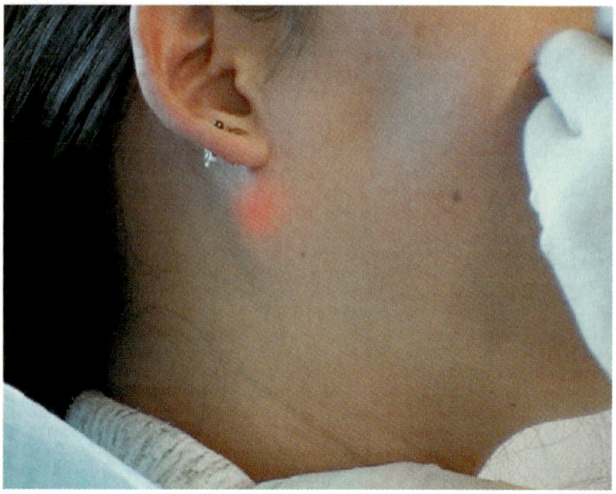

Fig. 6.3: External view of the tip of the endoscope during parotid sialendoscopy. The endoscope can be advanced to the anatomical limits of the gland

on admission figures in England, Escudier and McGurk [10] have estimated this incidence between 1/15,000 and 1/30,000. Personal data, based on consultations in both the private and public sectors, report an incidence between 1/5,000 and 1/10,000.

According to past autopsy studies [46] sialolithiasis is supposed to affect 1% of salivary glands. However, its frequency is most probably underestimated due to the poor sensitivity of outdated methods of detection and an absence of treatment options for intraglandular calculi, leading to more conservative approaches.

According to most published data [10, 28], salivary calculi are localized in the submandibular gland in 80–90% of cases. However, in our experience, parotid glands are affected more frequently (up to 40%), a difference possibly explained by the sensitivity of the new detection methods used [36, 37]. Probably for similar reasons, we found a high incidence of multiple calculi, with multiple sialolithiasis in 58% (29 out of 50) of parotid [37] and 29% (31 out of 106) of submandibular [36] glands.

The annual growth rate of established salivary calculi has been estimated to be 1 mm per year [46]. They vary in shape, being either round or irregular. The size ranges from 2 mm to 2 cm, the average being 3.2 mm and 4.9 mm, respectively, for parotid and submandibular stones, according to two recent studies [36, 37], a finding that emphasizes the need for fragmentation before extraction of these stones.

Pathophysiology

Calculi are composed of organic and inorganic substances, in varying ratios. The organic substances are glycoproteins, mucopolysaccharides, and cellular debris [4]. The inorganic substances are mainly calcium carbonates and calcium phosphates. Calcium, magnesium, and phosphate ions contribute each between 20% and 25%, with other minerals (Mn, Fe, Cu) composing the remaining. The chemical composition consists mainly of microcrystalline apatite, $Ca_5(PO_4)_3OH$, or whitlockite, $Ca_3(PO_4)_2$ [57]. Apatite is the most frequent component present throughout the calculus, while whitlockite is mainly found in the core [2, 57]. The formation of either form depends on the concentrations of calcium and phosphorus, with low concentrations favoring the formation of apatite, while whitlockite is formed when the concentrations are high [24]. Other crystalline forms include brushite and weddellite, which are present in small amounts, mainly at the periphery of calculi [57]. These forms might be the initial form of calcium deposition, followed by subsequent remodeling into apatite [57].

Often, the organic substances predominate in the center of the calculus, while the periphery is essentially inorganic [4, 57]. The presence of bacteria in calculi has been suggested by scanning electron microscopy aspects [26], where oval, elongated shapes are identified. A recent polymerase chain reaction (PCR) study found bacterial DNA, mainly of oral commensals belonging to the *Streptococcus* species, in all examined calculi [55].

The exact pathogenesis of sialolithiasis remains unknown, and various hypotheses have been proposed [4]. The first is based upon the existence of intracellular microcalculi which when excreted in the canal become a nidus for further calcification [8, 16]. The second possible hypothesis is that bacteria present within the oral cavity might migrate into the salivary ducts and become the nidus for further calcification [32]. Both hypotheses suppose an initial organic nidus that progressively grows by the deposition of layers of inorganic and organic substance.

The etiologic agents responsible for sialolithiasis have remained elusive. Sheman and McGurk attempted to correlate the geographic distribution of hard water and salivary calculi in the UK [54]. This study indicated that no link between hard water and sialolithiasis or sialadenitis could be demonstrated, suggesting that high calcium intake might not lead to salivary calculi. In rats, experimental hypercalcemia failed to result in sialoliths [9].

There is recent interest in the effects of tobacco on saliva. Tobacco smoking has been shown to affect saliva in chronic smokers resulting in an increased cytotoxic activity, a decreased polymorphonuclear phagocytic ability, a reduction of salivary amylase, as well as a reduction of salivary protecting proteins, such as peroxidase [41]. If cigarette smoke impairs the phagocytic and protective functions of saliva, the hypothesis of a link between infection and sialolithiasis could be supported. In a recent epidemiological study examining the nutrition and other behaviors of patients suffering from sialolithiasis, we have found tobacco smoking to be the only positive correlation.

Classic Treatment of Sialolithiasis

The classic management of sialolithiasis is antibiotic and anti-inflammatory treatment, hoping the calculi will be expelled spontaneously through the papilla. In cases of submandibular calculi located close to Wharton's papilla, a marsupialization (sialodochoplasty) is performed and the calculus removed [44, 50]. Interestingly, although sialolithiasis is the most frequent reason for excision of the submandibular gland [51], often the calculi are left in the Wharton's duct remnant [15]. In cases of posteriorly located submandibular or parotid calculi, a conservative approach is adopted whenever possible, probably because parotidectomy for infectious conditions is associated with a higher incidence of facial nerve complications [12].

It is commonly believed that a gland suffering from sialolithiasis is no longer functional [38]. Our recent clinical-pathological study of submandibular glands removed for sialolithiasis revealed the following: (1) no correlation between the degree of gland alteration and the number of infectious episodes; (2) no correlation between the degree of gland alteration and the duration of evolution; and (3) despite appropriate indications for removal of the submandibular gland, close to 50% of the glands removed were histopathologically normal or close to normal [38]. A conservative approach even in long-standing sialolithiasis therefore appears justified.

External lithotripsy, initially reported by Iro and colleagues in the early 1990s [17], was popular in Europe, but requires several sessions at intervals of a few weeks. Once fragmented, calculi are supposed to pass spontaneously, since no stone extraction is described with this technique. The remaining debris can be seen as the ideal nidus for further calcification and recurrence of sialolithiasis. Success rates up to 75% for the parotid, and up to 40% for the submandibular gland are reported [1, 14, 17, 19, 20, 45, 47]. The success rate seems similar for external and intraductal lithotripsy [3, 14, 21, 25]. While sialendoscopy might become an adjuvant procedure to external lithotripsy to retrieve the fragments, we see little utility in de novo investing in such expensive equipment (see below). In addition, these techniques could result in significant damage to the gland.

Since the first trials of retrieving stones blindly with a basket under radiological control [23, 53], other techniques for sialolithiasis fragmentation have been described, such as electrohydraulic [26] and pneumoblastic devices [18]. Electrohydraulic devices, initially described as promising [26], have been proven to be of low efficiency at low voltages. At higher voltages, although we have found that destruction was possible, injuries of the duct wall have been described and the technique criticized [20]. Pneumoblastic devices are based on the delivery of mechanical energy to the stone. While no clinical trials using this technique have been published for salivary gland calculi, in vitro studies tend to emphasize the risks of wall perforations of the duct [18].

Other Ductal Pathologies

The strictures of ductal systems in both glands can be divided into four types (Fig. 6.4). Type I consists of membranous strictures, thin and localized, usually located in second and higher generation branches. Type II consists of large (but less than 1 cm) strictures usually affecting the main ducts. Type III are diffuse strictures affecting the main duct with a normal intraglandular ductal system. Type IV are stenotic processes affecting the whole ductal system and can be divided into type IVa (diffuse reduction of caliber without other strictures) and type IVb (diffuse reduction of caliber associated with irregular strictures).

Indications and Contraindications

The indications for sialendoscopy are all salivary gland swellings of unclear origin [34], including swellings associated with calculi, strictures, inflammation, or tumor, and other processes that may cause obstruction of the duct [11, 29, 30]. Adults and children are both included.

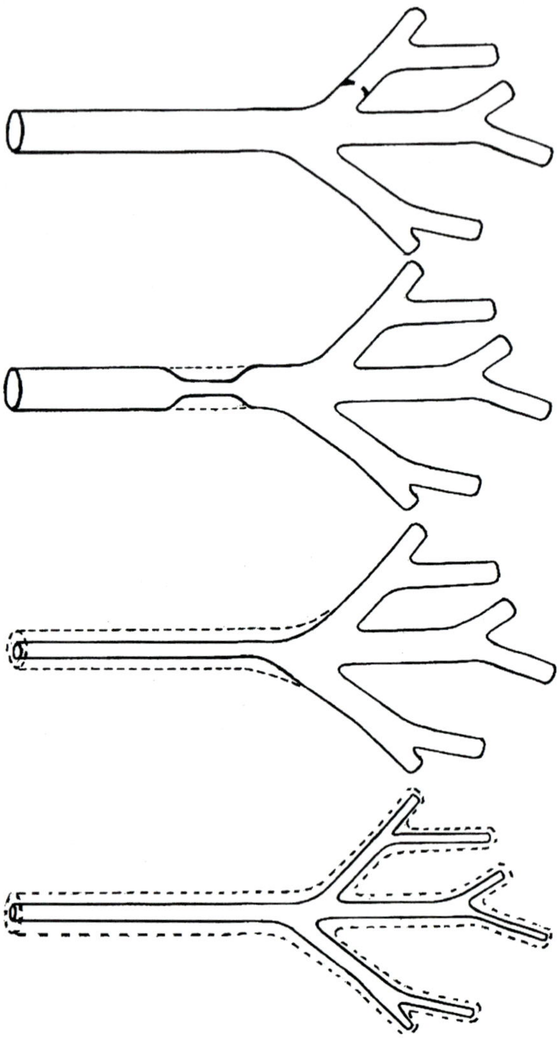

Fig. 6.4: Various types of stenotic processes. From *top* to *bottom*: type I: membranous stricture, type II: large stricture, type III: diffuse stenosis of main duct, type IV: diffuse generalized stenosis (type IVa without localized strictures, type IVb with multiple localized strictures)

Calculi are either grasped with the basket or forceps when they float in the lumen, or fragmented with a laser beam before retrieving the fragments. Strictures can be dilated with balloon catheters under endoscopic vision, or with metallic guides. A large calculus or a tight stricture might require extending the anesthesia and the surgical approach. Therefore, advanced age and poor medical condition of each patient and the severity of the disease might constitute relative contraindications.

Contraindications widely accepted are acute inflammatory processes. Salivary gland infection and inflammation leads to an increase of fragility of the ductal system, and increases the risk of perforation during sialendoscopy [29]. There are also technical contraindications, related to the equipment used (if a small diameter sialendoscope is not available in case of diffuse stenosis) or to the patient's anatomy (accessibility of stones and strictures). These factors constitute the main limitations of interventional sialendoscopy.

There are no other specific contraindications, mostly because diagnostic sialendoscopy is an outpatient procedure, performed under local anesthesia, and minimally invasive. Even elderly or unstable patients, unable to undergo a general anesthesia, can benefit from this technique.

The main technical limitations of interventional sialendoscopy alone (without combining an external approach) at the present time are calculi that are located far posterior or a duct with a stricture that renders the progression of the endoscope difficult and the dilatation impossible.

The course of the duct puts certain limitations on semirigid sialendoscopy, especially if sharp curvatures of the duct prevents the scope from being advanced. The main previously described limitation being the size of the sialendoscope has drastically changed since the development of the most recent generation of "all-in one" sialendoscopes. The variety in sizes now allows for exploration of almost all salivary ducts.

Manipulation of small-sized endoscopes in large channels is difficult, as well as introduction of an overly large endoscope into a stenotic duct. Maneuvering within the narrow salivary ducts has to be absolutely atraumatic because of the risk of ductal perforation and unpredictable secondary consequences. Significant trauma to the wall of the duct could result in later stenosis.

Equipment

Salivary Probes

Salivary probes are commercially available in 12 sizes. The tip design is extremely important to make the use of the probes as atraumatic as possible. Classic buttoned salivary probes are not suitable for this technique. Salivary probes should not be introduced too far to minimize trauma to the duct or perforation (Fig. 6.5a).

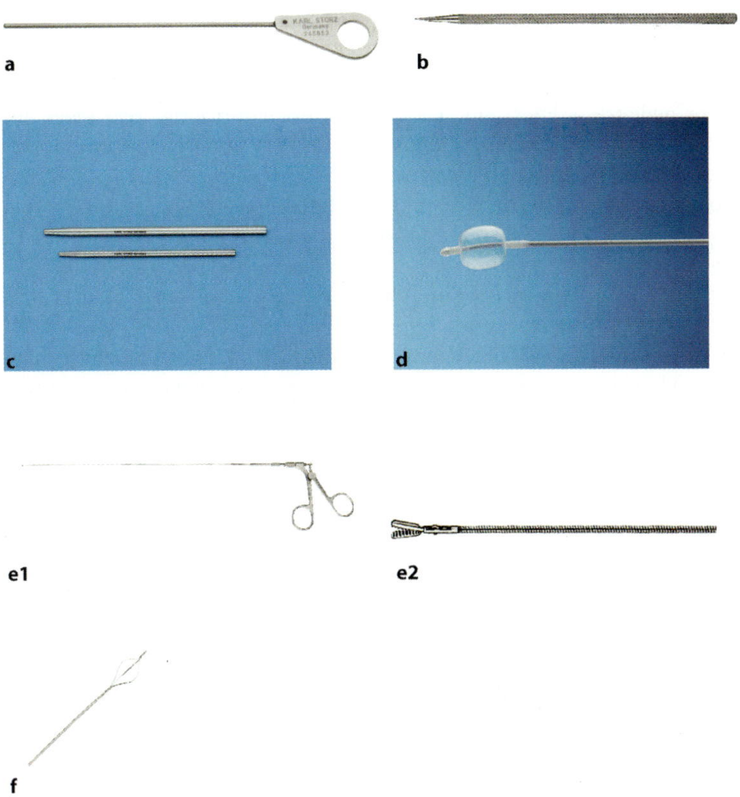

Fig. 6.5: Instruments. **a** Salivary probes. **b** Conic dilator. **c** Hollow rigid bougies. **d** Balloon dilators. **e** Forceps, 0.8 mm diameter. **f** Baskets for removal of calculus

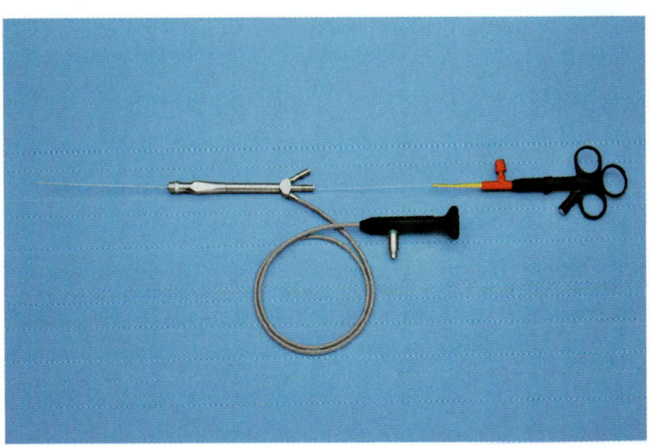

Fig. 6.6: All-in-one sialendoscope with basket in working channel

Conic Dilator

The specially designed dilator shown in Fig. 6.5b should be used intermittently between the uses of salivary probes for gentle dilation of the papilla. As it is a non-invasive procedure, there should be minimal trauma to the papilla, and the systematic use of marsupialization, as proposed by others [43], should be avoided.

Sialendoscopes

The technology of the endoscopes we developed over the last 10 years evolved over four generations: free optical fiber, flexible endoscopes, and two generations of semi-rigid endoscopic devices of various diameters (with The Karl Storz Company). The third-generation multipurpose endoscopes comprised two endoscopes of different sizes and various sheaths, allowing for diagnostic and interventional sialendoscopy. The last generation of sialendoscopes could be called "all-in-one" sialendoscopes because they have an integrated irrigation channel that may also be used for introducing small-sized operating instruments (Fig. 6.6).

Multipurpose Sialendoscopes

Diagnostic sialendoscopy requires that the miniature endoscope be available in two sizes, 0.75 mm for pediatric or stenosed ducts and 1 mm in diameter for adult/nonstenotic ducts. The irrigation channel is formed by the tiny gap between the scope and the lumen of the examination sheath.

Interventional sialendoscopy requires that the examination sheath be replaced by a special operating sheath with an irrigation channel and one integrated working channel. Operating sheaths are available in three sizes, with inner diameters of 0.65, 0.9, and 1.15 mm. Depending on their size, they allow the passage of balloon dilators, forceps, and baskets (Fig. 6.7).

All-in-one Sialendoscopes

These endoscopes may be used for both diagnostic and interventional procedures eliminating the need for changing the instrument. They are available in four different diameters:

1. The 0.89-mm sialendoscope allows for exploration of small pediatric ducts, or fibrous/stenotic ducts. The device is also used to perform dacryocystorhinostomies. The working/rinsing channel measures 0.3 mm.
2. The 1.1-mm sialendoscope is suited for both diagnostic and interventional procedures, with a working channel of 0.4 mm and a separate rinsing channel of 0.3 mm.

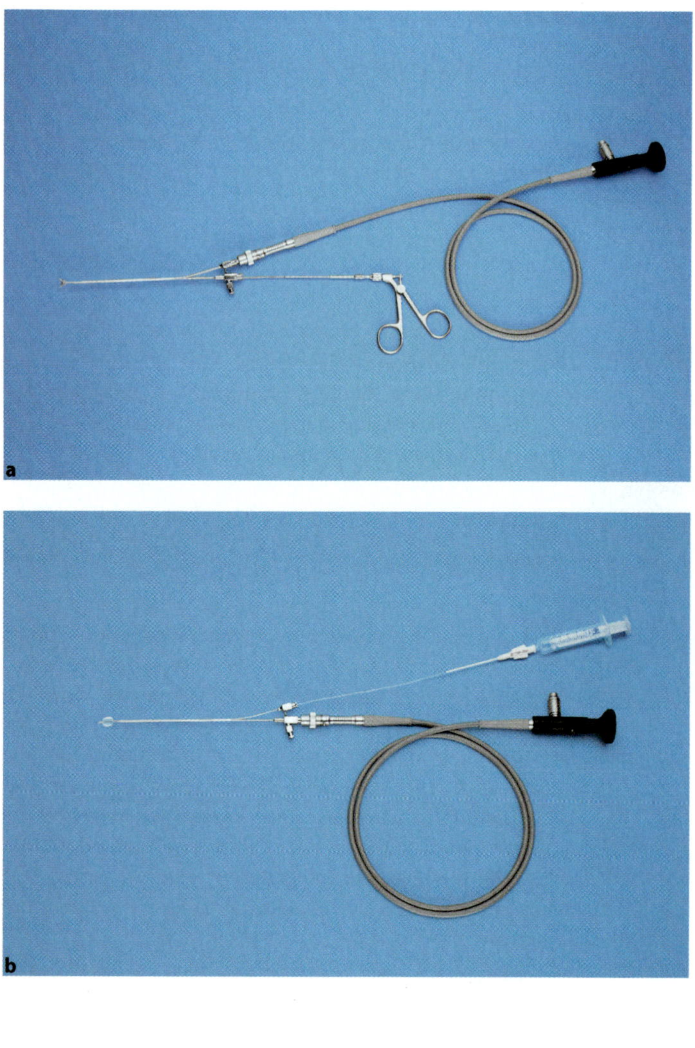

Fig. 6.7: Multipurpose sialendoscope. **a** With forceps in working channel. **b** With balloon catheter in working channel

3. The 1.3-mm sialendoscope is the "universal" sialendoscope, as its outer diameter is sized to allow for diagnostic and interventional sialendoscopy of the submandibular and parotid ducts. Its rinsing channel of 0.3 mm and its working channel of 0.6 mm allow the passage of baskets or laser fibers. However, this size of working channel does not permit the passage of balloon dilators or forceps (Fig. 6.6).
4. The 1.6-mm sialendoscope allows the use of forceps. Its outer diameter is sized to allow for endoscopic inspection and treatment of the parotid and submandibular ducts. Its rinsing channel of 0.3 mm and its working channel of 0.8 mm allow the use of baskets, laser fibers, and also forceps.

It is important to mention that the lumen of affected ducts is often narrowed due to inflammatory conditions, making the use of small-diameter sialendoscopes necessary. Therefore, the 1.6-mm sialendoscope may not be suitable in all cases. Due to its diameter, its introduction into the papilla is also more difficult than smaller endoscopes.

Calculus Retrieval Baskets

With time and experience we have been repeatedly improving and modifying the baskets needed for calculus retrieval, to allow optimum-sized prototypes to be produced. The baskets that are currently available come in three sizes, with either three, four, or six wires each, and diameters ranging from 0.4 to 0.6 mm, and lengths from 50 to 60 cm (Fig. 6.5f).

Hollow Rigid Bougies

These bougies allow a blind dilatation of gross stenoses of the main parotid or submandibular ducts (Fig. 6.5c). The guidewire is inserted first under endoscopic control, traversing the stenotic process, and the sialendoscope is then removed, having marked and noted the distance to the stenosis. The metal bougie is then gently inserted, using increasing diameters.

Forceps

Custom-made forceps measuring 0.8 mm have also been designed and may be used to retrieve small salivary calculi or for taking biopsies within the salivary ductal system (Fig. 6.5e). Care has to be taken when manipulating these instruments, since they are small, friable, and fragile. Thus, very little pressure should be exerted when grasping a sialolith to avoid resultant damage to the instrument.

Disposable Balloon Dilators

Disposable dilators allow for endoscopic-controlled dilatation of localized stenoses, mainly encountered in the parotid duct system. High-pressure balloons, as used in interventional cardiology to fragment arteriosclerosis, could damage and perforate the salivary duct if their inflating diameter should extend the dilatation capacity of the pathologic duct. Therefore, we prefer low-pressure inflatable balloons that are filled with saline under endoscopic vision (Fig. 6.5d).

Recommended Equipment for Beginners: Basic Set

The 1.3-mm Marchal sialendoscope is the universal scope that may be used for diagnosis and treatment in the majority of cases, in an outpatient setting as well as intraoperatively. It has received Food and Drugs Administration (FDA) approval.

The basic set consists of a conic dilator, bougies of various sizes, and the universal 1.3-mm sialendoscope.

Recommended Equipment: Advanced Set

The 0.75-mm sialendoscope in conjunction with various sheaths extends the technical options and may be applied in the entire field of interventional sialendoscopy (Fig. 6.6). It allows a customized bending of the scope, exploration of all sizes of ducts, and use of all interventional devices (basket, balloon catheter, laser fiber, forceps) to treat salivary pathologies.

Significance of the Tip Design

The small angulation at the end of all models of "all-in-one" sialendoscopes facilitates targeted catheterization of branches (Fig. 6.8), whereas a conventional on-axis tip usually poses some difficulties in advancing and entering the branch ahead. A slight bend may also be given to the sheaths of "multipurpose sialendoscopes": after inserting the obturator, the tip may be very slightly bent, allowing for the optimal curve. The endoscope itself follows the curve of the sheath and reverts to its former state after completion of the procedure.

Significance of the Beveled Tip

Catheterization of the papilla is a challenging procedure with a relatively long learning curve. Once adequate dilatation has been achieved by use of bougies of varying sizes, introduction of the operating sialendoscope is considerably facilitated by the beveled tip of the sheath. This design feature allows the tip to be used as a dilation probe.

Significance of Late Marsupialization

Marsupialization should be completely avoided, particularly at the beginning of the procedure. The irrigation fluid has a dilating effect that provides excellent vision of all ductal branches. Early marsupialization leads to poor visual conditions and makes the technique more difficult to master because of the irrigation liquid escaping from the ductal system at its opening (Fig. 6.9). Furthermore, marsupialization of the ductal papillae, especially in the parotid, should either be completely avoided, or kept as small as possible to prevent retrograde passage of air and oral contents.

Diagnostic Sialendoscopy

Diagnostic sialendoscopy [11, 13, 29–31, 35–37, 39, 40, 42, 43] is a minimally invasive, outpatient procedure performed under local anesthesia. Even the elderly or unstable patients who are unsuitable for a general anesthesia can safely undergo this technique. There is no contraindication related to a medication or medical condition. The need for a semirigid system has also been proved by the impossibility of directing a flexible system without a mobile tip, and its fragility and poor image quality [36, 37]. In a previous study, diagnostic sialendoscopy could be achieved in 98% of cases, while others report a success rate of 96% [43]. It aims to replace classic radiological investigations, such as sialography.

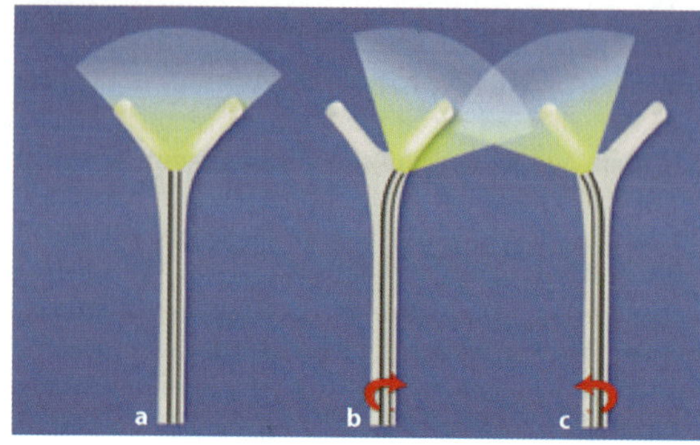

Fig. 6.8: Tip of the instrument. The small angulation facilitates targeted catheterization of branches (**b, c**), because an on-axis tip (**a**) usually poses some difficulties in advancing to the next branch

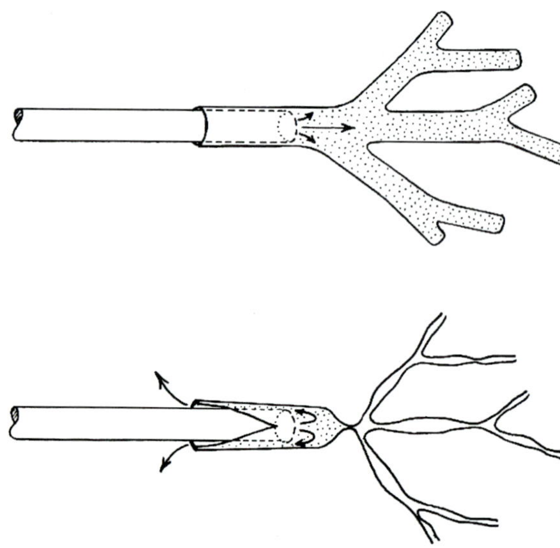

Fig. 6.9: Importance of non-marsupialization. *Top* Sialendoscope introduced in dilated papilla: rinsing produces adequate dilatation of ductal system. *Bottom* Sialendoscope introduced after marsupialization: rinsing flows back out without dilating ductal system

Preparation: Operating Room Set-up

Sialendoscopy can be done as an outpatient procedure in the clinic with the patient sitting in a chair, sitting partially recumbent, or supine (Fig. 6.10). The disadvantage of a fully upright sitting position is that it is associated with an increased risk of vasovagal syncope. To be readily prepared for sensitive patients or the incidence of difficulties while the interventional approach is performed, an anesthetic unit should be kept available with an experienced anesthetist on standby throughout the entire procedure. A mobile cart with connections for a video camera, video monitor, VCR, and printer are on the opposite side of the patient, allowing for direct observation of the surgical procedure. An assistant (physician, nurse, or technician) is located on that side and is responsible for performing the perioperative procedures.

Anesthesia

Sialendoscopy generally requires local anesthesia of the papilla and the ductal system. A topical anesthetic paste or spray (10% or 20%) is applied to either Stensen's or Wharton's papilla at the beginning of the procedure. After introduction of the sialendoscope, anesthesia of the ductal system is induced with an irrigation solution of Xylocaine, Lidocaine, or Carbostesin 0.5%. Depending on the age and weight of the patient, the total amount infiltrated should not exceed 40 cc, because of absorption risks. Diagnostic sialendoscopy can usually be performed under local anesthesia. Taking into account that interventional sialendoscopy is usually performed in the same sitting, sedation or even general anesthesia can be applied by the anesthesiologist. This largely depends on the level of difficulty of the individual case.

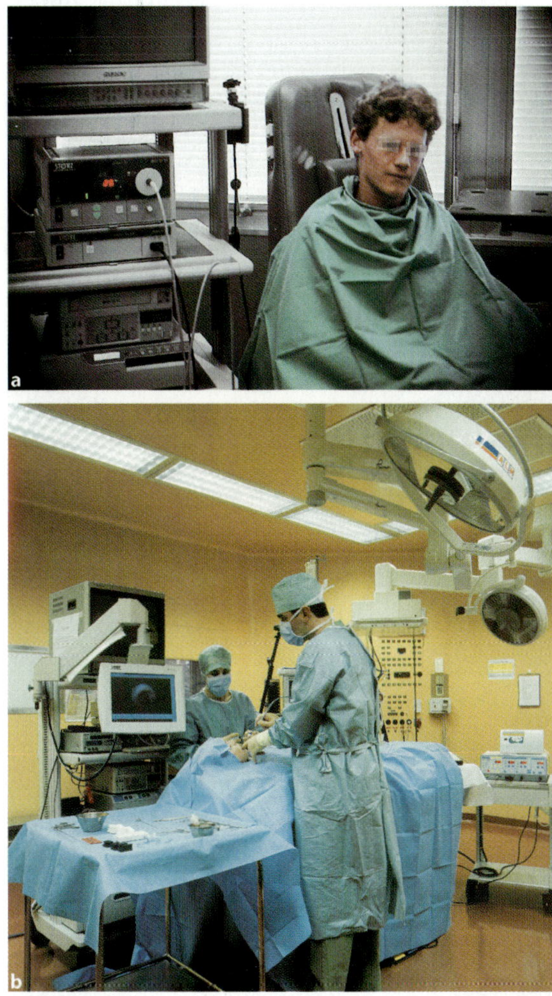

Fig. 6.10: Positioning. **a** Patient sitting (diagnostic sialendoscopy). **b** Patient lying in supine position (interventional sialendoscopy)

Step-by-step Technique: Parotid and Submandibular Sialendoscopy

1. Local anesthesia of the papilla with an anesthetic paste or spray (10% or 20%).
2. Introduction of salivary probes of increasing diameter (Fig. 6.11a).
3. Introduction of the dilator (Fig. 6.11b).
4. Placement of dental tampons in the posterior aspect of the vestibule and gingivobuccal sulcus. These will later be replaced with new dry ones during sialendoscopy.
5. Introduction of the sialendoscope (Fig. 6.11c).
6. Exploration of the ductal system under continuous rinsing. The introduction of a guidewire in the working channel is optional, depending on the experience of the surgeon; it facilitates introduction of the scope into the duct.

Postoperative Care

Patients are usually given anti-inflammatory medications (non-steroidal), to help decrease the swelling after a diagnostic procedure. Antibiotics, given at the beginning, are no longer dispensed for a simple procedure.

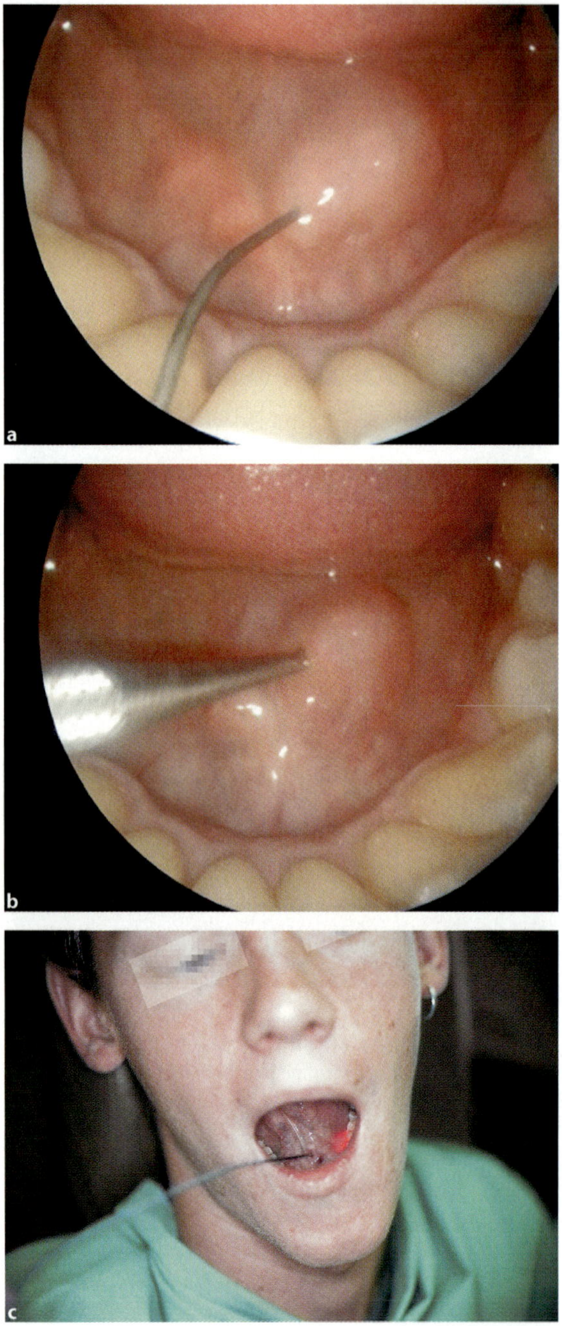

Fig. 6.11: Sialendoscopy step by step. **a** Introduction of salivary probes after Xylo-adrenalin infiltration. **b** Introduction of conic dilator. **c** Introduction of sialendoscope

Clinical Examples

Mucous Plugs

Floating mucous plugs can be seen alone or in conjunction with salivary stones or stenotic processes. It has been suggested that these "mucous plugs" present in the ductal system may represent the nidus for the development of calculi (Fig. 6.12).

Sialolithiasis

Salivary calculi can be either solitary or multiple (Fig. 6.13), particularly in the parotid gland. As seen before, their location can be proximal, distal, or intraglandular. They vary in shape, being either round or irregular (Fig. 6.14). The calculi in the parotid duct are often smaller, longer, and smoother than the more calcified calculi in the submandibular duct.

Depending on the size of the calculus, they can either float in the lumen, become partially fixed due to irregular shapes, or even become attached to the wall of the duct. In some cases, they are trapped behind a bifurcation.

Ductal Stenosis

Stenotic processes can be of four types, as previously described. Examples of the endoscopic appearance of these stenoses is shown in Fig. 6.15. Stenosis of the ducts can mimic the symptoms of sialolithiasis, being recurrent swellings of salivary glands. Stenotic processes are more frequent in the parotid gland than in the submandibular gland.

Limitations and Complications

Rare limitations include an extremely tortuous duct that could hamper endoscope progression and difficulties in directing the endoscope at the distal end of the ductal system. Complications of diagnostic sialendoscopy are immediate, such as perforation of the duct, which can cause swellings of the face or neck. There can also be late complications due to these perforations, such as sialoceles, which might become infected. If the endoscopy is not performed minimally invasively, and the floor of

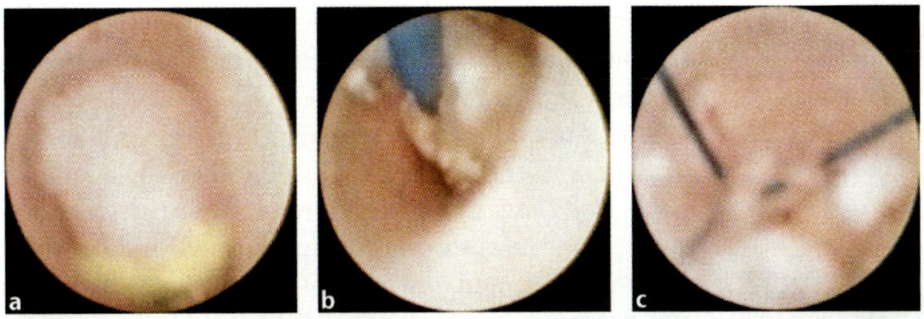

Fig. 6.12: Mucous plug. **a** Mucous plug is attached to the calculus which impairs intraductal vision. **b** The mucosal plug is mechanically detached by gently tapping on the calculus with the laser fiber tip. **c** Extraction of this plug using a wire basket

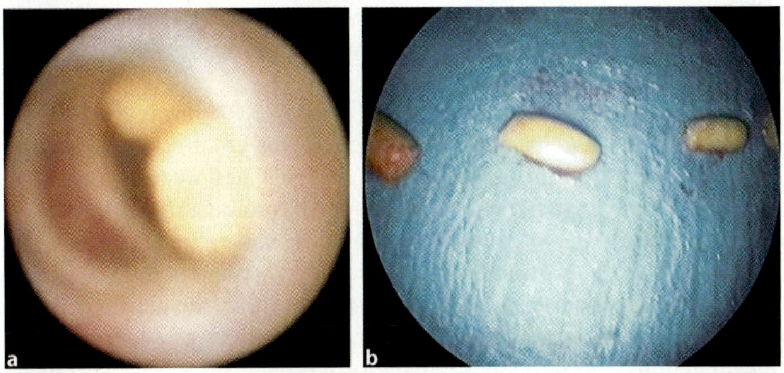

Fig. 6.13: Multiple calculi. **a** Endoscopic view. **b** Multiple calculi extracted from the parotid duct

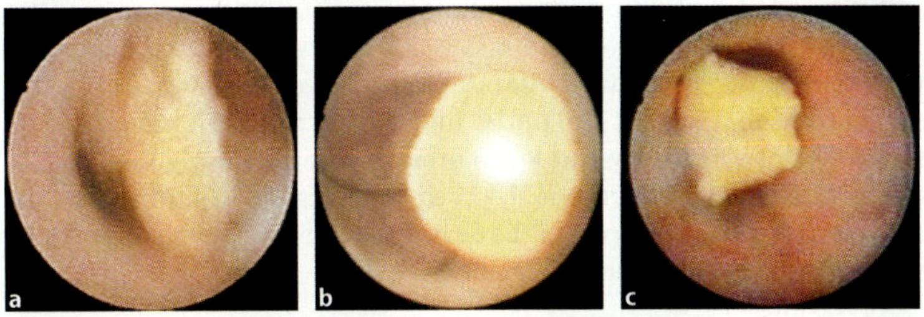

Fig. 6.14: Various morphologies of salivary calculi. **a** Disk shaped. **b** Round. **c** Irregular

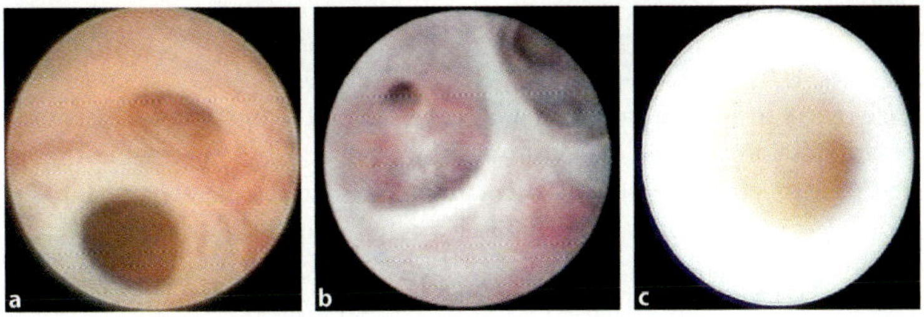

Fig. 6.15: Stenosis. **a** Membranous thin stricture of Stensen's duct. **b** Tight stenosis of Wharton's duct. **c** Diffuse stenosis of Stensen's duct

mouth or Stensen's papilla is largely dissected as proposed by others [11], it might lead to future stenosis.

Despite its apparent simplicity, diagnostic sialendoscopy is a technically challenging procedure with a long learning curve. Operating and ductal manipulation of the rigid sialendoscope is delicate, requires extensive experience, and may be hazardous due to theoretical risks of perforation and vascular or neural damage. The sialendoscope should only be advanced when distal vision is adequate and not obstructed. Perforations of the duct associated with ductal manipulation can lead to diffuse edema of the floor of the mouth or of the buccal area. Meticulous attention has to be given to this anatomical area because of rare but possible potential risks of a life-threatening enlargement of the swelling.

Interventional Sialendoscopy

Although many authors have reported on extraction of submandibular calculi, the literature on sialendoscopy of Stensen's duct is limited, since most series report on parotid as well as submandibular sialolithiasis [37]. Probably, the smaller diameter of the Stensen's duct [58] has made its exploration more challenging, and therefore previous authors [22] have performed an endoscopy, followed by the blind retrieval of the calculus with a Dormia basket, corresponding possibly to a "endoscopically-assisted calculus retrieval," but not to interventional sialendoscopy. While we initially used this method, we no longer recommend this procedure because of the limitations of the technique and the potential risks of perforation and stenosis.

We have developed and used five different generations of endoscopes [36, 37]. Our first real attempts to perform extraction of calculi under endoscopic control were done with a flexible fiberscope, which we have abandoned, not only because of difficult maneuvering and poor visualization, but also because of fragility, difficulty in sterilization of the instruments, and frequent "stripping" of the internal coating of the working channel of the endoscope by grasping the wire basket. Satisfying results were obtained with semirigid endoscopy, which initially consisted of the juxtaposition of two tubes. Because of the size of the instrument relative to the lumen of the duct, progression within the duct was difficult and has resulted in tears of the wall of the duct.

The results of interventional sialendoscopy are directly related to the size of the calculi and ducts in both submandibular and parotid glands. Calculi can have either a smooth surface or have sharp edges. In our hands, round and floating calculi are associated with a very easy retrieval, while calculi with sharp edges are often blocked in the duct and are more challenging. Size is probably the most important factor in predicting the success of classic interventional sialendoscopy in parotid calculi: for calculi smaller than 3 mm, 97% could be retrieved with the wire basket, while for calculi larger than 3 mm, the success of this technique was 35% [37] without fragmentation. For sharp-edged calculi, fragmentation prior to extraction is necessary.

In our opinion, the best system for fragmentation of calculi is a laser fiber, as initially described by Gundlach et al. [13]. The laser fiber is introduced in the sialendoscope, laser-sialolithotripsy is performed under direct visual control, and retrieval of fragments is achieved with grasping wire baskets. A distinct advantage of our technique is the retrieval of calculi and their fragments after lithotripsy, contrary to the majority of previously described methods.

The holmium:YAG laser at 2,104 nm is well known and has proven its efficiency for urolithiasis [27, 56]. Its use for salivary calculi is similar, and we have used it for many years. However, one has to be attentive to its potential dangers because of its absorption characteristics in the surrounding tissues and because of the heat generated from the fragmentation within the narrow salivary ducts. Laser irradiation may inadvertently cause damage to duct walls. Therefore, it is mandatory that the laser be operated only under clear direct vision, continuous flow irrigation, and in close contact with the stone, tangential to the duct, while carefully sparing the duct walls. The dye laser at 350 nm as initially described [3], has proven its efficacy and low morbidity because the high energy delivered is not absorbed by the tissues. Unfortunately, the actual cost of the device and its specificity may render its acquisition difficult.

Operating Room Layout and Anesthesia

The patient is placed supine on the operating table and is given either intravenous sedation or general anesthesia. In cases of large submandibular calculi, a nasal intubation is preferred as it might be necessary to go intraorally. General anesthesia is often preferred as laser fragmentation and dilatation of strictures can cause pain.

Step-by-step Technique: Parotid and Submandibular Interventional Sialendoscopy

The algorithm for approaching salivary calculi is shown in Fig. 6.16.

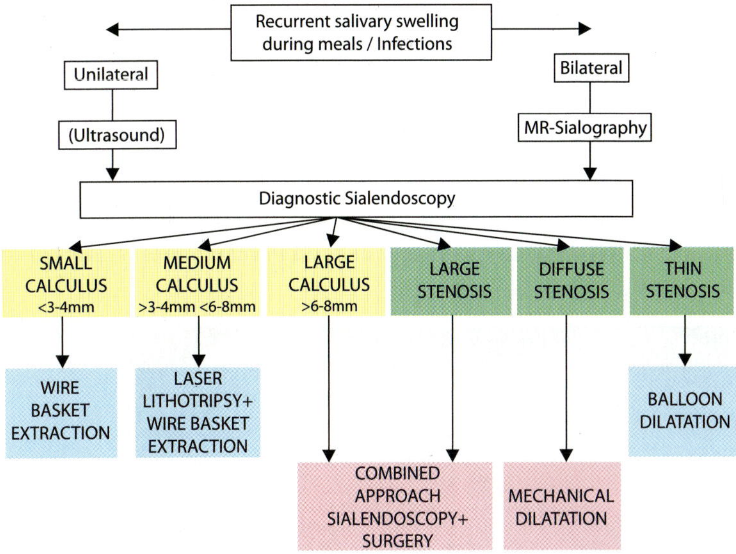

Fig. 6.16: Algorithm for diagnostic and interventional sialendoscopy

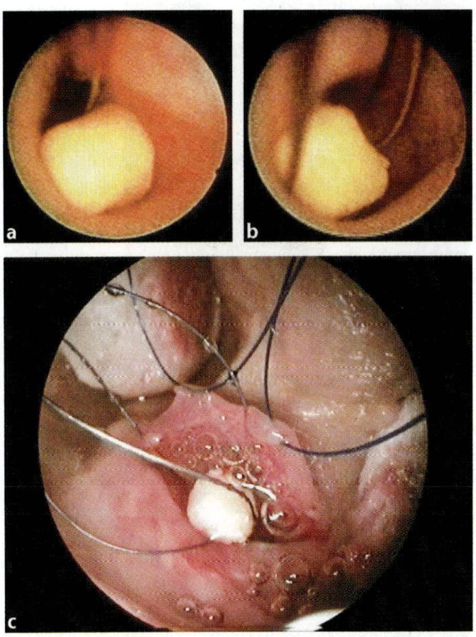

Fig. 6.17: Floating calculus extraction in Wharton's duct. **a** Opening of the basket behind the calculus. **b** Closure on the calculus. **c** Mini-marsupialization at the end of the procedure

Clinical Examples

Calculus Removal by Use of a Wire Basket

Following diagnostic sialendoscopy exposing the calculus, the approach is the same for the submandibular and parotid glands, although the diameter of the parotid duct is smaller [58].

For small calculi (less than 4 mm in diameter) in submandibular cases and less than 3 mm for parotid cases, extraction is performed with wire baskets of various sizes (Fig. 6.17). In cases of larger calculi, others have described fragmentation with forceps [11]. In our hands, it only led to the destruction of the forceps because of the hardness of the calculi.

Calculus Removal by Use of a Wire Basket, Preceded by Laser Fragmentation

Laser fragmentation and extraction of debris using a wire basket through a minimal incision of Wharton's papilla is followed by a complete clearance of the duct. Calculus removal should only be performed after complete fragmentation of the stone (Fig. 6.18). In attempting to retrieve large fragments of calculi, the surgeon runs the risk of being faced with a trapped wire basket, a situation that cannot be resolved by applying firm traction to the instrument and must be avoided under any circumstance.

Sialendoscopic Treatment of Stenosis

Although less frequently encountered than sialolithiasis, stenosis of the duct results in the same clinical symptoms. Endoscopic localization of the stenosis is essential for selecting the suitable dilation system. In cases of thick and long stenosis of the main salivary duct, the rigid dilator is used, as well as a larger sialendoscope under visual control.

Initially, the guidewire is introduced through the working channel of the endoscope, until it passes through the stenosis. Then, the endoscope is withdrawn proximally and the dilator is introduced. In the case of a thin, usually peripheral stenosis, dilatation may be performed

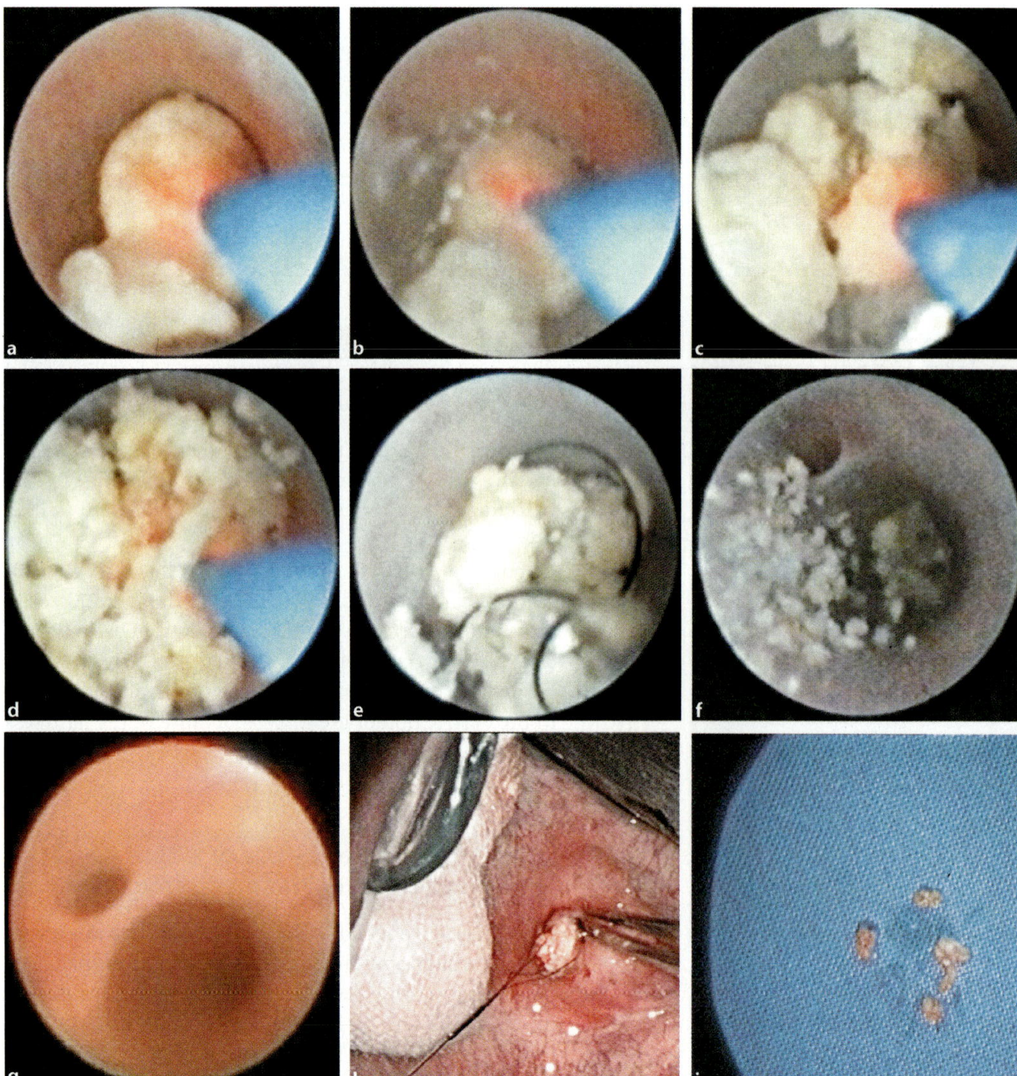

Fig. 6.18a–i: Laser fragmentation of salivary calculi and basket extraction of fragments

with a balloon-tipped catheter under endoscopic control (Fig. 6.19).

Postoperative Care

Interventional sialendoscopic procedures are usually conducted under prophylactic antibiotic medication administered 48 h or more prior to the procedure, depending on the individual case. Frequent self-massaging of the gland is recommended. Outpatient clinic follow-up visits are performed directly after the intervention. Patients with rupture of Wharton's duct or with deliberately extended marsupialization of the duct have to be subjected to careful clinical monitoring because of the risk of edema diffusion and/or infection of the floor of the mouth which might develop into a life-threatening emergency.

Limitations and Complications

Limitations and failures are caused by:

1. The traumatic handling of the papilla
2. The diameter of Stensen's or Wharton's duct
3. Distorted branching systems, impossible to explore
4. A calculus which is too large
5. A stenosis which is too tight

Having performed more than 900 sialendoscopies, both parotid and submandibular, over a 10-year period, we have not encountered any facial nerve palsies or hemorrhage. Those complications which did occur were perforations and blockage of baskets. Perforations and blockage of the basket occurred in our experience at the beginning of the learning curve. These complications can be avoided by not trying to retrieve non-floating stones

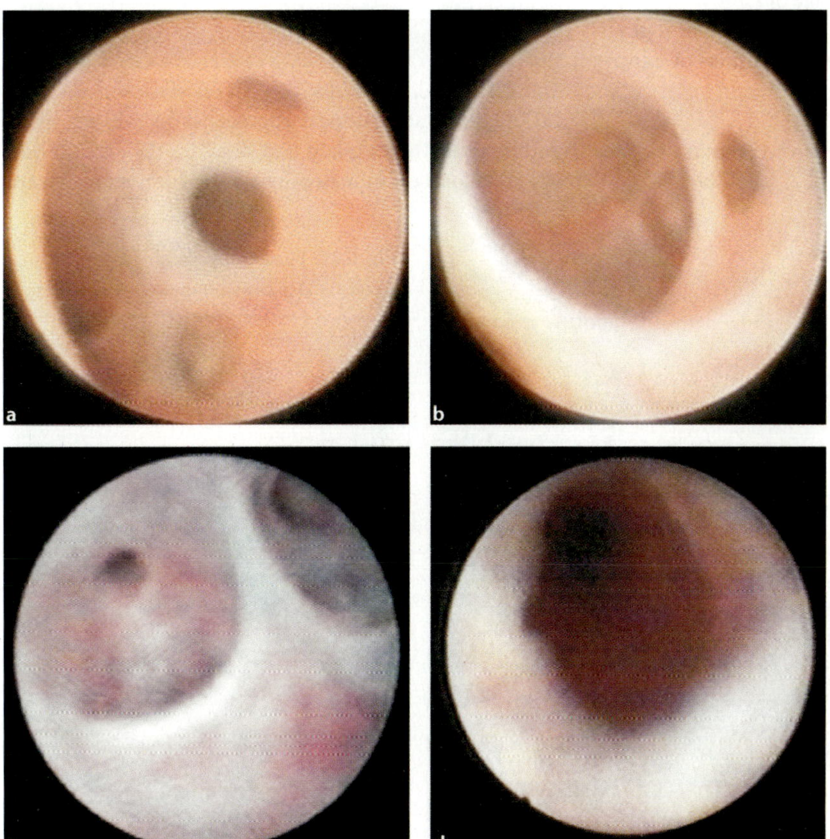

Fig. 6.19: Treatment of stenosis. **a** Endoscopic view of a thin stenosis before dilatation. **b** View of balloon dilatation. **c** Endoscopic view of a thick stenosis before dilatation. **d** Close-up view after rigid bougie dilatation

with the basket, and fragmenting them first with the laser or applying the double approach technique. As this technique has a steep learning curve, it needs a lot of cautious care at the beginning.

Training

Founded under the auspices of the International Salivary Gland Society in 2002, the European Sialendoscopy Training Center (ESTC) is located in Geneva, Switzerland.

The aims of the ESTC are:

1. To train clinicians in the indications and procedures associated with diagnostic and therapeutic sialendoscopy,
2. To organize and disseminate experience gained by clinicians in this field, and
3. To conduct international courses and conferences as appropriate, to facilitate exchange of knowledge, experiences, and advances gained by leading clinical physicians who focus on diseases and conditions of salivary glands.

The first Sialendoscopy Hands-on Training Course took place in Geneva, January 2002, after the "First International Congress on Salivary Gland Diseases." Since that time, more than 250 participants from more than 30 countries have received tuition and have gained experience in the technique of sialendoscopy (Fig. 6.20).

Hands-on Training

In Geneva, a specific training and demonstration model for sialendoscopy has been validated. The use of fresh pig heads has proven to be ideal, after extensive trials conducted with other animal models and human cadaveric specimens. During each course, participants are paired and work on one fresh pig head. The lectures held during the hands-on course are divided into two sessions, the first focusing on diagnostic and the second on interventional sialendoscopy.

Conferences

The international faculty reports on clinical, radiological, medical, and surgical approaches to salivary gland pathologies. They explain and describe their techniques of sialendoscopy in a step-by-step fashion using a vari-

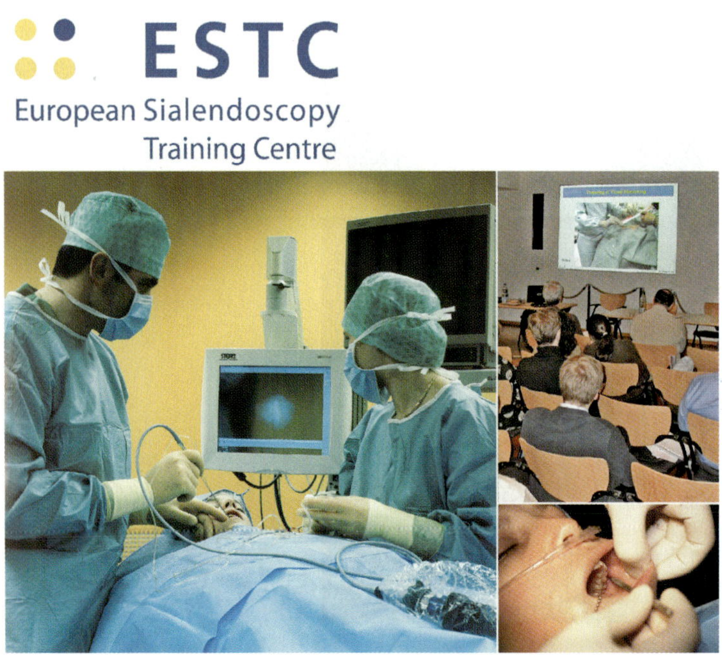

Fig. 6.20: European Sialendoscopy Training Center: video conference and live surgery

ety of videos and interactive presentations that allow for open discussion and comments. Recent developments in new equipment and designs combined with advances in instrumentation technology are presented during such conferences. Abstract sessions are an outstanding way to disseminate the results of clinical research or to present and discuss case histories. Round-table format and informal discussions facilitate reporting on advances and prospects of research that address the management of salivary gland duct pathologies.

Live Surgery

Owing to the availability of an excellent video-conference system linking the operating room to the conference room, live surgery can be viewed on a large central video screen. Participants are encouraged to ask questions and discuss with the surgeon during the operation. Through this real-time approach not only the steps of the procedure but also the risks and advantages are made tangible to the course participants. At the subsequent hands-on sessions, surgical tricks and tips are demonstrated, expanded upon, and taught.

Conclusion

Taking into consideration differences in instrumentation and video-endoscopic equipment, as well as complexity, duration, and potential complications of the procedures, a distinction has to be made between diagnostic and interventional sialendoscopy. Diagnostic sialendoscopy is a low morbidity minimally invasive technique that is intended to become the investigational procedure of choice for salivary duct pathologies. Interventional sialendoscopy allows for extraction and/or fragmentation in the majority of cases of sialolithiasis and can therefore prevent excision of salivary glands.

Over the past decade the role of sialendoscopy has been established in the management of major salivary gland, parotid and submandibular, disorders and diseases. Previously, these problems were either not treated or were treated with reluctance, and in the majority resulted in removal of part or all of the gland with its resultant morbidity and not infrequent persistence of the presenting symptoms.

Take Home Messages

- Sialendoscopy allows for complete exploration of the salivary ductal system and allows for a precise evaluation of its pathologies.
- Sialendoscopy allows for the division of non-neoplastic salivary gland diseases into parenchymal and ductal.
- Salivary glands suffering from ductal obstructive processes including stenoses or sialolithiasis can recover or maintain function after sialendoscopic treatment.
- Interventional sialendoscopy allows for significant reduction in excision of salivary glands.

References

1. Aidan P, De Kerviler E, LeDuc A, Monteil JP (1996) Treatment of salivary stones by extracorporeal lithotripsy. Am J Otolaryngol 17(4):246–250
2. Anneroth G, Eneroth CM, Isacsson G (1975) Crystalline structure of salivary calculi. A microradiographic and microdiffractometric study. J Oral Pathol 4(5):266–272
3. Arzoz E, Santiago A, Esnal F, Palomero R (1996) Endoscopic intracorporeal lithotripsy for sialolithiasis. J Oral Maxillofac Surg 54(7):847–850
4. Ashby RA (1995) The chemistry of sialoliths – stones and their homes. In: Norman JED, McGurk M, eds. Color atlas and text of the salivary glands. Diseases, disorders, and surgery. London: Mosby-Wolfe
5. Biffoni M, Marchesi M, Picchi P, Nuccio G, Faloci C, Tartaglia F, Mastropietro T, Millarelli M (1997) Excision of Submandibular Gland: Our Experience. Giorn Chir 18:477–480
6. Brady JM, McKinney L, Stanback JS (1989) Scanning electron microscopy of submandibular sialoliths: a preliminary report. Dentomaxillofac Radiol 18(1):42–44
7. Cawson RA, Gleeson MJ, Eveson JW (1997) Sialadenitis. In: Cawson RA, Gleeson MJ, Eveson JW, eds. Pathology and surgery of the salivary glands. Oxford: Isis Medical Media:33–63

8. Epivatianos A, Harrison JD, Dimitriou T (1987) Ultrastructural and histochemical observations on microcalculi in chronic submandibular sialadenitis. J Oral Pathol 16(10):514–517
9. Epivatianos A, Harrison JD, Garrett JR, Davies KJ, Senkus R. (1986) Ultrastructural and histochemical observations on intracellular and luminal microcalculi in the feline sublingual salivary gland. J Oral Pathol 15(10):513–517
10. Escudier MP, McGurk M (1999) Symptomatic sialoadenitis and sialolithiasis in the English population, an estimate of the cost of hospital treatment. Br Dent J 186(9):463–466
11. Giger R, Mhawech P, Marchal F, Lehmann W, Dulguerov P (2005) Mucoepidermoid carcinoma of Stensen's duct: a case report and review of the literature. Head Neck 27(9):829–833
12. Goh YH, Sethi DS (1998) Submandibular gland excision: a five-year review. J Laryngol Otol 112(3):269–273
13. Gundlach P, Scherer H, Hopf J, Leege N, Muller G, Hirst L, Scholz C (1990) Die endoskopisch kontrollierte Laserlithotripsie von Speichelsteinen. In-vitro-Untersuchungen und erster klinischer Einsatz. HNO 38:247–250
14. Gutmann R, Ziegler G, Leunig A, Jacob K, Feyh J (1995) Die endoskopische und extrakorporale Stosswellen-Lithotripsie von Speichelsteinen. Laryngorhinootologie 74(4):249–253
15. Hald J, Andreassen U. K. (1994) Submandibular gland excision: short- and long-term complications. ORL 56:87–91
16. Harrison JD, Epivatianos A, Bhatia SN (1997) Role of microliths in the aetiology of chronic submandibular sialadenitis: a clinicopathological investigation of 154 cases. Histopathology 31(3):237–251
17. Iro H, Schneider HT, Fodra C (1992) Shockwave lithotripsy of salivary duct stones. Lancet 339:1333–1336
18. Iro H, Benzel W, Gode U, Zenk J (1995) Pneumatische intrakorporale Lithotripsie von Speichelsteinen. In-vitro- und tierexperimentelle Untersuchungen. HNO 43(3):172–176
19. Iro H, Zenk J, Waldfahrer F, Benzel W, Schneider T, Ell C (1998) Extracorporeal shock wave lithotripsy of parotid stones. Results of a prospective clinical trial. Ann Otol Rhinol Laryngol 107(10 Pt 1):860–864
20. Iro H, Zenk J, Waldfahrer F, Benzel W (1996) Aktueller Stand minimal-invasiver Behandlungsverfahren bei der Sialolithiasis. HNO 44(2):78–84
21. Ito H, Baba S (1996) Pulsed dye laser lithotripsy of submandibular gland salivary calculus. J Laryngol Otol 1 110(10):942–946
22. Katz P (1997) Thérapeutiques non chirurgicales des lithiases salivaires. Endoscopie et lithotrypsie extra-corporelle. Rev Off Soc Fr ORL 45:47–52
23. Kelly I, Dick R (1990) Technical report: Interventional sialography; Dormia basket removal of Wharton's duct calculus. Clin Radiol 43:205
24. Koutsoukos PG, Nancollas GH (1981) Crystal growth of calcium phosphates – epitaxial considerations. J Crystal Growth 53:10–19
25. Konigsberger R, Feyh J, Goetz A, Schilling V, Kastenbauer E (1990) Die endoskopisch kontrollierte Laserlithotripsie zur Behandlung der Sialolithiasis. Laryngorhinootologie 69(6):322–323
26. Konigsberger R, Feyh J, Goetz A, Kastenbauer E (1993) Endoscopically-controlled electrohydraulic intracorporeal shock wave lithotripsy (EISL) of salivary stones. J Otolaryngol 22:12–13
27. Larizgoitia I, Pons JM (1999) A systematic review of the clinical efficacy and effectiveness of the holmium:YAG laser in urology. BJU Int 84(1):1–9
28. Lustmann J, Regev E, Melamed Y (1990) Sialolithiasis. A survey on 245 patients and a review of the literature. Int J Oral Maxillofac Surg 19(3):135–138
29. Marchal F (2005) Salivary gland endoscopy: new limits? Rev Stomatol Chir Maxillofac 106(4):244–249
30. Marchal F, Dulguerov P (2003) Sialolithiasis management: The state of the art. Arch Otolaryngol Head Neck Surg 129: 951–956
31. Marchal F, Dulguerov P, Lehmann W (1999) Interventional sialendoscopy. N Engl J Med 341:1242–1243
32. Marchal F, Kurt AM, Dulguerov P, Lehmann W (2001) Retrograde theory in sialolithiasis formation. Arch Otolaryngol Head Neck Surg 127(1):66–68
33. Marchal F, Becker M, Dulguerov P, Lehmann W (2000) How I Do It: Interventional sialendoscopy. Laryngoscope 110:318–320
34. Marchal F, Dulguerov P, Becker M, Lehmann W (2002) Interventional Sialendoscopy. In: Wackym PA, Rice DH, Schaefer SD, Minimally Invasive Surgery of the Head, Neck and Cranial Base. Philadelphia, Lippincott, Williams & Wilkins
35. Marchal F, Becker M, Vavrina J, Dulguerov P, Lehmann W (1997) Diagnostic et traitement des sialolithiases. Bull Med Suisses 79:1023–1027
36. Marchal F, Dulguerov P, Becker M, Barki G, Disant F, Lehmann W (2002) Submandibular diagnostic and interventional sialendoscopy: new procedure for ductal disorders. Ann Otol Rhinol Laryngol 111(1):27–35
37. Marchal F, Dulguerov P, Becker M, Barki G, Disant F, Lehmann W (2001) Specificity of parotid sialendoscopy. Laryngoscope 111(2):264–271

38. Marchal F, Kurt AM, Dulguerov P, Becker M, Oedman M, Lehmann W (2001) Histopathology of submandibular glands removed for sialolithiasis. Ann Otol Rhinol Laryngol 110(5 Pt 1):464–469
39. Marchal F, Dulguerov P, Becker M, Kurt AM, Guyot JP, Lehmann W (1998) Traitement ambulatoire de la lithiase salivaire. Med Hyg 56: 1961–1962
40. Marchal F, Dulguerov P, Guyot JP, Lehmann W (1999) Sialendoscopie et lithotripsie intracanalaire. ORL Nova 8:262–264
41. Nagler RM, Klein I, Zarzhevsky N, Drigues N, Reznick AZ (2002) Characterization of the differentiated antioxidant profile of human saliva. Free Radic Biol Med 32(3):268–277
42. Nahlieli O, Baruchin AM (1997) Sialoendoscopy: three years' experience as a diagnostic and treatment modality. J Oral Maxillofac Surg 55:912–918
43. Nahlieli O, Baruchin AM (1999) Endoscopic technique for the diagnosis and treatment of obstructive salivary gland diseases. J Oral Maxillofac Surg 57:1394–1401
44. Oedman M, Marchal F (2002) Relationship between calcium intake and sialolithiasis formation. Proceedings of the 1st International meeting on Salivary Gland Diseases, pp 128–130
45. Ottaviani F, Capaccio P, Campi M, Ottaviani A (1996) Extracorporeal electromagnetic shock-wave lithotripsy for salivary gland stones. Laryngoscope 106(6):761–764
46. Rauch S, Gorlin RJ (1970) Diseases of the salivary glands. In: Gorlin RJ, Goldmann HM (1970) Thomas' Oral Pathology. eds. Mosby, St. Louis pp 997–1003
47. Reimers M, Vavrina J, Schlegel C (2000) Results after shock wave lithotripsy for salivary gland stones. Schweiz Med Wochenschr Suppl (125):122S–126S
48. Rice DH (1999) Noninflammatory, non-neoplastic disorders of the salivary glands. Otolaryngol Clin North Am 32:835–843
49. Rice DH (1999) Chronic inflammatory disorders of the salivary glands. Otolaryngol Clin North Am 32:813–818
50. Rice DH (1993) Diseases of the salivary glands – non neoplastic. In: Bailey B, Pillsbury HC (1993) Head and Neck Surgery – Otolaryngology Vol I. Philadelphia: eds. J.B. Lippincott. pp 475–484
51. Rice DH (1999) Noninflammatory, non-neoplastic disorders of the salivary glands. Otolaryngol Clin North Am 32(5):835–843
52. Rontal M, Rontal E (1987) The use of sialodochoplasty in the treatment of benign inflammatory obstructive submandibular gland disease. Laryngoscope 97:1417–1421
53. Sharma RK, Al Khalifa S, Paulose KO, Ahmed N (1994) Parotid duct stone removal by a Dormia basket. J Laryngol Otol 108:699–701
54. Sheman JA, McGurk M (2000) Lack of correlation between water hardness and salivary calculi in England. Br J Oral Maxillofac Surg 38(1):50–53
55. Teymoortash A, Wollstein AC, Lippert BM, Peldszus R, Werner JA (2002) Bacteria and pathogenesis of human salivary calculus. Acta Otolaryngol 122(2):210–214
56. Wollin TA, Denstedt JD (1998) The holmium laser in urology. J Clin Laser Med Surg 16(1):13–20
57. Yamamoto H, Sakae T, Takagi M, Otake S (1984) Scanning electron microscopic and X-ray microdiffractometeric studies on sialolith-crystals in human submandibular glands. Acta Pathol Jpn 34(1):47–53
58. Zenk J, Hosenmann WG, Iro H (1998) Diameters of the main excretory ducts of adult human submandibular and parotid gland: a histologic study. Oral Surg Oral Med Oral Pathol Oral Radiol Endod 85:576–580

Chapter 7

Removal of Calculi or Strictures in Salivary Ducts that Cannot be Removed by Sialendoscopy

7

Francis Marchal

Contents

Core Features

- Patients with large calculi require specialists who have special expertise to evaluate and treat their symptoms.
- The treatment of each patient must be individualized.
- Combined surgical expertise using interventional sialendoscopy and conventional salivary gland surgery may avoid removal of the gland.

Complications to Avoid

- Careful selection of patients will avoid disappointment.
- Magnified loupes and a neurostimulator will compliment careful dissection and avoid damage to the facial nerve.
- Check the distal ductal system after the calculus is removed to ensure that no calculi have been missed!
- The insertion of a stent for 3 weeks will aid with healing and minimize restenosis.
- Ductoplasty, using a vein graft, needs to be sutured "watertight" to avoid salivary leak.

Introduction

The management of large salivary gland calculi has always been a therapeutic challenge: when they cannot be accessed easily by a simple marsupialization [18, 19] the removal of the gland becomes mandatory. The advent of external lithotripsy in the early 1990s [7] gave hope for conservative treatment of all calculi, with success rates ranging from 40% in the submandibular gland to 75% in the parotid gland. Unfortunately, results were poor specifically in patients with large calculi [1, 3, 6, 8]. Interventional sialendoscopy, first described in the 1990s, became popular when technological improvements made interventions reproducible for hundreds of patients in the years after 2000 [10–14, 16]. Nevertheless, success rates of interventional sialendoscopy with intraductal laser fragmentation and basket extraction of calculi remained attainable in only 80% of patients [10]. The remaining 20% of patients treated unsuccessfully was not only due to large-sized calculi (6 mm and larger) but also many of these patients had associated ductal stenosis, mostly in the parotid gland [9].

In all cases, when the calculus was considered too large to be fragmented, and/or when the stenosis was too tight to be dilated, the only solution was to remove the gland, with its associated significant morbidity [1, 3, 8]. To avoid excision of these salivary glands, we report two recently developed techniques combining sialendoscopy and external surgery [9].

Parotid Gland

Technique

7

Sialendoscopy is performed classically with sialendoscopes, which range from 0.89 to 1.6 mm in diameter. Once the calculus or stenosis is located endoscopically (Fig. 7.1), the sialendoscope is stabilized in position proximal to the lesion, and fixed at the angle of the mouth. Alternatively, a flexible light fiber, which is less cumbersome, may be introduced along the working channel of the sialendoscope. Once the light is in position, the sialendoscope is retrieved by sliding it along the light fiber which is then stabilized at the angle of mouth. The patient is positioned for a classic external parotid approach, with facial nerve monitoring attached (Fig. 7.2). Saline and adrenaline 1:200,000 solution is infiltrated into the planned incision and lateral to the intraparotid illuminated area (Fig. 7.3).

The surgical approach used may be either classic or face-lift type (Fig. 7.4), depending on the age and desires of the patient. The length of the incision is calculated on whether the surgical access required is to explore the anterior or posterior part of Stensen's duct. The skin is elevated as for a classic face-lift approach, and the light source is activated in order to localize the calculus or the stenotic process. The light source must be intermittently disconnected to avoid burning the mucosa of the duct, which may lead to subsequent stenosis. AU-SMAS flap is prepared and dissected around the illuminated area (Fig. 7.5).

When the parotid is exposed, the salivary tissue is dissected very carefully with the help of loupes or an operating microscope, in order to access Stensen's duct. Since the duct crosses several branches of the facial nerve, one must be extremely cautious with the dissection. The use of the nerve stimulator may help with the identification of the facial nerve and minimize the possibility of local trauma and subsequent nerve damage. When the duct is prepared (Fig. 7.6), the use of two colored lengths of Silastic tubing will help with stabilizing the duct and also to localize the pathologic target (Fig. 7.7). The duct is then incised over the calculus or the stenotic segment using microsurgical instruments (Fig. 7.7).

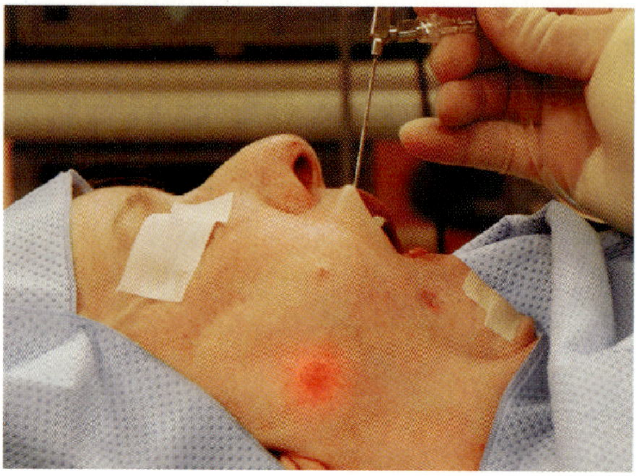

Fig. 7.1: Localization of the calculus with the endoscope

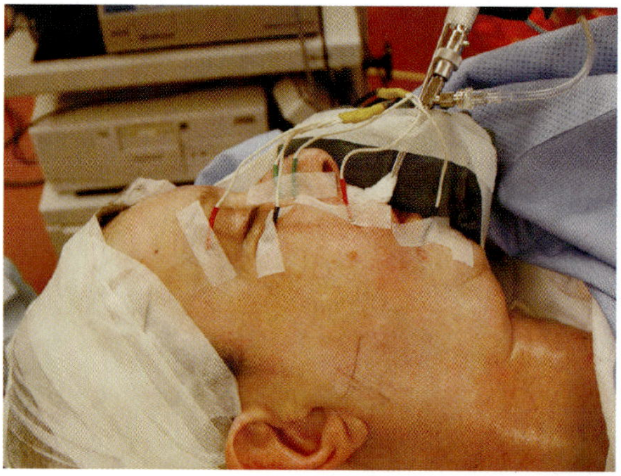

Fig. 7.2: Fixation of the endoscope and facial nerve monitoring

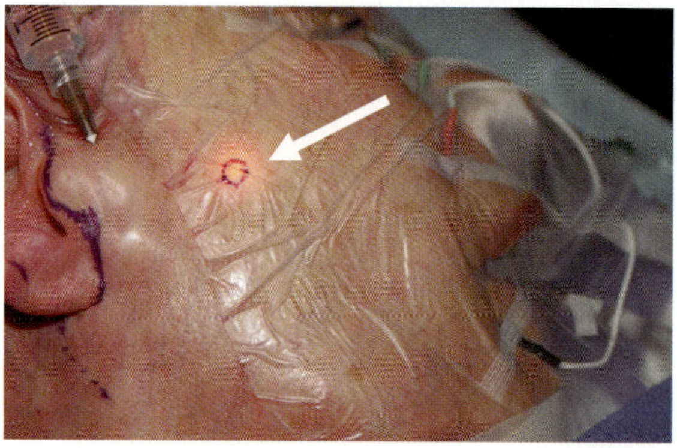

Fig. 7.3: Saline-adrenaline infiltration of the area. Light spot showing calculus (*white arrow*)

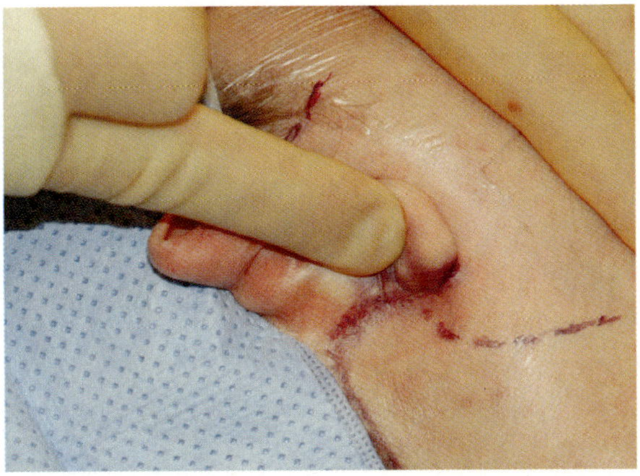

Fig. 7.4: Types of incisions

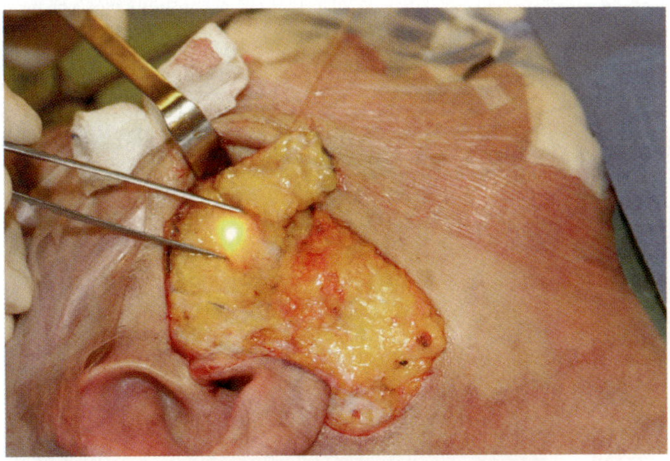

Fig. 7.5: U-SMAS preparation around the light spot

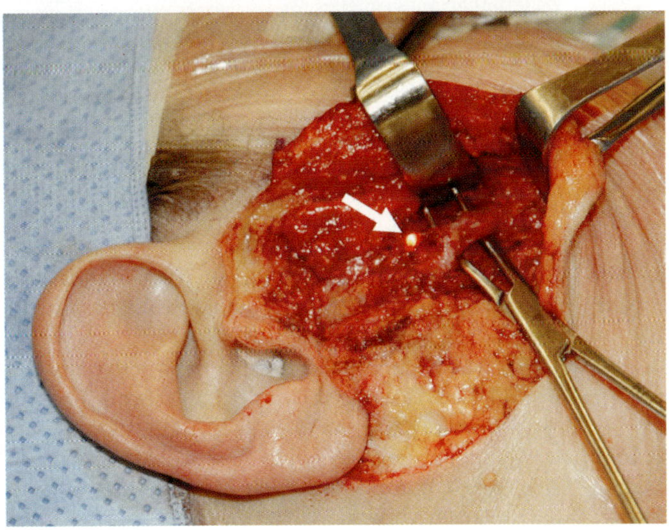

Fig. 7.6: Preparation of Stensen's duct (*white arrow*: tip of endoscope)

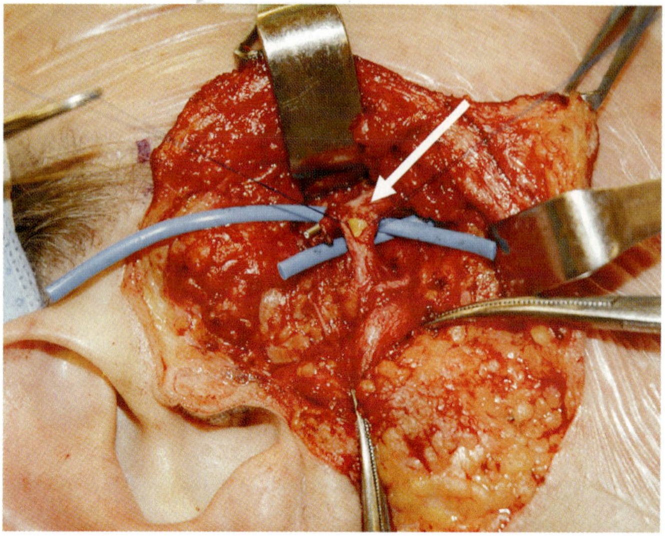

Fig. 7.7: Incision of the duct over the calculus (*white arrow*)

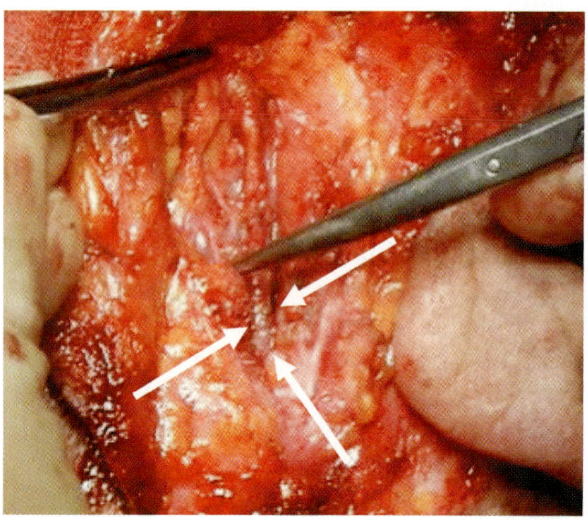

Fig. 7.8: Vein graft patch sutured onto Stensen's duct

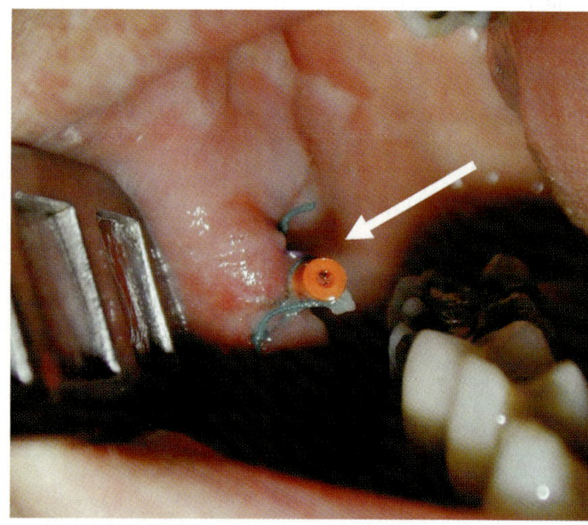

Fig. 7.9: Stent (*white arrow*) positioned in Stensen's duct

After the calculus has been removed, the distal part of the duct must be examined with the sialendoscope to ensure that a second stenosis or another calculus has not been overlooked. After endoscopic verification that no other pathology is present, the duct is closed using 7-0 or 8-0 Prolene sutures.

When large calculi are present, they cause pressure dilatation of the normal duct. A microsurgical reduction of the resultant enlargement of the duct should be performed. In cases of stenosis, the use of a vein graft as a ductoplasty patch will possibly reduce the chance that the stenosis will persist or recur (Fig. 7.8).

In cases of stenosis, a stent may be introduced either from the external approach or via a sialendoscope forwarded on the guidewire transorally. The stent is attached with a non-absorbable suture close to Stensen's papilla (Fig. 7.9). In our experience, the ideal duration of stenting should be 3 weeks.

After completion of the closure, either primary or when a vein graft has been used, it is recommended that the repaired duct is irrigated using the sialendoscope to ensure that a "watertight" closure of the suture line has been achieved to avoid leakage of saliva. The use of fibrin glue may also aid in securing a salivary seal (Fig. 7.10). The U-SMAS patch is then sutured back with interrupted 4-0 or 5-0 Vicryl sutures. The skin is sutured with either intradermal 4-0 or separate 6-0 Prolene sutures (Fig. 7.11).

Discussion

Classically when the patients were symptomatic, i.e., recurrent pain and swelling of the gland, the only solution for those with large calculi or tight stenoses was a parotidectomy with ligation of Stensen's duct [2, 4, 15, 18, 19]. Our technique described here allows for removal of parotid calculi of any size, using an external approach with preservation of the parotid gland. After performing this procedure several times, the average time duration for each subsequent procedure should not exceed 90 min. To date, 37 cases have been treated as described using this combined technique, with a mean follow-up period of 19 months, and with improvement of symptoms in 92% (33/37) of patients [9]. Of the three cases which were

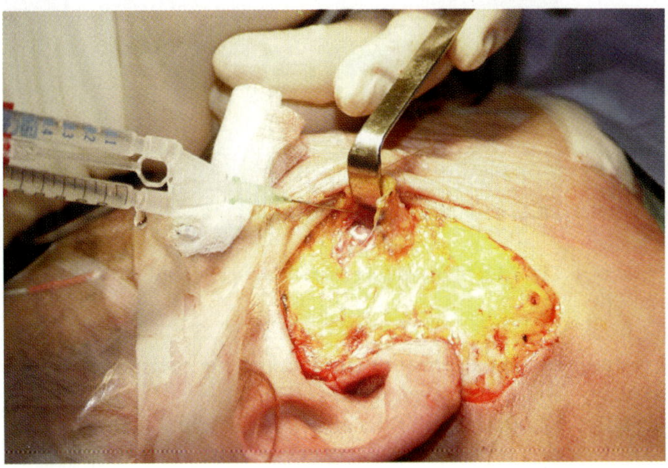

Fig. 7.10: Fibrin glue applied around Stensen's duct

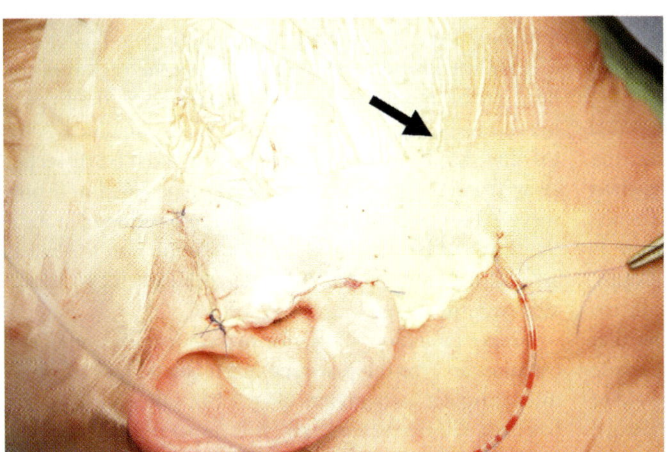

Fig. 7.11: Skin closure with intradermal Prolene 4-0 sutures

unsuccessful, one had polycystic ductal disease, another patient had a mega Stensen's duct, and the third had a mixture of the above pathology; all were subsequently treated by the ligation of the duct. In the last case, no vein graft had been interposed on a tight stenotic process of the initial portion of Stensen's duct, and it restenosed despite stenting.

Stenotic processes which cannot be handled endoscopically—either because they are too tight or because of recurrence following previous dilatations—can be treated using this approach with the suture of a vein patch over the stenosis.

The cosmetic results are excellent, as with this surgical approach no glandular tissue is removed and the scar is hidden (Fig. 7.12: 1 week postoperatively; Fig. 7.13: 3 months postoperatively). The risks of injuring the facial nerve are minimal and in our patient group no patient experienced weakness or paralysis of any facial nerve branch.

Frey's syndrome was not reported and no patient required division of the greater auricular nerve or the restitution of the soft tissue over the parotid gland and its coverage with the SMAS.

Other authors [17] have described the direct approach for removing calculi in the parotid glands, through a direct incision in the jaw. This approach allows a minimal scar, which might be visible. As branches of the facial nerve cross the duct, there might be a greater risk of facial palsy. Also, a short external incision over the jaw may lead to a non-closure of the duct, and might lead to a salivary fistula. In our experience the complications seen at the beginning of the procedure were related to less than watertight suturing of the duct, leading to salivary fistula.

Submandibular Gland

Technique

Sialendoscopy is preferentially performed using the 1.3-mm sialendoscope, until the calculus is reached (Fig. 7.14), usually found or located embedded in the intraglandular portion of the duct, or rarely a stricture is found. The endoscope is fixed to the floor of the mouth, or as mentioned above, a flexible light fiber can be introduced along the working channel and stabilized so that the surgical access to the floor of the mouth can be made without risk of disturbing the light fiber. With the help of an assistant, the floor of the mouth can be pushed upward

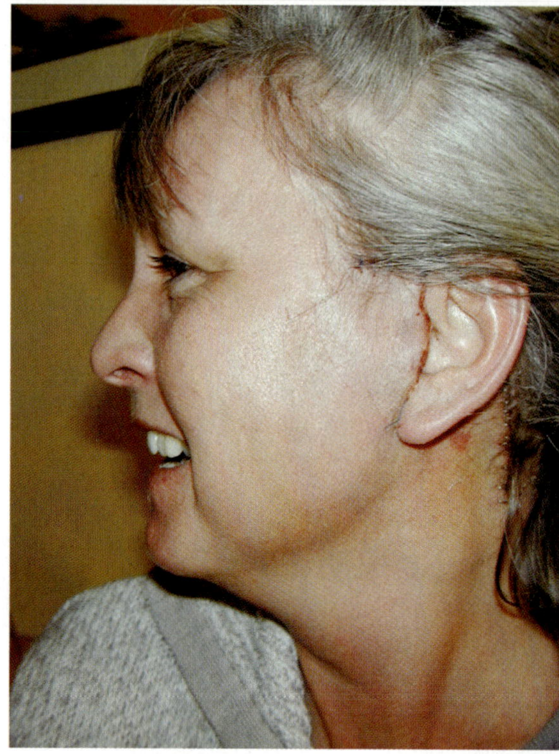

Fig. 7.12: Minimal scar 1 week postoperatively

by digital pressure from below the patients mandible, which aids surgical access (Fig. 7.15).

Infiltration of the anterior and lateral floor of mouth area is performed using xylo-adrenalin 1% with adrenalin 1:200,000 saline (Fig. 7.16). The size and location of the incision is guided by the location of the illuminated area, and is usually about 2 cm in length (Fig. 7.17).

Extreme caution while dissecting in the region of the floor of the mouth needs to be exercised as the lingual nerve can be injured as it crosses Wharton's duct. After the duct has been clearly identified, it must be dissected away from the lingual nerve which is isolated and preserved. Two colored Silastic bands are positioned around the duct and the nerve (Fig. 7.18). Traction on the bands around the duct allows the duct to be stretched which aids with the dissection.

Finger palpation allows for precise localization of the calculus, and for the planning of the ductal incision with microsurgical instruments (Fig. 7.19). Once the calculus has been removed (Fig. 7.20), it is imperative that the en-

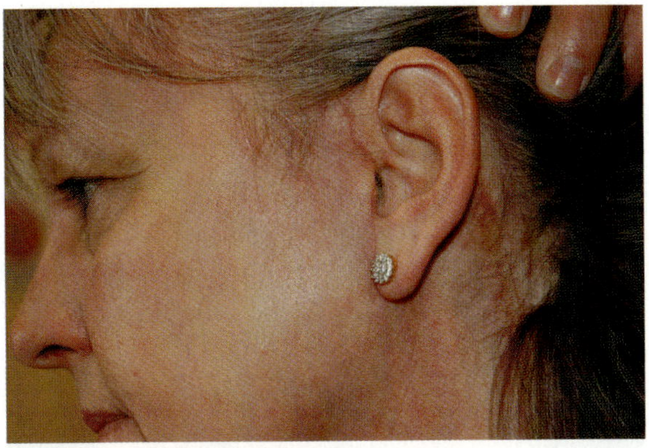

Fig. 7.13: Scarring 3 months postoperatively

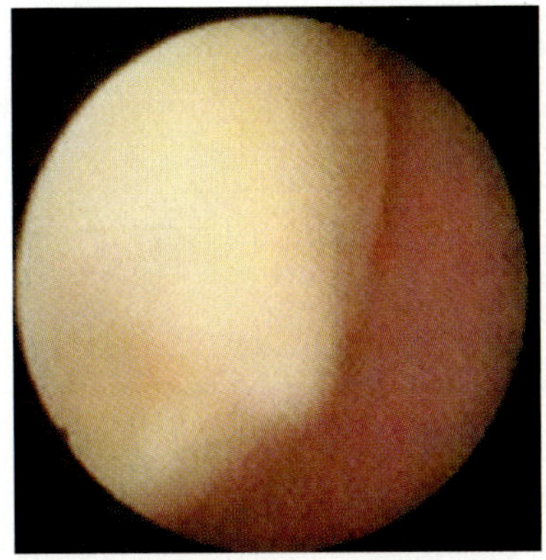

Fig. 7.14: Obstructive submandibular calculus blocked in the intraglandular part of Stensen's duct

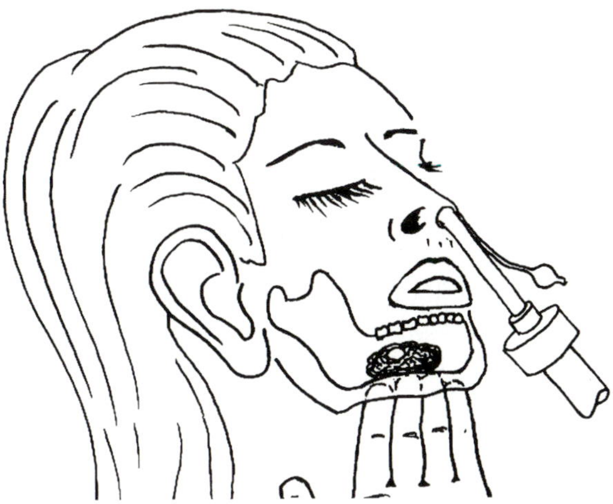

Fig. 7.15: Positioning of the assistant during the procedure

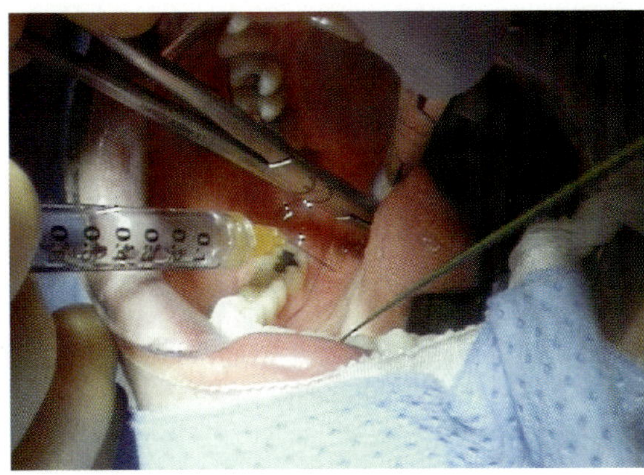

Fig. 7.16: Xylo-adrenalin infiltration

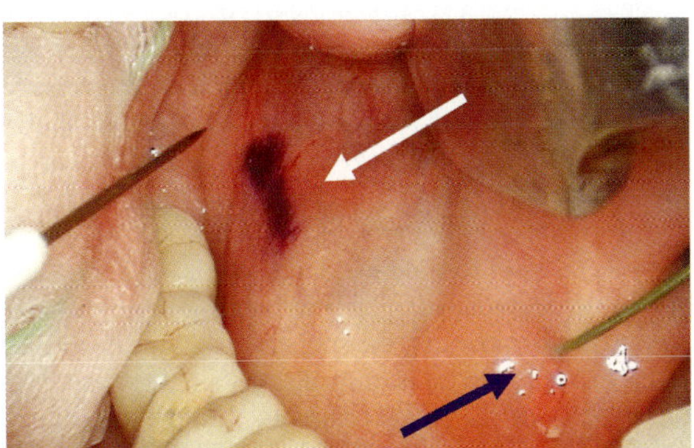

Fig. 7.17: Incision in floor of mouth (*white arrow*). Guidewire in Wharton's duct (*blue arrow*)

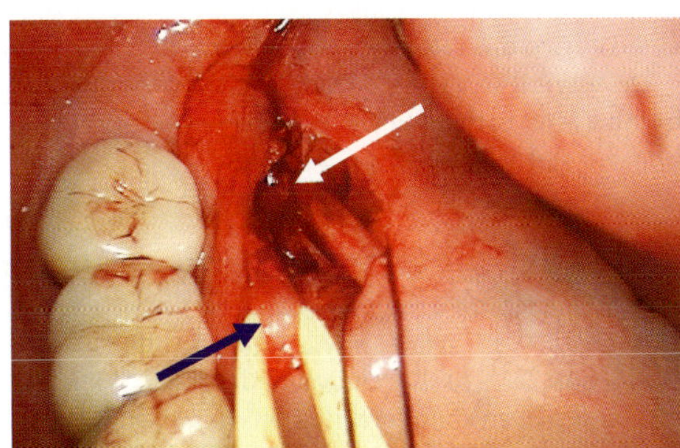

Fig. 7.18: Lingual nerve (*blue arrow*), and Wharton's duct (*white arrow*) dissection

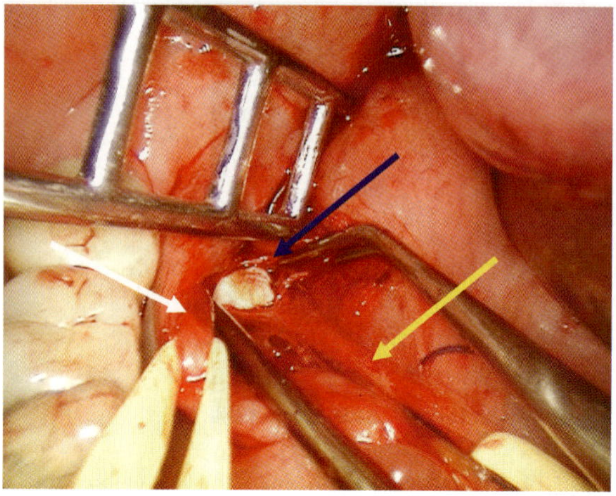

Fig. 7.19: Preparation of lingual nerve (*white arrow*); open duct (*yellow arrow*) showing calculus (blue arrow)

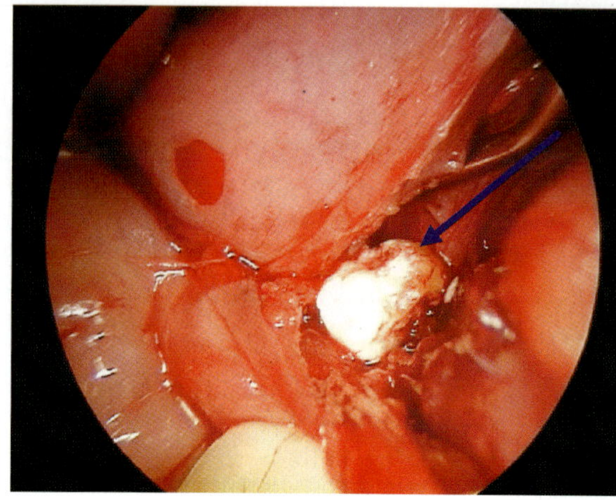

Fig. 7.20: Retrieval of calculus (*blue arrow*)

doscope allows for completion of the exploration of the remaining distal duct to ensure that residual calculi or other pathologies have not been overlooked.

A 0.45-mm-diameter guidewire should be inserted using the endoscope through the repaired ductotomy to lie in a position in the posterior portion of the duct (Fig. 7.21). The sialendoscope is removed and the guidewire left in position. The stent is introduced over the guidewire and positioned to ensure stenting of the ductoplasty area (Fig. 7.22). The stent is then sutured with a non-resorbable suture close to Wharton's papilla. The stent should be kept in position for about 3 weeks, depending on the tolerance of the patient to the foreign body. The stent and suture should be removed as indicated, but the patient needs to be encouraged and supported during this recovery period.

The surgical area is closed, one layer onto the duct and the other layer to the submucosal and mucous membrane using 5-0 or 4-0 Vicryl (Fig. 7.23).

Discussion

Historically, large symptomatic submandibular calculi lead in most cases to the removal of the gland. When the calculus is palpable intraorally, even if intraglandular, an intraoral approach is often used [18, 19]. However, our data show a relatively high incidence of postoperative stenotic scarring of Wharton's duct, even after stenting.

Minimal posterior incision of the duct reduces the risk of further stenosis, and also provides a quicker recovery for the patient. The use of the guidewire technique, which has also been used in positioning of the scope in the duct [5], may be used to position the stent in the distal part of the duct.

To date, with optimizing this combined technique in 29 cases, patients have experienced a symptomatic success rate of 69% with a mean follow-up of 22 months.

Conclusion

The combined endoscopic and external approaches represent a new treatment for large salivary calculi and salivary duct strictures of both the parotid and the submandibular glands. This operation results in a significant reduction in the number of salivary gland excisions.

Interventional sialendoscopy requires the use of an intraductal laser to fragment large stones, and this type of laser is not readily available in the majority of departments. In this situation, the surgical technique described can also be used in cases of smaller calculi that cannot be retrieved using the basket technique through the natural salivary duct orifice.

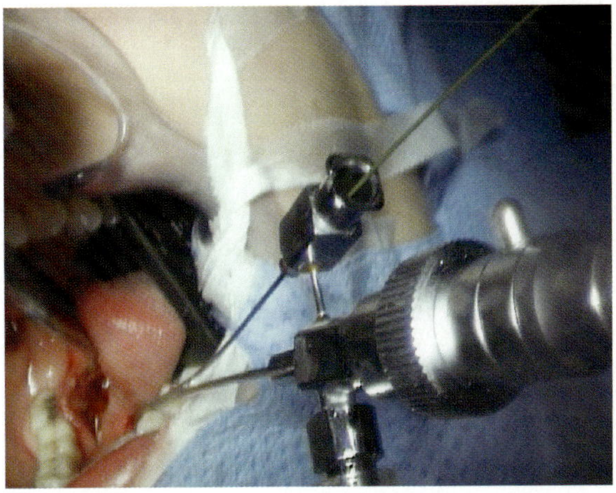

Fig. 7.21: Introduction of guidewire into the distal portion of duct

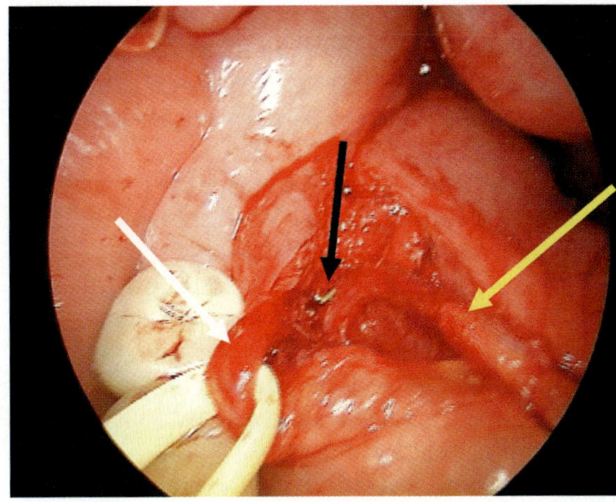

Fig. 7.22: Stent is forwarded on guidewire (*black arrow*). (*White arrow*: lingual nerve, *yellow arrow*: Wharton's duct)

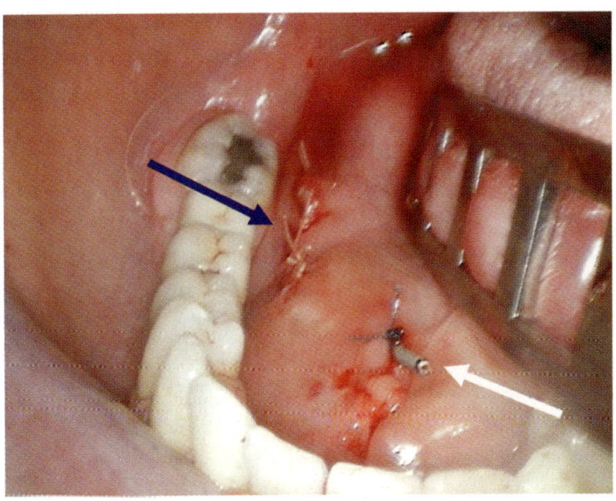

Fig. 7.23: Posterior aspect is sutured (*blue arrow*), and the stent fixed near Wharton's papilla (*white arrow*)

Lastly, it is important to emphasize that these techniques require salivary gland surgical expertise and procedures such as sialendoscopy should be performed by surgeons who are able to convert sialendoscopy into classic salivary gland surgery and have the ability to be able to handle the possible sequelae and complications.

Take Home Messages

- The management of large salivary duct calculi requires expertise in sialendoscopy and conventional salivary gland surgery, to achieve patient satisfaction following removal of the calculus, to minimize the postoperative complications, and to avoid return of their symptoms.
- The combined endoscopic-external approach allows precise control of the ductal pathology, retrieval of calculi of any size, and microsurgical enlargement of ductal stenosis.
- The microsurgical sutures of the duct are essential in this approach to avoid salivary stenosis and fistula.
- Watertight closure of the duct is essential in avoiding salivary fistula and to facilitate healing.

References

1. Aidan P, De Kerviler E, LeDuc A, Monteil JP (1996) Treatment of salivary stones by extracorporeal lithotripsy. Am J Otolaryngol 17(4):246–250
2. Bates D, O'Brien CJ, Tikaram K, Painter DM (1998) Parotid and submandibular sialadenitis treated by salivary gland excision. Aust N Z J Surg 68(2):120–124
3. Capaccio P, Ottaviani F, Manzo R, Schindler A, Cesana B (2004) Extracorporeal lithotripsy for salivary calculi: a long-term clinical experience. Laryngoscope 114(6):1069–1073
4. Cawson RA, Gleeson MJ, Eveson JW (1997) Sialadenitis. In: Cawson RA, Gleeson MJ, Eveson JW (1997) eds. Pathology and surgery of the salivary glands. Oxford: Isis Medical Media 33–63
5. Chossegros C, Guyot L, Richard O, Barki G, Marchal F (2006) A technical improvement in sialendoscopy to enter the salivary ducts. Laryngoscope May 116(5):842–844
6. Gutmann R, Ziegler G, Leunig A, Jacob K, Feyh J (1995) Die endoskopische und extrakorporale Stosswellen-Lithotripsie von Speichelsteinen. Laryngorhinootologie 74(4):249–253
7. Iro H, et al. (1992) Shockwave lithotripsy of salivary duct stones. Lancet 339(8805):1333–1336
8. Iro H, Zenk J, Waldfahrer F, Benzel W, Schneider T, Ell C (1998) Extracorporeal shock wave lithotripsy of parotid stones. Results of a prospective clinical trial. Ann Otol Rhinol Laryngol. 107(10 Pt 1):860–864
9. Marchal F. (2007) A combined endoscopic and external approach for extraction of large stones with presentation of parotid and submandibular glands. Laryngoscope 117(2):373–377
10. Marchal F, Dulguerov P (2003) Sialolithiasis management: the state of the art. Arch Otolaryngol Head Neck Surg 129(9):951–956
11. Marchal F, Becker M, Dulguerov P, Lehmann W (2000) Interventional sialendoscopy. Laryngoscope 110(2 Pt 1):318–320
12. Marchal F, Dulguerov P, Lehmann W (1999) Interventional sialendoscopy. N Engl J Med 341(16):1242–1243
13. Marchal F, Dulguerov P, Becker M, Barki G, Disant F, Lehmann W (2001) Specificity of parotid sialendoscopy. Laryngoscope 111(2):264–271
14. Marchal F, Dulguerov P, Becker M, Barki G, Disant F, Lehmann W (2002) Submandibular diagnostic and interventional sialendoscopy: new procedure for ductal disorders. Ann Otol Rhinol Laryngol 111(1):27–35
15. Marchal F, Kurt AM, Dulguerov P, Becker M, Oedman M, Lehmann W (2001) Histopathology of submandibular glands removed for sialolithiasis. Ann Otol Rhinol Laryngol 110(5 Pt 1):464–469
16. Nahlieli O, Baruchin AM (1999) Endoscopic technique for the diagnosis and treatment of obstructive salivary gland diseases. J Oral Maxillofac Surg 57(12):1394–1401
17. Nahlieli O, London D, Zagury A, Eliav E (2002) Combined approach to impacted parotid stones. J Oral Maxillofac Surg 60(12):1418–1423
18. Rice DH (1999) Non-inflammatory, non-neoplastic disorders of the salivary glands. Otolaryngol Clin North Am 32(5):835–843
19. Rice DH (1993) Diseases of the salivary glands – non neoplastic. In: Bailey B, Pillsbury HC, eds. Head and Neck Surgery – Otolaryngology. Vol I. Philadelphia: J.B. Lippincott 475–484

Chapter 8

Fine-needle Aspiration Biopsy

Grace C.H. Yang

8

Contents

Core Features

- Minimally invasive biopsy
- Simple but not trivial
- Accurate diagnosis depends mostly on meticulous technique
- Immediate test turnaround time possible
- Cost effective

Complications to Avoid

- Minor bleeding (intralesional or subcutaneously). This complication can be avoided by advising patients to avoid blood thinners 5 days prior to biopsy; by compression immediately following withdrawal of the needle; or by using 27-gauge needles.
- Infection. This complication can be avoided by using an alcohol wipe and a needle finer than 22 gauge.

Introduction

Fine-needle aspiration (FNA) biopsy is similar to bone marrow aspiration. The samples are aspirated, deposited on microscopic slides, and smeared. Hematologists interpret aspiration smears of bone marrow and peripheral blood, while cytopathologists interpret aspiration smears of the remaining body sites. In addition to the Romanowsky stain used by hematologists, cytopathologist also use Papanicolaou stain for additional nuclear and cytoplasmic details.

The Needle

Conventional wisdom says "the larger the needle, the more abundant the sample obtained." However, it does not apply to FNA, because blood is the biggest enemy of a satisfactory FNA sample. Blood dilutes the cells and makes the sample unsatisfactory (100 cells/0.1 ml of blood is satisfactory, but 100 cells/1 ml of blood is unsatisfactory). Unlike paraffin sections used in histopathology, FNA smears require just a few cells to be diagnostic, but blood aspirated from needles larger than 22 gauge will not only ruin a good sample, but also ruin subsequent samples, because now the blood vessels are ruptured flooding the surrounding area. Optimally, one uses the finest needle possible to obtain a minimally bloody sample which will be diagnostic. Needles smaller than a critical cross-sectional luminal area (Table 8.1) can go in and out of blood vessels as if nothing happened. The elasticity of the blood vessel smooth muscle wall snaps back and seals the puncture holes as soon as the needle passes. One example is acupuncture which can penetrate the human body in various places without causing pain, bleeding, or infection. Acupuncture uses a 27-gauge needle, the same gauge needle most frequently used for thyroid FNA by cytopathologists at the New York University (NYU) Medical Center. The needle is so fine that there is no need to press the puncture site to prevent hematoma. In Fig. 8.1 there is no 22-gauge needle because no 22-gauge needle can be found anywhere in the three FNA clinics at the NYU Medical Center.

8

Fine-needle Sampling Without Syringe

Fine-needle sampling without syringe can obtain cells and tissue particles into the needle hub and is used most frequently by cytopathologists at the NYU Medical Center. This technique was first described in 1987 by Zajdela et al. of Institute Curie in France [17]. This method gives one greatest sensitivity to the changes in the texture of tissues through which the needle passes. The mass is stabilized with the left hand. The fine needle is held by the right thumb and index finger. After the needle is advanced into the nodule, it is moved about in a cone-shaped tissue volume. The needle tip acts like cork borer to cut tiny cores of tissue, which pushed each other into the needle hub. The needle is moved as fast as the needle of a sewing machine. As soon as the sample shows up in the needle hub, the sampling stops. A 10-ml syringe filled with air is attached and the sample is expelled onto microscope slides and smeared. Needle sampling without a syringe is best for small lesions. Although this technique yields less quantity of sample, the quality of sample is better due to minimal dilution with blood. However, the time to obtain an adequate sample is longer than aspiration with suction from a syringe. In addition, it is difficult to sample mesenchymal lesions without suction.

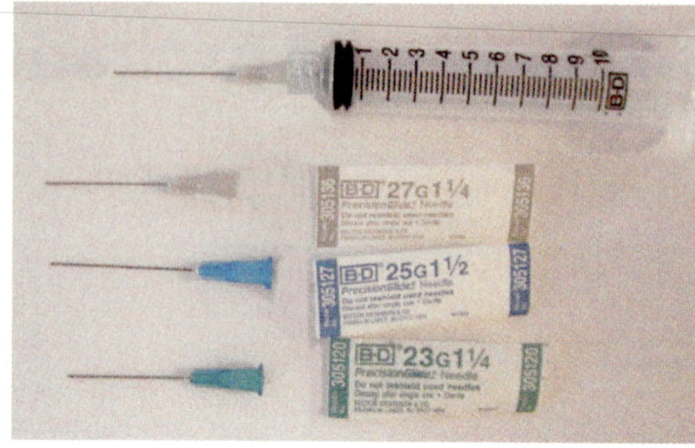

Fig. 8.1: Needles and syringe used for fine-needle aspiration (FNA) biopsy

Table 8.1. Diameter of needles used for fine-needle aspiration

Needle gauge	Outside diameter (mm)	Inside diameter (mm)	Cross-sectional lumen area (mm^2)
22	0.71	0.41	0.13
23	0.64	0.33	0.09
25	0.51	0.25	0.05
27	0.41	0.20	0.03

The Syringe

Single use, sterile, disposable plastic 10-ml syringes with a Luer-Lok tip are used in FNA. Larger syringes do not yield larger samples. It is important not to attach the needle too tightly to the syringe, because it slows the removal of the needle and delays smear preparation leading to clotting of the sample.

Syringe Holders

Until late 1990s, the pistol-grip syringe holder, developed in Sweden, was popular. In recent years, the pencil-grip syringe holder [10] (Fig. 8.2) has become popular for clinicians. It is equipped with a release button for automatically drawing back the syringe plunger, and a regulating knob for setting a predetermined amount of negative pressure for the aspiration. It places the hand much closer to the target than the pistol-grip syringe holder, and uses hand movement rather than arm movement. After the needle is advanced into the nodule, a button is pushed and the syringe holder rises automatically to a preset position. Similar to needle sampling without a syringe, the needle tip is moving back and forth cutting fine cores of tissue within the nodule in a cone-shaped imaginary space. The succession of fine-needle cores cut by the needle tip will push each other into the hub of the needle. The vacuum in the syringe facilitates moving of the sample into the needle hub. After the sample appears in the needle hub, the syringe along with the needle is removed from the holder. Surprisingly, the 2- to 3-ml vacuum does not suck the sample from the needle hub into the syringe, because the needle hole has been sealed by the sample. The syringe is then detached from the syringe holder and the needle is separated from the syringe. The plunger is raised all the way up, the syringe is reattached to the needle containing the sample, and the sample is expelled from the needle hub onto the microscopic slides and smears made.

Labeling the Microscopic Slides

Prior to the performance of aspiration, one must label the microscopic slides. Using #2 lead pencil, the frosted end of the slide is labeled with the patient's last name and the number of the nodule. Labeling slides just before aspiration not only eliminates the possibility of confusing patients, but also avoids depositing the sample on the wrong side of the microscopic slide, with the possibility of having the specimen wiped off in the cytology laboratory.

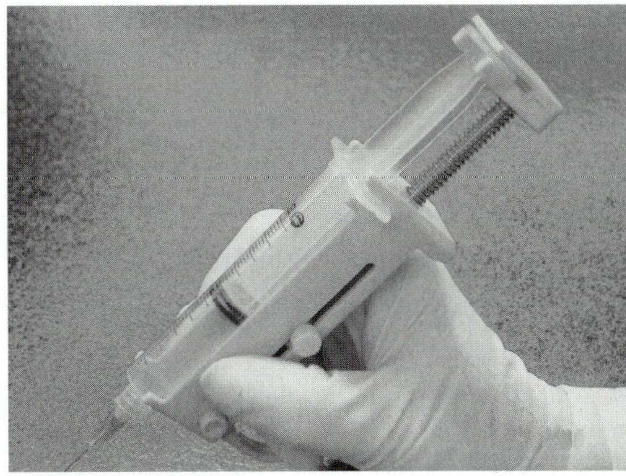

Fig. 8.2: Syringe holder for FNA procedure

The Basic Aspiration Procedure

Fine-needle aspiration biopsy can be adapted to many clinical settings and problems, but the basic procedure remains the same [9]. While the number of passes performed on a given nodule varies, the actual performance of puncture takes less than 10 s per pass in the majority of the cases due to the rapid movement of the needle (as rapid as the needle movement in a sewing machine). The majority of time is spent in locating the lesion, preparing the skin, recovering the sample from the needle hub, and making smears. Despite the procedure's simplicity, individuals new to FNA biopsy should practice the basic procedure using a fruit, such as an orange, until it goes smoothly, quickly, and becomes second nature. The basic aspiration procedure can be broken down into the following steps:

1. Wipe the skin with an alcohol pad.
2. Locate, palpate, and stabilize the nodule.
3. Pass the needle through the skin.
4. Advance the needle into the nodule.
5. Apply suction by raising the plunger, if a syringe holder is used.
6. Move the needle rapidly back and forth, sampling different areas of the nodule.
7. Remove the needle from the patient.
8. Detach the needle from the syringe.
9. Fill the syringe with air.

10. Reattach the needle with the sample onto the syringe.
11. Touch the needle tip to a microscope slide with bevel side down.
12. Express the specimen onto the microscope slide.
13. Make oval smears.

Locate, Palpate, and Stabilize the Target Lesion

Two fingers of the left hand outline and immobilize the mass. In the case of large nodules, only a portion of the nodule is spanned by the fingertips. In the cases of smaller nodules, the entire nodule is encompassed by the fingertips. This approach allows the operator to immobilize the target for the needle to aim. The fingers are arched and extend from the hand, which is poised above a point near the palpable nodule. This makes use of the sensitive fingertips in localizing the target. In this position, the small intrinsic muscles of the hand are relaxed and the fine movements of the fingertips ensure accurate puncture of small targets. Once the nodule is stabilized, the needle is passed through the skin to the lesion. It is helpful to think of the needle as an extension of the index finger of the right hand and the nodule as an extension of the palpating fingers of the left hand. Aiming at a small target is analogous to touching the tip of one index finger with the other. After the needle enters the lesion and suction is applied, the needle is moved back and forth through the mass almost as fast as the needle in the sewing machine. The actual motion causes the needle tip to describe a cone, with its base in the mass and its apex at the entry point of the skin. Always move the needle in a straight line, and change direction at the top of the cone, i.e., near the entry point of the skin. The rapid motion of the needle cuts loose numerous tiny cores of tissue that move up to the hub of the needle. This activity takes only a few seconds. The operator needs to have split vision, monitoring the transparent needle hub as well as watching the reaction of the patients. As soon as material appears in the needle hub, aspiration stops. Depending on the nature of the lesion, in some instances, larger volumes of cyst fluid or blood may be obtained.

Recovery of the Sample from Needle Hub

Hold the air-filled syringe with the left hand and place the needle tip on the glass slide with the bevel side down. Then, using the right hand, carefully push the plunger to deposit a small droplet on each slide, approximately 1 cm from the label. After the sample is deposited onto the slides and smears made, an effort should be made to recover the residual sample adhered to the needle hub by the following maneuver. Holding the needle upward with the left thumb and index finger, use the right thumb and index finger to lift the open end of the needle hub upward and let go, allowing the open end of the needle hub to bounce back onto the microscopic slide so that the adhering material is dislodged onto the glass slide for another smear. One should practice this technique with unused needles filled with creamy hand lotion before applying it to needles containing potentially infectious patient material. The needle can also be gripped with a hemostat, to reduce the danger of an accidental needle-stick injury. The material in the needle hub could be the purest part of the specimen without contamination with blood or fluid. Therefore, recovery, smearing, and study of the needle hub material is important.

Frequently, a small droplet of the sample may be left in the tip of the syringe. It can be recovered in the following manner. The plunger is gently raised all the way up to fill the syringe with air. The plastic tip of the syringe is placed on the glass slide and the plunger is rapidly, forcefully, and audibly pushed all the way down. This maneuver can be rapidly repeated several times so that the droplet at tip of the syringe can be recovered and smeared.

The Fine Art of Smear Preparation

Preparation of smears is the most important steps of FNA. Unless high-quality smears are created, it does not matter how good the samples are, they will be challenging to interpret, because the criteria used for diagnosis by cytopathologists depends on a properly executed smear. First and foremost is to stop aspirating as soon as the sample appears in the needle hub and immediately transfer the sample to the slide and smear, since specimens may dry and a bloody sample may clot.

The smearing technique for FNA is similar to making smears for bone marrow aspirates by hematologists, but more refined. At the NYU Medical Center, the direct smears are made in the Swedish method as taught by the late Torsten Löwhagen of Karolinska Institute in Sweden [9]. The aspirate was deposited 1 cm from the frosted end of the bottom slide. Holding the frosted end with the left thumb and index finger and the rest of the slide supported by the remaining three fingers, the bottom slide remains horizontal and motionless. Another slide is held by the right thumb and index finger at a right angle to the bottom slide; the top slide is placed on the bottom slide at 45° at a distance so that when the top slide is lowered to 0° in a hinge-like fashion, the majority, but not all, of the droplet will be touched. The untouched area of the droplet serves as an anchor, so that the entire droplet will not roll with the top slide. The top slide then moves over the entire length of the bottom slide toward the preparer in a gentle, quick, and steady fashion. In fact, the top slide glides over the bottom slide along a parallel space filled with air without actually touching the bottom slide. The sample is suspended in a liquid meniscus between the top and bottom slides, so that the cells will be spread apart but not crushed.

Preparation of Multiple Smears from a Single Aspiration by DAB Technique

Sometimes, especially from aspiration of carcinoma or lymphoma, a single pass yields too much sample for one slide and the smear will be too thick for examination. One needs to split the sample into several slides by the DAB technique [11]. These tiny smears will be thin enough for microscopic examination. After depositing a large drop of the sample on the slide, take another slide (the spreader slide) and hold it with right thumb and index finger parallel to the aspirator. The sample deposited on the bottom slide, which is perpendicular to the aspirator, is lightly touched (dabbed) with outer edge of the spreader slide at different spots, starting from the far end of the spreader slide and moving toward the fingers holding the spreader slide. The spreader slide with the newly dabbed droplets can be transferred to three new slides to make three small smears. The last smear is made by flipping over the spreader slide to obtain a new edge, and smear the original slide. In this way, four small high-quality smears can be prepared from one pass.

Although the above descriptions may seem tedious to the reader, they can be mastered with practice and can be executed within a few seconds. Just as the basic motions of the FNA procedure should be mastered before the patient is approached, so should the handling of aspirated material. Smear making can be practiced using droplets of creamy hand lotion. The aspiration can be simulated by material aspirated from an orange.

Gross Examination of the Smears for Specimen Adequacy

Gross examination of the smears is often the ignored step for FNA. Even without a microscope, the operator can gather important information regarding the adequacy of the sample, because the physical features of the aspirates correlate to microscopic findings [16]. Is the sample easy or difficult to expel to the slide? Is the smear easy to make or felt viscous? Typically, the aspirate of pleomorphic adenoma is thick and viscous due to chondromyxoid stroma and Warthin's tumor is thin due to lymphocytes and rare sheets of oncocytic epithelium. Does the smear appear shiny like glazed honey (colloid nodule), thin like water (cystic degeneration), thick like dried tooth paste (epidermal inclusion cyst), or bloody like peripheral blood. Can one observe particles on the smear? If blood appears in the syringe as soon as the needle enters the nodule, make a smear and empty the blood into a test tube containing CytoRich Red and try a different area of the nodule. Never submit slides that the operator already knows by gross examination are unsatisfactory, because cytology laboratories are obligated by regulations to process every single slide that is submitted. Frequently, the cytology laboratory receives a dozen slides, out of which, ten slides appear empty by gross examination. It is the operator's duty to select the satisfactory slides to transport to the cytology laboratory based on gross examination (Fig. 8.3). If the first pass is unsatisfactory, take additional passes until satisfactory, while the patient is still available.

Air Drying the Smears to Create Large, Flat Cells

In the older methods, wet smears were plunged immediately into a coplin jar containing 95% ethanol or sprayed by spray fixative. Air drying was considered bad for cells. In 1988, it was discovered by Chan and Kung [2] that air-dried cells within a certain time period can be restored to transparency by simply soaking in normal saline for 30 s. Ultrafast Papanicolaou stain [14] incorporates this air-drying rehydration by saline technique [13] as the first step, because it allows cytopathologists to examine large, flat, and transparent cells, maximizing the resolution of nuclear and cytoplasmic details and increasing the sensitivity of cancer detection [12]. Figure 8.4 illustrates the cytologic details that can be achieved by this method

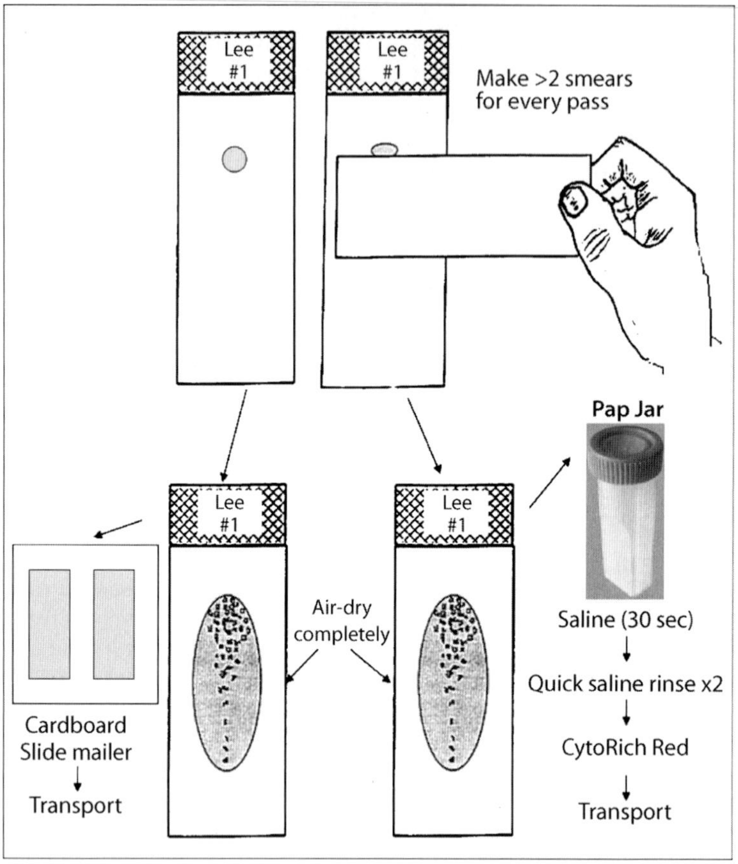

Fig. 8.3: Preparation of FNA smears for transport

and difficult diagnostic problems that can be solved. It is known that approximately 5% of pleomorphic adenomas [3, 4, 7] and some basal cell adenomas [8], share the cylindromatous stroma of adenoid cystic carcinoma on smears. This pitfall is the reason cytopathologists are reluctant to diagnose adenoid cystic carcinoma, and often report "Salivary gland neoplasm with cylindromatous stroma: adenoid cystic carcinoma versus pleomorphic adenoma." This kind of report makes FNA of salivary gland useless to the surgeons, since the former requires radical surgical with wide margins, while the latter uses a conservative approach [1]. The distinction is possible [15] using large, flat, and transparent cells by allowing the smears to air dry followed by rehydration in saline, a simple and elegant technique. In 30 s the saline enters the air-dried cells by osmosis, making nucleated cells transparent and red blood cells hemolyzed. The leaked hemoglobin particles may cover the cells on the smear; therefore, it must be removed by two quick rinses in saline. If left in saline for more than 30 s, the cells will start to detach from the glass surface, so precise timing is important. The cellular details are suboptimal when there is a delay in rehydration by saline. That is why one must rehydrate the smears in saline before transporting the slides in CytoRich Red solution to the cytology laboratory. Figure 8.3 illustrates the steps from the preparation of smears to transport. The air-dried opaque cells transported in cardboard slide holders will be stained in the cytology laboratory for Romanowsky stain to highlight the metachromatic stroma and background substance. The large, flat, and transparent cells transported in Pap jars will be processed for Papanicolaou stain for additional nuclear and cytoplasmic details.

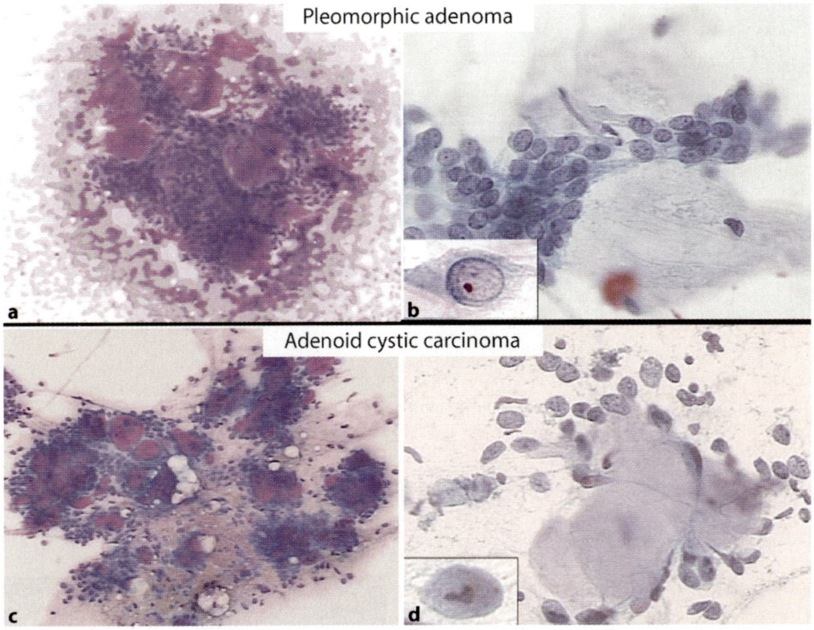

Fig. 8.4: Distinguishing adenoid cystic carcinoma from pleomorphic adenoma in salivary gland aspirates, processed with the method described in Fig. 8.3. **a** Pleomorphic adenoma with metachromatic cylindromatous stroma covered by tumor cells. Romanowsky stain, 100×. **b** The oval neoplastic cells of pleomorphic adenoma have visible cytoplasm. Ultrafast Papanicolaou stain, 400×. Inset Close-up of a tumor cell shows pale nucleus with small round nucleolus and abundant cytoplasm. 1,000×. **c** Adenoid cystic carcinoma with metachromatic cylindromatous stroma. Romanowsky stain, 100×. **d** The cytoplasm of neoplastic cells of adenoid cystic carcinoma measures <1 μm, which is beyond the resolution of the light microscope, thus the neoplastic cells look like naked nuclei. Ultrafast Papanicolaou stain, 400×. *Inset* Close-up of a tumor cell shows no cytoplasm, darker chromatin, and the irregular nucleolus. 1,000×

CytoRich Red is the Cytology Fixative for the Twenty-first Century

All of the previous fixatives, such as 95% ethanol, fix everything in the sample, including nucleated cells, red blood cells, and the background protein. In 1996, an innovative fixative, CytoRich Red, was developed by Maksem [5, 6]. This solution selectively fixes nucleated cells, while paradoxically dissolving red blood cells and background protein. One milliliter of CytoRich Red can lyse 25 μl of whole blood. It is important to know that CytoRich Red will only hemolyze red blood cells when they are wet, and not when they are dried. That is why the air-dried smears must first be immersed in saline before transporting in CytoRich Red, which will dissolve residual hemoglobin particles covering the cells on the smears, providing a clean background for optimal cytologic examination. The rehydrated air-dried cells received in the cytology laboratory can be stained with the standard Papanicolaou stain, and show flat, large, and transparent cells in a clean background for optimal analysis of cellular details.

Liquid Fixation is for Operators Who Cannot Master the Art of Smearing

The sample obtained by aspiration can be directly expressed into liquid fixatives, such as CytoRich Red. Liquid fixation relieves the aspirators from learning to how to make FNA smears, however, the resolution of cellular details is markedly decreased. Using an egg as an analogy (Fig. 8.5), egg yolk is the nucleus of the cell and egg white is the cytoplasm of the cell. The water is boiling in the pot, the eggshell is broken, and the egg is dropped into the boiling water and immediately

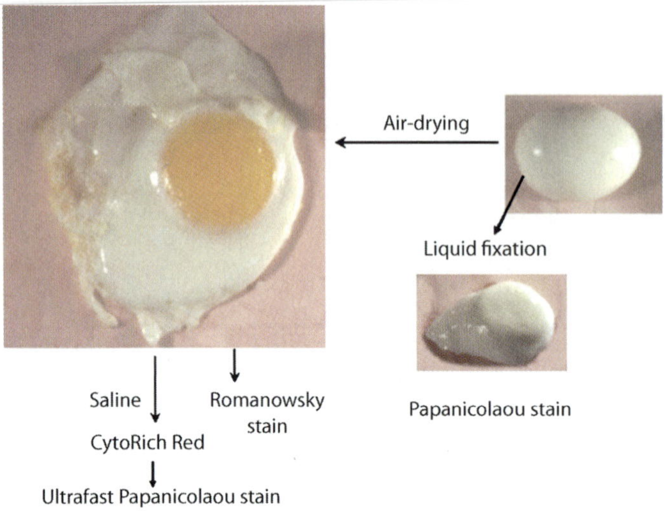

Fig. 8.5: Cytology preparation is analogous to preparation of eggs. Highest resolution of cytologic details is possible only with air drying, which provides the largest cytoplasm and nucleus for cytomorphologic analysis. Cells placed in liquid fixation are like poached eggs with smaller nuclei and cytoplasm, making it difficult to distinguish look-alike entities

cooked into poached egg. Liquid-fixed cells are analogous to "poached egg" with smaller nuclei and smaller cytoplasm under the microscope. Air-dried cells are like "sunny-side up egg." The eggshell is cracked and the egg is dropped over a flat pan. The egg flattens by gravity and is then cooked into sunny-side up egg. Air-drying allows the cells to flatten by gravity. The flattened cells appear larger under the microscope for higher resolution of cytoplasmic and nuclear details. In addition, liquid fixation precludes the use of Romanowsky stain, the most popular stain for cytopathologists, and the use of Ultrafast Papanicolaou stain, the stain that provides the highest resolution of nuclear and cytoplasmic details. Placing fine-needle aspirates in liquid fixation for cytopathologists is like placing bone marrow aspirates into liquid fixative for hematologists. The exquisite cellular details shown in Fig. 8.4 for optimal cytomorphologic analysis and to distinguish look-alike entities will not be possible in liquid fixation.

Needle-rinse Material Contributes Little to FNA Diagnoses

Although routine preparation and examination of slides from needle-rinse material may be unnecessary and inefficient, collecting this material at the bedside requires very little additional time or effort. Thus, some operators routinely rinse the needle and syringe at the time of FNA and then process this rinse-material specimen only in rare cases in which additional material is needed.

Role of FNA Biopsy to Diagnose Lymphoma of the Parotid Gland

With the advent of sophisticated cellular immunological methods, such as flow cytometry, characterization of different cellular subsets within the aspirate population can be achieved by staining for surface markers using fluorescent antibodies. Collection of a least two needle passes in Hanks' basic salt solution or Roswell Park Memorial Institute (RPMI) medium for immunophenotyping by flow cytometry addresses some of the concerns with adequacy of FNA biopsy specimens. Immunophenotyping by flow cytometry detects cell surface antigens using a variety of monoclonal antibodies that indicate differentiation, lineage (B or T ells), and whether there is a monoclonal production of the light chains or the heavy chains. Immunophenotyping also confirms the reactive nature of the lymph node because there will be a polyclonal pattern of immunoglobulins with production of both light chains with a kappa:lambda ratio of 2:1. Gene rearrangement studies can be performed when immunophenotyping is equivocal, and this has resulted in a substantial increase in accuracy for typing lymphomas. These are the genes for cell surface antigen receptors, and arrangement of these genes is the earliest genetic event in the development of lymphomas. The gene rearrangement can be detected using the Southern blot technique or polymerase chain reaction. Even if an open biopsy of a lymph node has to be performed following a FNA biopsy, reactive, inflammatory, and metastatic lesions have been eliminated and the diagnostic possibilities are narrowed down.

Take Home Messages

- BLOOD IS THE ENEMY: use the finest needle possible to avoid dilution of tumor cells by a tsunami of blood.
- LESS IS MORE: a scanty undiluted sample is better than an abundant blood diluted sample.
- THE CLOCK IS TICKING: work fast to avoid clotting of the sample before smearing.
- GROSS INSPECTION of smears for adequacy and correlation with final diagnosis.
- METICULOUSLY FOLLOW DIRECTIONS which will ensure success of FNA.

Supplies for FNA Biopsy

Alcohol pads:
- Sterile, alcohol prep pad, reorder #:122
- PSS Select, Jacksonville, FL 32216

Needles:
BD PrecisionGlide needles, single use
- Cat# 302136 27 gauge, 1-1/4"
- Cat# 302127 25 gauge, 1-1/2"
- Cat# 302120 23 gauge, 1-1/4"

Syringes:
BD 10-ml plastic disposable syringe with Luer-Lok tip
- Ref 309604
- Becton-Dickinson, Franklin Lakes, NJ 07417
- Becton-Dickinson, http://www.bd.com

Pencil-grip syringe holder:
- Tao aspirator, Tao & Tao Technology, 886 Sands Lane, Camano Island, WA 98282; Tel.: +1-360-3876186, http://www.taoaspirator.com

Pistol-grip syringe holder:
- Cameco Syringe holder, Belpro Medical, 9915 Place York, Anjou, Quebec, Canada Tel.: +1-888-2301010, http://www.belpro.ca/com

Microscopic slides:
- Newcomer Supply, 2505 Parview Road, Middleton, WI 53562; Tel.: +1-800-3837799
- Cat# 6215 Microscopic slides with frosted ends, 3×1×0.1 cm

Saline:
- Baxter Healthcare., One Baxter Parkway, Deerfield, IL 60015; Tel.: +1-800-4229837, http://www.baxter.com/
- Cat# 2F7124 0.9% NaCl, irrigation saline, USP

CytoRich Red preservative:
- TriPath Imaging, 780 Plantation Drive, Burlington, NC 27215; Tel.: +1-866-8747284, http://www.tripathimaging.com/
- Cat# CytoRich Red preservative 3600 ml/bottle

Pap jars:
- Evergreen Scientific, 2300 East 49th St., PO Box 58248, Los Angeles, CA 90058; Tel.: +1-800-4216261, http://www.evergreensci.com/ch/pfp.htm
- Cat# 240-5420-G8K Pap jars w/ green caps, empty, pack of 200

Cardboard slide mailers:
- Richard-Allan Scientific, Kalamazoo, MI 49008; Tel.: +1-800-5227270, http://www.rallansci.com/
- Cat#2500 Slide Mailer

References

1. Casler JD, Conley JJ (1992) Surgical management of adenoid cystic carcinoma in the parotid gland. Otolaryngol Head Neck Surg 106:332–338
2. Chan JKC, Kung ITM (1988) Rehydration with air-dried smears with normal saline. Application in fine needle aspiration cytologic examination. Am J Clin Pathol 89:30–34
3. Kapadia SB, Dusenbery D, Dekker A (1997) Fine needle aspiration of pleomorphic adenoma and adenoid cystic carcinoma of salivary gland origin. Acta Cytol 41:487–492
4. Löwhagen T, Tani EM, Skoog L Salivary glands and rare head and neck lesions. In: Bibbo M (1991) Comprehensive Cytopathology. Philadelphia, Saunders, pp 621–648
5. Maksem JA (1996) The CytoRich Fixation System. Cytology preparation manual of TriPath Imaging Inc. Burlington, North Carolina

6. Maksem J, Sager F, Bender R (1997) Endometrial collection and interpretation using Tao brush and CytoRich fixative system: A feasibility study. Diagn Cytopathol 17:339–346
7. Schindler S, Nayer R, Dutra J, Bedrossian CW (2001) Diagnostic challenges in aspiration cytology of salivary glands. Semin Diagn Pathol 18:124–146
8. Stanley MW (2002) Selected problems in fine needle aspiration of head and neck masses. Mod Pathol 15:342–350
9. Stanley MW, Löwhagen T (1993) Fine needle aspiration of palpable masses. Butterworth-Heinemann. Boston
10. Tao LC, Smith JW (1999) Fine-needle aspiration biopsy using a newly developed pencil-grip syringe holder. Diagn Cytopathol 20:99–104
11. Vazquez MF (1991) Manual of applied aspiration pathology. New York State Society of Pathologists. XXII Annual CME Meeting. Poughkeepsie, NY
12. Yang GCH (1994) The mathematical basis for the increased sensitivity in cancer detection on air-dried cytopreparation. Mod Pathol 7:681–684
13. Yang GCH (1995) Ultrafast Papanicolaou stain: A superior stain for fine needle aspiration cytology applied in conjunction with the rehydration of air-dried smear with normal saline solution technique. Adv Anat Pathol 2:208–211
14. Yang GCH, Alvarez II (1995) Ultrafast Papanicolaou stain: An alternative preparation for fine-needle aspiration cytology. Acta Cytol 39:55–60
15. Yang GCH, Waisman J (2006) Distinguishing adenoid cystic carcinoma from cylindromatous adenomas in salivary fine-needle aspirates: The cytologic clues and ultrastructural basis. Diagn Cytopathol 34:284–288
16. Yang GCH, Yang G-Y, Tao L-C (2004) Distinguishing well-differentiated hepatocellular carcinoma from benign liver by the physical features of fine needle aspirates. Modern Pathol 17:789–802
17. Zajdela A, Zillhardt P, Voillemot N (1987) Cytological diagnosis by fine needle sampling without aspiration. Cancer 59:1201–1205

Chapter 9

Management of Infections of the Salivary Glands

9

Francis Marchal and Patrick J. Bradley

Contents

Core Features

- Infections of the salivary gland most commonly affect the major glands.
- Infections may present as an acute, chronic, or acute and chronic problem.
- The most common pathogens identified are viral and bacterial.
- Children are affected with the same diseases as adults.
- Adults most commonly present with total gland obstruction associated with sialolithiasis, ductal stenosis, or sialectasis.
- Patients with recurrent symptoms should be investigated electively.
- Total gland swelling is more likely ductal disease, as distinct to partial gland swelling which may be neoplastic or inflammatory disease.

Complications to Avoid

- Investigation should be considered in all patients, children and adults, who have recurrent symptoms, swelling ± pain, to exclude reversible disease or a neoplastic process.

Introduction

Infection of the salivary glands is best defined as an acute and/or a chronic condition which presents as swelling, with or without pain, with or without systemic involvement, and which affects the major and minor salivary glands. The most common pathogens identified are viral and bacterial. The most frequent clinical problem is that of an adult who presents with a swelling of the parotid or submandibular gland, with a diagnosis of obstructive sialadenitis associated with sialolithiasis, ductal stenosis, or sialectasis. The probable cause for the obstructive sialadenitis is associated with a bacterial infection. One of the theories proposed for such infectious processes is the retrograde theory of bacterial infection from the oral cavity.

In the general population, mumps is associated with acute swelling of the parotid gland. It is a specific viral disease, contagious and epidemic, which typically affects school-age children. It can also affect adults, mainly the elderly. It is associated with fever, malaise, myalgia, and headache. Most children who present with an isolated acute painful parotid swelling do not have mumps as a diagnosis, but similar symptoms can be caused by other viruses. These viral infections are not epidemic and are non-infectious, but are sporadic and are commonly and erroneously labeled as mumps. Frequently, parents and General Medical Practitioners consider that when an acute parotid gland swelling episode arises it is mumps, but one can only be infected with the mumps virus once because antibodies are precipitated and this prevents a second infection.

Recurrent parotitis of childhood is the most frequent non-viral affection of salivary glands in children, and these distressing symptoms, swelling, pain, and systemic upset, usually resolve around puberty. Its precise origin remains unclear, and as a result no specific treatment exists. Sialendoscopy, when performed, has proven until now to be partly effective.

Swelling of the parotid, acute and chronic, present in two fashions: swelling of the whole gland (such as mumps) or partial swelling of the gland (such as tuberculosis, cat-scratch disease, benign and/or malignant neoplasms).

In the case of submandibular swelling, the whole gland is considered swollen and a swelling of part of the gland is difficult to differentiate clinically. Also, differentiating submandibular gland from adjacent lymph nodes is sometimes difficult and requires the use of radiological imaging. Not infrequently, discrete inflammatory swellings of the parotid or submandibular gland are in fact infections of peri- or intraglandular lymph nodes.

Infectious processes of the minor salivary glands including sublingual, generally present as a painless non-ulcerative swelling similar to that of a neoplasm. The diagnosis frequently requires a tissue diagnosis.

In the past, the classic division of salivary gland diseases and infections relied on a differential diagnosis. A different concept proposed is to classify these diseases according to their clinical presentation, considering the frequency of the episodes and the combinations of the associated symptoms. This understanding necessitates separating glands into submandibular and parotid because of their different etiologies and frequencies of these disorders.

Infectious salivary swellings have to be differentiated into acute and progressive (chronic). Acute is defined as a patient who had a previously normal gland, with a sudden onset of a diffuse ill-defined swelling of the entire gland or a localized swollen area with indiscrete margins associated with pain, and more rarely erythema, and purulent exudate visible at the papilla. Chronic presentation is a gradual awareness of a diffuse swelling of the entire gland or a discrete well defined mass or swelling, most usually not associated with pain, sometimes presenting with skin involvement (which might be a sign of a neoplasm or tuberculosis).

Algorithms

The algorithms in Figs. 9.1 and 9.2 show the differential diagnosis of parotid and submandibular swellings.

Investigations of Infectious and Inflammatory Conditions

Most patients who present with an acute swelling irrespective of age are considered to have an inflammatory or infectious course. Such patients are usually treated empirically by antibiotics, even though many such presentations include viral conditions. Therefore, investigation of these patients when the symptoms, most frequently pain, resolve is in the non-acute resolved phase. However, should purulent exudates be evident at the papilla, then it would seem appropriate to take a sample and send it for culture and sensitivity.

In the resolved acute clinical presentation, investigations, if facilities are available, would be in ranked order: ultrasound, followed by sialendoscopy. In the acute unresolved cases (after approximately 2 weeks of treatment), a magnetic resonance (MR) sialogram or plain computed

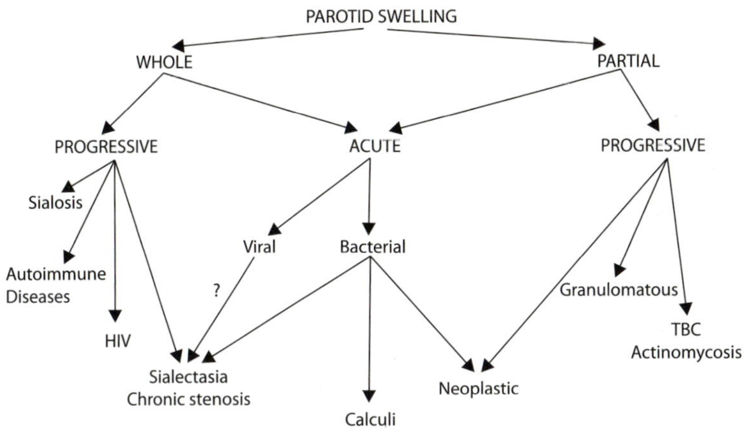

Fig. 9.1: Differential diagnosis of parotid swellings

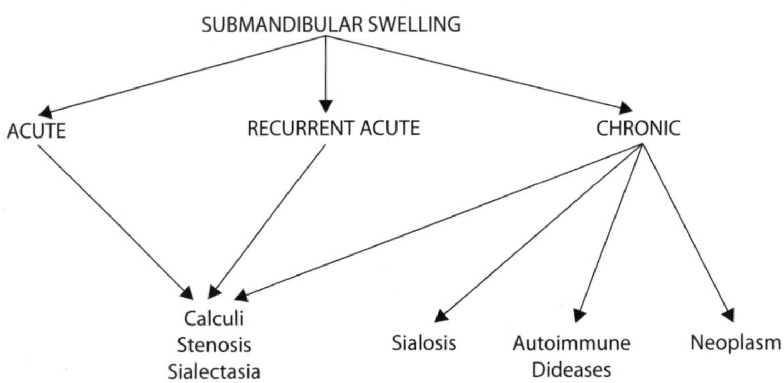

Fig. 9.2: Differential diagnosis of submandibular swellings

tomographic (CT)-MR image would be appropriate. In the chronic situation, a plain CT-MR image, ultrasound (US)-guided fine-needle aspiration cytology (FNAC), or MR sialogram is mandatory.

Treatment of Infectious and Inflammatory Conditions

In the child or infant in an acute situation, the most frequent diagnosis is viral infection. As the child will be toxic and pyrexial and suffers pain, antibiotics, analgesics, and hydration are recommended. In the recurrent acute situation occurring at frequent intervals, anti-inflammatory with analgesia treatment should be given. The parents anticipate a treatment, but its effectiveness in preventing recurrence is much debated and frequently does not shorten or prevent further episodes. In adults, the acute situation is most usually associated with a bacterial infection. They require hydration, antibiotics, anti-inflammatories, and analgesia. In the chronic situation, the patient should be treated according to the result of the previous investigations, described above, including the results of a culture if performed.

Viral Diseases

Mumps

Mumps is the most common viral infection of the salivary glands [1] and presents with unilateral or bilateral swelling of the parotid glands. In 85% of cases, it affects children under the age of 15 years. Stensen's papilla may be irritated and swollen, but no purulent exudate is visible or expressible. Glandular symptoms are often preceded by 1–3 days of a prodromal period, where the patients complaints might include malaise, discomfort, loss of appetite, chills, fever, and sore throat. The swelling usually lasts from a couple of days to one week, and there is no purulent exudate at the papilla on examination [2, 3]. Laboratory findings include leukocytopenia, with relative lymphocytosis. Serum amylase can be analyzed: it peaks in the first week and normalizes by the second or third week. Soluble antibodies directed against the nucleoprotein core of the virus appear within the final week of the infection, and disappear within 8 months [4]. Antibodies directed against the outer surface appear several weeks after soluble antibodies, and persist for 5 years [5].

Mumps is due to a paramyxovirus, an RNA virus related to the influenza and parainfluenza viruses. Mumps is spread by aerosol droplets from the saliva and nasopharyngeal secretions of an infected individual and spreads easily in highly populated urban areas. Incubation lasts from 2 to 3 weeks and the patient is infectious from 3 days before the onset of salivary swellings to 7 days after [6]. The peak incidence is at age 4–6 years, but the incidence has dropped in the last decades because of the systematic introduction of mumps vaccine. Studies have shown that more than 95% of adults have antibodies against mumps. Complications include orchitis (25% in young males), pancreatitis, sensorineural hearing loss (1/20,000 in children, being the first cause of acquired sensorineural hearing loss in children), and meningoencephalitis [6]. Mumps might be a cause of abortion during the first trimester of pregnancy because of fetal endocardial fibroelastosis.

Classic treatment includes antibiotics, sialagogues, and rehydration, the treatment depending on the clinical course and on the extent of the disease.

Non-mumps

Other viruses may mimic clinical mumps, such as influenza and parainfluenza viruses (type 1 and 3), Coxsackie viruses (A and B), echovirus, and lymphocytic choriomeningitis virus [4, 7, 8]. Cytomegalovirus and adenoviruses have also been described, mostly in human immunodeficiency virus (HIV) patients. Patients will have the same symptoms as described for classic mumps.

Human Immunodeficiency Virus

Parotid HIV manifestations present as an enlargement of the gland due to multiple lymphoepithelial cysts [9]. These cysts can be assessed by the use of ultrasound and fine-needle aspiration, which reveals serous fluid with the presence of lymphocytes and macrophages. Their presentation has not been associated with the prognosis of the disease [10]. As the parotid gland contains many lymph nodes at different levels, they might be enlarged as HIV virus mainly affects lymphoid tissue. One should not forget the differential diagnosis with solid tumors which also have an increased incidence in the parotid of HIV patients [9]. Infectious causative agents are *Pneumocystis carinii*, adenovirus, histoplasma, and cytomegalovirus (CMV), which can be found in the saliva [11].

Thirty percent of HIV-infected children have proven to have enlargement of their parotid glands [12]

Bacterial Diseases

Clinical Course

The illness is of acute onset, with tender painful swelling of the salivary gland. Parotids are affected more frequently than submandibular glands. One of the possible reasons would be that the bacteriostatic activity of the parotid saliva is inferior to that of submandibular saliva. Palpation of the gland is painful and causes purulent discharge at the papilla. Massaging the gland and expressing purulent exudate and saliva—even though this is painful—relieves the pressure pain of the patient by diminishing the pressure in the ductal system.

Localized infections of minor salivary glands including sublingual glands can be seen, and have the same causative agents. Calculi are also encountered [13].

Management consists of broad-spectrum antibiotics, after having performed a culture looking for the precise etiology of the infection. Associated anti-inflammatory medication may help to reduce the pain and swelling symptoms of the patient. In cases of severe swelling, corticosteroids do diminish the inflammation, and have a rapid effect in relieving the symptoms. The geriatric population is affected by marantic parotitis, caused by dehydration [14].

Small children can also be affected by this disease, in the first 2 weeks of life, in the parotid [15] and more rarely in the submandibular gland [16, 17], and these episodes affect most frequently premature infants who are often dehydrated, showing the importance of dehydration as a probable pathogenic factor.

Type of Bacteria

The contamination mode of the parotid gland in cases of suppurative parotitis is unknown. The retrograde contamination of the gland by bacteria from the oral cavity, and the stasis of salivary flow or a reduced salivary flow might be the main causes. Penicillin-resistant coagulase-positive staphylococcus is commonly encountered, but the flora is usually mixed, containing not only *Streptococcus pneumoniae* and beta-hemolytic streptococcus, but also gram-negative germs, such as coli. Anaerobic bacteria also play a role, and studies have shown the presence of 30–40% of anaerobic bacteria (bacteroides, peptostreptococcus, fusobacteria) [18–21].

Bacteria that affect infants are the same as those that affect adults [7, 22, 23], and *Pseudomonas aeruginosa*, *Neisseria catarrhalis*, and methicillin-resistant *Staphylococcus aureus* (MRSA) have been reported [24]. In South-East Asia, *Pseudomonas pseudomallei* has also been reported [4].

Cat-scratch Disease

This disease involves lymph nodes adjacent to salivary glands and the salivary glands may be involved by continuous spread. Patients usually remember being exposed to cats, and children or young adults are most often involved. *Bartonella henselae*, a gram-negative bacteria, is the pathogen [25]. Laboratory findings include specific polymerase chain reaction (PCR) or serology. Although generally prescribed, antibiotics seem not to be effective in shortening the course of the disease. The affected lymph node disappears spontaneously within a few months.

Actinomycosis

Actinomycosis affects lymph nodes adjacent to salivary glands, masquerading as a salivary gland infection. The pathogen is Actinomyces israelii [26]. Other pathogens include *Actinomyces proprionica*, *A. viscosus*, and *A. odontolyticus*. There are three forms of infections. The first is acute, associated with suppuration. The second is chronic, slowly progressive, with marked induration and may be mistakenly diagnosed as a neoplasm. The third form is subacute and is represented by a slightly tender and tumor-like mass attached to the mandible. The finding of "sulfur grounds" on pathological evaluation are pathognomonic of this condition. Treatment of the acute phase is surgical, with eventual drainage of the exudates. Broad-spectrum antibiotics are administered.

Other Diseases

Recurrent Parotitis in Children

The disease is characterized by recurrent episodes of acute or subacute swellings of the parotid glands, unilateral or bilateral, associated with fever and pain. Mucopurulent saliva can be expressed from the papilla, which is often red. Episodes recur every several months, sometimes more often, but the child is free of symptoms between the episodes. The age of presentation has been described from 8 months to 16 years [5], but more frequently from 5 to 7 years [3], and the symptoms usually decrease or cease at puberty (92% of symptom-free adults at 22 years, independent of treatment) [27]. The histological appearance of the salivary gland reveals massive infiltration with lymphocytes with lymphoid follicle formation, and cystic ductal formations (sialectasis) [27, 28]. No therapy is available for this disease, but antibiotics are usually given. Anti-inflammatory medication also reduces the severity of the attacks. Among etiological factors considered are congenital malformation of the parotid ducts [29, 30], familial background and impaired rates of secretion [31–35], primary or secondary infections, and local manifestations of systemic immunological disease [36]. The sialographic changes remain until adult life [27]. Recently, sialendoscopy has proven to be effective in these cases [37–40]. The sialendoscopic appearance of the duct shows diffuse reduction of the caliber of Stensen's duct [41], associated sometimes with multiple localized stenosis, and sometimes with salivary calculi (personal data). Parotid surgery has been described, as well as ligation of the duct [36, 42] which in our opinion should be absolutely avoided.

Granulomatous Sialadenitis

They are of different types of granulomatous diseases affecting salivary glands (Table 9.1). Ductal obstruction secondary to calculi or more rarely to tumor is the commonly identified cause [29]. The parotid gland is involved in most of cases. Symptoms include painless firm nodules in the parotid area. Histological confirmation of the disease include typical non caseous granulomas.

Mycobacteria

Mycobacterium tuberculosis and atypical mycobacterium both affect lymph nodes adjacent to salivary glands or intraglandular lymph nodes [43–47]. Usually, they are contaminated by the local infection affecting the mouth, the pharynx, or the lungs [43, 44, 48, 49]. The clinical presentation can be an acute inflammatory lesion or a chronic tumor-like lesion.

Diagnosis of *Mycobacterium tuberculosis* is best made by a purified protein derivative (PPD) skin test followed by a fine-needle aspiration to avoid unnecessary surgery. Treatment relies on medical management using a combination of antibiotics including isoniazid, rifampicin, and pyrazinamide.

In cases of atypical mycobacteria, adults and infants can be infected, but it is commonly seen in children between 2 and 5 years, and adults suffering from immunodeficiency disorders [50]. *Mycobacterium avium-intracellulare* and *M. scrofulaceum* are the organisms responsible [51], and the diagnosis is made either by culture performed after therapeutic excisional biopsy of the lymph node or by a specific PPD test. Its diagnosis is often delayed, as the classic PPD test remains negative. Treatment is surgical and excision but sometimes curettage may eradicate the localized infection depending on its location, but chemotherapy may play a role in suboptimal surgery.

Sarcoidosis

Sarcoidosis is a systemic disease involving multiple organs. Its etiology remains unclear, but several hypotheses have been made, including autoantigens and infectious organisms [52]. Salivary glands are usually affected, and specifically the parotid glands. Symptoms include swellings and dry mouth. Laboratory findings include amylase and kallikrein diminishing during the acute phase of the disease, and the finding of angiotensin-converting enzyme (ACE test). Diagnosis is confirmed if there is radiological and histological evidence of non-caseous epithelial granulomas. Biopsies can be obtained either from minor salivary glands with a less good sensitivity than parotid biopsies [53, 54]. Corticosteroids are the best therapeutic option.

Heerfordt's disease, also called uveoparotid fever, associates parotid enlargement with uveitis and facial palsy. It is a rare form of sarcoidosis occurring in young patients in their 20s.

Hydatic Disease

This diagnosis is suspected in endemic areas and is extremely rare. Salivary glands suffer from a cystic condition and the diagnosis is usually made postoperatively [55].

Take Home Messages

- Mumps is the most common viral cause of parotid swelling in children, but is a "once in a lifetime" infection.
- Recurrent parotitis in children should be treated symptomatically.
- Antibiotics should only be given when a specific bacterial infectious diagnosis is suspected or proven.
- Partial salivary gland swellings, after investigation, may require excision to prove the likely pathogens if infection is the cause, or to exclude the possibility of a malignant neoplastic process.

Table 9.1. Types of granulomatous sialadenitis

Tuberculosis
Crohn's disease
Melkersson-Rosenthal syndrome
• Cheilitis granulomatosa Miescher
Granulomatous giant cell sialadenitis
• Submandibular or sublingual
Xanthogranulomatous sialadenitis
Wegener's granulomatosis
Churg-Strauss granulomatosis
Sialadenitis after sialography
Inflammatory pseudotumors
• Eosinophilic granuloma
• Kimura's disease
• Angiolymphoid hyperplasia with eosinophilia
• Lymphomatous granulomatosis
• Rosai-Dorfman disease

References

1. Bann SG, Litman N (1979) Mumps virus. In: Mandell GL, Douglas RG, Bennett JE, eds. Principles and practice of infectious diseases, 2nd Edition. New York: John Wiley & Sons: 971–977
2. Bradley P J (2002) Microbiology and management of sialadenitis. Curr Infect Dis Rep 4:217–224
3. Bradley P J (1997) Salivary Gland Diseases in Children, Chapter in Scott-Brown's Diseases of the Ear, Nose and Throat 6th Edition, Volume Paediatrics. Editied by Cinnamond M. and Adams D. Publishers Blackwell, London
4. Mc Quone S (1999) Acute viral and bacterial infections of the salivary glands. Otolaryngol Clin North Am 32(5):793–811
5. Woolley AL, MD (1996) Salivary gland diseases in children. Curr Opin Otolaryngol Head Neck Surg 4:385–391
6. Johnson A (1989) Inflammatory conditions of the major salivary glands. Ear Nose Throat J 68:94–102
7. Rice DH (1982) Non-neoplatic salivary gland disorders. In Current Therapy in Otolaryngology Head and Neck Surgery. Edited by Gates GA. Trenton, NJ: BC Dekker: 178–183
8. Zollar LM, Muffson MA (1970) Acute parotitis associated with parainfluenza 3 virus infection. Am J Dis Child 119: 147–148
9. Huang RD, Pearlman S, Friedman WH, Loree T (1991) Benign cystic vs. solid lesions of the Parotid Gland in HIV Patients. Head Neck 13: 522–527
10. Seibert RW (1996) Diseases of the salivary glands, In Pediatric Otolaryngology, Vol 2, Edn 3. Edited by Bluestone CD, Stool SE, Kenna MA. Philadelphia: WB Saunders 1093–1107
11. Scott GB, Buck BE, Leterman JG (1984) Acquired immunodeficiency syndrome in infants. N Engl J Med 310:76–81
12. Schiodt M, Greenspan D, Levy JA, Nelson JA, Chernoff D, Hollander H, Greenspan JS (1989) Does HIV cause salivary gland disease ? AIDS 3:819–822
13. Alcure ML, Della Coletta R, Graner E, Di Hipolito O Jr, Lopes MA (2005) Sialolithiasis of minor salivary glands: a clinical and histopathological study. Gen Dent 53: 278–281
14. Wang S, Zou Z, Wu Q, Sun K, Ma X, Zhu X (1996) Chronic suppurative parotitis: a proposed classification. Chin Med J (Engl) 109: 555–560
15. Chiu CH, Lin TY (1996) Clinical and microbiological analysis of six children with acute suppurative parotitis. Acta Paediatr 85:106–108
16. Ungkanont K, Kolatat T, Tantinikorn W (1998) Neonatal suppurative submandibular sialadenitis: a rare clinical entity. Int J Paediatr Otolaryngol 43:141–145
17. Bafaqeeh SA (1998) Complicated neonatal submandibular suppurative sialadenitis. Int J Paed Otolaryngol 44:267–271
18. Brook I, Frazier EH, Thompson DH (1991) Aerobic and anaerobic microbiology of acute suppurative parotitis. Laryngoscope 101:170–172
19. Brook I (1992) Diagnosis and management of parotitis. Arch Otolaryngol Head Neck Surg 118, 469–471
20. Brook I (2002) Aerobic and Anaerobic Microbiology of Suppurative Sialadenitis. J Med Microbiol 51:526–529
21. Brook I (2003) Acute bacterial suppurative parotitis: microbiology and management. J Craniofac Surg 14:37–40
22. Myer C, Cotton RT (1986) Salivary gland disease in children: a review: part 1: acquired non-neoplastic disease. Clin Pediatr 25:314–322
23. Wilson WR, Eavey RD, Lang DW (1980) Recurrent parotitis during childhood. Clin Pediatr 19:235–236
24. Takahashi R, Chikaoka S, Ito T, Yamada M, Matsuatani S, Nakae S (2000) Neonatal submandibular suppurative sialadenitis. Eur J Paediatr 159:868
25. Malatskey S, Fradis M, Ben-Davis J, Podoshin L (2000) Cat-scratch disease of the parotid gland. Ann Otol Rhinol Laryngol 109:679–682
26. Belmont MJ, Behar PM, Wax MK (1999) Atypical presentation of actinomycosis. Head Neck 21:264–268
27. Geterud A, Lindvall AM, Nyten O (1988) Follow up study of recurrent parotitis in children. Ann Otol Rhinol Laryngol 97:341–346
28. Cohen HA, Gross S, Nussinovitch M, Frydman M, Varsano I (1992) Recurrent parotitis. Arch Dis Child 67:1036–1037
29. Ericson S, Zetterlund B, Ohman J (1991) Recurrent parotitis and sialectasis in childhood: clinical radiological, immunologic, bacteriologic, and histologic study. Ann Otol Rhinol Laryngol 100:527–535
30. Bailey H (1945) Congenital parotid sialectasis. J Int Coll Surg 8:109–112
31. Smith M (1953) Familial incidence of sialectasis. BMJ 2:1359
32. Jones HE (1953) Recurrent parotitis in children. Arch Dis Child 28:182–186
33. Katezem M (1969) Recurrent parotitis in children. S Afr J Surg 7:37–42
34. Galili D, Marmay Y (1986) Juvenile recurrent parotitis: clinicoradiologic follow up study and the beneficial effects of sialography. Oral Surg Oral Med Oral Pathol 61:550–556

35. Maynard JD (1965) Recurrent parotid enlargement. Br J Surg 52:784–789
36. Konno A, Ito E (1978) A study on the pathogenesis of recurrent parotitis in childhood. Ann Otol Rhinol Laryngol 88:1–20
37. Nahlieli O, Baruchin AM (1997) Sialoendoscopy: three years' experience as a diagnostic and treatment modality. J Oral Maxillofac Surg 55:912–918
38. Marchal F, Dulguerov P, Lehmann W (1999) Interventional sialendoscopy. N Engl J Med 341:1242–1243
39. Marchal F, Dulguerov P, Becker M, Barki G, Disant F, Lehmann W (2002) Submandibular diagnostic and interventional sialendoscopy: new procedure for ductal disorders. Ann Otol Rhinol Laryngol 111:27–35
40. Marchal F, Dulguerov P, Becker M, Barki G, Disant F, Lehmann W (2001) Specificity of parotid sialendoscopy. Laryngoscope 111:264–271
41. Marchal F, Dulguerov P (2003) Sialolithiasis management: The state of the art. Arch Otolaryngol Head Neck Surg 129: 951–956
42. Diamant H (1958) Ligation of the parotid duct in chronic recurrent parotitis. Acta Otolaryngol (Stockh) 49:375–380
43. Holmes S, Gleeson MJ, Cawson RA (2000) Mycobacterial disease of the parotid gland. Oral Surg Oral Med Oral Pathol Oral Radiol Endod 90:292–298
44. Handa U, Kumar S, Punia RS, Mohan H, Abrol R, Saini V (2001) Tuberculuous parotitis: a series of five cases diagnosed on FNAC. J Laryngol Otol 115: 235–237
45. Perlman DC, D'Amico R, Salomon N (2001) Mycobacterial infections of the head and neck. Curr Infect Dis Rep 3: 233–241
46. Kanlikama M, Mumbuc S, Bayazit Y, Sirikci A (2000) Management strategy of mycobacterial cervical lymphadenitis. J Laryngol Otol 114: 274–278
47. Cleary K, Batsakis JG (1995) Mycobacterial disease of the head and neck: current perspective. Ann Otol Rhinol Laryngol 104(10 Pt 1):830–833
48. Jervis PN, Lee JA, Bull PD (2001) Management of non-tuberculous mycobacterial perisialadenitis in children. Clin Otolaryngol 26:243–248
49. Pransky SM, Reisman BK, Kearns DB, SEID AB, Collins D, Krous NF (1990), Cervicofacial Mycobacterial adenitis in children endemic to San Diego. Laryngoscope 100:920–925
50. Roland N, Jackson SR (2004) Non-neoplastic disease of the salivary glands. Surgery 8:173–175
51. Falworth MS, Simpson MT (1996) Cervical lymphadenitis in children: the role of Mycobacterium avium-intracellulare. Br J Oral Maxillofac Surg 34(6):511–514
52. Balal H, Chou L, Cottrell DA (1999) Sarcoidosis: medical and dental implications. Oral Surg Oral Med Oral Pathol Oral Radiol Endod 88:386–390
53. Cahn L, Eisenbud LR, Blake MN, Stern D (1964) Biopsies of normal-appearing palates of patients with known sarcoidosis. Oral Surg Oral Med Oral Pathol 18:342–345
54 Marx RE, Hartman KS, Retman KA (1988) A prospective study comparing incisional labial to incisional parotid biopsies in the detection and confirmation of sarcoidosis, Sjogrens disease, sialosis and lymphoma. J Rheumatol 15:621–629
55. de Norman JE, Mitchell RD (1998) Unusual conditions of the major and minor salivary glands. Int J Oral Maxillofac Surg 7:157–171

Chapter 10

Management of Mucocele and Ranula

Paul D. Kim and Alfred Simental

10

Contents

Core Features

- Epidemiology of mucoceles and ranulas.
- Anatomy of the minor salivary, sublingual and submandibular glands.
- Pathophysiology of mucocele and ranula formation.
- Clinical findings of mucoceles and ranula.
- Management of mucoceles and ranula.
- Surgical procedure for mucocele, ranula, and plunging ranula.
- Complications of surgical treatment of mucocele and ranula.

Complications to Avoid

- Failure to identify Wharton's duct, lingual nerve, and hypoglossal nerve may result in injury to these structures.
- Marginal mandibular nerve injury.
- Failure to use imaging studies may result in understaging of a plunging ranula.
- Recurrent ranulas may be scarred and adherent to surrounding structures.
- Failure to remove the sublingual gland may result in recurrence.

Introduction

Three paired major salivary glands as well as hundreds of minor salivary glands drain directly into the mouth providing moisture and lubrication to the oral cavity. This lubrication facilitates speech and swallowing, and keeps the mucosa moist. Obstruction of the outflow tract of the salivary glands and extravasation of mucus into the surrounding tissues may result in a mucocele or a ranula which is unique to the sublingual gland. The term "ranula" has its derivation traced to the oral anatomy of the frog.

Mucus-filled pseudocysts are non-epithelial-lined collections that are visible in the floor of the mouth and may be due to mucoceles, ranulas, or plunging ranulas. Mucoceles arise most often secondary to injury of one of the minor salivary glands that causes small areas of mucus extravasation into the soft tissues (Fig. 10.1). The mucus then becomes walled off and forms a pseudocyst. The ranula is clinically described as a painless mucus pseudocyst on the floor of the mouth. Simple and complex ranulas occur secondary to injury of one the sublingual ducts. Simple ranulas have mucus that is walled off above the mylohyoid muscle. Complex or plunging ranulas develop when mucus extravasation spreads deep to the mylohyoid muscle and presents as a mass in the neck.

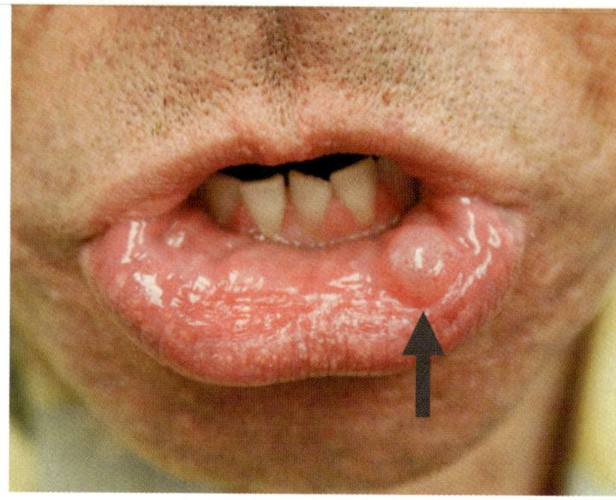

Fig. 10.1: Clinical photograph of mucocele on lower lip

Anatomy

There are estimated to be approximately 600 to 1,000 minor salivary glands in the mucosa of the oral cavity. They are found along the buccal mucosa, floor of mouth, ventral tongue, hard and soft palate, and pharynx. These minor salivary glands have their own individual ducts through which the saliva passes into the oral cavity.

The sublingual gland measures approximately 3 cm in a sagittal plane [1] and is bound medially by the genioglossus muscle, laterally by the inner cortex of the mandible, inferiorly by the mylohyoid muscle, and superiorly by the mucosa of the floor of mouth. There are up to 20 minor ducts of Rivini that drain into the floor of the mouth. The largest duct, called Bartholin's duct, can empty into Wharton's duct or it empties into the posterior floor of the mouth.

The submandibular gland is located inferior to the mandible and is bordered by the lingual and hypoglossal nerves medially which lie on the hyoglossus muscle and track under the mylohyoid, laterally by the platysma muscle and facial vein, and superiorly by the mandible. The drainage path of the submandibular gland is Wharton's duct which is approximately 5 cm in length, coursing between the hypoglossal and lingual nerves, under the mylohyoid and into the anterior floor of the mouth.

Pathophysiology

The origin of a ranula is thought to be due to obliteration of a minor duct of the sublingual gland, while the main excretory duct remains patent [2]. Unlike the parotid and submandibular glands that are stimulated by the parasympathetic system to express saliva during deglutition, the sublingual glands exhibit a more constant production of saliva.

Extravasation of saliva moves throughout the sublingual gland and into the submucosa via hydrostatic pressure as the sublingual gland continues to produce saliva. The extravasated mucus can then spread around or through the mylohyoid muscle into the submental or submandibular spaces.

When the ranula spreads to occupy the submental or submandibular space and has penetrated deep to the mylohyoid muscle, it is referred to as a plunging ranula. Ectopic sublingual gland tissue in the neck may also cause a plunging ranula.

Injury to Wharton's duct may also result in the formation of a ranula, however this is an uncommon mechanism. This would require a very focal area of scarring in the duct that affects the sublingual drainage, such as the Bartholin's duct, while allowing the submandibular gland to freely drain.

Epidemiology

Zhao et al. [3], in a review of 580 cases, reported that ranulas are most prevalent in the second decade of life and are slightly more common in females (male to female ratio of 1:1.2), but a distinct male predilection was noted for the plunging ranula (male to female ratio of 1:0.74). Oral ranulas most commonly involved the left side (left to right ratio of 1:0.62), while the plunging and mixed ranula commonly involved the right side.

Patients with a plunging ranula tend to report the presence of a mass in the neck for greater than 6 months, indicating that with time a simple ranula may eventually dissect by hydrostatic pressure into the neck and become a plunging ranula.

Chidzonga and Rusakaniko [4], in a review of 83 cases of ranulas in Zimbabwe, reported a concomitant positive serology for human immunodeficiency virus (HIV) in 88%, with most of the patients in the 0–10 year age group. They suggested that sublingual ranulas in Zimbabwe be considered another HIV/AIDS-associated lesion, especially when found in children.

Clinical Diagnosis

The clinical history of a mucocele and ranula may include a soft, compressible, painless mass that may be translucent. These frequently form on the lower lip and the floor of the mouth. It may be associated with previous oral surgery, intraoral injury, or tumor growth. They usually enlarge slowly and may be ballotable on bimanual palpation of the neck and floor of mouth. Neurologic changes such as numbness or weakness of the tongue, or numbness of the lip, a hard and indurated surface, or loose teeth should alert the practitioner to suspect underlying malignancy.

The usual presentation of a plunging ranula is a soft, compressible, mass in the submandibular or submental region. These may be initially misdiagnosed as sialadenitis or a salivary tumor. Transillumination of the mass may be feasible in the larger ranula. Intraoral examination should demonstrate an intraoral component combined with the cervical component. Isolated cervical plunging ranula can rarely occur and is confirmed postsurgically by histologic verification of the pseudocyst [5]. Plunging ranula may be quite large and extend to the inferior aspect of the neck or the chest wall.

Imaging

Magnetic resonance imaging (MRI) can show herniation of the sublingual tissue and cystic material through the mylohyoid muscle(s) (Figs. 10.2, 10.3). T1-weighted images are usually low enhancing while T2-weighted images are bright. If the mucocele or ranula is infected, the signal findings may vary.

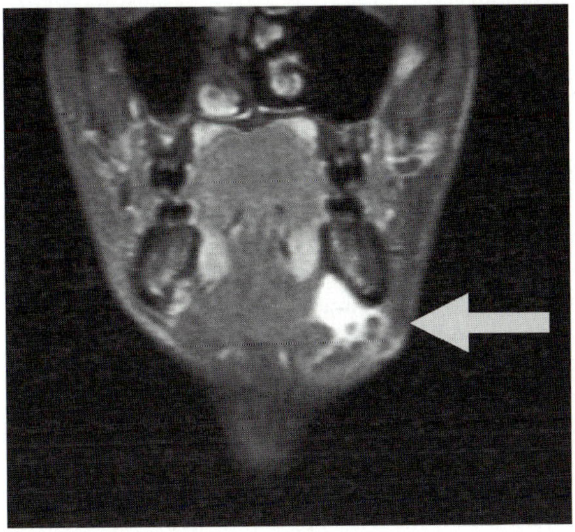

Fig. 10.2: Coronal T2-weighted MRI of plunging ranula

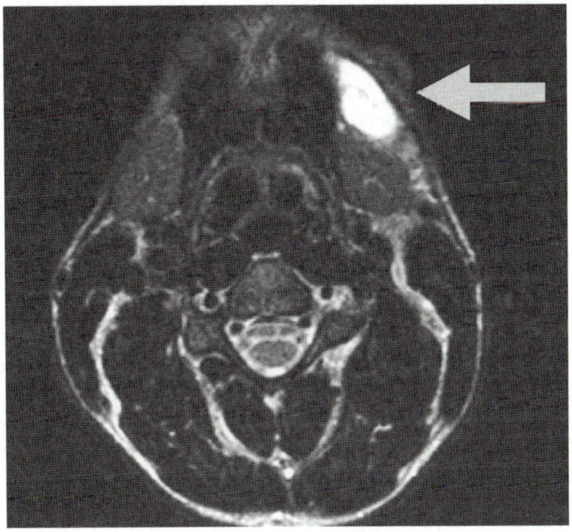

Fig. 10.3: Axial T2-weighted MRI of plunging ranula

The imaging can be augmented during a modified Valsalva maneuver to evaluate whether there is a neoplasm, fluid, or normal anatomy. A Valsalva maneuver may make a plunging ranula more prominent during the imaging process. Coronal images are particularly suited to demonstrate this [6]. With coronal images, the mylohyoid muscle can be seen which may help to differentiate a ranula from a plunging ranula. The use of gadopentetate dimeglumine (Gd-DTPA) enhancement improves visualization of the extent of the salivary glands in relation to the pseudocyst [7, 8]. The contrast enhancement may help enhance the rim of the pseudocyst.

The use of ultrasound of the neck in the evaluation of a plunging ranula may also reveal deficiencies in the mylohyoid muscle with herniation of the sublingual gland [1]. Ultrasonography can provide good visualization of the sublingual space and the relation to the ranula.

10

With computed tomography (CT), a plunging ranula can be readily identified preoperatively as a cystic mass in the suprahyoid anterior neck [9] (Fig. 10.4). The ranula is usually unilocular, which makes it different than most lymphangiomas [10]. The differential diagnosis of a mass in this area on CT scan includes a branchial cleft cyst which has a more prominent wall, a thyroglossal duct cyst which is usually found as a midline structure, a lymph node with a necrotic center, or a salivary gland cystic tumor. Coronal images can assist in differentiating a large ranula from a plunging ranula, as the plunging ranula will extend below the level of the mylohyoid.

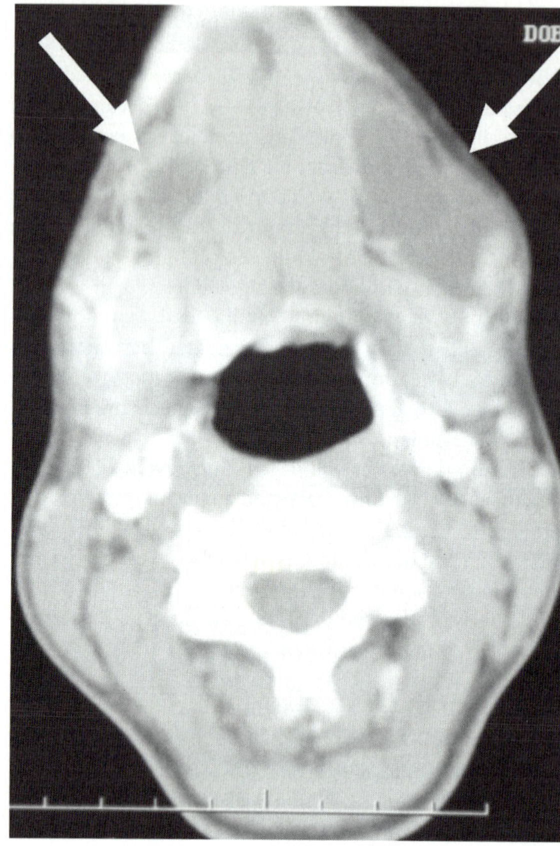

Fig. 10.4: Axial view contrast-enhanced CT scan of bilateral plunging ranula

Management

Some patients may experience spontaneous resolution or rupture of their mucocele or ranula [11]. Many different treatment options exist such as sclerotherapy, marsupialization, and excision with or without combined excision of the involved salivary tissue. Treatment efficacy usually increases when the ranula or mucocele is most prominent.

Kim et al. [12] reported the use of sclerotherapy in 9 patients with ranulas. OK-432 sclerotherapy was also applied in 9 patients with plunging ranula with complete resolution [12]. Lee et al. [13] used OK-432 sclerotherapy with 13 patients and had 9 patients completely regressed. There were no complications encountered. Fukase et al. [14] reported a series of 32 patients treated with OK-432 sclerotherapy, including 21 patients with simple ranula and 11 with plunging ranula. Thirty-one patients (97%) demonstrated a disappearance or marked improvement. The most common side effects were pain at the injection site and fever in almost half of the patients. While the first 4 patients were observed in the hospital for 4–5 days, the remaining 28 patients were safely managed on an outpatient basis.

Marsupialization of the mucocele or ranula has also been used with varying success and variation in utilized methods. A simple intraoral incision over the mucocele with subsequent drainage, placement of a silk suture seton, and carbon dioxide laser vaporization of the ranulas have all been described [15, 16]. Each of these techniques includes a method to allow the pseudocyst to drain and communicate into the oral cavity. Yuca et al. [17], in a review of 9 pediatric patients with intraoral ranulas less than 2 cm, reported that marsupialization was successful in 6 of the patients.

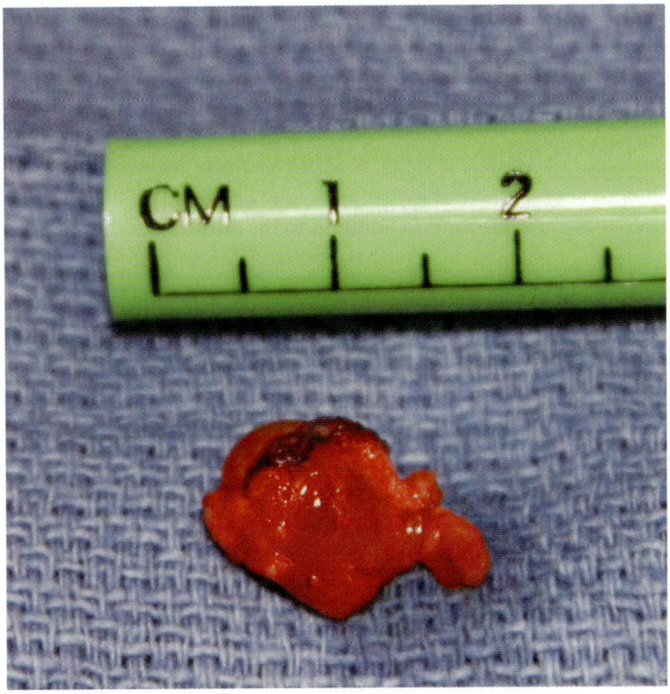

Fig. 10.5: Removal of a mucocele with involved minor salivary gland tissue

Takagi et al. [18] described a method of fenestration with continuous pressure as a simple noninvasive method for plunging ranulas in a series of four patients with no recurrences. This method includes making an incision into the floor of mouth overlying the ranula and suturing a Penrose drain into place. Continuous pressure is then applied using an external pressure dressing taped to the neck for 3 weeks.

Transoral excision of the ranula or mucocele has become common practice in the USA. Great care should be taken to prevent rupture of the pseudocyst's thin wall during surgery, as incomplete resection of the cyst wall may occur inadvertently once the mucus has dissipated [19].

In order to lessen the complication and occurrence of rupture, Choi [20] recommended hydrodissection with saline and lidocaine with 1:100,000 epinephrine. Hydrodissection may allow improved visual distinction between the mucocele and the surrounding normal mucosa and other structures. Compared with other techniques, he found that hydrodissection was associated with less bleeding, fewer incidents of neural and soft tissue damage, and a lower recurrence rate in a series of 38 patients [20].

Baurmash has advocated that removal of the sublingual gland is not always necessary and reported four cases to illustrate his approach. All the patients were treated successfully with conservative management by removing the cyst only and retained normal functioning sublingual glands [21].

Recurrence rates are felt to depend upon the complete removal of the cyst and the involved sublingual gland [3] (Fig. 10.5). Other authors also believe that transoral excision of the ranula and sublingual gland is the recommended method [7, 22]. Residual cysts in the floor of the mouth after excision of the sublingual gland often regress. Dissection and identification of the lingual nerve and submandibular duct are often necessary to accomplish a complete and thorough excision of the sublingual gland [11]. In addition, identification and preservation of the hypoglossal nerve is required. Transoral endoscopic assisted excision of plunging ranulas is advocated by Guerrissi et al. [23].

Some authors feel that excision of the pseudocyst is probably unnecessary and places surrounding structures at risk of damage, but a biopsy of the pseudocyst wall is important to confirm the diagnosis [24–26]. Zhao et al. also concur that recurrence rates of ranulas of any type are excessive unless the involved sublingual gland is removed [3].

Transcervical excision of the ranula (and sometimes the submandibular gland) and intraoral excision of the sublingual gland is necessary in the complete treatment of plunging ranula. It is important to identify the lingual and hypoglossal nerves during this procedure and to identify the course of the pseudocyst through or deep to the mylohyoid muscle.

Special Consideration: Neonatal Ranula

Neonatal ranula may cause oral or oropharyngeal obstruction resulting in life-threatening airway compromise upon delivery. Kolker et al. [27] reported a patient with a prenatal ultrasound that identified a ranula in the developing fetus encompassing the entire oral cavity. The cystic mass displaced the tongue anterosuperiorly against the palate. Anticipating airway obstruction, an ex utero intrapartum treatment (EXIT) team was created and at 38 weeks gestation, a caesarian section and EXIT procedures were performed leaving the umbilical cord attached to the baby for continued placental oxygenation. The large sublingual mass was then excised intraorally followed by intubation and transection of the umbilical cord. The mass was consistent with a congenital ranula. There was no recurrence or complication noted at 6 months.

An additional report by Onderglu et al. [28] reported a similar EXIT procedure at 38 weeks gestation and management by simple aspiration of the cyst fluid prior to ligation of the umbilical cord, again with no recurrence at 6 month follow-up. While rare, neonatal ranula can be safely managed with the EXIT procedure technique.

Surgical Approach to Mucocele and Ranula Excision

Local anesthesia is usually well tolerated by patients with a small mucocele of the oral cavity. After informed consent is obtained, 1% lidocaine with epinephrine is used to infiltrate the area surrounding the mucocele. It is advised to first delineate the boundaries of the mucocele because hydrodissection from the local infiltration may distort the anatomy. An elliptical incision is made around the mucocele to include the sublingual salivary gland that is the underlying cause of ranula. Hemostasis is achieved with an electrocautery device and the wound closed with absorbable suture. Frequently there is no tension on the wound which allows for a single-layer interrupted closure.

We feel strongly that the definitive treatment for simple and plunging ranulas require resection of the involved salivary gland in addition to the resection of the pseudocyst. General anesthesia with nasal intubation is required for excision of the mucocele because of the difficulty in keeping the mouth open and controlling bleeding in an awake patient. The floor of the mouth is palpated and Wharton's duct is identified in relation to the ranula. This duct is stented to allow identification and prevent injury during the resection.

An elliptical excision is performed in the floor of the mouth and tapered over the sublingual gland. Dissection lateral to the sublingual gland and ranula is carefully performed. The medial dissection consists of dissecting close to the ranula, and between the sublingual gland and Wharton's duct. Great caution with posterior dissection is taken while identifying and preserving the lingual and hypoglossal nerves, and completing the resection of the ranula and sublingual gland.

Upon completion of the dissection and removal of the gland, careful hemostasis is achieved. If Wharton's duct is injured, it may be marsupialized to the floor of mouth mucosa to allow for drainage. Closure of the wound is performed with absorbable sutures in a single layer.

Excision of plunging ranulas may be completed in the same manner if ideal retraction and delivery are performed with bimanual palpation. Some patients may require an incision on the neck for exposure and delivery of the ranula. In addition to identifying the submandibular duct and lingual nerve during the dissection, care must be taken not to rupture the pseudocyst as the ranula is followed through or around the mylohyoid muscle.

If transoral visualization is poor, a neck incision is performed three finger breadths below the inferior margin of the mandible in a skin crease and the submandibular gland is identified and mobilized away from the ranula. Completion of the posterior and inferior extent of the plunging ranula is performed after careful identification of the facial artery and veins to prevent bleeding in the operative site. The intraoral incisions are closed, a suction drain is placed in the neck after thorough irrigation, and the neck is closed in layers. A subcutaneous absorbable suture is used for the skin closure.

Complications/Morbidity

In a clinical review of 571 patients with surgical treatment of ranulas, the most commonly reported complications were recurrence (5.8%), sensory deficit of tongue (4.9%), and injury to Wharton's duct (1.82%) [29]. Neurologic deficits are more likely to be sensory in nature involving the lingual nerve. These present immediately and commonly resolve within 2–7 months. However, weakness of the tongue can occur from injury to the hypoglossal nerve, which is also usually transient. Permanent injury is best prevented by precise identification of the nerve branches and maintenance of a dry surgical field with the use of ultrasonic cutting shears or bipolar electrosurgical technology. Injury to Wharton's duct may not always be preventable due to the location of the ranula, but may be prevented by routine identification. In addition, caution should be taken to prevent inadvertent ligation of a preserved duct when repairing the mucosal defect after resection of the mucocele. If the duct does require transection and is irreparable, ipsilateral submandibular gland excision may be required to prevent obstructive complications.

Recurrence is usually delayed, as mucus will slowly accumulate, or scarring from previously resected mucoceles results in formation of a mucocele from other salivary tissue. Haberal et al. reported recurrence of ranulas in 6.25% of pediatric patients undergoing marsupialization [19].

The recurrence rates of ranulas were not related to swelling patterns or surgical approaches, but intimately related to the methods of surgical procedures. The recurrence rates for marsupialization, excision of ranula, and excision of the sublingual gland or gland combined with lesion were 66.67%, 57.69%, and 1.20%, respectively [3].

Plunging ranula can be associated with the additional risk of injury to the marginal mandibular nerve, as the ranula may infiltrate around the mandibular periosteum and submandibular gland capsule. This is especially true in cases where the plunging ranula has been previously infected. Surgical excision of ranula presents a greater technical challenge than would seem on initial evaluation due to their infiltrative nature. Nonetheless, surgical treatment of ranula, especially in adults, continues to be a successful venture.

Take Home Messages

- Ranulas should be excised together with the involved sublingual salivary gland.
- CT scans or MRI is helpful in defining the extent of the ranula.
- Transoral excision must be carried out with preservation of the Wharton's duct, lingual nerve, and hypoglossal nerve.
- Plunging ranula is best treated with a combination transoral excision of the cyst and sublingual gland and a cervical approach to excise the plunging ranula portion.

References

1. Windisch G, Weiglein AH, Kiesler K (2004) Herniation of the mylohyoid muscle. J Craniofac Surg 15:566–569
2. Beck C (1985) [How is a ranula formed?] Laryngol Rhinol Otol (Stuttg) 64:535–536
3. Zhao YF, Jia Y, Chen XM, Zhang WF (2004) Clinical review of 580 ranulas. Oral Surg Oral Med Oral Pathol Oral Radiol Endod 98:281–287
4. Chidzonga MM, Rusakaniko S (2004) Ranula: another HIV/AIDS associated oral lesion in Zimbabwe? Oral Dis 10:229–232
5. Kovacic M (2003) [Plunging ranula.] Acta Med Croatica 57:305–308
6. Keberle M, Eulert S, Relic A, Hahn D (2005) Functional MR imaging of submandibular herniation of sublingual tissues through a gap of the mylohyoid muscle in two cases of submandibular masses. Eur Radiol 15:59–65
7. Hidaka H, Oshima T, Kakehata S, Watanabe K, Toshima M, Suzuki H, Kobayashi T (2003) Two cases of plunging ranula managed by the intraoral approach. Tohoku J Exp Med 200:59–65
8. Asaumi J, Shigehara H, Konouchi H, Yanagi Y, Hisatomi M, Matsuzaki H, Kishi K (2002) Assessment of carcinoma in the sublingual region based on magnetic resonance imaging. Oncol Rep 9:1283–1287

9. Charnoff SK, Carter BL (1986) Plunging ranula: CT diagnosis. Radiology 158:467–468
10. Macdonald AJ, Salzman KL, Harnsberger HR (2003) Giant ranula of the neck: differentiation from cystic hygroma. AJNR Am J Neuroradiol 24:757–761
11. Pandit RT, Park AH (2002) Management of pediatric ranula. Otolaryngol Head Neck Surg 127:115–118
12. Kim KH, Sung MW, Roh JL, Han MH (2004) Sclerotherapy for congenital lesions in the head and neck. Otolaryngol Head Neck Surg 131:307–316
13. Lee HM, Lim HW, Kang HJ, Chae SW, Hwang SJ, Jung KY, Woo JS (2006) Treatment of ranula in pediatric patients with intralesional injection of OK-432. Laryngoscope 116:966–969
14. Fukase S, Ohta N, Inamura K, Aoyagi M (2003) Treatment of ranula with intracystic injection of the streptococcal preparation OK-432. Ann Otol Rhinol Laryngol 112:214–220
15. Mintz S, Barak S, Horowitz I (1994) Carbon dioxide laser excision and vaporization of nonplunging ranulas: a comparison of two treatment protocols. J Oral Maxillofac Surg 52:370–372
16. Niccoli-Filho W, Morosolli AR (2004) Surgical treatment of ranula with carbon dioxide laser radiation. Lasers Med Sci 19:12–14
17. Yuca K, Bayram I, Cankaya H, Caksen H, Kiroglu AF, Kiris M (2005) Pediatric intraoral ranulas: an analysis of nine cases. Tohoku J Exp Med 205:151–155
18. Takagi S, Mizukawa N, Kimura T, Asaumi JI (2003) Treatment of a plunging ranula with fenestration and continuous pressure. Br J Oral Maxillofac Surg 41:410–413
19. Haberal I, Gocmen H, Samim E (2004) Surgical management of pediatric ranula. Int J Pediatr Otorhinolaryngol 68:161–163
20. Choi TW, Oh CK (2003) Hydrodissection for complete removal of a ranula. Ear Nose Throat J 82:946–947, 951
21. Baurmash HD (2002) Treating oral ranula: another case against blanket removal of the sublingual gland. Br J Oral Maxillofac Surg 40:455–456
22. Kobayashi T, Ochi K, Komatsuzaki Y, Sugiura N, Saito S (2003) Blanket removal of the sublingual gland for treatment of plunging ranula. Laryngoscope 113:386–388
23. Guerrissi JO, Taborda G (2001) Endoscopic excision of the submandibular gland by an intraoral approach. J Craniofac Surg 12:299–303
24. Davison MJ, Morton RP, McIvor NP (1998) Plunging ranula: clinical observations. Head Neck 20:63–68
25. Yoshimura Y, Obara S, Kondoh T, Naitoh S (1995) A comparison of three methods used for treatment of ranula. J Oral Maxillofac Surg 53:280–282
26. Mizuno A, Yamaguchi K (1993) The plunging ranula. Int J Oral Maxillofac Surg 22:113–115
27. Kolker MT, Batti JS, Schoem SR (2004) The extero intrapartum treatment procedure for congenital ranula in a Jehovah's Witness. Otolaryngol Head Neck Surg 130:508–510
28. Onderglu L, Saygan-Karamuvsel B, Deren D, Bozdag G, et al. (2003) Prenatal diagnosis of ranula at 21 weeks of gestation. Ultrasound Obstet Gynecol 22:399–401
29. Zhao YF, Jia J, Jia Y (2005) Complications associated with surgical management of ranulas. J Oral Maxillofac Surg 63:51–54

Chapter 11

Xerostomia

Mark S. Chambers, Ioli-Ioanna Artopoulou, and Adam S. Garden

11

Contents

Core Features

- Pathogenesis of radiation-induced xerostomia
- Xerostomia and quality of life
- Treatment
- Stringent oral and dental care
- Radiation therapy protectants
- Salivary gland transfer techniques
- Gene therapy
- Pharmacologic options
- Emerging parotid gland-sparing techniques

Introduction

Saliva is an essential body fluid. It is important in maintaining oral health, taste acuity, mastication, deglutition and digestion, regulation of oral flora, oral cleansing, voice acuity, and speech articulation. Saliva is composed largely of water but also contains minerals, electrolytes, buffers, enzymes, growth factors, cytokines, immunoglobulins, proteins, and metabolic waste products, with the concentrations and compositions of these components varying with the individual. Many systemic disorders, medications, and oncologic therapies can affect salivary function, greatly compromising oral health.

There are numerous minor salivary glands in the lining of the upper aerodigestive tract and the respiratory system. However, most of the saliva is produced by the three pairs of major salivary glands: the parotid, the submandibular, and the sublingual glands. The paired major salivary glands have a basic anatomic structure that features acini with a specialized row of myoepithelial cells and a ductal system [1–3]. The acinar cells are the secretory end pieces and are responsible for the initial transport of fluid into the glandular ductal system [4]. The parotid glands consist mainly of serous acinar cells, which are highly radiosensitive, and secrete mainly under stimulation (e.g., gustatory, mastication). The submandibular glands consist of both mixed mucous and serous cells, whereas the sublingual glands consist mainly of mucinous cells, which are less radiosensitive. The ductal cells of each gland form a branching system that moves saliva into the respective glandular duct within the oral cavity [2–4].

The major glands combined produce up to 1.5 l of saliva a day [1]. This accounts for up to 90% of salivary secretions [5]. The parotid glands contribute between 52% and 70% of the salivary constituent upon stimulation (i.e., gustatory, masticatory) [2–4, 6]. The majority of the salivary flow from the parotid gland, however, is only induced during mastication and occurs for less than 1 h over the course of a day. The submandibular glands mainly provide resting saliva. More importantly, most of the protective function of the saliva is attributable to the effect of the submandibular glands. The submandibular glands contribute between 70% to 82% to the balance of resting whole saliva [2–4, 6].

The role of saliva in maintaining oral homeostasis is underappreciated and has not been fully elucidated. Saliva protects and lubricates the oral cavity and serves as an antibacterial, antiviral, and antifungal agent [1, 6]. Saliva is also an important facilitator of digestion, particularly the early breakdown of food, as well as taste acuity and articulation. Clinically, when the salivary glands are functionally deficient ("hypo" function), observable effects include difficulty speaking, difficulty chewing, difficulty swallowing, and impaired ability to taste. Other results of salivary gland hypofunction include an increased incidence of caries and periodontal disease with the presence of opportunistic organisms. The increased incidence of caries is caused by an increase in caries-forming organisms, which flourish in an acidic environment; therefore, even minimally functioning salivary glands can maintain an increase in the pH of the saliva and decrease the harmful effects of caries-forming organisms [2–4, 6–10]. Any increase in saliva, no matter how small, with concomitant increases in the production of salivary constituents may benefit patients with xerostomia [1].

The volume of salivary secretion may be decreased by a number of disease processes and other factors. Xerostomia is defined as the perception of dry mouth and is estimated to affect 22–26% of the general population [7]. It reportedly occurs more commonly in the elderly [10] and in patients with advanced cancer (29–77%) [7]. Xerostomia may also be associated with immunotherapy [9, 11], chemotherapy [6, 7], and radiation treatment involving the major salivary glands [12, 13].

Virtually all patients who undergo radiation therapy of the head and neck have some degree of xerostomia as a result of damage to the salivary glands [13–16]. Xerostomia may also be caused or exacerbated by the concomitant or sequential use of chemotherapy agents and other drugs [5]. Xerostomia is associated with oral discomfort and pain, increased rates of dental caries and oral infection, difficulty speaking and swallowing, and, ultimately, decreased nutritional intake and weight loss [13, 26] (Fig. 11.1). Thus, xerostomia significantly impairs the

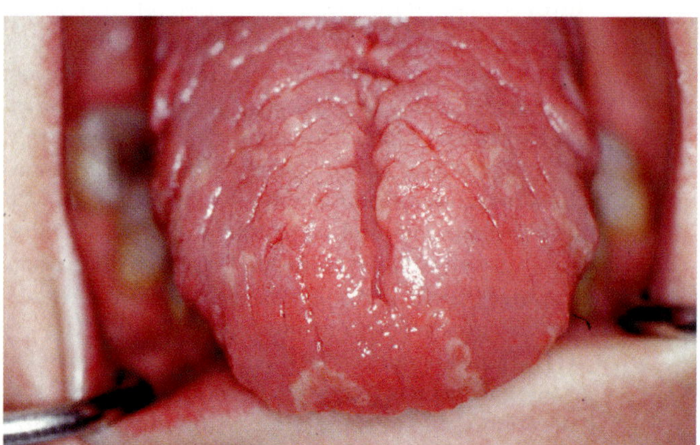

Fig. 11.1: Radiation-induced xerostomia of the oral tongue with fissuring of the dorsal anatomy, crenations, and leukoplakia

quality of life (QOL) and can compromise the continuity of cancer treatment.

The remainder of this chapter will be devoted to current knowledge of radiation-induced xerostomia and its sequelae.

Pathogenesis of Radiation-induced Xerostomia

A number of disease processes and other factors may decrease salivary secretion. Xerostomia has been reported in association with rheumatoid conditions, particularly Sjögren's syndrome [1, 17], human immunodeficiency virus infection [11], diabetes [12, 18], hypertension [12], and hematopoietic cell or bone marrow transplantation or graft-versus-host disease [19]. Medications also associated with xerostomia include many chemotherapy agents [20], antihypertensives [21], overactive-bladder agents [22], pain medications [21, 23], and psychiatric agents (Table 11.1) [21, 24]. Xerostomia has also been reported in association with some types of immunotherapy [25]. Radiation therapy, particularly directed at the oral mucosa and salivary glands can cause severe xerostomia [13, 26].

During therapy for head and neck cancer, the appropriate daily and total radiation doses are based on tumor size and individual clinical situations. Typically, daily radiation doses are 1.8–2 Gy, with subclinical microscopic cancer requiring at least 50 Gy over a 5-week period; smaller lesions (T1), 60–66 Gy; intermediate lesions (T2), 66–70 Gy; and large tumors (T3 and T4), more than 70 Gy [13, 14]. Radiation portals often include delivery of high doses to the parotid and submandibular glands bilaterally [27] and in some cases a large proportion of the minor salivary glands [28]. Clinically, xerostomia has been reported with as little as two or three doses of 2 Gy each, although many changes occurring with less than 60 Gy may be reversible [29, 30]. However, in some patients, doses greater than 30 Gy can cause permanent xerostomia [27].

Damage to the salivary glands results in reduced salivary flow, changes in the electrolyte and immunoglobulin composition of saliva, reduction of salivary pH, and re population of the mouth by cariogenic microflora [13]. When the major salivary glands are included in the radiation field, salivary function often decreases by 50–60% in the first week, with basal salivary flow reaching a measurable minimum 2–3 weeks after 23 Gy of fractionated radiation [13, 27, 30]. The extent of glandular change is generally directly related to the dose of radiation to the salivary glands, with the most severe and irreversible forms of salivary dysfunction resulting from damage to or loss of salivary acinar cells [13, 29].

The pathogenesis of radiation-induced xerostomia involves more than damage to the salivary glands, however, a lack of lubrication reduces the ability of chemoreceptors on the tongue and palate to accept stimuli presented with foods or liquids, resulting in failure of the salivary response. The minimal volume and thickened mucinous saliva that is produced may form a barrier to dietary, thermal, and mechanical stimulation of the taste buds. This, in turn, affects the pathway of salivary gland stimulation and ultimate secretion. The mucosa of the tongue may be atrophied, with decreased surface area for taste buds. Significant loss of appetite may occur, along with mucositis. As dietary intake decreases, weight loss alone may become a significant factor in the continuity of cancer therapy [31]. Methods for assessing radiation-induced

Table 11.1. Drugs that may cause or exacerbate xerostomia [7, 13, 23]

Anorexiants
Antiacne agents
Antianxiety agents
Anticholinergic/antispasmodic agents
Anticonvulsants
Antidepressants
Antidiarrheal agents
Antihistamines
Antihypertensive agents
Anti-inflammatory analgesic agents
Antiemetic agents
Antiparkinsonian agents
Antipsychotic agents
Bronchodilators
Chemotherapy agents
Decongestants
Diuretics
Muscle relaxants
Narcotic analgesics
Sedatives

xerostomia include clinical examination; subjective measures, such as patient self-report instruments and visual analog scales; and objective measures, such as assessment of stimulated and unstimulated salivary flow rates [32]. Metrics for describing xerostomia have been poor. The most recent version of the Common Terminology Criteria for Adverse Events v3.0 (CTCAE v3.0) has been developed and represents an important improvement as a comprehensive, multimodality grading system to include both acute and late effects [33, 34].

Quality of Life

Radiation-induced xerostomia can be an acute complication that improves with time but is often a permanent condition that seriously impairs the patient's well-being. Xerostomia predisposes patients to an altered oral microflora with increased virulent bacteria and fungal activity [35]. Loss of salivary function usually results in the appearance of an increased number of caries-forming bacteria (mutans Streptococci and Lactobacillus) in the oral cavity, with resultant "radiation caries" caused by a loss of buffering capacity, lowered salivary pH, elimination of mechanical flushing, and decreased production of salivary immunoglobulins (i.e., IgA, IgG, IgM), lysozymes, and peroxidases (Fig. 11.2) [6, 29, 35]. Xerostomia may result in mucositis; oral pain or discomfort; and difficulty with mastication, deglutition, and articulation; and it is associated with increased caries, dysgeusia, ageusia, soft tissue breakdown, bone loss, and chronic infection [15, 26]. When not monitored and controlled, xerostomia may lead to accumulation of plaque and other debris on teeth and periodontal tissues [6]. Cariogenic plaque buildup on teeth may lead to tooth decay, gingivitis, and periodontitis. According to Berger and Kilroy [31], elevated plaque matrix resulting from xerostomia may pose the greatest risk of osteoradionecrosis. Ill-fitting removable prostheses in patients with xerostomia, causing tissue irritation, can compound mucositis and result in fenestration of supporting mucosa and post-treatment osteoradionecrosis. In addition, recent evidence suggests a potential link between oral and dental disease and systemic illnesses, such as atherosclerosis, coronary artery disease, and cerebrovascular ischemia [36].

Saliva plays a significant role in taste acuity, although the interaction is not completely understood [37]. It is known that a diminished salivary flow can markedly affect this interaction [6]. Saliva has modulating effects on the basic taste modalities: sour, sweet, salty, and bitter. Saliva strongly influences salty taste threshold levels and provides the ionic environment necessary for signal transduction by taste cells. The type of taste stimuli can also influence salivary flow rate and composition. Sour taste induces the highest flow rate and sodium concentrations, whereas salt gives rise to high protein and calcium concentrations [37]. Chemoreceptors on the dorsal tongue anatomy are markedly affected by xerostomia with a diminished acuity, therefore decreasing the effect of taste and affecting the patient's QOL [6, 26, 37].

Patients with cancer of the head and neck must sometimes choose between treatment options that provide equivalent cure rates but potentially differing effects on QOL. Several recent studies have reported on the preva-

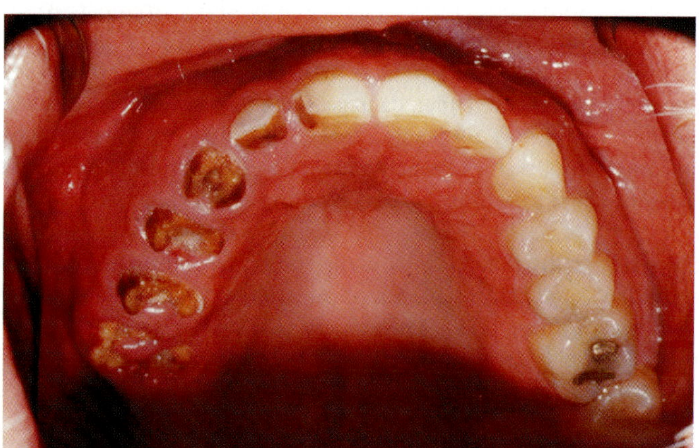

Fig. 11.2: Fifty-year-old male patient with history of adenocarcinoma of the parotid gland status post-parotidectomy and radiation therapy presenting with unilateral caries (1.5 years post-radiation therapy)

lence of xerostomia symptoms and their impact on QOL in persons treated for cancer of the head and neck [13].

Hughes et al. [38] investigated the prevalence of long-term dysphagia after radiation for carcinoma of the nasopharynx. These researchers assessed 50 patients, aged 26–75 years, who had received radiation 12–119 months earlier, and showed that 96% of patients had xerostomia and 76% had dysphagia. In another study, Logemann et al. [26] evaluated perception and performance of the swallow function in 36 patients, aged 40–76 years, who received radiation of at least 40 Gy to the oral cavity or oropharyngeal areas over a 6-week period, with or without concurrent chemotherapy. Each patient underwent pretherapy and post-therapy testing, including a questionnaire on the global perception of dry mouth, measurement of stimulated saliva production, and videofluorographic study of oropharyngeal swallow. After radiation therapy, significantly more patients reported swallowing difficulty, dry mouth, needing water while eating, food sticking to the mouth or throat, and change in taste. Mean saliva weight decreased from 5.1 g before treatment to 1.4 g after treatment ($p < .0001$) and generally was lower in patients who reported swallowing difficulty. The researchers concluded that chemoradiation therapy results in xerostomia and a significant increase in patient perception of swallowing difficulty.

Harrison et al. [39] treated 36 patients, aged 35–71 years, with primary radiation for squamous cell carcinoma of the base of the tongue; all received external beam radiation therapy (45–54 Gy) to the primary site and the neck, followed by an electron boost (up to 60 Gy) to involved neck nodes and an iridium-192 implant boost to the primary site (20–30 Gy). After a median follow-up of 5 years, 29 long-term survivors completed four surveys, including validated QOL instruments. From these results, the researchers concluded that most of the patients had excellent functional status and QOL and were able to maintain prediagnosis income and employment status. However, the results of the Memorial Symptom Assessment Scale indicated that xerostomia occurred in all patients and was rated as causing moderate to severe distress by 89%. Other commonly reported symptoms included difficulty swallowing (76%; moderate to severe distress in 90% of those affected) and decreased energy (48%; moderate to severe distress in 64%). Although only 34% of patients reported change in taste, 70% of these found this effect to cause moderate to severe distress.

Epstein et al. [40] used the European Organization for Research and Treatment of Cancer (EORTC) Quality of Life Questionnaire, with an addendum to assess oral symptoms and function, to measure QOL of 65 patients, aged 21–79 years, who more than 6 months earlier had undergone radiation therapy with or without surgery for head and neck and oral cancers. Results showed that 91.8% of patients reported xerostomia; 75.4%, change in taste; 63.1%, dysphagia; 50.8%, altered speech; 48.5%, difficulty with dentures; 43%, difficulty chewing or eating; and 38.5%, increased tooth decay (in dentate patients). In addition, pain was common (58.4%), interfering with daily activities in 30.8%. The frequency of oral side effects was correlated with radiation treatment fields and dose. Most patients reported their overall QOL and overall physical condition to be less than excellent.

In a similar study, Epstein et al. [13, 40] found that xerostomia, change in taste, dysphagia, speech difficulties, and oral pain were commonly reported oral symptoms, and that oral QOL did not return to pretreatment levels by 6 months after treatment. Development of further general, disease-specific, and region-specific QOL studies are needed to help guide cancer treatment choices, assess QOL and function after treatment, and assess the management of oral complications after radiation for cancer of the head and neck [39, 40].

Treatment

Stringent Oral and Dental Care

To minimize the severity of xerostomia and oral complications, it is important to begin aggressive oral care prior to starting radiation therapy. Appropriate nutritional intake, effective oral hygiene, and early detection of oral lesions are important pretreatment practices. Evaluation by a dental team experienced in oral oncology, ideally weeks in advance of therapy, is essential to determine oral health status, perform necessary dental and oral interventions, and allow for healing from any invasive procedures that may be required. Greater attention will be required in identifying mucosal lesions, dental caries and endodontic disease, periodontal disease, ill-fitting dentures, orthodontic appliances, temporomandibular dysfunction, and salivary abnormalities. A stringent program of oral hygiene is crucial and should be performed before, during, and after therapy (Table 11.2) [6, 13, 15, 41].

Table 11.2. Management steps for patients with radiation-induced xerostomia [6, 13, 15, 41]

Function	Treatment options
Plaque removal	Tooth brushing (nontartar controlled)
	Flossing
	Other oral hygiene aids
Remineralization	Topical high-concentration prescription fluorides
	Children: topical and systemic
	Adults: topical
Prevention/treatment of infection	Antimicrobials, such as chlorhexidine rinses, povidone-iodine oral rinses, tetracycline oral rinses
Temporary relief of dryness	Salivary substitutes or rinses containing hydroxyethyl-, hydroxypropyl-, or carboxymethylcellulose
Stimulation of remaining salivary gland tissue	Sialogogic agents (cholinergic agonists)
	FDA-approved: pilocarpine
	Investigational: cevimeline, bethanechol chloride, others

Radiation Therapy Protectants

Agents have been developed to ameliorate or eliminate toxicities associated with chemotherapy and radiation [42]. Amifostine, an agent studied for its selective protection of normal tissue from damage induced by radiation and chemotherapy, was approved by the US Food and Drug Administration (FDA) as a cytoprotective agent with cisplatin-based chemotherapy for ovarian cancer and, later, for prevention of xerostomia in patients treated with radiation for head and neck cancer [43]. This recommendation was based on the results of a phase III multi-institutional randomized study reported by Brizel et al. [44]. The incidence of grade 2 or higher chronic xerostomia was reduced from 57% in the control arm to 34% in patients receiving amifostine. There were no differences in survival or disease control, suggesting that amifostine protected salivary function without protecting the cancer. Clinical practice guidelines of the American Society of Clinical Oncology, published in 1999, indicate that amifostine may be considered for use in patients who undergo fractionated radiation in the head and neck region to decrease the incidence of acute and late xerostomia [42]. The recommended dose of amifostine is 200 mg/m^2 per day administered as a slow intravenous push over 3 min, 15–30 min before each fraction of radiation. Patients require close monitoring for side effects, including hypotension and nausea, and some patients may require antiemetics [42, 43]. Investigations with a subcutaneous administration of amifostine are ongoing, because this form of administration may be more practical and lower the toxicity of the drug.

Salivary Gland Transfer Techniques

Although the radiation ports used in treating cancer of the head and neck generally deliver 60–65 Gy to the major salivary glands, the submental region is regularly shielded, receiving only scatter radiation of 5% of the total dose [13, 16]. Several animal studies [45–47] have demonstrated the feasibility of microvascular autotransplantation of submandibular and parotid gland tissue. In a recent human study, Seikaly et al. [16] transferred the submandibular gland to the submental space in patients undergoing surgery and radiation for head and neck cancer. The glands survived transfer and continued to function after radiation with appropriate shielding. This continues to be an area of investigation in multicenter settings.

Table 11.3. Xerostomia: pharmacologic options [1]

	Product	Manufacturer
Saliva substitutes	Oral Balance	Laclede Research Labs, Gardena, CA
	Salivart	Gebauer Company, Cleveland, OH
	MouthKote	Parnell Pharmaceuticals, Larkspur, CA
	Saliva Substitute	Roxane Laboratories, Columbus, OH
	MoistPlus	Medical Warehouse, Stormville, NY
	MedOral spray	BHM Labs, Port Richey, FL
	Oasis	Glaxo Smith Kline, Philadelphia, PA
Fluoride	Gel Kam (0.4% SnF)	Colgate Oral Pharmaceuticals, Canton, MA
	Prevident Gel (1.1% NaF)	Colgate Oral Pharmaceuticals, Canton, MA
	NeutraCare (1.1% NaF)	Oral-B Laboratories, Belmont, CA
	Omni Gel (0.4% SnF)	Omni Gel, Gravette, AR
	Prevident 5000 plus dentifrice	Colgate Oral Pharmaceuticals, Canton, MA
Cholinergic agonists	Pilocarpine (Salagen)	MGI Pharma, Minnetonka, MN
	Cevimeline (Exovac)	Daiichi Sankyo, Montvale, NJ

Gene Therapy

Emerging research and medical technology are providing specificity and sensitivity methods to determine the roles of human salivary components. Gene transfer may be potentially useful for treating inherited single-gene deficiency disorders and malignancies refractory to other therapies, as well as restoring function to irradiated salivary glands [48, 49]. There are no published reports examining a prophylactic gene transfer approach to reducing or eliminating radiation damage of the salivary glands [48]. Translational studies involving plasmid-mediated gene transfer for reducing radiation-induced damage have been conducted, and results of in vivo animal studies in lung and esophageal tissue are quite promising [50, 51]. Research in nonviral gene-mediated therapeutics for restoring radiation-induced salivary gland dysfunction may prove beneficial [8].

Pharmacologic Options

Current therapies for the pharmacologic management of radiation-induced xerostomia include the use of prescription fluoride agents to maintain optimal oral hygiene, antimicrobials to prevent dental caries and oral infection, saliva substitutes to relieve dryness, and sialogogic agents, i.e., cholinergic agents, to stimulate saliva production from remaining intact salivary gland tissues (Table 11.3) [13, 15, 40].

Proper oral care before, during, and after radiation is essential, with the use of topical 0.4% stannous fluoride or 1.1% sodium fluoride gel once daily to minimize dental caries [6]. Oral antimicrobial agents may also be beneficial in preventing oral infection. Chlorhexidine gluconate, for example, provides broad-spectrum activity in vitro against gram-positive, gram-negative, and fungal pathogens and binds well to oral surfaces (minimizing gastrointestinal absorption). However, the desiccating effect of the alcohol in some chlorhexidine solutions may exacerbate xerostomia; therefore, an aqueous-based solution may be beneficial [6, 41].

Saliva substitutes containing hydroxyethyl-, hydroxypropyl-, or carboxymethylcellulose may be beneficial as palliative agents to relieve the discomfort of xerostomia by temporarily wetting the oral mucosa [52]. One recent study investigated the use of a xanthan gum-based saliva substitute [28]. Patient reports showed similar improvement with the xanthan gum-based saliva substitute and placebo (of similar composition, without xanthan gum), but with a trend toward increased improvement in speech and sensory problems with the xanthan gum agent. The researchers concluded that this agent was not of greater benefit than other saliva substitutes for patients with radiation-induced xerostomia [28]. Other new saliva substitutes (moisturizing gels) with enzymatic and protein components (e.g., glucose oxidase and lactoperoxidase), which present prospective antibacterial effectiveness and increased oral moisture, are under study.

For patients with residual salivary gland function, cholinergic agonists may produce symptomatic improvement [18, 28]. Pilocarpine is currently the only sialogogic agent approved by the FDA for radiation-induced xerostomia. Pilocarpine functions primarily as a muscarinic-cholinergic agonist with mild β-adrenergic activity. Muscarinic agonists in sufficient dosage can increase secretion of exocrine glands, such as salivary and sweat glands, as well as the tone of smooth muscle in the gastrointestinal and urinary tracts. Studies have shown oral pilocarpine to have efficacy in patients with Sjögren's syndrome, radiation-induced xerostomia, and opioid-induced xerostomia, as well as increasing salivary flow and restoring salivary composition in those with graft-versus-host disease caused by allogeneic bone marrow transplantation [5, 25, 29, 53–56]. The role of pilocarpine during radiation to decrease xerostomia requires further investigation. Preliminary data from a randomized Radiation Therapy Oncology Group (RTOG) study suggest some improvement in objective saliva measurements in patients receiving pilocarpine during radiation compared with patients receiving placebo. However, there were no differences in patients' perception of their xerostomia when patients receiving active drug were compared with the placebo control arm [57]. Warde et al. [58] from Canada revealed in a smaller phase III trial that there was no beneficial effect of pilocarpine on radiation-induced xerostomia when administered during radiation for patients with cancer of the head and neck.

In October 2002, Hodson et al. [59] updated their Cancer Care Ontario Practice Guidelines (CCOPG) for the Symptomatic Treatment of Radiation-Induced Xerostomia in Head and Neck Cancer Patients. The group's recommendations were based largely on evidence from four randomized, placebo-controlled studies of oral pilocarpine [52, 60–62], one comparison trial of pilocarpine mouthwash versus artificial saliva [63], and one study of long-term efficacy [64]. In a crossover study by Greenspan and Daniels [61] including 12 patients who had severe xerostomia 6 months after radiation therapy, nine patients showed marked improvement after 3 months of treatment with 15–30 mg of pilocarpine daily, whereas none showed meaningful improvement while taking placebo. Schuller et al. [62] administered an oral solution containing 3 mg of pilocarpine or placebo to patients who had undergone surgery and postoperative radiation therapy an average of 21 months earlier; the pilocarpine solution produced no improvement in dry mouth, taste, or swallowing compared with placebo. LeVeque et al. conducted a randomized, placebo-controlled dose escalation study, and Johnson et al. conducted a three-arm randomized, placebo-controlled trial (placebo, pilocarpine 5 mg three times a day, and pilocarpine 10 mg three times a day) [52, 60]. In both studies, significantly more patients treated with pilocarpine than those subjects receiving placebo reported improvement in xerostomia. In addition, LeVeque et al. found that treatment with pilocarpine led to a significant decrease in the use of oral comfort agents such as artificial saliva, hard candies, and water [52].

In a randomized crossover study of pilocarpine mouthwash versus mucin-based artificial saliva, Davies and Singer [63] found a mean change in the xerostomia score after 3 months of 22.5% with pilocarpine and 15.2% with artificial saliva. For 36 months, Jacobs and van der Pas [64] followed patients with radiation-induced xerostomia who were treated with pilocarpine, 2.5–10 mg twice a day or three times a day (starting dose, 5 mg three times a day). They found improvements at the last visit in dryness of the mouth and tongue, oral comfort, ability to sleep, ease of speaking, and ability to eat. In these studies, no serious adverse events were associated with pilocarpine treatment. The most frequently reported adverse event was excessive sweating; others included chills, nausea, dizziness, rhinitis, and asthenia. Largely on the basis of these studies, the authors of the CCOPG [59] reached the following conclusions: (1) for patients with cancer of the head and neck with symptomatic xerostomia after radiation therapy using conventional fractionation schedules, pilocarpine 5 mg three times a day is recommended; (2) patients must have evidence of preexisting salivary function; (3) the ideal duration of treatment with pilocarpine is undefined, and the decision to extend treatment beyond 3 months can be made on the basis of clinical judgment only; (4) it is highly reasonable to use pilocarpine for patients with symptomatic xerostomia after hyperfractionated or accelerated-fractionation radiation [59]; and (5) pilocarpine is contraindicated in patients with uncontrolled asthma, acute iritis, or narrow-angle glaucoma. It should be used with caution in patients with controlled asthma, chronic bronchitis, chronic obstructive pulmonary disease, or cardiovascular disease [65].

Other cholinergic agents with sialogogic properties, such as cevimeline hydrochloride, may prove beneficial for cancer patients with xerostomia. Cevimeline is a newer muscarinic agonist that has been found to be safe and effective in treating xerostomia associated with Sjögren's syndrome and has received FDA approval for that use [66, 67]. In addition, cevimeline has shown efficacy in animal studies by increasing saliva secretions after X-ray exposure of the head and neck [68] and is currently under study for use in patients with cancer of the head and neck who have radiation-induced xerostomia. A randomized, double-blind, placebo-controlled study was conducted with cevimeline in patients with Sjögren's syndrome, and most of the subjects receiving active drug had a global improvement in their xerostomia. The effects of cevimeline at 15 mg three times a day (45 mg/day) and 30 mg three times a day (90 mg/day) were compared with those of placebo, and statistically significant global improvement in the symptoms of dry mouth ($p = .0004$) was seen for the 30 mg three times a day group than the placebo group. Salivary flow rates increased at both doses of cevimeline compared with placebo [69]. The incidence of serious adverse events was low in all treatment groups. The most common drug-related adverse events were excessive sweating, nausea, rhinitis, and diarrhea [70].

In addition to these currently available and emerging pharmacotherapies, the use of chewing gums made with noncariogenic sweeteners may help stimulate saliva secretion and reduce oral mucosal friction [71]. Humidification may also be helpful; in a recent study, however, hyperthermic supersaturated humidification by way of a nasal cannula in patients with radiation-induced xerostomia yielded little or no additional relief compared with a standard bedside humidifier [15].

Emerging Parotid Gland-sparing Techniques

Recent efforts have focused on the use of conformal radiation or other newer radiotherapy techniques to spare a portion of the major salivary glands [27]. Intensity-modulated radiotherapy (IMRT) is a form of conformal radiation that allows for sculpting dose distributions that conform specifically to a three-dimensional shape of the target. The clinical advantages to using IMRT are numerous and include improvement in radiation dose uniformity, creation of concave dose patterns conforming to the shape of the tumor, assignment of weightings to targets and critical structures, treatment of multiple targets simultaneously, and lowering of complication rates. The desire for conformal doses and the lack of internal organ motion make IMRT attractive for patients with cancer of the head and neck [72–74]. Several studies have demonstrated the significant benefit of IMRT over conventional treatment with respect to dosimetric superiority compared with more conventional approaches [75–77]. Recently, IMRT has been used for treatment of cancers of the head and neck and studied for improved tumor coverage with resultant increased rates in locoregional control and decreased short-term toxicity [76]. Longitudinal data on the therapeutic efficacy of IMRT are lacking with regard to long-term tumor outcome and late radiation toxicity [76]. However, a substantial number of studies have documented the reduction of radiation-induced xerostomia following IMRT for squamous cell carcinoma of the pharynx and larynx [13, 27, 72–77].

Conventional Parotid Doses and Sparing

Dreizen et al. [78] quantified saliva production in patients undergoing radiotherapy for cancer of the head and neck. In this study, after a dose of 10 Gy, patients had already developed a 50% reduction in salivary flow. After receiving 50 Gy, patients had less than 10% of their salivary flow remaining, and few patients regained salivary function. Emami et al. [79] defined the tolerance dose of the saliva glands to radiation, stating the minimum tolerance dose of 5/5 (tumor dose causing 5% complication rate at 5 years) as 30 Gy, and the tolerance dose 50/5 as 50 Gy. Leslie and Dische [80] described high rates of xerostomia in patients whose parotid glands were irradiated with 40 Gy but negligible rates in patients who received less than 14 Gy. Thus, the tolerance doses of the glands lie somewhere within this wide range.

Parotid-sparing Techniques

Reducing the radiation dose to the major salivary glands is achievable with IMRT [72, 77]. Reddy et al. investigated the use of parotid-sparing irradiation techniques in patients with cancer of the oral cavity. Thirty-one patients were treated with two-dimensional techniques sparing at least one parotid gland from radiation beams, whereas 83 patients were treated with bilateral opposed photon beams, including both parotid glands. Patients treated with the parotid-sparing technique were able to maintain nutritional intake and baseline body weight during and after radiation therapy. In contrast, those treated with the bilateral technique had poor nutritional intake and lost more than 10% of body weight, which was not regained during the 2 years after treatment. When analyzed according to tumor stage, primary tumor control rates with the parotid-sparing and bilateral techniques were similar (93% and 87%, respectively, for early-stage tumors; 42% and 36%, respectively, for advanced-stage tumors); therefore, the authors noted that selection of patients who might benefit from this technique requires consideration of the risk of contralateral cervical lymph node metastases [30].

In another study, O'Sullivan et al. used an ipsilateral technique to restrict irradiation to the primary tumor and neck on the same side in patients with carcinoma of the tonsillar region. From 1970 to 1991, these researchers treated 228 of 642 patients with carcinoma of the tonsillar region (mainly T1 and T2, N0 and N1) with this technique. After a mean follow-up of 7 years, the 3-year actuarial local control rate was 77% and the cause-specific survival rate was 76%, with failure in the opposite side of the neck in eight patients. Difficulties with primary coverage early in the study resulted in higher rates of local failure. The researchers concluded that, in appropriately selected patients with carcinoma of the tonsil, the risk of failure in the opposite side of the neck is minimal with ipsilateral therapy, but CT planning is necessary to ensure adequate target coverage [81].

While the above suggest that a subset of patients requiring radiation therapy can be treated unilaterally, and avoid a high likelihood of developing xerostomia, most patients with mucosal cancer of the head and neck still require radiation to both sides of the neck. In order to diminish xerostomia in patients undergoing bilateral radiation therapy, conformal techniques and eventually IMRT were tested as methods to decrease the dose to the parotid glands [82–84]. Unfortunately, while it was recognized that the parotid glands are sensitive to radiation, the precise tolerance dose was unclear. To begin to answer the question of whether parotid gland sparing was feasible and efficacious, the dose, volume, and functional relationships in parotid salivary glands following conformal and multisegmental IMRT of the head and neck were studied by Eisbruch et al. [85]. Eighty-eight patients with cancer of the head and neck participated in the study. Unstimulated and stimulated saliva was measured from each parotid gland before radiotherapy and 1, 3, 6, and 12 months afterward. Glands receiving a mean dose below or equal to a threshold of less than 25% of the pretreatment level (24 Gy for unstimulated and 26 Gy for stimulated saliva) revealed preservation of the flow rates after radiotherapy. More importantly, and contrary to the belief that xerostomia was irreversible, these patients continued to improve over time [85]. The glands receiving doses below the threshold had functional recovery over time, whereas glands receiving higher doses did not recover [77, 85]. Age, sex, preradiotherapy surgery, chemotherapy, and specific intercurrent illnesses were not found to affect the salivary flow rates. Eisbruch et al. [82, 85, 86] concluded that a mean dose of less than 26 Gy to the parotid gland should be the planning goal for substantial sparing of gland function.

Besides objective measures of xerostomia (parotid flow rates) the University of Michigan team also performed subjective assessments. The group developed and validated the xerostomia questionnaire (XQ). This is an eight-item instrument in which subjects rate their own assessment of dryness with regards to talking, eating, sleeping, and the need for water for comfort in differing scenarios. Eisbruch et al. [27] then demonstrated that if the mean parotid dose was kept below 21 Gy, patients experienced lower scores (i.e., less subjective xerostomia). However, when compared to patients who were treated with unilateral techniques, despite improvement in xerostomia, patients treated to the bilateral neck still had more complaints of dry mouth. In addition, the oral cavity mean radiation dose was found to be significantly correlated with xerostomia scores, indicating that it may be beneficial to spare the uninvolved oral cavity to further reduce xerostomia [27].

These University of Michigan researchers also studied the parotid salivary function up to 12 months after radiotherapy in 20 patients undergoing bilateral neck parotid-sparing irradiation to determine if parotid preservation improves xerostomia-related QOL [84]. Salivary sampling and a 15-item xerostomia-related QOL scale were completed by each patient. The salivary flow from spared and treated glands significantly decreased at the completion of radiotherapy. After radiotherapy, unstimulated and stimulated function increased and was not significantly different from baseline figures; therefore, these authors concluded that, with the use of parotid-sparing radiotherapy, contralateral glands are preserved 12 months after treatment with parallel improvement in xerostomia-related QOL [84]. This same group of researchers [86, 87] also tested QOL and xerostomia in patients treated with IMRT compared to patients treated with conventional radiotherapy. Twelve months after parotid-sparing IMRT, statistical significance was found between patient-reported xerostomia and four domains of QOL: eating, communication, pain, and emotion [87].

Using mathematical modeling, Chao et al. [88] concluded that the functional outcome of salivary flow using inverse-planning IMRT could be modeled as a function of dose, and therefore the mean dose to each parotid gland is a reasonable indicator for the functional outcome of each gland. The entire parotid volume was used to compute dose-volume histograms in this trial evaluating 41 patients with head and neck cancer. Stimulated saliva production at 6 months reduced exponentially for each gland independently, at a rate of approximately 4% per Gy of mean parotid dose [88].

In another study by the same authors, acute toxicity, late toxicity, and tumor control were retrospectively compared in 430 patients with cancer of the oropharynx who underwent radiotherapy with a conventional beam arrangement or IMRT [89]. These investigators concluded that the dosimetric advantage of IMRT translated into significant reduction of late salivary toxicity, with no adverse impact on tumor control or disease-free survival [89, 90]. After IMRT, only 17–30% of patients had late grade 2 xerostomia. Although the majority had moderate to severe dry mouth during therapy, the spared salivary glands showed recovery over time. The dosimetric conformity of IMRT for normal tissue sparing in patients with oropharyngeal cancer was studied by Chao et al. [91] in assessing the therapeutic outcomes of IMRT as it relates to the impact on gross tumor volume (GTV) and nodal gross tumor volume (nGTV). A multivariate analysis revealed that GTV and nGTV were important independent risk factors predictive of therapeutic outcome for definitive treatment of oropharyngeal IMRT [91].

In delineating the target volume for radiation in parotid gland-sparing techniques, Eisbruch et al. [92] recently published results of a longitudinal clinical investigation assessing patients treated with parotid-sparing IMRT for non-nasopharyngeal squamous cell carcinomas of the head and neck; furthermore, patients were examined for locoregional failures near the base of the skull and their relationships to the target delineation in the upper neck. The results reported in this study confirmed that defining level II in the contralateral node-negative neck so that the targets included the subdigastric nodes, yet not to extend as cranial as in conventional radiotherapy, allowed substantial sparing of the contralateral parotid glands and, hence, reduced salivary dysfunction. Another study evaluating the radiotherapy target volume and organs at risk in oropharyngeal carcinoma defined the lowering of the cranial border of the level II lymph nodes from C1 to C2 in patients with bilateral cervical radiotherapy and found reduced toxic effects on major salivary gland tissue, as proposed by Astreinidou et al. [93]. The lowering of the cranial border to C2 with IMRT could be considered on the contralateral side if the risk of metastasis on that side is significantly low, thus reducing the average mean dose to the contralateral parotid gland. Astreinidou et al. [93] calculated that the reduction of the normal tissue complication probability for xerostomia 1 year after radiotherapy could be up to 68% (lowering the cranial border to C2), compared with conventional radiotherapy when treating C1.

Munter et al. [94] evaluated salivary gland function after IMRT for cancer of the head and neck using quantitative pertechnetate scintigraphy. The mean dose to the primary planning target volume was 61.5 Gy, and the median follow-up was 23 months. This study revealed that it was possible to protect the parotid glands and reduce the incidence of xerostomia in patients with cancer of the head and neck if mean parotid doses were less than 30 Gy.

Conclusions

Xerostomia has been reported as the most common late effect of radiation for cancer of the head and neck [13, 27]. Despite current preventive and treatment efforts, xerostomia remains a common complication of radiation, causing significant impairment of QOL. Several investigational interventions are promising. First, advanced radiation delivery techniques, such as IMRT, potentially deliver a higher dose to the tumor target without increasing the dose to normal tissues, such as salivary glands, thereby allowing a higher dose per fraction and improved physical and biologic therapeutic ratios. Emerging data indicate that IMRT and other new parotid-sparing techniques hold promise for the treatment of cancer of the head and neck, potentially offering reduced severity of xerostomia without compromised tumor control for appropriately selected patients [76, 95]. Second, early studies have demonstrated the feasibility of the transfer of the submandibular gland to the submental space in patients undergoing radiation, preserving salivary function and preventing xerostomia [16]. Third, sialogogic agents that have been effective in treating xerostomia associated with other disease processes, such as Sjögren's syndrome, hold promise of improved relief for patients radiated for cancer of the head and neck. Finally, the use of gene therapy and tissue engineering to restore salivary gland water pathways—or even the creation of an artificial salivary gland—may be on the horizon [13, 66]. Together with careful assessment, monitoring, and management of radiation-induced xerostomia, these emerging treatment strategies may significantly improve the QOL for future patients undergoing radiation for cancer of the head and neck.

Take Home Messages

- Saliva is a complex bodily fluid that has multiple properties: protective, digestive, lubrication, remineralizing, and facilitating speech, eating, and swallowing.
- Damage to the salivary glands results in reduced salivary flow, changes in the electrolyte and immunoglobulin composition of saliva, reduction of salivary pH, and repopulation of the mouth by cariogenic microflora.
- Xerostomia is defined as the perception of dry mouth and is estimated to affect 22–26% of the general population.
- Xerostomia is associated with oral discomfort and pain, increased rates of dental caries and oral infection, difficulty speaking and swallowing, and, ultimately, decreased nutritional intake and weight loss.
- Current therapies for the pharmacologic management of radiation-induced xerostomia include the use of prescription fluoride agents to maintain optimal oral hygiene, antimicrobials to prevent dental caries and oral infection, saliva substitutes to relieve dryness, and sialogogic agents, i.e., cholinergic agents, to stimulate saliva production from remaining intact salivary gland tissues.
- Emerging data indicate that IMRT and other new parotid-sparing techniques hold promise for the treatment of cancer of the head and neck, potentially offering reduced severity of xerostomia without compromised tumor control for appropriately selected patients.
- Parotid gland mean dose of less than 26 Gy should be the planning goal for substantial sparing of gland function.

References

1. Chambers MS (2004) Sjögren's Disease. ORL Head Neck Nurs 22:22–30
2. Dawes C (1987) Physiological factors affecting salivary flow rate, oral sugar clearance, and the sensation of dry mouth in man. J Dent Res 66(Spec Issue):648–653
3. Percival RS, Challacombe SJ, Marsh PD (1994) Flow rates of resting whole and stimulated parotid saliva in relation to age and gender. J Dent Res 73:1416–1420
4. Fox PC, Eversole R (2001) Diseases of the salivary glands. In: Silverman S, Eversole LR, & Truelove E (Eds.) Essentials of oral medicine (pp. 260–276). Hamilton: BC Decker
5. Mercadante S, Calderone L, Villari P (2000) The use of pilocarpine in opioid-induced xerostomia. Palliat Med 14:529–531
6. Chambers MS, Toth BB, Martin JW, et al. (1995) Oral and dental management of the cancer patient: Prevention and treatment of complications. Support Care Cancer 3:168–175
7. Peterson DE (2000) Oral problems in supportive care: No longer an orphan topic? Support Care Cancer 8:347–348
8. Chambers MS (2003) Clinical commentary on prophylactic treatment of radiation-induced xerostomia. Arch Otolaryngol Head Neck Surg 129:251–252
9. Davies AN, Singer J (1994) A comparison of artificial saliva and pilocarpine in radiation-induced xerostomia. J Laryngol Otol 108:663–665
10. Narhi TO (1994) Prevalence of subjective feelings of dry mouth in the elderly. J Dent Res 73:20–25
11. Schiodt M (1992) HIV-associated salivary gland disease: A review. Oral Surg Oral Med Oral Pathol Oral Radiol Endod 73:164–167
12. Sreebny LM, Valdini A, Yu A (1989) Xerostomia. Part II: Relationship to nonoral symptoms, drugs, and diseases. Oral Surg Oral Med Oral Pathol Oral Radiol Endod 68:419–427
13. Chambers MS, Garden AS, Kies MS, et al. (2004) Radiation-induced xerostomia in patients with head and neck cancer: Pathogenesis, impact on quality of life, and management. Head Neck 26:796–807
14. Shaha AR, Patel S, Shasha D, Harrison LB (2001) Head and neck cancer. In: Lenhard RE Jr, Osteen RT, Gansler T, editors. Clinical oncology. Atlanta, Ga: American Cancer Society; pp 297–330
15. Criswell MA, Sinha CK (2001) Hyperthermic, supersaturated humidification in the treatment of xerostomia. Laryngoscope 111:992–996

16. Seikaly H, Jha N, McGaw T, et al. (2001) Submandibular gland transfer: a new method of preventing radiation-induced xerostomia. Laryngoscope 111:347–352
17. Davies AN, Broadley K, Beighton D (2001) Xerostomia in patients with advanced cancer. J Pain Symptom Manage 22:820–825
18. Kao CH, Tsai SC, Sun SS (2001) Scintigraphic evidence of poor salivary function in type 2 diabetes. Diabetes Care 24:952–953
19. Nicolatou-Galitis O, Kitra V, Vliet-Constantinidou C, et al. (2001) The oral manifestations of chronic graft-versus-host disease (cGVHD) in paediatric allogeneic bone marrow transplant recipients. J Oral Pathol Med 30:148–153
20. Kies MS, Haraf DJ, Rosen F, et al. (2001) Concomitant infusional paclitaxel and fluorouracil, oral hydroxyurea, and hyperfractionated radiation for locally advanced squamous head and neck cancer. J Clin Oncol 19:1961–1969
21. Bergdahl M, Bergdahl J (2000) Low unstimulated salivary flow and subjective oral dryness: association with medication, anxiety, depression, and stress. J Dent Res 79:1652–1658
22. Malone-Lee JG, Walsh JB, Maugourd MF (2001) Toltero dine: a safe and effective treatment for older patients with overactive bladder. J Am Geriatr Soc 49:700–705
23. California Dental Hygienists Association. Xerostomia: drymouth. Available at: http://www.cdha.org/articles/drymouth.htm. Accessed February 7, 2003
24. Sjogren R, Nordstrom G (2000) Oral health status of psychiatric patients. J Clin Nurs 9:632–638
25. Nagler RM, Gez E, Rubinov R, et al. (2001) The effect of low-dose interleukin-2-based immunotherapy on salivary function and composition in patients with metastatic renal cell carcinoma. Arch Oral Biol 46:487–493
26. Logemann JA, Smith CH, Pauloski BR, et al. (2001) Effects of xerostomia on perception and performance of swallow function. Head Neck 23:317–321
27. Eisbruch A, Kim HM, Terrell JE, et al. (2001) Xerostomia and its predictors following parotidsparing irradiation of head-and-neck cancer. Int J Radiat Oncol Biol Phys 50:695–704
28. Jellema AP, Langendijk H, Bergenhenegouwen L, et al. (2001) The efficacy of Xialine in patients with xerostomia resulting from radiotherapy for head and neck cancer: a pilot-study. Radiother Oncol 59:157–160
29. Leek H, Albertsson M (2002) Pilocarpine treatment of xerostomia in head and neck patients. Micron 33:153–155
30. Reddy SP, Leman CR, Marks JE, et al. (2001) Parotid sparing irradiation for cancer of the oral cavity: maintenance of oral nutrition and body weight by preserving parotid function. Am J Clin Oncol 24:341–346
31. Berger AM, Kilroy TJ (1998) Oral complications of cancer therapy. In: Berger AM, Portenoy RK, Weissman DE, editors. Principles and practice of supportive oncology. Philadelphia: Lippincott-Raven Publishers; pp 223–236
32. Cox JD, Stetz J, Pajak TF (1995) Toxicity criteria of the Radiation Therapy Oncology Group (RTOG) and the European Organization for Research and Treatment of Cancer (EORTC). Int J Radiat Oncol Biol Phys 31:1341–1346
33. Trotti A, Colevas D, Setser A, et al. (2003) CTCAE v3.0: Development of a comprehensive grading system for the adverse effects of cancer treatment. Semin Radiat Oncol 13:176–181
34. Common Terminology Criteria for Adverse Events v3.0 (CTCAE): http://ctep.cancer.gov/forms/CTCAEv3.pdf; published December 12, 2003
35. Chambers MS, Keene HJ, Toth BB, et al. (2002) Mutans Streptococci in xerostomic cancer patients after pilocarpine therapy. J Dent Res 81, Special Issue A (IADR/AADR Abstract 3609); 443
36. Slavkin HC, Baum BJ (2000) Relationship of dental and oral pathology to systemic illness. JAMA 284:1215–1217
37. Spielman AI (1990) Interaction of saliva and taste. J Dent Res 69:838–843
38. Hughes PJ, Scott PM, Kew J, et al. (2000) Dysphagia in treated nasopharyngeal cancer. Head Neck 22:393–397
39. Harrison LB, Zelefsky MJ, Pfister DG, et al. (1997) Detailed quality of life assessment in patients treated with primary radiotherapy for squamous cell cancer of the base of the tongue. Head Neck 19:169–175
40. Epstein JB, Robertson M, Emerton S, et al. (2001) Quality of life and oral function in patients treated with radiation therapy for head and neck cancer. Head Neck 23:389–398
41. Schubert MM, Peterson DE, Lloid ME (1999) Oral complications. In: Thomas ED, Forman SJ, editors. Hematopoietic cell transplantation. 2nd ed. Malden, Ma: Blackwell Science Inc.; pp 751–763
42. Hensley ML, Schuchter LM, Lindley C, et al. (1999) American Society of Clinical Oncology clinical practice guidelines for the use of chemotherapy and radiotherapy protectants. J Clin Oncol 17:3333–3355
43. Lindegaard JC, Grau C (2000) Has the outlook improved for amifostine as a clinical radioprotector? Radiother Oncol 57:113–118
44. Brizel DM, Wasserman TH, Henke M, et al. (2000) Phase III randomized trial of amifostine as a radioprotector in head and neck cancer. J Clin Oncol 18:3339–3345
45. Spiegel JH, Deschler DG, Cheney ML (2001) Microvascular transplantation and replantation of the rabbit submandibular gland. Arch Otolaryngol Head Neck Surg 127:991–996

46. Spiegel JH, Zhang F, Levin DE, et al. (2000) Microvascular transplantation of the rat submandibular gland. Plast Reconstr Surg 106:1326–1335
47. Greer JE, Eltorky M, Robbins KT (2000) A feasibility study of salivary gland autograft transplantation for xerostomia. Head Neck 22:241–246
48. Nagler RM, Baum BJ (2003) Treatment reduces the severity of xerostomia following radiation therapy for oral cavity cancer. Arch Otolaryngol Head Neck Surg 129:245–251
49. Delporte C, O'Connell BC, He X, et al. (1997) Increased fluid secretion after adenoviral-mediated transfer of the aquaporin-1 cDNA to irradiated rat salivary glands. Proc Natl Acad Sci USA 94:3268–3273
50. Epperly MW, Gretton JA, DeFilippi SJ, et al. (2001) Modulation of radiation-induced cytokine elevation associated with esophagitis and esophageal stricture by manganese superoxide dismutase-plasmid/liposome (SOD2-PL) gene therapy. Radiat Res 155:2–14
51. Epperly MW, DeFelippi SJ, Sikora CA, et al. (2000) Intratracheal injection A manganese superoxide dismutase (MnSOD) plasmid/liposomes protects normal lung but not orthotopic tumors from irradiation. Gene Ther 7:1011–1018
52. LeVeque FG, Montgomery M, Potter D, et al. (1993) A multicenter, randomized, double-blind, placebo-controlled, dosetitration study of oral pilocarpine for treatment of radiation-induced xerostomia in head and neck cancer patients. J Clin Oncol 11:1124–1131
53. Fox PC, van der Ven PF, Baum BJ, et al. (1986) Pilocarpine for the treatment of xerostomia associated with salivary gland dysfunction. Oral Surg Oral Med Oral Pathol 61:243–248
54. Chambers MS, Toth BB, Payne R, et al. (1997) Mutans streptococci and salivary flow rates in cancer patients attending a pain clinic [abstract]. J Dent Res 76:358. Abstract 2755
55. Chambers M, Martin C, Toth B, et al. (1997) Assessment of functional improvement in cancer patients with oral pilocarpine as treatment for analgesia-induced xerostomia [abstract]. Support Care Cancer 5:164. Abstract 45
56. Chambers M, Toth B, Martin C, et al. (1997) Assessment of salivary flow improvement in cancer patients with oral pilocarpine as treatment for analgesia-induced xerostomia [abstract]. Proc Am Soc Clin Oncol 16:50a. Abstract 174
57. Scarantino CW, Leveque F, Scott C, et al. (2001) A phase III study on the concurrent use of oral pilocarpine to reduce hyposalivation and mucositis associated with radiation therapy in head and neck cancer patients [abstract]. Int J Radiat Oncol Biol Phys 51(suppl 1):85–86. Abstract 152
58. Warde P, Aslanidis J, Kroll B, et al. (2001) A phase III placebo controlled trial of oral pilocarpine in patients undergoing radiation therapy for head and neck cancer [abstract]. Int J Radiat Oncol Biol Phys 51(suppl 1):86. Abstract 153
59. Cancer Care Ontario Practice Guideline Initiative. Hodson DI, Haines T, Berry M, et al. and the Head and Neck Cancer Disease Site Group. Symptomatic treatment of radiation-induced xerostomia in head and neck cancer patients (Practice Guideline Report No. 5-5). Available at: http://www.ccopebc.ca/guidelines/head/cpg5_5f.html. Accessed February 7, 2003
60. Johnson JT, Ferretti GA, Nethery WJ, et al. (1993) Oral pilocarpine for post-irradiation xerostomia in patients with head and neck cancer. N Engl J Med 329:390–395
61. Greenspan D, Daniels TE (1987) Effectiveness of pilocarpine in postradiation xerostomia. Cancer 59:1123–1125
62. Schuller DE, Stevens P, Clausen KP, et al. (1989) Treatment of radiation side effects with oral pilocarpine. J Surg Oncol 42:272–276
63. Davies AN, Singer J (1994) A comparison of artificial saliva and pilocarpine in radiation-induced xerostomia. J Laryngol Otol 108:663–665
64. Jacobs CD, van der Pas M (1996) A multicenter maintenance study of oral pilocarpine tablets for radiation-induced xerostomia. Oncology (Huntingt) 10(suppl):16–20
65. Wiseman LR, Faulds D (1995) Oral pilocarpine: a review of its pharmacological properties and clinical potential in xerostomia. Drugs 49:143–155
66. Atkinson JC, Baum BJ (2001) Salivary enhancement: current status and future therapies. J Dent Educ 65:1096–1101
67. Al-Hashimi I (2001) The management of Sjögren's syndrome in dental practice. J Am Dent Assoc 132:1409–1417
68. Iga Y, Arisawa H, Ogane N, et al. (1998) (F)-cis-2-methylspiro[1,3-oxathiolane-5,3(-quinuclidine] hydrochloride, hemihydrate (SNI-2011, cevimeline hydrochloride) induces saliva and tear secretions in rats and mice: the role of muscarinic acetylcholine receptors. Jpn J Pharmacol 78:373–380
69. Petrone D, Condemi JJ, Fife R, et al. (2002) A double-blind, randomized, placebo-controlled study of cevimeline in Sjögren's syndrome patients with xerostomia and keratoconjunctivitis sicca. Arthritis Rheum 46:748–754
70. Evoxac Capsules (cevimeline hydrochloride). In: Physician's desk reference. 55th ed. Montvale, NJ: Medical Economics Co; 2001:1110–1112
71. Olsson H, Spak CJ, Axell T (1991) The effect of a chewing gum on salivary secretion, oral mucosal friction, and the feeling of dry mouth in xerostomic patients. Acta Odontol Scand 49:273–279

72. Chambers MS, Garden AS, Rosenthal DI, et al. (2005) Intensity-modulated radiotherapy: Is xerostomia still prevalent? Curr Oncol Rep 7:131–136
73. Eisbruch A, Foote RL, O'Sullivan B, et al. (2002) Intensity-modulated radiation therapy for head and neck cancer: emphasis on the selection and delineation of the targets. Semin Radiat Oncol 2:238–249
74. Ozyigit G, Yang T, Chao KS (2004) Intensity-modulated radiation therapy for head and neck cancer. Curr Treat Options Oncol 5:3–9
75. Eisbruch A, Dawson LA, Kim HM, et al. (1999) Conformal and intensity modulated irradiation of head and neck cancer: the potential for improved target irradiation, salivary gland function, and quality of life. Acta Otorhinolaryngol Belg 53:271–275
76. Garden AS, Morrison WH, Rosenthal DI, et al. (2004) Target coverage for head and neck cancers treated with IMRT: review of clinical experiences. Semin Radiat Oncol 14:103–109
77. Chao KS (2002) Protection of salivary function by intensity-modulated radiation therapy in patients with head and neck cancer. Semin Radiat Oncol 12(Suppl 1):20 25
78. Dreizen S, Brown LR, Daly TE, et al. (1977) Prevention of xerostomia related dental caries in irradiated cancer patients. J Dent Res 56:99–104
79. Emami B, Lyman J, Brown A, et al. (1991) Tolerance of normal tissue to therapeutic irradiation. Int J Radiat Oncol Biol Phys 21:109–122
80. Leslie MD, Dische S (1991) Parotid gland function following accelerated and conventionally fractionated radiotherapy. Radiother Oncol 22:133–139
81. O'Sullivan B, Warde P, Grice B, et al. (2001) The benefits and pitfalls of ipsilateral radiotherapy in carcinoma of the tonsillar region. Int J Radiat Oncol Biol Phys 51:332–343
82. Eisbruch A, Ship JA, Kim HM, et al. (2001) Partial irradiation of the parotid gland. Semin Radiat Oncol 11:234–239
83. Webb S (2001) IMRT: General considerations. In Intensity-modulated Radiation Therapy. Edited by Webb S. Philadelphia: Institute of Physics Publishing; pp 1–34
84. Henson BS, Inglehart MR, Eisbruch A, et al. (2001) Preserved salivary output and xerostomia-related quality of life in head and neck cancer patients receiving parotid-sparing radiotherapy. Oral Oncol 37:84–93
85. Eisbruch A, Ten Haken RK, Kim HM, et al. (1999) Dose, volume, and function relationships in parotid salivary glands following conformal and intensity-modulated irradiation of head and neck cancer. Int J Radiat Oncol Biol Phys 45:577–587
86. Eisbruch A, Ship JA, Dawson LA, et al. (2003) Salivary gland sparing and improved target irradiation by conformal and intensity modulated irradiation of head and neck cancer. World J Surg 27:832–837
87. Lin A, Kim HM, Terrell JE, et al. (2003) Quality of life after parotid sparing IMRT for head-and-neck cancer: a prospective longitudinal study. Int J Radiat Oncol Biol Phys 57:61–670
88. Chao KS, Deasy JO, Markman J, et al. (2001) A prospective study of salivary function sparing in patients with head-and-neck cancers receiving intensity-modulated or three-dimensional radiation therapy: initial results. Int J Radiat Oncol Biol Phys 49:907–916
89. Chao KS, Majhail N, Huang CJ, et al. (2001) Intensity-modulated radiation therapy reduces late salivary toxicity without compromising tumor control in patients with oropharyngeal carcinoma: a comparison with conventional techniques. Radiother Oncol 61:275–280
90. Chao KS, Low DA, Perez CA, et al. (2000) Intensity-modulated radiation therapy in head and neck cancers: the Mallinckrodt experience. Int J Cancer 90:92–103
91. Chao KS, Ozyigit G, Blanco AI, et al. (2004) Intensity-modulated radiation therapy for oropharyngeal carcinoma: impact of tumor volume. Int J Radiat Oncol Biol Phys 59:43–50
92. Eisbruch A, Marsh LH, Dawson LA, et al. (2004) Recurrences near base of skull after IMRT for head-and-neck cancer: implications for target delineation in high neck and for parotid gland sparing. Int J Radiat Oncol Biol Phys 59:28–42
93. Astreinidou E, Dehnad H, Terhaard CH, et al. (2004) Level II lymph nodes and radiation-induced xerostomia. Int J Radiat Oncol Biol Phys 58:124–131
94. Munter MW, Karger CP, Hoffner SG, et al. (2004) Evaluation of salivary gland function after treatment of head-and-neck tumors with intensity-modulated radiotherapy by quantitative pertechnetate scintigraphy. Int J Radiat Oncol Biol Phys 58:175–184
95. Eisbruch A (2002) Clinical aspects of IMRT for head-and-neck cancer. Med Dosim 27:99–104

Chapter 12

Diagnosis and Management of Autoimmune Salivary Gland Disorders

12

Philip C. Fox, Catherine H. Hong, Andre G. Brun, and Michael T. Brennan

Contents

Core Features

- Sjögren's syndrome and graft-versus-host-disease (GVHD) are autoimmune diseases affecting the salivary glands, as well as many other organ systems.
- The effects of these disorders on the salivary glands have a profound impact on oral health and functions.
- Dryness of the mouth (xerostomia) is the most common symptom associated with salivary gland dysfunction.
- Evaluation methods for xerostomia and salivary gland function are presented.
- Management of autoimmune salivary gland disorders combines palliative agents, secretagogues, and disease-modifying drugs.

Introduction

In this chapter we will discuss the most prominent autoimmune salivary gland diseases: Sjögren's syndrome and graft-versus-host disease (GVHD). Both may have profound affects on salivary gland performance and subsequently on oral health and function.

Sjögren's syndrome is an autoimmune exocrinopathy, which affects between 2 and 4 million persons in the USA, 90% of whom are women [1]. The most common manifestations are dysfunction of the salivary and lacrimal systems, which typically present as complaints of oral and ocular dryness, respectively. Xerostomia is the term used to describe the symptom of dryness of the mouth. Sjögren's syndrome, however, is a systemic disorder and dryness may affect other mucosal areas (nose, throat, trachea, vagina) and the skin, and may also involve many organ systems including the thyroid, lung, and kidney.

There are primary and secondary forms of the syndrome. Secondary Sjögren's syndrome occurs in conjunction with another autoimmune connective tissue disease, such as rheumatoid arthritis, systemic lupus erythematosus, systemic sclerosis, or primary biliary cirrhosis, while patients with primary Sjögren's syndrome have no other autoimmune disorder. Patients with both primary and secondary Sjögren's syndrome usually have prominent serologic signs of autoimmunity, including hypergammaglobulinemia, autoantibodies, an elevated sedimentation rate, decreased white blood cells, monoclonal gammopathies, and hypocomplementemia. Patients have an increased risk of developing malignant lymphoma, most typically mucosal-associated B-cell lymphomas (MALTomas) involving the salivary glands. It has been estimated that patients with primary Sjögren's syndrome have a 20- to 40-fold increased risk of lymphoma [2, 3]. Recently, factors have been identified to recognize those patients at greatest risk. These include vasculitis, low C4, and salivary gland enlargement at initial presentation [3–5].

Graft-versus-host disease is a recognized complication of allogeneic transplantation caused by the interaction of immunocompetent donor cells with cells of the immunodeficient host [6]. GVHD frequently involves the salivary glands, more commonly in chronic GVHD (>100 days post-transplant) [7]. The complaints of xerostomia are much the same as in Sjögren's syndrome and the histopathologic pattern in the minor salivary glands of the lip is similar as well. Due to the accessibility of tissue from this site, biopsy of the labial minor salivary glands is used to diagnose and monitor chronic GVHD [8].

We will review the oral and systemic manifestations of these conditions, available diagnostic methods will be discussed, and current management approaches will be presented.

Manifestations of Autoimmune Salivary Gland Diseases

Sjögren's Syndrome

Sjögren's syndrome is an autoimmune disease characterized primarily by decreased lacrimal and salivary gland secretions. In addition, patients may also present with a variety of other manifestations. For simplicity and organizational purposes, clinical manifestations of Sjögren's syndrome have been categorized into exocrine (glandular) and nonexocrine (extraglandular).

Exocrine (Glandular) Involvement

Salivary Glands

Persistent or intermittent enlargement of the salivary glands has been reported in 30–50% of Sjögren's syndrome patients at some point during the course of the disease [9]. Biopsy of the parotid gland demonstrates a pathognomonic lymphocytic infiltration [10] surrounding the ducts, eventually replacing the glandular epithelium. The parotid gland frequently harbors what are termed benign lymphoepithelial lesions, which can resemble lymphoid structures. Biopsy of the minor salivary glands reveals focal mononuclear cell sialadenitis [11], described in greater detail in the next section. As a consequence of these histologic changes, and possibly other immune-mediated activity, there is diminished salivary flow and possibly alteration of the composition of the saliva.

The parotid gland is the salivary gland most frequently enlarged, however, the submandibular glands may also be affected. Inspection and palpation of the glands usually will reveal bilateral, non-tender, firm, and diffuse swelling. Although enlarged salivary glands are a fairly typical and benign presentation in patients with Sjögren's syndrome, it is prudent for the clinician to carry out a thorough examination, as patients with Sjögren's syndrome are known to have a significantly increased risk of developing B-cell lymphoma [2, 3]. This often involves the salivary glands and patients must be questioned in detail about any recent changes to the character of the glands. A particularly hard

12

or nodular gland may require further investigation to rule out lymphoma and any persistent enlargement of the gland should be viewed with alarm and followed carefully.

The most common oral symptom in Sjögren's syndrome is xerostomia, a direct consequence of salivary dysfunction [9]. Since the extent of salivary dysfunction is variable in Sjögren's syndrome and patients vary in their tolerance of dryness, symptoms of dry mouth are variable in this patient population. In addition to complaints of dry mouth, dysphagia, adherence of food to the buccal or palatal surfaces, problems with dentures, a feeling of burning when eating spicy foods, an inability to eat dry foods, difficulty speaking for extended periods, and taste changes are common subjective complaints [9].

As described in the next section, salivary flow can be collected and measured to quantify salivary output. A rate of less than 0.1 ml/min of whole unstimulated saliva reflects salivary gland hypofunction [12]. Other clues to suggest reduced salivary flow are production of thick, frothy, mucus-like saliva and absence of saliva pooling in the floor of the mouth. Observation of Stensen's duct while pressing the parotid gland will reveal that no saliva or a small amount of clear "glue-like" material will appear. A tongue blade touched to the buccal mucosa may adhere, rather than releasing easily as expected with normally hydrated mucosa. Infrequently, acute bacterial sialadenitis may occur due to retrograde tracking of bacteria via the salivary duct into the salivary gland due to very low outward saliva flow and the absence of normal concentrations of antimicrobial proteins present in saliva.

Soft Tissue

In addition to saliva's antimicrobial and remineralizing properties, it also protects the soft tissues with its cleansing and lubricating properties. With diminished or no saliva production, chapped lips and dry, flaky perioral skin are common findings on an extraoral examination. Cracking and fissuring of the corners of the mouth, known as perlèche or angular cheilitis, are also noted in these patients. Intraorally, it is not unusual to find an erythematous, dry, atrophic, or cobblestone appearance to the oral mucosa (Fig. 12.1). The tongue may appear furrowed, atrophic, and devoid of papillae.

Opportunistic fungal infections are common and occur in about 30–70% of Sjögren's syndrome patients [13]. Chronic erythematous candidiasis is the most frequent type of fungal infection observed and may be responsible for the burning sensation and intolerance to spicy food. It is important to recognize that this form of candidiasis appears not as the white, curd-like lesions of thrush, but as reddened areas of the mucosa. It therefore may be overlooked and undertreated in this population.

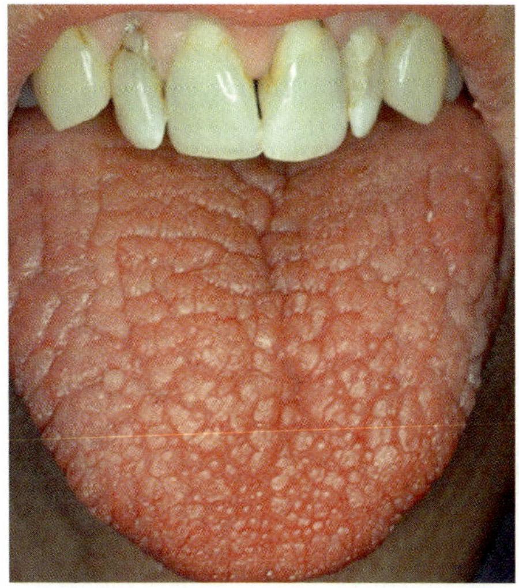

Fig. 12.1: Mucosal alterations in Sjögren's syndrome. Dry, furrowed, cobblestone appearance of the tongue of a patient with severe salivary gland dysfunction from Sjögren's syndrome. Note also the extensive restored dental caries

Hard Tissue

Salivary gland dysfunction predisposes patients to developing dental caries. Soto-Rojas et al. [14] found cervical or incisal caries at 83% of patients with Sjögren's syndrome, a very high number for adults. In another study, Christensen and coauthors found a higher number of decayed, missing, or filled teeth (DMFT) in both younger and older patients with primary Sjögren's syndrome compared with the respective control groups [15]. In this study, patients also reported having had more teeth extracted and more trouble with their teeth compared to the control group.

Keratoconjunctivitis Sicca

Keratoconjunctivitis sicca is the term used to describe the ocular surface changes found in Sjögren's syndrome as a result of lacrimal gland involvement. These changes are attributed to a reduction in the aqueous component of tears and changes in tear constituents. Patients with dry eyes often complain of a gritty, scratchy sensation, especially during eye blinking [16]. Other symptoms include irritation, a dull ache, blurred vision, photophobia, and discharge at the inner canthus of the eye, especially on awakening. Corneal ulceration is a serious complication of severe dry eyes if the problem is not addressed.

Nonexocrine (Extraglandular) Involvement

Cutaneous

Dryness of the skin (xerosis) and pruritis are common cutaneous symptoms of Sjögren's syndrome. Xerosis tends to be worse in the winter months, when humidity is lower, and manifests as dry scaly skin, affecting the lower extremities and axillary creases, in particular. Scratching in response to pruritis may result in hyperpigmentation of the skin. The pathophysiology behind xerosis is not well investigated. Studies have linked xerosis with the decrease in sebaceous or sweat gland secretion, however, many investigators believe that a specific alteration of the function of stratum corneum may also be responsible for skin xerosis [17]. Other cutaneous manifestations include alopecia, photosensitivity lesions, erythema nodosum, lichen planus, vitiligo, cutaneous B-cell lymphoma, granuloma annulare, and granulomatous panniculitis. Dryness and decreased luster of the hair are also common complaints.

Patients with Sjögren's syndrome may develop vascular disease. Approximately 13–20% have a reaction of the extremities to cold temperature known as Raynaud's phenomenon [18]. Raynaud's phenomenon is in general innocuous and does not cause any significant consequences, although it may be painful. In addition to the vasospastic response to cold, Sjögren's syndrome patients may suffer from inflammatory vascular disease, which is by the far the most severe cutaneous complication. The skin manifestations of inflammatory vasculitis are varied and are dependent on the extent of blood vessel involvement in the skin and the magnitude of the host's inflammatory response. Vasculitis most frequently presents with palpable and nonpalpable purpura of the lower extremities [19], which can mimic Waldenström's hyperglobulinemic purpura. Urticaria-like lesions, erythema multiforme-like eruptions, and nodular vasculitis are also observed.

Respiratory Involvement

A dry and persistent cough is a common symptom in patients with Sjögren's syndrome. This is due to the involvement of exocrine glands in the airway, which results in decreased mucosal secretions and subsequent dryness of the upper airway. This condition has been labeled xerotrachea as it is the tracheobronchial equivalent of xerostomia.

Ito et al. [20] found that nonspecific interstitial pneumonia (NSIP) was the most frequent diagnosis in 31 lung biopsies and two autopsies obtained from patients with Sjögren's syndrome. Eight patients had bronchiolar disease and four were diagnosed with malignant lymphoma. Patients often will have bibasilar crepitations before they complain of cough and dyspnea on exertion. Pulmonary hyperinflation and recurrent pulmonary infections have also been reported.

Musculoskeletal Involvement

More than half of patients with primary Sjögren's syndrome complain of arthralgia with or without evidence of arthritis. The hands and knees are most frequently affected and complaints usually have a symmetric distribution. Unlike rheumatoid arthritis, the arthropathy is typically nonerosive and does not result in any deformation. Myalgia is also common in both primary and secondary Sjögren's syndrome.

Gastrointestinal Involvement

Dysphagia is a frequent complaint in Sjögren's syndrome, most probably related to the lack of saliva and esophageal dryness. However, the presence of esophageal dysmotility has also been thought to be a possible contributing cause [21]. Other common gastrointestinal complaints include nausea, dyspepsia, and epigastric pain. Gastroscopy performed on Sjögren's syndrome patients who present with gastrointestinal symptoms will occasionally reveal an atrophic gastric mucosa with a cobblestone appearance. A biopsy of the gastric mucosa may also reveal chronic atrophic gastritis with or without intestinal metaplasia. Testing for *Helicobacter pylori* should be performed in patients who have gastritis, because this organism has been shown to be associated with MALT lymphomas in Sjögren's syndrome patients.

A few case reports have associated celiac disease [21] with Sjögren's syndrome, however, more research is needed to verify the relationship between the two conditions.

Peripheral and Central Neuropathies

Peripheral neuropathy is an extensively documented complication in primary Sjögren's syndrome [22]. This slowly progressive condition usually has a symmetric distribution and is characterized by anesthesia and dysesthesias of the extremities.

Cranial nerve neuropathies are also known occurrences in patients with Sjögren's syndrome, especially in those with a pre-existing peripheral neuropathy. Trigeminal neuropathy is the most common cranial nerve neuropathy, but other cranial nerves may also be affected, e.g., the facial nerve (Bell's palsy).

The prevalence of central nervous system (CNS) involvement in Sjögren's syndrome is debatable. Some studies have suggested that involvement of the CNS occurs in as many as 25% of patients with primary Sjögren's syndrome [23], while others feel this is a great overestimation. In spite of this dispute, the serious consequences of CNS involvement make early diagnosis and treatment of this condition extremely important.

The clinical presentations of CNS disease in Sjögren's syndrome are extremely diverse. CNS involvement can range from focal lesions to widespread neurologic disease affecting the brain and the spinal cord. Focal lesions result in motor or sensory deficits that can manifest as hemiparesis, monoparesis, seizures, multiple sclerosis-like symptoms, or cerebellar syndromes e.g., tremors, dyskinesia. Widespread disease of the brain may present as subacute or acute encephalopathy, psychiatric disorders, and dementia. Spinal cord involvement can lead to acute transverse myelopathy, chronic progressive myelopathy, and neurogenic bladder. These more severe CNS manifestations are very uncommon in Sjögren's syndrome.

Other Organ System Involvement

Cristiansson first noted the presence of liver disease in patients with Sjögren's syndrome in 1954 and since then this relationship has been proven in many studies. Abnormal liver function tests (elevated alkaline phosphatase and serum aminotransferases) and biopsy features of primary biliary cirrhosis, portal tract fibrosis, or chronic active hepatitis are some of the frequent findings in Sjögren's syndrome patients with hepatic involvement [24].

There is evidence to demonstrate that patients with Sjögren's syndrome have a higher incidence of heart disease. In one report [25], one third of patients had increased pericardial echogenicity, which is suggestive of a history of pericarditis. However, acute pericarditis is a rare complication of Sjögren's syndrome.

Heart block in neonates of mothers with Sjögren's syndrome has also been reported and may be attributed to the presence of anti-SS-A (Ro) autoantibodies in the maternal circulation [26]. Adult onset heart block can also occur in Sjögren's syndrome patients and has been postulated to be associated with the production of antibodies against cardiac muscle and muscarinic receptors.

The reported prevalence of renal involvement in Sjögren's syndrome is extremely variable, ranging from 2% to 67%. Interstitial nephritis is the most common type of renal pathology and laboratory results include elevation in the plasma creatinine concentration and hypokalemia [27]. Dysuria, urinary frequency, nocturia, and urgency symptoms in Sjögren's syndrome patients are thought to be due to interstitial cystitis if there is no evidence of infection. Renal tubular acidosis has also been reported as a manifestation of the syndrome.

Depression and personality disorders have been found to be more common in patients with Sjögren's syndrome. The literature suggests that this could be either a direct consequence of CNS pathology, or a reaction to the stress of being afflicted with a chronic illness. Patients with Sjögren's syndrome often suffer from significant fatigue [28], and researchers continue to puzzle over the pathogenesis of this symptom. This is a debilitating condition because it can interfere with daily chores and social activities, thus reducing the quality of life of many patients. Fatigue has been postulated to be a consequence of sleep deprivation as a result of frequent awakening at night due to the discomfort from xerostomia which necessitates frequent drinking of fluids. The resultant polydipsia leads to polyuria and more awakening. Chronic inflammation, mediated by cytokines such as IL-1 and IL-6, autonomic nervous system dysfunction, and low blood pressure have also been suggested as possible etiologies for the fatigue [29].

Lymphoma

The lymphocytic proliferation observed in Sjögren's syndrome may progress from a polyclonal infiltration to a monoclonal gammopathy to a frank lymphoma. Malignant lymphoproliferative disorders are known to occur at a higher frequency in patients with Sjögren's syndrome. Increased frequency of circulating monoclonal immunoglobulins, increased mixed monoclonal cryoglobulins, non-Hodgkin's lymphoma (NHL) and the MALT (mucosa-associated lymphoid tissue) lymphomas (MALTomas) have been reported to occur at a higher rate.

A meta-analysis published in 2005 by Zintzaras et al. [4] concluded that there is a higher risk of developing non-Hodgkin's lymphoma (NHL) in patients with primary Sjögren's syndrome compared to other autoimmune diseases such as systemic lupus erythematosus and rheumatoid arthritis. The risk of NHL (primarily B-cell MALTomas) in patients with Sjögren's syndrome is about 20 times higher than that in the general population, with a lifetime risk of approximately 4–10% [3]. The presence of persistently enlarged or nodular parotid or submandibular glands, regional or generalized lymphadenopathy, pulmonary infiltrates, hepatomegaly, vasculitis, or a monoclonal gammopathy may be signs of malignancy.

Graft-versus-host Disease

Graft-versus-host disease (GVHD) is a major complication following bone marrow transplantation (BMT). The disease is classified into acute and chronic forms based on the time of onset.

Acute Graft-versus-host Disease

Oral Changes

Studies on acute oral GVHD are limited and its prevalence is unknown. Woo et al. [6] estimated that about 60–70% of patients with grade III–IV acute GVHD would develop oral changes consistent with GVHD. These changes may present as painful desquamative and ulcerative lesions, white papular eruptions, or lichenoid changes which can involve the entire oral cavity. Hsiao et al. [30] reported that lichenoid changes appeared later in acute GVHD compared to mucosal erythema, atrophy, and ulceration, which were observed more often in early acute GVHD.

The diagnosis of acute GVHD can be challenging, as many of its presentations imitate the effects of chemoradiotherapy, antibiotic reactions, or complications from infections. Acute oral GVHD may be extremely difficult to distinguish clinically from herpes simplex virus (HSV) infections or chemotherapy-induced mucositis. Worsening of an existing HSV culture negative mucositis after day 21, worsening of xerostomia and pain, and the late onset of oral ulcers beyond day 21 are features that may help to differentiate between acute GVHD and chemotherapy-induced mucositis [6].

Systemic Changes

The primary target organs in acute GVHD are the skin, liver, and gastrointestinal tract. The earliest and most common presentation of acute GVHD is a pruritic maculopapular rash. This is first noted on the palms of the hands, soles of the feet, ears, shoulders, and nape of the neck. The rash can spread to involve the whole body, and in severe GVHD may form bullous lesions and toxic epidermal necrolysis-like desquamation. Hepatic GVHD is characterized by a rise in serum levels of conjugated bilirubin, alkaline phosphatase, and aminotransferase. Gastrointestinal involvement in acute GVHD is often severe and consists of nausea, vomiting, bloody diarrhea, and abdominal cramps. Other organ systems, including the kidney and hematopoietic system may also be involved.

Chronic Graft-versus-host Disease

Chronic GVHD occurs between 100 and 400 days post BMT. The condition can progress from acute GVHD (progressive onset), follow previous resolution of acute GVHD (quiescent), or have a de novo late onset without prior acute GVHD. Chronic GVHD is graded as either limited or extensive depending on the clinical severity and target organs affected. Limited disease is characterized by localized skin involvement and/or evidence of hepatic dysfunction. Extensive disease presents either with generalized skin involvement, or with localized skin involvement or hepatic dysfunction plus at least one of the following:

1. Liver histology showing progressive hepatitis, bridging necrosis, or cirrhosis.
2. Involvement of the eye.
3. Involvement of minor salivary glands or mucosa of the oral cavity.

4. Involvement of any other target organ.

Chronic GVHD is the single most important factor that determines long-term outcome and quality of life of a patient following a bone marrow transplant.

Oral Changes of Chronic GVHD

Salivary Glands

Salivary glands are known targets of GVHD and destruction of these glands results in salivary gland dysfunction leading to xerostomia and disruption of oral mucosal integrity. Due to the resemblance of pathologic changes in GVHD animal models to Sjögren's syndrome, the term "Sjögren's-like syndrome" has been coined to describe patients with chronic GVHD who display both salivary gland dysfunction and keratoconjunctivitis sicca. Histologic examination of the salivary glands in the lip in patients with chronic GVHD reveals periductal lymphocytic infiltration of both intralobular and major excretory ducts with pronounced ductal damage, eventually leading to acinar damage and fibrosis [31].

Izutsu et al. [32] collected whole saliva samples from 12 allogeneic BMT recipients with chronic GVHD and 10 healthy BMT recipients without GVHD. The study showed elevated sodium and decreased concentrations of IgA in the whole saliva of patients with chronic GVHD when compared to those without GVHD. The authors suggested that the reduction in IgA may be a contributing factor to frequent sinobronchial infections reported in patients with chronic GVHD.

Soft Tissue

The most common changes in the oral mucosa associated with chronic GVHD are erythema, mucosal atrophy, and lichenoid reactions [33]. These lesions can involve any site in the oral and perioral region (Fig. 12.2).

Lichenoid reactions are the most distinctive oral change and have the highest positive predictive value [6, 34]. Schubert and Sullivan found that 81–100% of patients with an oral lichenoid reaction had chronic GVHD [34]. Lichenoid reactions appear as lacy striations of the oral mucosa that are clinically similar to the striations of Wickham in oral lichen planus. These lesions can be faint and only affect limited patches of oral mucosa or can present as thick and confluent areas affecting the entire oral cavity.

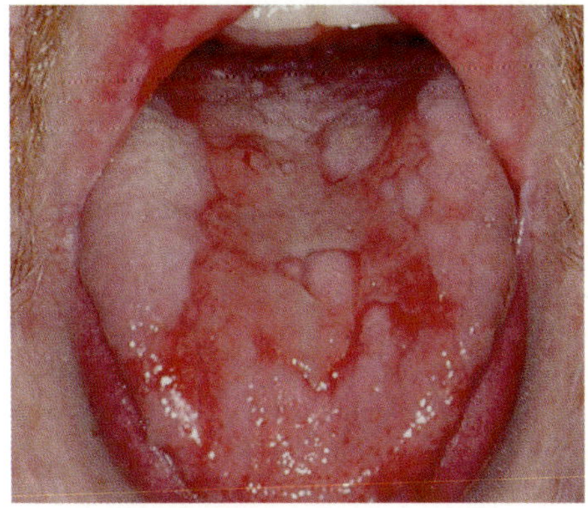

Fig. 12.2: Tongue lesions in chronic graft-versus-host disease in a 25-year-old patient treated with bone marrow transplantation 7 months earlier

Erosive lesions are generally associated with more severe oral involvement. These lesions are often accompanied by pain in the oral cavity (which may be the first presenting symptom), which significantly impedes eating and oral hygiene measures.

Scleroderma-like changes also may be observed in chronic oral GVHD, resulting in trismus due to perioral fibrosis. Schubert et al. [34] reported that 73% of patients with chronic GVHD versus 26% of patients without GVHD developed trismus and fibrosis. Fibrosis can also affect the tongue, causing decreased mobility, which may interfere with speech and mastication.

Hard Tissue

There have been conflicting reports concerning the incidence of dental caries in patients with chronic GVHD [35–37]. However, as there is compelling evidence that saliva provides the principal defense for teeth against dental caries [38], patients with chronic GVHD with decreased salivary function are considered to be at risk for developing dental caries. It is thus reasonable for the dentist to implement a home fluoride regimen and to advise patients to maintain excellent oral hygiene and to avoid cariogenic foods in their diet.

Systemic Changes of Chronic Graft-versus-host Disease

Numerous articles on chronic GVHD have described its systemic manifestations as resembling those found in autoimmune diseases such as systemic lupus erythematosus, progressive systemic sclerosis, primary biliary cirrhosis, and rheumatoid arthritis. Chronic GVHD has also been reported to arise or worsen after an infectious insult or when there are changes to the patient's immune status. Based upon these observations, chronic GVHD is viewed as an autoimmune phenomenon.

The skin, liver, gastrointestinal tract, and lungs are the principal target organs in chronic GVHD [33]. The two most common skin changes are lichen planus-like lesions and cutaneous manifestations of scleroderma. Skin involvement may first present with varying degrees of erythema, hypo- and hyperpigmentation, plaques, and areas of desquamation. If untreated, the skin may become indurated and fixed to the underlying fascia, resulting in development of joint contractures and debility similar to scleroderma.

Liver biopsy in chronic GVHD may reveal lobular hepatitis, chronic persistent hepatitis, chronic active hepatitis, or a reduction or absence of small bile ducts with cholestasis. Liver function tests are abnormal, such as elevations in the serum alkaline phosphatase and bilirubin levels.

Involvement of the esophagus has been reported in patients with chronic GVHD and this can cause dysphagia, painful ulcers, and malnutrition. Webs, ring-like narrowing, and strictures of the mid and upper esophagus have been observed in radiographic examinations. Fibrosis of the gastrointestinal submucosa and sclerosis of the intestine have also been associated with chronic GVHD. Also, obstructive lung disease has been reported to occur in patients with chronic GVHD. A feeling of dyspnea and a nonproductive cough are common complaints.

Diagnosis of Autoimmune Salivary Gland Disease

Methods for judging salivary gland performance are the same regardless of the etiology. Diagnosis utilizes a combination of subjective and objective assessments, including an assessment of symptoms such as oral dryness and objective measures of salivary function. In the following section we will review methods for assessment of salivary gland function, with a focus on the diagnosis of Sjögren's syndrome.

Sjögren's Syndrome

Xerostomia is the most common symptom associated with salivary gland dysfunction and the most frequent complaint of patients with Sjögren's syndrome. In addition to asking if the mouth is dry, one should delve more fully into the complaint. Is dryness periodic or constant, mild or severe, does it interfere with oral functions such as eating and speaking? Fox et al. showed that specific questions relating to dryness while eating, difficulty swallowing foods, or the need to drink fluids to ease swallowing, and the perception of too little saliva in the mouth were strongly correlated with objective measures of salivary gland performance [39]. In contrast, the complaints of dryness at night or on awakening or keeping water at the bedside were not predictive of salivary gland dysfunction. Patients with complaints of dryness should be questioned in greater detail to help determine if the symptom likely is related to objective salivary gland disease.

Another method of subjective assessment of dry mouth is to use a validated scale such as that developed by the National Cancer Institute (NCI) as a part of the Common Terminology Criteria for Adverse Events (CTCAE) reporting forms. The scale assesses dry mouth symptoms based on dietary alterations (Table 12.1). While relatively insensitive, it gives information on the severity of dry mouth related to its impact on diet and nutrition. Increased sensitivity can be achieved by combining whole unstimulated salivary flow measurements (see below) with the subjective component of the assessment scale.

It is important to recognize that xerostomia may be caused by many conditions other than Sjögren's syndrome. Medications, radiotherapy to the head and neck region, and other medical conditions such as cystic fibrosis, HIV infection, or poorly controlled diabetes can all lead to salivary gland dysfunction and the feeling of dry mouth [40, 41].

In addition to being a major factor in oral comfort, saliva is critical for proper oral function and to maintain oral health. Sialometry is the measurement of saliva production in a given individual. Saliva can be measured as whole saliva, which is the total fluid contents of the mouth, usually obtained by expectoration. Individual gland saliva

Table 12.1. Common Terminology Criteria for Adverse Events (CTCAE) scale for dry mouth

Grade	Symptoms
0	No changes
1	Symptomatic (dry or thick saliva) without significant dietary alterations
2	Symptomatic and significant dietary alteration (e.g., copious water, other lubricants, diet limited to purees and/or soft, moist foods)
3	Symptoms leading to inability to adequately aliment orally; IV fluids, tube feedings, or total parenteral nutrition (TPN) indicated

Source: CTCAE accessed at http://ctep.cancer.gov/forms/ CTCAEv3.pdf

production can also be measured. A collector is used in the Stensen's duct to isolate the parotid gland secretions, while special collectors placed in the Wharton's duct in the floor of mouth isolate the submandibular/sublingual saliva. Saliva can be collected in a resting (unstimulated) state or following stimulation, which may increase output by a factor of 10. Whole saliva is generally collected by the drooling or the spitting method. Resting flow requires that the subject not eat, drink, smoke, or have any oral stimulation for at least 1 h prior to collection. Stimulation is usually by chewing paraffin or application of 2–5% citric acid to the tongue [42]. Resting whole salivary flow rates below 0.1 ml/min and stimulated rates of less than 0.7 ml/min are generally accepted as abnormally low. The great majority of Sjögren's syndrome patients demonstrate decreased salivary output [43] and resting whole saliva flow rate is one criterion in the widely used classification criteria for the disorder (see below).

Many studies have shown that resting flow rates decrease with age. However, carefully controlled studies of healthy older individuals demonstrate that salivary function does not decline as a consequence of aging per se. The decline in salivary output found with aging can be explained by the effects of medications and medical conditions which compromise salivary function and is more common in older individuals [44]. Further, the response of older subjects to stimulation or sialagogues is unchanged [45].

Saliva is a highly complex fluid containing over sixty components and it may be analyzed based on its molecular or biochemical components. In Sjögren's syndrome, studies have examined electrolytes, immunoglobulins, cytokines, and autoantibody levels in saliva. Markers of inflammation have been routinely isolated, as well. Common findings in the saliva of patients with Sjögren's syndrome include increased levels of sodium, immunoglobulins (particularly IgA), anti-Ro and La autoantibodies, lactoferrin, lysozyme, β2 microglobulin, prostaglandin E2, thromboxane B2, IL-6, and hyaluronic acid [46, 47]. Unfortunately, none of the above markers has proved sensitive or specific enough to serve as a diagnostic criterion for Sjögren's syndrome.

Sialography is another useful diagnostic modality for salivary gland disorders. A contrast agent is injected into the ductal system of the major glands via the major secretory ducts and visualized using conventional or computed tomography (CT) radiography (Fig. 12.3). Sialograms of salivary glands affected by Sjögren's syndrome show punctate, globular, cavitary, or destructive sialectasia, depending on the stage of the disease [48]. Sialographic findings may be supportive of the diagnosis, but are not highly specific. Other radiographic modalities used for assessment of salivary glands include CT and

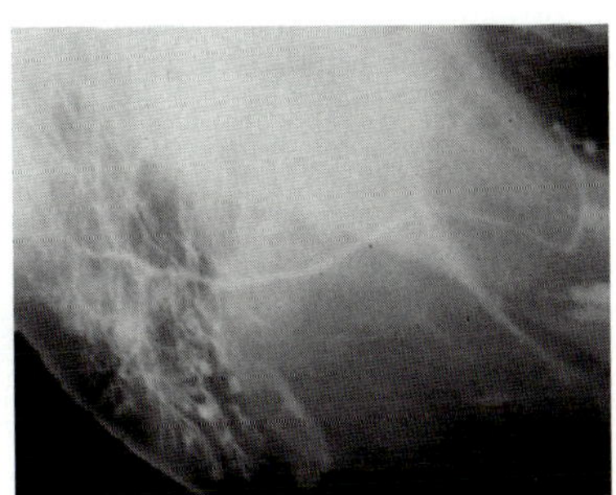

Fig. 12.3: Parotid gland sialogram showing punctuate changes in a patient with Sjögren's syndrome

magnetic resonance imaging (MRI). While MRI and CT are best used for salivary tumors and inflammatory disease, respectively, neither clearly show the early punctate changes seen in sialograms in Sjögren's syndrome [49]. Therefore, in the earliest stages, the involved glands appear normal on both CT and MRI. When the disease progresses, CT shows a honeycomb glandular appearance that is considered nondiagnostic for Sjögren's syndrome, as it is seen also in granulomatous diseases [49]. In later stages, as acini are lost, MRI may reveal diffuse cysts. It is important to note that this pattern, in the presence of cervical adenopathy, is most indicative of HIV/AIDS. In the absence of adenopathy, the likely diagnosis is Sjögren's syndrome.

Salivary gland scintigraphy is another objective imaging method to assess salivary gland function. This method utilizes the radionuclide technetium pertechnetate (Tc99m) which is injected intravenously. Using a gamma detector, one can quantify and time the uptake of tracer from the blood into the major salivary glands and then spontaneous excretion into the oral cavity (Fig. 12.4). This activity is considered indicative of resting (basal) salivary function. At the conclusion of the study, a strong salivary stimulus is given orally to measure stimulated response capability. Time-activity curves can be constructed. Scintigraphy is an accurate measure of salivary gland function, but the changes seen in Sjögren's syndrome lack diagnostic specificity. In early Sjögren's syndrome, with minimal salivary gland dysfunction, there is usually normal Tc99m uptake, but significantly decreased excretion. With increasing dysfunction, one sees significant decreases in both uptake and excretion [50].

Biopsy of minor salivary glands has been shown to be the best single criterion used to diagnose the salivary component of Sjögren's syndrome [11]. Minor salivary glands are usually biopsied through normal-appearing mucosa of the lower lip between the midline and commissure. Local infiltration with anesthetic containing vasoconstrictor is followed by a single incision of 1.5–2 cm horizontally to just penetrate epithelium. The minor salivary glands are then removed by blunt dissection, while avoiding sensory nerves [51]. Typically, specimens should include five or more glands to yield enough tissue for focal scoring.

Characteristic histopathologic changes include loss of acinar cells, a relative preservation of ductal structures, and the presence of an intense, focal periductal/vascular mononuclear cell infiltrate (Fig. 12.5). A focus is defined as the localized aggregation of inflammatory cells containing 50 or more lymphocytes, plasma cells, or macrophages. A "focus score" is derived by determining the biopsy surface area and the number of foci. A positive biopsy for Sjögren's syndrome requires a focal score of ≥1 focus per 4 mm^2.

Classification criteria for Sjögren's syndrome were developed and validated between 1989 and 1996 by the European Study Group on Classification for Sjögren's syndrome. These criteria were reviewed by the American-European Consensus Group (AECG), who suggested some modification, defined clearer classification rules for primary versus secondary disease, and provided more precise exclusion criteria [52]. The most recent results were published in 2002. The widespread acceptance of these classification criteria in the research community has greatly aided standardization of diagnosis and definition of patients.

There are six criteria: two dealing with symptoms of ocular and oral dryness; one measuring lacrimal function; one quantifying salivary function; the labial minor salivary gland biopsy; and the presence of autoantibodies against anti-SS-A (Ro) and anti-SS-B (La). Four of these six criteria are required for positive case classification. Critically, either a positive labial minor salivary gland biopsy or the presence of autoantibodies is required to establish a definitive case.

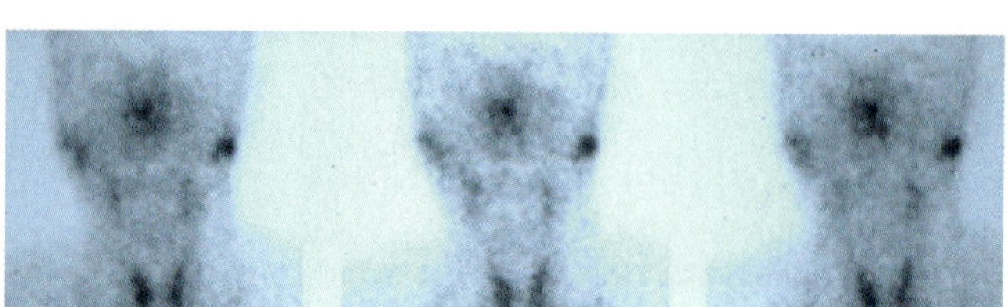

Fig. 12.4: A sequence of scintigraphic images showing asymmetric uptake of the tracer technetium pertechnetate into the major salivary glands (parotid>submandibular; left parotid>right) and progressive secretion of tracer into the oral cavity. The thyroid gland is visible at the bottom of the images

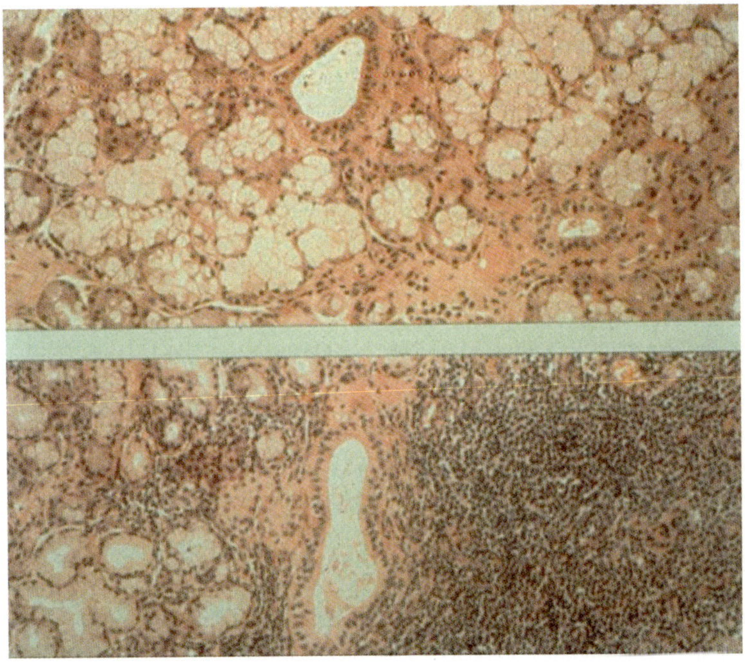

Fig. 12.5: Labial minor salivary glands from a healthy individual (*top*) and a patient with Sjögren's syndrome (*bottom*). Note the presence of a dense, focal mononuclear cell infiltrate and a loss of acinar cells with preservation of ducts in the Sjögren's syndrome specimen (H&E stain of formalin-fixed tissue)

Graft-versus-host Disease

As noted earlier, biopsy of the labial minor salivary glands is one method commonly used to diagnose and monitor chronic GVHD. The medical history and clinical presentation will guide diagnostic evaluation.

Management of Autoimmune Salivary Gland Diseases

Management strategies for autoimmune salivary gland disease are dependent on the extent of glandular and extraglandular manifestations. As previously discussed, the exocrine involvement most often results in symptoms of dry mouth and dry eyes. Patients also may experience other oral manifestations such as fungal infections, mucosal burning and pain, swelling of the salivary gland, or dental caries. The following sections will present an overview of management strategies for the various glandular and extraglandular manifestations of Sjögren's syndrome, which serve as a prototype for treatment of salivary gland dysfunction of any etiology.

Xerostomia Management

Treatment of xerostomia is the same regardless of the underlying disease process. Therapeutic modalities for xerostomia may be categorized as topical agents, secretagogues, and disease-modifying drugs.

Topical Agents

The primary rationale of topical agents is palliation; to provide symptomatic relief of dry mouth. A wide range of interventions have been evaluated to include the following: many saliva substitutes ("artificial salivas") [53], mucin-containing lozenges and gum [54, 55], and evening primrose oil or the essential omega-6 fatty acid gamma-linolenic acid (GLA), which is extracted from primrose oil [56, 57]. Formal systematic reviews have been conducted and have shown most of these trials were of poor quality with only a few of even moderate quality [58, 59]. Therefore, due to the high level of bias in the literature regarding topical therapies, it is difficult to determine with confidence the efficacy of topical agents in the moderation of dryness symptoms.

Two studies with moderate levels of bias have been published that evaluated topical therapies in Sjögren's syndrome. The first examined the efficacy of Efamol (evening primrose oil) in a randomized, double-blind, crossover study, and found no significant differences versus a placebo solution in the moderation of xerostomia [56]. Another study examined topical anhydrous crystalline maltose lozenges administered three times a day. Improvement in salivary output and moderation of dry mouth complaints were reported, although the effects were modest [60]. Despite the paucity of clinical data to demonstrate the efficacy of topical agents, these agents must not be overlooked clinically and remain a mainstay in the management strategy of the dryness component of Sjögren's syndrome. As significant side effects have not been reported with these agents, patients should be encouraged to try topical therapies as an initial management approach.

Secretagogues

Stimulation of the salivary glands has been attempted by physical and pharmacologic means. Electrostimulation of the salivary glands has been attempted [61–63], but practical long-term application is a challenge and the results have been modest. Presently, newer approaches are being investigated and show promise [64].

Parasympathomimetic medications have shown the most success for xerostomia relief. The Food and Drug Administration (FDA) has approved two medications for the relief of dry mouth in Sjögren's syndrome: pilocarpine (Salagen) and cevimeline (Evoxac) [64–67]. Both medications are muscarinic agonists, resulting in a transient increase in salivary output and statistically significant improvement in complaints of oral dryness. Cevimeline has a reported increased specificity to M3 muscarinic receptors compared to pilocarpine, which might suggest the potential for fewer side effects. However, clinical trials have not confirmed a lower side effect profile with cevimeline. Common side effects of both medications include sweating, flushing, urinary incontinence, and gastrointestinal discomfort. Side effects are frequent, but are rarely severe or serious. Parasympathomimetics are contraindicated in patients with uncontrolled asthma, narrow-angle glaucoma, and acute iritis and should be used with caution in patients with significant cardiovascular disease, Parkinson disease, asthma, and chronic obstructive pulmonary disease. Pilocarpine is currently recommended at a dosage of 5 mg up to four times daily, while cevimeline is commonly prescribed at 30 mg three times daily. These medications are widely used and provide significant relief of dryness complaints in many patients. Pilocarpine has also been approved for treatment of xerostomia related to head and neck radiotherapy.

Disease-modifying Agents

A wide range of treatments have been studied that attempt to address the underlying disease process in Sjögren's syndrome and therefore improve salivary gland dysfunction. Therapeutic strategies have included hormone moderation, general and targeted anti-inflammatory approaches, blunting of the B-cell response, and treatment of potential viral etiologies.

Hormones

Sex hormones are known to influence autoimmune activity. However, hormonal treatments have shown minimal success on the glandular and extraglandular manifestations of Sjögren's syndrome. Dehydroepiandrosterone (DHEA) demonstrated no benefit compared to placebo in a randomized double-blind trial [68]. A small pilot study did show some benefit in the relief of xerostomia with nandrolone decanoate, although there were no differences compared to placebo in any objective dryness measures [69]. As these medications are both androgen-type hormones, adverse effects of acne and hirsutism are common and limit patient acceptance in this primarily female patient population.

Nonspecific Disease-modifying Agents

Generalized moderation of the inflammatory response in Sjögren's syndrome using anti-rheumatic agents has shown minimal success for the management of dryness symptoms. Trials of prednisone, azathioprine, and hydroxychloroquine have shown minimal benefit for dry mouth [70–72]. Although not helpful for the management of xerostomia, these medications may be useful for treatment of some of the extraglandular manifestations of Sjögren's syndrome, such as vasculitis and fatigue.

Specific Disease-modifying Agents

More recent studies have attempted to target specific biologic pathways to modify the underlying disease process. One study examined the efficacy of very low dose interferon-alpha, 150 or 450 IU once or three times a day in primary Sjögren's syndrome. Although no changes were found in the primary endpoint of symptomatic oral dryness and unstimulated whole saliva, a secondary analysis showed a significant benefit of 150 IU interferon-alpha three times daily over placebo, with increased stimulated whole salivary flow rates at 12 weeks [73]. A subsequent phase 3 trial at this dose found increased unstimulated salivary function compared to placebo at 24 weeks. However, the co-primary endpoints of stimulated whole saliva flow and oral dryness were not significantly improved relative to placebo [74].

Another approach has been to modify the inflammatory cytokine pathway, specifically targeting tumor necrosis factor alpha (TNFα). Anti-TNFα agents, including infliximab, entanercept, and thalidomide have shown no significant efficacy in randomized controlled trials in Sjögren's syndrome [75–77]. Interestingly, biologic measures of cell activation were decreased with thalidomide use, although clinical outcomes were not clearly impacted in this clinical trial which was discontinued due to an unacceptably high side effect profile in primary Sjögren's syndrome patients [78].

Recently, there has been interest in modulation of B-cell activation. As there is well documented B-cell hyperreactivity in Sjögren's syndrome, this approach may have an impact on the underlying disease. Rituximab binds specifically to the CD20 antigen which is present on B cells and involved in activation. In an open-label study, improvement in symptoms of dry mouth and salivary gland function was demonstrated with a concomitant decrease of peripheral B cells. Serum sickness symptoms were found in 20% of patients. Although these results are promising, a randomized controlled trial is necessary before recommendation of this treatment option for Sjögren's syndrome [79].

Antiviral Agents

The potential of a viral etiology for Sjögren's syndrome has been proposed. A randomized clinical trial was conducted with an anti-retroviral medication for the treatment of Sjögren's syndrome. In this trial, primary Sjögren's syndrome patients were randomized to 150 mg of lamivudine, a reverse transcriptase inhibitor, given two times daily or placebo [80]. No significant clinical improvements were noted.

Summary for Management of Dry Mouth

The quality of published studies of management of dry mouth approaches varies widely, from poorly documented case reports to well-controlled randomized trials. This complicates comparison and assessment of the results. Based on the current literature and best clinical practice, the overall management strategy for oral dryness should include a combination of topical palliative agents and secretagogues. Due to the potential for side effects from disease-modifying agents, clearer evidence of clinical efficacy must be demonstrated before these can be recommended. Additional symptomatic approaches for dry mouth include use of water throughout the day, gustatory and masticatory stimulation of salivary flow, and increased humidification.

Management of Dry Eye

Artificial tears remain the cornerstone of treatment of dry eye. In general, appropriate referral to an ophthalmologist is important for appropriate diagnosis and long-term management of dry eyes.

Recent clinical trials have demonstrated the benefit of Restasis (cyclosporine ophthalmic emulsion, 0.05%) [81]. This medication has been approved by the FDA to increase tear production in patients whose tear production is presumed to be suppressed due to ocular inflammation associated with keratoconjunctivitis sicca. The mechanism of action is thought to be related to anti-inflammatory and immunomodulatory effects. Restasis is prescribed as one drop in each eye two times a day. A common side effect is ocular burning, which often decreases with long-term use.

Parasympathomimetics have also improved symptoms of dry eye in Sjögren's syndrome patients. Pilocarpine at a dose of 5 mg twice daily demonstrated significant improvement of subjective ocular dryness compared to placebo. No differences in objective measures of lacrimal flow (i.e., Schirmer's I test) were seen [82]. Cevimeline has also been shown to improve dry eye symptoms at a dose of 20 mg three times a day [83].

Omega-6 essential fatty acid therapy has also been evaluated for the treatment of dry eyes in Sjögren's syndrome. A randomized, controlled trial compared oral administration of 112 mg of linoleic acid and 15 mg of gamma-linolenic acid to placebo. Significant improvement in symptoms of dry eye and objective measures of dryness was found in the active intervention group [84].

Similar to management of dry mouth symptoms, the overall therapeutic approach to dry eye in Sjögren's syndrome depends on appropriate symptomatic relief with a combination of topical agents (i.e., eye drops) and systemic agents. Use of Restasis is a newer therapeutic option, with additional treatment choices of parasympathomimetics and omega-6 essential fatty acid therapy. Successful management of dry eyes is best provided by referral to an ophthalmologist or optometrist familiar with the treatment of dry eye.

Other Oral Manifestations

Salivary Gland Enlargement

As previously noted, salivary gland swelling is a common manifestation of Sjögren's syndrome. Patients may experience a wide range of clinical presentations of salivary gland swelling, from sporadic exacerbations to chronic enlargement of the glands.

Acute exacerbations of rapid onset swelling and pain are most often caused by chronically compromised salivary output with a concomitant retrograde bacterial infection. Treatment in this setting includes the following: antibiotics; massage of the gland to help remove accumulated debris in the ductal system; and the use of gustatory (sugar-free sour candies), masticatory (sugar-free gum), or pharmaceutical stimulation (parasympathomimetics) of the glands.

Patients with Sjögren's syndrome who present with asymptomatic, chronic swelling of the gland should be followed with routine clinical and radiographic re-evaluations. The primary concern with this clinical situation is the potential of a lymphoma. A fine-needle aspiration or open biopsy may be indicated, depending on the clinical and radiographic appearance. Removal of the gland surgically may be an option for patients with an aesthetic compromise due to a chronically enlarged gland.

Oral Candidiasis

Saliva contains natural anti-fungal molecules (e.g., histatins). With less saliva present in the oral cavity in Sjögren's syndrome, a decrease in the ability to control oral fungal populations and prevent fungal infections often occurs. As previously noted, the clinical appearance of fungal infections (most commonly *Candida albicans*) in the oral cavity in Sjögren's syndrome is variable and ranges from pseudomembranous (white plaques that can be rubbed off), to erythematous, hyperplastic, and angular cheilitis (at the corners of the mouth).

Few clinical trials have been completed in Sjögren's syndrome to provide guidance for the therapeutic efficacy of the different anti-fungal therapies. Many treatment options exist for the treatment of fungal infection, as listed in Table 12.2. For patients with very low levels

Table 12.2. Therapies for oral fungal infections

	Dose/application
Topical agents:	
• Clotrimazole troches	10 mg 5×/day × 10 days
• Nystatin rinse	100,000 units/ml; 5 ml swish and spit q.i.d.
• Nystatin-triamcinolone acetonide (Mycolog II) ointment	Dab on corners of mouth q.i.d.
• Nystatin ointment	Thin layer applied inside denture t.i.d.
• Chlorhexidine rinse	10 ml swish and spit b.i.d.
Systemic agents:	
• Diflucan (Fluconazole)	200 mg loading dose followed by 100 mg/day for 1 week

of stimulated salivary flow, liquid suspensions are easier to use. Clotrimazole troches are often beneficial, but patients must be able to dissolve these for clinical efficacy and they may increase the caries risk due to high sucrose content. Nystatin rinse may be beneficial as an anti-fungal, but also may increase the caries risk. Angular cheilitis can be treated with nystatin-triamcinolone ointment or a similar anti-fungal ointment four times daily until the lesion clears.

Oral Burning

A subjective complaint of oral burning is often related to an underlying fungal infection, therefore treatment with anti-fungals should be considered. If a fungal infection is not present, other etiological factors include oral trauma from poor mucosal lubrication and parafunctional oral movements (e.g., rubbing tongue or lips against teeth), hematinic deficiencies (e.g., vitamin B_{12} or folic acid), and burning mouth syndrome (BMS).

Empirical anti-fungal therapy is often prescribed with a complaint of oral burning. Treatment options for poor mucosal lubrication with an associated parafunctional movement include oral lubricants and/or relief of sharp tooth edges. Hematinic deficiencies confirmed by laboratory tests can be managed by appropriate vitamin replacement. BMS by definition is a diagnosis of exclusion, with treatment options including clonazepam, alpha-lipoic acid, and cognitive therapy [85].

Dental Caries

A common oral manifestation of salivary gland dysfunction is an increased rate of dental caries. Appropriate routine dental care is vital to provide preventive therapy and early diagnosis and treatment. Supplemental fluoride therapy is the mainstay of preventive therapy, including over the counter (OTC) formulations and prescription fluoride formulations.

Management of caries is based on an assessment of each patient's caries risk. For patients with a stable to low caries rate, an OTC fluoride rinse (e.g., ACT) may be sufficient. If a patient has a moderate to high caries rate, prescription fluoride gels should be prescribed. Other preventive options include chlorhexidine rinse or varnish, xylitol-containing products (e.g., mints and gum), and fluoride varnishes [86].

Extraglandular Manifestations

Appropriate medical specialty referral is vital for the management of the numerous extraglandular manifestations of Sjögren's syndrome. Detailed information on the management of these extraglandular manifestations is beyond the scope of the present chapter. As previously noted, the use of disease-modifying agents may be appropriate for the management of some extraglandular manifestations of Sjögren's syndrome.

Take Home Messages

- Autoimmune salivary gland disorders may have a profound impact on oral health and functions. Dryness of the mouth (xerostomia) is the most common presentation of these disorders and is most often a manifestation of salivary gland dysfunction.
- Management combines palliation of symptoms, prevention of complications, stimulation of exocrine function with secretagogues, and therapy directed at the underlying autoimmunity with disease-modifying drugs.

References

1. Kassan SS, Moutsopoulos HM (2004) Clinical manifestations and early diagnosis of Sjogren syndrome. Arch Intern Med 164:1275–1284
2. Kassan SS, Thomas TL, Moutsopoulos HM, Hoover R, Kimberly RP, Budman DR, Costa J, Decker JL, Chused TM (1978) Increased risk of lymphoma in sicca syndrome. Ann Intern Med 89:888–892
3. Theander E, Henriksson G, Ljungberg O, Mandl T, Manthorpe R, Jacobsson LT (2006) Lymphoma and other malignancies in primary Sjogren's syndrome: a cohort study on cancer incidence and lymphoma predictors. Ann Rheum Dis 65:796–803
4. Zintzaras E, Voulgarelis M, Moutsopoulos HM (2005) The risk of lymphoma development in autoimmune diseases: a meta-analysis. Arch Intern Med 165:2337–2344

5. Ioannidis JP, Vassiliou VA, Moutsopoulos HM (2002) Long-term risk of mortality and lymphoproliferative disease and predictive classification of primary Sjogren's syndrome. Arthritis Rheum 46:741–747
6. Woo SB, Lee SJ, Schubert MM (1997) Graft-vs.-host disease. Crit Rev Oral Biol Med 8:201–216
7. Nagler R, Marmary Y, Krausz Y, Chisin R, Markitziu A, Nagler A (1996) Major salivary gland dysfunction in human acute and chronic graft-versus-host disease (GVHD). Bone Marrow Transplant 17:219–224
8. Sale GE, Shulman HM, Schubert MM, Sullivan KM, Kopecky KJ, Hackman RC, Morton TH, Storb R, Thomas ED (1981) Oral and ophthalmic pathology of graft versus host disease in man: predictive value of the lip biopsy. Hum Pathol 12:1022–1030
9. Daniels TE, Fox PC (1992) Salivary and oral components of Sjogren's syndrome. Rheum Dis Clin North Am 18(3):571–589
10. Pijpe J, Kalk WW, van der Wal JE, Vissink A, Kluin PM, Roodenburg JL, Bootsma H, Kallenberg CG, Spijkervet FK (2007) Parotid gland biopsy compared with labial biopsy in the diagnosis of patients with primary Sjögren's syndrome. Rheumatology 46(2):335–341
11. Daniels TE (1984) Labial salivary gland biopsy in Sjogren's syndrome: Assessment as a diagnostic tool criterion in 362 suspected cases. Arthritis Rheum 27(2):147–156
12. Sreebny L (1992) Saliva-salivary gland hypofunction (SGH). FDI Working Group 10. J Dent Assoc S Afr 47:498–501
13. Hernandez YL, Lindahl G (1989) Oral candidiasis in Sjogren's syndrome: Prevalence, clinical correlations and treatment. Oral Surg Oral Med Oral Pathol 68(3):324–329
14. Soto-Rojas AE, Villa AR, Sifuentes-Osornio J, Alarcon-Segovia D, Kraus A (1998) Oral manifestations in patients with Sjogren's syndrome. J Rheumatol 25:906–910
15. Christensen LB, Petersen PE, Thorn JJ, Schiodt M (2001) Dental caries and dental health behavior of patients with primary Sjogren syndrome. Acta Odontol Scand. 59(3):116–120
16. Friedlaender MH (1992) Ocular manifestations of Sjogren's syndrome: Keratoconjunctivitis sicca. Rheum Dis Clin North Am 18(3):591–608
17. Rogeudas AM, Misery L, Sassolas B, Le Masson G, Pennec YL, Youinou P (2004) Cutaneous manifestations of primary Sjogren's syndrome are underestimated. Clin Exp Rheumatol 22:632–636
18. Provost TT, Watson R (1992) Cutaneous manifestations of Sjogren's syndrome. Rheum Dis Clin North Am 18(3):609–616
19. Alexander E, Provost T (1987) Sjogren's syndrome. Arch Dermatol 123:801–810
20. Ito I, Nagai S, Kitaichi M, Nicholson AG, Johkoh T, Noma S, Kim DS, Handa T, Izumi T, Mishima M (2005) Pulmonary manifestations of primary Sjogren's syndrome. A clinical, radiographic and pathologic study. Am J Respir Crit Care Med 171:632–638
21. Constantopoulos SH, Tsianos EV, Moutsopoulos HM (1992) Pulmonary manifestations and gastrointestinal manifestations of Sjogren's syndrome. Rheum Dis Clin North Am 18(3):617–635
22. Hietaharju A, Yli-Kerttula U, Hakkinen V, Frey H (1990) Nervous system manifestation in Sjogren's syndrome. Acta Neurol Scand 81:144–152
23. Alexander E (1992) Central nervous system disease in Sjogren's syndrome. Rheum Dis Clin North Am 18(3):637–672
24. Kaplan MJ, Ike RW (2002) The liver is a common non-exocrine target in primary Sjogren's syndrome: a retrospective review. BMC Gastroenterol 13(2):21
25. Edhag O, Helmers C, Samnegard H, Sjogren A, Vallin H (1997) Two cases of myocardial disease simulating constrictive pericarditis. Scand J Thorac Cardiovasc Surg 11(3):225–227
26. Borda E, Sterin-Borda L (2001) Autoantibodies against neonatal heart M1 muscarinic acetylcholine receptor in children with congenital heart block. J Autoimmun 16(2):143–150
27. Bossini N, Savoldi S, Franceschini F, Mombelloni S, Baronio M, Cavazzana I, Viola BF, Valzorio B, Mazzucchelli C, Cattaneo R, Scolari F, Maiorca R (2001) Clinical and morphological features of kidney involvement in primary Sjogren's syndrome. Nephrol Dial Transplant 16(12):2328–2336
28. Barendregt PJ, Visser MR, Smets EM, Tulen JH, Van den Meiracker AH, Boomsma F, Markusse HM (1998) Fatigue in primary Sjogren's syndrome. Ann Rheum Dis 57:291–295
29. Chao NJ (2006) Clinical manifestations of Sjogren's syndrome. www.uptodate.com
30. Hsiao M, Schubert MM, Thornquist M (1988) Oral manifestations of acute graft-versus-host disease following marrow transplantation (abstract). J Dent Res 67(Spec Iss):202
31. Soares AB, Faria PR, Magna LA, Correa ME, de Sousa CA, Almeida OP, Cintra ML (2005) Chronic GVHD in minor salivary glands and oral mucosa: histopathological and immunohistochemical evaluation of 25 patients. J Oral Pathol Med 34:368–373

32. Izutsu KT, Sullivan KM, Schubert MM, Truelove EL, Shulman HM, Sale GE, Morton TH, Rice JC, Witherspoon RP, Storb R, Thomas ED (1983) Disordered salivary immunoglobulin secretion and sodium transport in human chronic graft-versus-host disease. Transplantation 35(5):441–451
33. Chao NJ (2006) Clinical manifestations and diagnosis of chronic graft-versus-host disease. www.uptodate.com
34. Schubert MM, Sullivan KM (1990) Recognition, incidence, and management of oral graft-versus-host disease. NCI Monogr 9:135–43
35. Uderzo C, Fraschinia D, Balduzzi A., Galimberti S, Arrigo G, Biagi E, Pignanelli M, Nicolini B, Rovelli A (1997) Long term effects of bone marrow transplantation on dental status in children with leukemia. Bone Marrow Transplant 20:865–69
36. Majorana A, Schubert MM, Porta F, Ugazio AG. Sapelli PL (2000) Oral complications of pediatric hematopoietic cell transplantation: diagnosis and management. Support Care Cancer 8:353–65
37. Berkowitz RJ, Jones P, Barsetti J, Cheung NK, Coccia PF (1987) Stomatologic complications of bone marrow transplantation in a pediatric population. Pediatr Dent 9(2):105–10
38. Featherstone JD (1999) Prevention and reversal of dental caries: role of low level fluoride. Community Dent Oral Epidemiol 27(1):31–40
39. Fox PC, Busch KA, Baum BJ (1987) Subjective reports of xerostomia and objective measures of salivary gland performance. J Am Dent Assoc 115:581–84
40. Guggenheimer J, Moore PA (2003) Xerostomia Etiology, Recognition and Treatment. J Am Dent Assoc 134:61–69
41. Atkinson JC, Fox PC (1992) Salivary gland dysfunction. Clin Geriatr Med 8:499–511
42. Navazesh M (1993) Methods for collecting saliva. Ann N Y Acad Sci 694:72–7
43. Sreebny LM, Zhu WX (1995) The use of whole saliva in the differential diagnosis of Sjogren's Syndrome. Adv Dent Res 10:17–24
44. Baum BJ (1986) Salivary gland function during aging. Gerodontics 2:61–64
45. Percival RS, Challacombe SJ, Marsh PD (1994) Flow rates of resting whole and stimulated parotid saliva in relation to age and gender. J Dent Res 73:1416–1420
46. Tishler M, Yaron I, Shirazi I, Yaron M (1997) Saliva: An additional diagnostic tool in Sjogren's Syndrome. Semin Arthritis Rheum 27:173–9
47. Atkinson JC (1993) The Role of Salivary Measurements in the diagnosis of salivary autoimmune diseases. Ann N Y Acad Sci 694:238–51
48. Saito T, Fukuda H, Arisue M, Matsuda A, Shindoh M, Amemiya A, Ohmori K (1991) Relationship between sialographic findings of parotid glands and histopathologic findings of labial glands in Sjogren's Syndrome. Oral Surg Oral Med Oral Pathol 72:675–80
49. Silvers AR, Som PM (1998) Salivary glands. Radiol Clin North Am 36:941–66
50. Wang S, Zou Z, Zhu J (1992) Sequential quantitative scintigraphy of parotid glands with chronic inflammatory diseases. 50:456–65
51. Fox PC (1985) Simplified biopsy technique for labial minor salivary glands. Plastic Reconstr Surg 75:592–3
52. Vitali C, Bombardieri S, Jonsson R, Moutsopoulos HM, Alexander EL, Carsons SE, Daniels TE, Fox PC, Fox RI, Kassan SS, Pillemer SR, Talal N, Weisman MH; European Study Group on Classification Criteria for Sjögren's Syndrome (2002) Classification criteria for Sjögren's syndrome: a revised version of the European criteria proposed by the American-European Consensus Group. Ann Rheum Dis 61:554–558
53. van der Reijden WA, van der Kwaak JS, Vissink A, Veerman EC, Amerongen AV (1996) Treatment of xerostomia with polymer-based saliva substitutes in patients with Sjögren's syndrome. Arthritis Rheum 39:57–63
54. Gravenmade EJ, Vissink A (1993) Mucin-containing lozenges in the treatment of intraoral problems associated with Sjögren's syndrome. A double-blinded crossover study in 42 patients. Oral Surg Oral Med Oral Pathol 75:466–71
55. Aagaard A, Godiksen S, Teglers PT Schiodt M, Glenert U (1992) Comparison between new saliva stimulants in patients with dry mouth: a placebo-controlled double-blinded crossover study. J Oral Pathol 21:376–80
56. Manthorpe R, Hagen-Petersen S, Prause JU (1984) Primary Sjögren's syndrome treated with Efamol/Efavlt. A double-blinded cross-over investigation. Rheumatol Int 4:165–7
57. Theander E, Horrobin DF, Jacobsson LT, Manthorpe R. (2002) Gammalinolenic acid treatment of fatigue associated with primary Sjogren's syndrome. Scand J Rheumatol 31:72–79
58. Brennan MT, Shariff G, Lockhart PB, Fox PC (2002) Treatment of xerostomia: A systematic review of therapeutic trials. Dent Clin North Am 46(4):847–856
59. von Bültzingslöwen I, Sollecito TP, Fox PC, Daniels T, Jonsson R, Lockhart PB, Wray D, Brennan MT, Carrozzo M, Gandera B, Fujibayashi T, Navazesh M, Rhodus NL, Schiødt M (2007) Salivary dysfunction associated with systemic diseases: systematic review and clinical management recommendations. Oral Surg Oral Med Oral Pathol Oral Radiol Endod 103 Suppl:S57:e1–15

60. Fox PC, Cummins MJ, Cummins JM (2002) A third study on the use of orally administered anhydrous crystalline maltose for relief of dry mouth in primary Sjogren's syndrome. J Altern Complement Med 8(5):651–659
61. Steller M, Chou L, Daniels TE (1988) Electrical stimulation of salivary flow in patients with Sjögren's syndrome. J Dent Res 67:1334–1337
62. Talal N, Quinn JH, Daniels TE (1992) The clinical effects of electrostimulation on salivary function of Sjögren's syndrome patients. A placebo controlled study. Rheumatol Int 12:43–45
63. Hargitai IA, Sherman RG, Strother JM (2005) The effects of electrostimulation on parotid saliva flow: a pilot study. Oral Surg Oral Med Oral Pathol Oral Radiol Endod 99(3):316–320
64. Strietzel FP, Martin-Granizo R, Fedele S, Lo Russo L, Mignogna M, Reichart PA, Wolff A (2007) Electrostimulating device in the management of xerostomia. Oral Dis 13:206–213
65. Vivino FB, Al-Hashimi I, Khan Z, LeVeque FG, Salisbury PL 3rd, Tran-Johnson TK, Muscoplat CC, Trivedi M, Goldlust B, Gallagher SC (1999) Pilocarpine tablets for the treatment of dry mouth and dry eye symptoms in patients with Sjögren syndrome: A randomized placebo-controlled fixed-dose multicenter trial. Arch Intern Med 159:174–181
66. Fife RS, Chase WF, Dore RK, Wiesenhutter CW, Lockhart PB, Tindall E, Suen JY (2002) Cevimeline for the treatment of xerostomia in patients with Sjogren syndrome: a randomized trial. Arch Intern Med 162(11):1293–1300
67. Petrone D, Condemi JJ, Fife R, Gluck O, Cohen S, Dalgin P (2002) A double-blind, randomized, placebo-controlled study of cevimeline in Sjogren's syndrome patients with xerostomia and keratoconjunctivitis sicca. Arthritis Rheum 46(3):748–754
68. Pillemer SR, Brennan MT, Sankar V, Leakan RA, Smith JA, Grisius M, Ligier S, Radfar L, Kok MR, Kingman A, Fox PC (2004) Pilot clinical trial of dehydroepiandrosterone (DHEA) versus placebo for Sjogren's syndrome. Arthritis Rheum 51(4):601–604
69. Drosos AA, van Vliet-Dascalopoulou E, Andonopoulos AP, Galanopoulou V, Skopouli FN, Moutsopoulos HM (1988) Nandrolone decanoate (deca-durabolin) in primary Sjogren's syndrome: a double blind pilot study. Clin Exp Rheumatol 6(1):53–57
70. Fox PC, Datiles M, Atkinson JC, Macynski AA, Scott J, Fletcher D, Valdez IH, Kurrasch RH, Delapenha R, Jackson W (1993) Prednisone and piroxicam for treatment of primary Sjögren's syndrome. Clin Exp Rheumatol 11:149–156
71. Price EJ, Rigby SP, Clancy U, Venables PJ (1998) A double blind placebo controlled trial of azathioprine in the treatment of primary Sjögren's syndrome. J Rheumatol 25:896–899
72. Kruize AA, Hene RJ, Kallenberg CG, van Bijsterveld OP, van der Heide A, Kater L, Bijlsma JW (1993) Hydroxychloroquine treatment for primary Sjögren's syndrome: a two year double blind crossover trial. Ann Rheum Dis 52:360–364
73. Ship JA, Fox PC, Michalek JE, Cummins MJ, Richards AB (1993) Treatment of primary Sjögren's syndrome with low-dose natural human interferon-alpha administered by the oral mucosal route: a phase II clinical trial. IFN protocol study group. J Interferon Cytokine Res 19:943–951
74. Cummins MJ, Papas A, Kammer GM, Fox PC (2003) Treatment of primary Sjogren's syndrome with low-dose human interferon alfa administered by the oromucosal route: combined phase III results. Arthritis Rheum 49:585–593
75. Mariette X, Ravaud P, Steinfeld S, Baron G, Goetz J, Hachulla E, Combe B, Puechal X, Pennec Y, Sauvezie B, Perdriger A, Hayem G, Janin A, Sibilia J (2004) Inefficacy of infliximab in primary Sjogren's syndrome: results of the randomized, controlled Trial of Remicade in Primary Sjogren's Syndrome (TRIPSS). Arthritis Rheum 50(4):1270–1276
76. Sankar V, Brennan MT, Kok MR, Leakan RA, Smith JA, Manny J, Baum BJ, Pillemer SR (2004) Etanercept in Sjogren's syndrome: a twelve-week randomized, double-blind, placebo-controlled pilot clinical trial. Arthritis Rheum 50(7):2240–2245
77. Pillemer SR, Leakan RA, Sankar V, Manny J, Baum BJ, Smith J, Chaudhry U, Fox PC, Radfar L, Ligier S, Brennan MT (2004) Prominent adverse effects of thalidomide in primary Sjogren's syndrome. Arthritis Rheum 51(3):505–506
78. Moutsopoulos NM, Angelov N, Sankar V, Leakan RA, Pillemer S, Wahl SM (2006) Immunological consequences of thalidomide treatment in Sjogren's syndrome. Ann Rheum Dis 65(1):112–114
79. Pijpe J, van Imhoff GW, Spijkervet FK, Roodenburg JL, Wolbink GJ, Mansour K, Vissink A, Kallenberg CG, Bootsma H (2005) Rituximab treatment in patients with primary Sjogren's syndrome: an open-label phase II study. Arthritis Rheum 52(9):2740–2750
80. Gescuk B, Wu AJ, Whitcher JP, Daniels TE, Lund S, Fye K, Davis JC Jr (2005) Lamivudine is not effective in primary Sjogren's syndrome. Ann Rheum Dis 64(9):1326–1330

81. Stevenson D, Tauber J, Reis BL (2000) Efficacy and safety of cyclosporin A ophthalmic emulsion in the treatment of moderate-to-severe dry eye disease: a dose-ranging, randomized trial. The Cyclosporin A Phase 2 Study Group. Ophthalmology 107(5):967–974
82. Tsifetaki N, Kitsos G, Paschides CA, Alamanos Y, Eftaxias V, Voulgari PV, Psilas K, Drosos AA (2003) Oral pilocarpine for the treatment of ocular symptoms in patients with Sjogren's syndrome: a randomised 12 week controlled study. Ann Rheum Dis 62(12):1204–1207
83. Ono M, Takamura E, Shinozaki K, Tsumura T, Hamano T, Yagi Y, Tsubota K (2004) Therapeutic effect of cevimeline on dry eye in patients with Sjogren's syndrome: a randomized, double-blind clinical study. Am J Ophthalmol 138(1):6–17
84. Aragona P, Bucolo C, Spinella R, Giuffrida S, Ferreri G (2005) Systemic omega-6 essential fatty acid treatment and pgel tear content in Sjogren's syndrome patients. Invest Ophthalmol Vis Sci 46(12):4474–4479
85. Zakrzewska JM, Forssell H, Glenny AM (2005) Interventions for the treatment of burning mouth syndrome. Cochrane Database Syst Rev 25(1):CD002779
86. Steinberg S (2002) A paradigm shift in the treatment of caries. Gen Dent 50(4):333–338

Chapter 13

Disorders of the Salivary Glands in Children

13

David L. Mandell

Contents

Core Features

- Primary lesions arising from the salivary glands in children are rare.
- Salivary gland disorders in the pediatric age group can be divided into two general categories: (1) salivary gland masses and (2) sialorrhea in neurologically disabled children.
- Salivary gland masses in the pediatric age group are more likely to consist of vascular anomalies and infectious and inflammatory lesions than epithelial glandular tumors.
- When oral motor therapy either fails or is not feasible for neurologically devastated children with sialorrhea, management options include pharmacotherapy or surgery designed to either redirect the flow of saliva or to decrease saliva production.

Complications to Avoid

- Parotidectomy can inadvertently be performed in children for lesions that typically do not require the operation, such as hemangioma, non-tuberculous mycobacterial infection, cat-scratch disease, and lymphoma. Remember that although solid tumors of salivary glandular origin do occur, they are rare in the pediatric age group. Imaging, fine-needle aspiration biopsy, and serology can help determine the diagnosis prior to committing to parotidectomy.
- When functions such as vision or hearing are at risk from eyelid or ear canal extension of a parotid hemangioma, systemic steroids and laser therapy are reasonable and less invasive options than parotidectomy, which is generally discouraged during the proliferative phase for this benign neoplasm that is expected to eventually involute on its own.
- When pursuing surgical excision or debulking for lymphatic malformations, remember that these lesions are benign and non-neoplastic; incomplete excision is a preferred alternative to inadvertent sacrifice of important neurovascular structures and the facial nerve.
- A first branchial anomaly must be considered in the differential diagnosis of an intraparotid cyst or recurrent parotid abscess. Failure to appreciate that these cystic lesions may be branchial in origin is a common cause of incomplete excision and recurrence. Appreciate the intimate relationship the anomalous tract can have with the facial nerve and consider a superficial parotidectomy approach.
- When relocating the submandibular ducts for neurologically impaired children with sialorrhea, leaving behind the sublingual glands invites a high risk of postoperative ranula formation.
- For chronic sialorrhea, the submandibular glands are more important to address than the parotid glands, since the majority of resting saliva production comes from the submandibular glands.
- Parotidectomy is generally considered too aggressive an approach for sialorrhea, and relocation of the parotid duct is associated with a high complication rate; ligation of the parotid duct is the most acceptable surgical option when the parotid glands need to be addressed.

Pediatric Salivary Gland Masses

Special Pediatric Considerations

When evaluating a child presenting with a mass within a major salivary gland, several distinct features unique to the pediatric population should be taken into consideration. Salivary tumors of glandular origin in the pediatric age group are rare, with only approximately 1.7% of all epithelial salivary tumors occurring in children [6]. In addition, masses arising within the pediatric salivary glands are more likely to consist of vascular anomalies such as hemangiomas and lymphatic malformations, or infectious and inflammatory lymphadenopathy, rather than glandular tumors of salivary origin. When true glandular epithelial tumors do occur, their extremely low incidence has often prevented any one pediatric institution from being able to report a definitive treatment algorithm. Thus, the same protocols used to treat adults with salivary glandular tumors, as thoroughly described through the rest of this textbook, are often employed for children. It is believed that the behavior of major salivary gland tumors in children is related to histologic type and clinical grade, similar to adults [36].

Traditional Beliefs Regarding the Etiology of Salivary Masses in the Pediatric Age Group

Approximately 50% of all parotid masses in the pediatric age group represent malignancy, which is a higher rate than that found in adults [27, 34]. Similar to adults, the most common glandular epithelial parotid tumor is pleomorphic adenoma [27, 34]. The most common malignant glandular neoplasm in children is mucoepidermoid carcinoma, followed by adenocarcinoma and acinic cell carcinoma [27, 34]. When mucoepidermoid carcinoma of the parotid gland is encountered in children, the histologic grade is typically low, and long-term outcome with appropriate treatment is favorable [38].

Modern Beliefs Regarding the Etiology of Parotid Masses in the Pediatric Age Group

When all pediatric salivary masses are considered (and not just those for which a parotidectomy specimen was obtained), recent reports have suggested that benign lesions overwhelmingly predominate.

For example, in a case series from the Massachusetts Eye and Ear Infirmary of 22 children who presented with an unknown, solid parotid mass over an 8-year period, only 1 patient had a malignancy (mucoepidermoid carcinoma) [5]. Eight patients (36%) had pleomorphic adenoma, and 13 patients (59%) had an inflammatory process such as cat-scratch disease, non-tuberculous mycobacterial infection, or toxoplasmosis.

In a review of all 118 children who had surgical treatment for a parotid mass from 1970 to 1997 at the Mayo Clinic in Rochester, Minnesota, 84% had benign lesions, whereas only (16%) had malignant tumors [36]. The most common benign parotid mass was pleomorphic adenoma (48% of benign masses). Other benign lesions included hemangiomas, branchial cleft cysts, lymphatic malformations, and neurofibromas. If vascular lesions were excluded, tumors of the parotid gland were malignant in 35% of patients. Since a greater number of parotid hemangiomas were observed (rather than excised) in the later years of the study, the number of parotid hemangiomas included in the analysis was likely underestimated.

In a recent survey of 324 masses in the salivary gland region, from Children's Memorial Hospital in Chicago, 87% of all salivary gland masses in children represented vascular anomalies (59% of all masses were hemangiomas and 27.5% were lymphatic malformations) [3]. Only 43 patients (13%) had solid masses, and most benign solid salivary masses were not of glandular origin, but rather included non-salivary tumors and inflammatory processes. Only 10 of 324 of all pediatric salivary masses (3%) were malignant tumors, with low-grade mucoepidermoid carcinoma being most common, followed by rhabdomyosarcoma.

Modern Beliefs Regarding the Etiology of Masses in the Submandibular Triangle

Most submandibular triangle masses in the pediatric age group represent inflammatory lesions or lesions of vascular origin, and glandular tumors are rare. In a review of 67 surgically excised masses in the submandibular triangle, from Children's Hospital of Philadelphia from 1987 to 2001, only 6 lesions (9%) were of primary salivary origin, including 4 pleomorphic adenomas and 2 mucoepidermoid carcinomas [19] (see Fig. 13.1). More common indications for submandibular triangle surgery included chronic submandibular gland inflammation, lymphatic malformations, hemangiomas, and a wide variety of infectious, inflammatory, and neoplastic submandibular lymph node disorders occurring adjacent to the submandibular gland (such as Hodgkin's lymphoma and post-transplant lymphoproliferative disorder).

General Approach to Salivary Gland Masses in the Pediatric Age Group

Since malignant salivary tumors are rare in children, inflammatory conditions are common, and clinical examination often cannot easily distinguish between intra- and extrasalivary masses, some authors have advocated an initial trial of antibiotics for the solitary mass in the vicinity of a major salivary gland, followed by other evaluations including fine-needle aspiration biopsy and imaging only if the mass persists [3, 19]. When true epithelial glandular tumors do occur in children, they should be treated according to the same principles as outlined for similar tumors in adults, as found throughout this textbook. What makes children, especially in the prepubescent years, particularly unique with regard to solid glandular salivary tumors is not the treatment or prognosis, but rather the rarity of the disease.

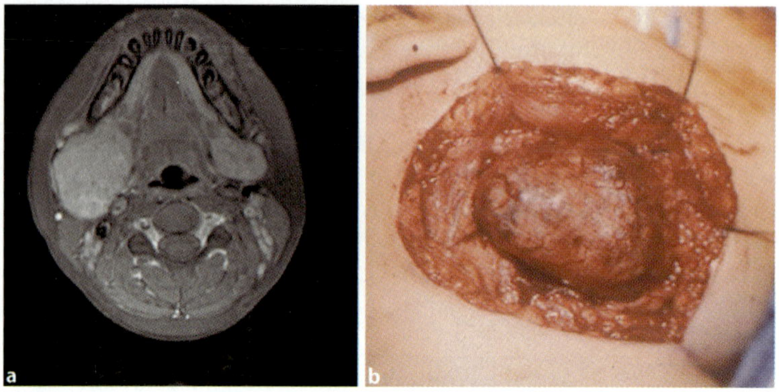

Fig. 13.1: Pleomorphic adenoma of the submandibular gland in a 10-year-old boy. **a** MRI demonstrating solid right submandibular mass. **b** Submandibular gland tumor excision

13

Hemangiomas of the Parotid Gland

Hemangioma, the most common tumor of the parotid gland in childhood, is a true benign epithelial neoplasm which typically proliferates during the first year of life and then begins to spontaneously involute over the course of several years. Now that the favorable natural history of hemangiomas of the parotid gland is more widely understood, parotidectomy is generally not performed during the proliferative phase of the disease, and in most cases observation has become the standard treatment [14].

The diagnosis of a hemangioma of the parotid gland is most commonly made by history and physical examination, with the lesion typically presenting as a soft, spongy, non-tender mass that is noticed during the first months of life and continues to enlarge for about a year. Nearly half of all patients have an associated vascular mark over the cheek. Radiographic confirmation with magnetic resonance imaging (MRI) is recommended for deep tumors with no cutaneous involvement in which the clinical diagnosis is less certain (see Fig. 13.2). The female to male ratio is approximately 4.5:1, and up to 24% of cases are bilateral [14]. Involvement of adjacent structures such as the lip, eyelids, and nose occurs with regularity. Approximately 21% of patients with hemangioma of the parotid gland can also have a separate focus of subglottic hemangioma, which can lead to progressive biphasic stridor and respiratory distress; 7% of children with hemangiomas of the parotid gland underwent tracheotomy in one recent large series from Children's Hospital in Boston [14].

During the first year of life, when the lesion is actively proliferating, observation is the treatment of choice. However, systemic high-dose steroids, given typically for a mean of 8–9 months, can be offered in cases of skin ulceration, respiratory distress, visual axis impairment from eyelid involvement, congestive heart failure, or conductive hearing loss from external auditory canal compression. With high-dose steroid therapy, regression or stabilization of the tumor occurs in approximately 84% of tumors [14].

In cases of hemangioma in the pediatric age group where the skin overlying the parotid gland has become ulcerated, pulsed dye laser therapy has been advocated by some authors, although potential complications such as pigmentation changes, severe hemorrhage, and long-term scarring have to be carefully considered [26, 49]. Pediatric ophthalmology consultation should be pursued if the periorbital soft tissues are involved. Other ancillary treatments such as interferon therapy and selective surgical debulking can be very carefully considered when vital functions are at risk [14].

Although caregivers are counseled that the tumor will eventually involute, up to 66% of patients will remain with cosmetic issues such as residual fibrofatty tissue and redundant or damaged skin, all of which could require future surgical procedures that would typically be deferred until the ages of 3–5 years [14]. This topic is dealt with in greater detail in Chapter 19, Vascular Lesions of Salivary Glands.

Lymphatic Malformations

Lymphatic malformations are non-neoplastic, congenital vascular anomalies composed of cystically dilated lymphatics. Approximately 47% of lymphatic malformations present as a mass in the head and neck [1]. The parotid gland may be directly involved in 2–18% of all lymphan-

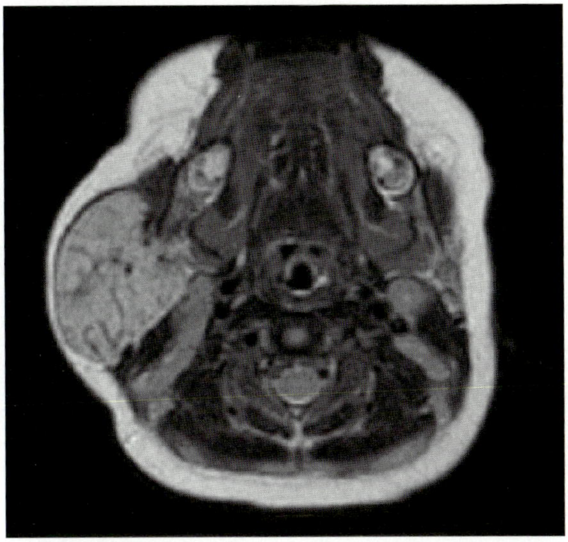

Fig. 13.2: MRI demonstrating a hemangioma of the right parotid gland in a 6-month-old infant diagnosed radiographically and managed successfully with observation

giomas of the head and neck [1, 17]. The average age of presentation is approximately 3 years [1], with 54% of the diagnoses established by the age of 1 year [17]. The diagnosis and the extent of the malformation are often confirmed with computed tomography (see Fig. 13.3). The malformations tend to grow slowly with the child, sometimes acutely enlarging in the setting of an upper respiratory infection or minor trauma. Rare cases of spontaneous regression have been reported, but in most instances, surgical excision has traditionally been the treatment of choice [1]. Many cases are asymptomatic and the primary concern is cosmetic, but larger lymphatic malformations can lead to compression of the neonatal airway and esophagus, and microcystic lesions involving the oral cavity, floor of mouth, and submandibular region can also lead to respiratory distress and dysphagia. Up to 32% of children with lymphatic malformations of the head and neck may develop respiratory and digestive tract symptoms [1].

Lymphatic malformations are often found to be insinuated between and around many vital structures. Given the benign nature of the disease, sacrifice of important neurovascular structures should be avoided during surgery, and as such, incomplete excision, or surgical "debulking," is considered reasonable and even advisable, especially in cases of microcystic disease or extensive infiltration. The overall recurrence rate after surgical excision of lymphatic malformations of the head and neck ranges from 13% to 33% [1], but can be as high as 85% for suprahyoid (versus infrahyoid) disease, where the submandibular and parotid glands are located [39]. Superficial and total parotidectomy have been performed as part of the surgical approach [17], but facial paresis and paralysis have been reported after excision of the lymphangioma in the region of the parotid gland [37].

To reduce morbidity and to try to decrease recurrence rates, recent interest has focused on the sclerosing effect of OK-432 (Picibanil) [12]. This agent is a potent immunostimulant made from a lyophilized mixture of a low-virulence strain of *Streptococcus pyogenes* incubated with benzylpenicillin. In a recent multi-institutional study consisting of 30 pediatric patients with lymphatic malformations, 29 of which were in the head and neck (including 1 within the parotid gland), OK-432 sclerotherapy led to either a complete or substantial response in 66% of patients; the response rate was higher (86%) in cases of macrocystic disease [12]. No significant side effects were noted. The results with OK-432 sclerotherapy are generally considered

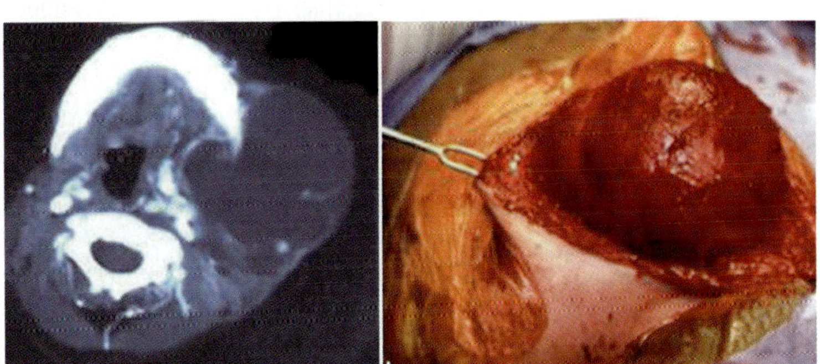

Fig. 13.3: Lymphatic malformation involving the submandibular gland in a 3-year-old girl. **a** CT scan with intravenous (IV) contrast showing a large, cystic lesion originating from the left submandibular triangle. **b** Surgical excision

to be similar to that expected from surgery. Sclerotherapy may be preferred in cases of salivary gland involvement so as to try to decrease the surgical risk of injury to the facial nerve. This topic is dealt with in greater detail in Chapter 19, Vascular Lesions of Salivary Glands.

Ranulas

A ranula typically presents as a unilateral cyst in the floor of the mouth, has a bluish hue, and is believed to result from an obstructed sublingual gland, or from extravasation of mucus after sublingual gland trauma [52]. The plunging ranula, which extends beyond the posterior border of the mylohyoid muscle, presents as a soft, painless, non-mobile swelling in the neck, whereas the mixed ranula has both intraoral and cervical swelling. Ranulas often present in children, with the peak incidence in the second decade of life; they can even be seen in infancy [52]. Intraoral ranulas confined to the oral cavity account for approximately 67% of cases; plunging ranulas occur in 21%, and mixed in 12% [52]. In infants, the diagnosis of intraoral ranula can be confused with foregut duplication cysts of the tongue, and plunging ranulas can be easily confused with lymphatic malformations. Computed tomography or magnetic resonance imaging can sometimes help clarify the etiology. A high amylase level in aspirated fluid can be diagnostic. For intraoral ranulas, excision of the ranula along with the associated sublingual gland is most likely to be curative, whereas simple marsupialization may yield a recurrence rate as high as 60% [52]. The plunging ranula is generally approached with both cervical and trans-oral incisions, with removal of the ranula and the associated sublingual gland, although intraoral removal of the sublingual gland alone has also been reported to be effective [52]. This topic is dealt with in greater detail in Chapter 10, Management of Mucocele and Ranula.

First Branchial Cleft Anomalies

Anomalies of the first branchial cleft are typically intimately involved with the pediatric parotid gland, and should be considered in the differential diagnosis of salivary gland masses in the pediatric age group.

The branchial apparatus, an embryonic structure that begins to develop during the fourth week of gestation, consists of four paired mesodermal arches of tissue that resemble fish gills and ultimately develop into the structures of the head and neck [30]. The arches are numbered in a craniocaudal direction, separated from each other on the external surface by ectoderm-lined grooves or clefts, and internally within the pharynx by endoderm (mucosa)-lined pouches. The first branchial cleft, between the first and second arches, normally persists in the newborn as the external auditory canal. First branchial cleft defects, however, can result in so-called duplication anomalies of the external auditory canal, and account for approximately 8–10% of all branchial anomalies [30].

Type I first branchial cleft lesions are considered to be duplication anomalies of the membranous external auditory canal that are purely ectodermal in origin, and thus free of cartilage [50]. In contrast, type II lesions represent duplication anomalies of both the membranous and cartilaginous external auditory canal, being both ectodermal and mesodermal in origin and grossly containing both skin and cartilage [50]. Anatomically, type I lesions tend to run parallel to the external auditory canal, whereas type II lesions run inferiorly through the substance of the parotid gland toward the neck, and are more closely involved with the facial nerve, sometimes even splitting through the main trunk.

Clinically, first branchial anomalies present as cysts or sinus tracts in the periauricular region or in the upper neck, anterior to the sternocleidomastoid muscle. The internal tract most commonly ends at the bony-cartilaginous junction of the external auditory canal. Cysts can become repeatedly infected, so a history of recurrent incision and drainage procedures in the parotid region in a child should raise suspicion for the presence of a congenital branchial cyst (see Fig. 13.4). Complete surgical excision of the anomaly is the treatment of choice, and in order to protect the facial nerve, a standard superficial parotidectomy approach should be employed with full exposure of the main trunk of the facial nerve [30]. This topic is dealt with in Chapter 14, Superficial Parotidectomy.

Infectious and Inflammatory Salivary Gland Disease in the Pediatric Age Group

Acute, Recurrent, and Chronic Parotitis

Acute parotitis in children is often recurrent in nature, characterized by repeated episodes of recurrent unilateral or bilateral swelling of the parotid gland with decreased

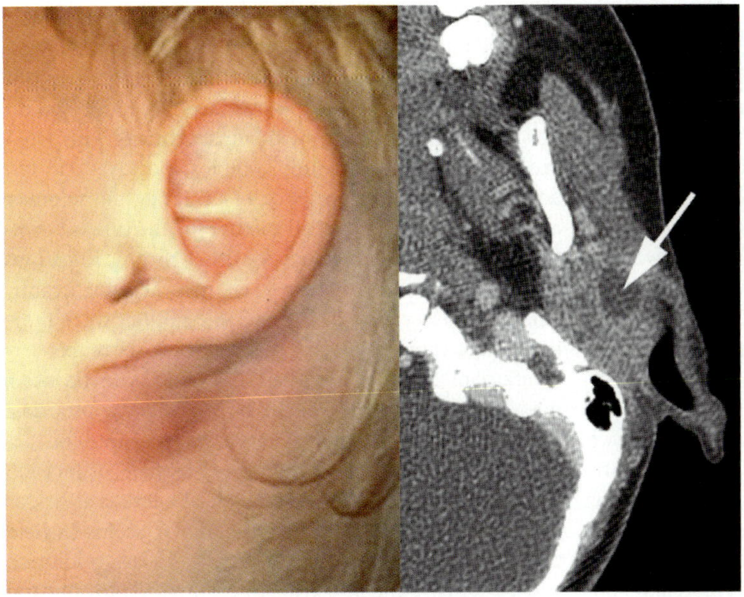

Fig. 13.4: Infected first branchial cleft cyst in a 3-year-old boy. **a** Acutely infected cystic mass near tail of parotid. **b** CT scan with IV contrast demonstrating the anomalous sinus tract coursing through the parotid gland (*arrow*), beyond the actual site of the abscess

saliva production and purulent discharge, with spontaneous improvement often noted when puberty is reached [11]. The etiology is unknown, but has been postulated to occur from retrograde infection through Stensen's duct by microorganisms in the oral cavity, or from canalicular system malformations. Computed tomography is often indicated to rule out underlying intraparotid lymphadenitis, a congenital cystic lesion, or a ductal stone. The mean age of affected children is 6 years, with a range of 2–11 years, and affected children are typically otherwise healthy [11]. Saliva samples yield positive bacterial cultures in up to 91% of cases, with the most commonly isolated bacteria including *Hemophilus influenzae* (40%), *Streptococcus pneumoniae* (38%), and *Streptococcus viridans* (35%), followed by *Moraxella catarrhalis* (4%) and anaerobes (1%) [11]. Antibiotic therapy targeting the expected gram-positive and gram-negative aerobic organisms is a mainstay of treatment, with parotidectomy rarely required.

In a review of 376 children diagnosed with parotitis, 43 (11%) were eventually treated surgically due to recurrent swelling that was not responding to antibiotics [36]. Histologic diagnoses included chronic sialadenitis (60%), chronic sialadenitis with abscess (21%), inflammatory lymphadenopathy (16%), and one case of Castleman disease, a histologically benign lymphoproliferative disorder. Of 35 patients with chronic sialadenitis, 9 had granulomatous lesions suspicious for disorders such as non-tuberculous mycobacterial infection [36].

Neonatal Suppurative Parotitis

Another related entity that is distinctly pediatric in nature is neonatal suppurative parotitis, an uncommon disease of the newborn characterized by acute swelling of the parotid gland and purulent exudate from Stensen's duct, typically occurring during the first month of life [42]. The disease is typically unilateral, sometimes with erythema of the skin over the cheek. Premature delivery is considered a major risk factor, probably due to an increased risk of dehydration with subsequent reduced salivary secretion, and it is presupposed that the infection ascends from the oral cavity. The most commonly isolated pathogen is *Staphylococcus aureus*, found in 55% of patients, followed by other gram-positive cocci (*Streptococcus viridans*, *Streptoccocus pyogenes*), occasional gram-negative bacilli (16% of cases), and rarely anaerobes [42]. Antibiotic treatment with anti-staphylococcal coverage is recommended; in 78% of cases, antibiotic therapy alone is sufficient to achieve disease resolution, usually within 24–48 h [42]. Surgical drainage may be required if clinical improvement does not occur, especially in the presence of a parotid abscess.

Non-tuberculous ("Atypical") Mycobacterial Disease

In children, non-tuberculous mycobacterial infections have a propensity to present as a mass in the region of the major salivary glands [31]. Prior to the 1950s, it was thought that most mycobacterial infections of the head and neck were due to *M. tuberculosis* (i.e., scrofula), and the other members of the mycobacteria family were thought to mainly cause disease in animals. Thus, when non-tuberculous mycobacteria became isolated as pathogens in humans, they were initially called "atypical." However, today over 95% of mycobacterial infections in children in the USA are due to these non-tuberculous organisms, most commonly from the *Mycobacterium avium* complex. Non-tuberculous mycobacteria organisms are ubiquitous in the environment, including the soil. The propensity for toddlers to put objects in their mouth, especially when the gingiva is ruptured from teething, is likely to account for the typical age range (1–5 years) and location (submandibular) of the lymphadenopathy seen with this disease.

Non-tuberculous mycobacterial disease typically presents in healthy, immunocompetent children as a painless mass that slowly increases in size over weeks to months, followed by discoloration and thinning of the overlying skin, sometimes with spontaneous drainage. In a study of 30 children with this disease at Children's Hospital of Pittsburgh, the most common location was in the submandibular triangle (50%), with another 15% occurring in the preauricular region [31]. Due to the inflamed, matted nature of the lymphadenopathy, along with the lack of any pain or fever, it can be difficult, even with computed tomography, to distinguish extrasalivary versus intrasalivary disease, and occasionally these infections can be mistaken for invasive neoplasms (see Fig. 13.5). The diagnosis can be made from tissue specimens with DNA probe testing for M. avium complex, positive acid-fast bacilli staining, and presence of caseating granulomas, along with a typical clinical picture for the disease combined with negative serology for other chronic infections such as cat-scratch disease [31]. In otherwise healthy children, observation is a reasonable option, since these lesions are thought to eventually resolve spontaneously (average of 20 months). If an antibiotic is to be used, macrolides are considered to be the most appropriate choice, although the clinical effectiveness of antibiotics is questionable. Surgical excision when feasible, or incision and curettage in cases where the facial nerve is at risk or there has been excessive skin breakdown, seems to yield the best results in terms of hastening disease resolution and avoiding months to years of cosmetic deformity and spontaneous discharge [31].

Cat-scratch Disease

Cat-scratch disease represents another example of a slow-growing, often asymptomatic infection of children that can involve peri- and intrasalivary gland lymph nodes and can lead to a great deal of confusion regarding diagnosis and treatment. The causative organism has been identified as *Bartonella henselae*, an intracellular gram-negative bacillus for which domestic cats are the natural

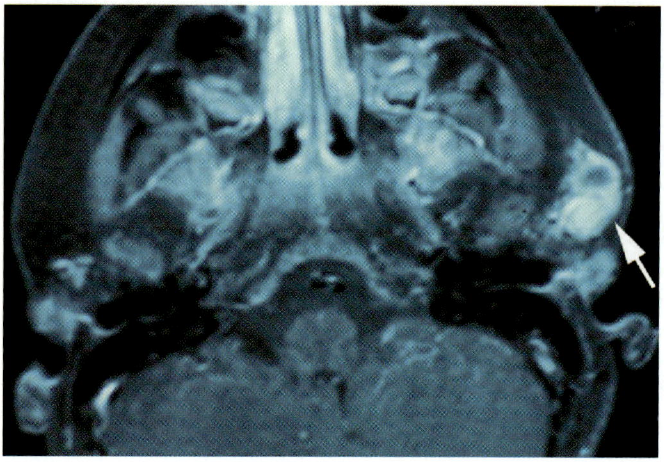

Fig. 13.5: MRI of the neck showing an invasive left parotid mass in a 4-year old boy, suspicious for malignancy (*arrow*). Tissue specimen revealed atypical mycobacterial infection

reservoir [32]. Transmission of *B. henselae* among cats is thought to occur through fleas, and transmission from cats to humans usually occurs by a scratch or bite. The disease typically presents as solitary or regional lymphadenopathy 1–3 weeks after a cat scratch or bite in an immunocompetent host. One or more red-brown papules may be visible at the site of inoculation. Cervical and submandibular lymph nodes are involved in 26% of cases, and preauricular lymph nodes are involved in 7% of cases [32]. Symptoms are usually minor and children usually do not appear to be sick. The overlying skin may appear erythematous and warm. The lymphadenopathy usually resolves spontaneously within 9 weeks, but sometimes can remain up to 12 months, with up to 10% of lesions requiring surgical drainage for suppuration [32]. The diagnosis is suspected based upon patient history and clinical examination, and can be confirmed most easily with serology, in which an indirect fluorescent antibody test and an enzyme immunoassay can detect specific serum antibodies to *B. henselae*. The bacteria can also be identified in tissue specimens with the Warthin-Starry stain reaction, and granulomas with multiple microabscesses are typical histologic features. Although the bacteria are sensitive to many antibiotics in vitro, antibiotics are less effective in clinical practice, due to the intracellular nature of the bacteria. If an antibiotic is used, azithromycin for 5–10 days is recommended, although most authors only recommend an antibiotic for significant morbidity, failure to resolve, or systemic complications [32].

Mumps

One of the classic causes of infectious parotitis in children is mumps, a single-stranded RNA virus belong to the Paramyxoviridae family [16]. The virus is transmitted by droplet spread, with an incubation period of 2–3 weeks, followed by parotid swelling and tenderness (usually bilaterally) in 95% of symptomatic cases. The parotitis is due to direct infection of ductal epithelium, and can be associated with a rise in serum amylase concentrations. During periods of mumps epidemics, the diagnosis can be easily made based upon clinical features alone. However, in the present era of widespread immunization, the disease is uncommon, and may have to be confirmed with serologic testing for mumps-specific IgM antibodies, nearly always detectable by the time of clinical illness. Although at least half of all cases of mumps may involve the central nervous system on the basis of cerebrospinal fluid analysis, significant neurologic complications such as meningitis and encephalitis are fortunately uncommon, as are orchitis and pancreatitis. Before widespread immunization, mumps happened to be one of the most common causes of acquired pediatric sensorineural hearing loss [16]. The outcome for mumps is usually favorable, and even in the presence of neurologic symptoms the fatality rate is only approximately 1%. Treatment is supportive.

Sjögren's Syndrome

Sjögren's syndrome is an idiopathic systemic autoimmune disease that affects the exocrine glands. Classic symptoms in adults include dry eyes (keratoconjunctivitis sicca) and dry mouth (xerostomia) [20]. The disorder is most prevalent in women in their fourth and fifth decades, and has been uncommonly reported in childhood. The presentation in childhood differs from that in adults, in that pediatric cases have a high incidence of recurrent parotitis and parotid gland enlargement (59% of cases) [20]. In adults with Sjögren's syndrome, parotitis is so rare that it is not even included in the diagnostic criteria for the disorder. Children also happen to have a much lower incidence of sicca symptoms (44% of cases), while in adults, sicca symptoms are a hallmark of the disease [20]. Accurate diagnosis in children is difficult, but in recalcitrant cases of recurrent pediatric parotitis, the diagnosis of Sjögren's syndrome should be considered. Diagnosis can be suggested by assessing for SSA or SSB autoantibodies, by obtaining a minor salivary gland biopsy to look for the classic histopathologic changes of chronic lymphocytic infiltration, and via pediatric rheumatology referral [20].

Bulimia Nervosa

Swelling of either the parotid or submandibular glands, usually of a bilateral nature, can be found transiently in up to 29% of bulimia nervosa patients [35]. Bulimia nervosa, in which patients induce vomiting after an episode of binge eating followed by periods of fasting, characteristically begins during the teenage years in young women with a self-image of obesity. The etiology of parotid enlargement is unclear, but may be related to autonomic neuropathy with a resultant build-up of zymogen storage within the acinar cells of the gland [29]. Bulimia nervosa should be considered in the differential diagnosis of unexplained parotid swelling in an otherwise healthy adolescent female patient.

Human Immunodeficiency Virus

Parotid gland hypertrophy is common in children infected with human immunodeficiency virus (HIV), being noted in 25% of cases [13]. The parotid gland enlargement is most likely due to lymphocytic infiltration. Hypertrophy of the parotid gland is much less frequently seen in adults with HIV.

Sialorrhea in the Neurologically Impaired Child

Drooling in the neurologically impaired child represents a major category among the spectrum of salivary gland disorders in the pediatric age group, occurring in up to 50% or more of children with cerebral palsy [45]. Cerebral palsy is a non-progressive disorder of neuromuscular function which occurs in approximately 1 of every 300 newborns [8]. In this setting, typically the salivary glands themselves are free of any intrinsic abnormalities, but rather poor oral motor control and swallowing dysfunction lead to an inability to handle what would otherwise be considered normal production of saliva. Since the underlying neuromuscular deficits are usually incurable, much of the therapy offered for this disorder focuses on either decreasing or redirecting salivary gland secretions.

Sialorrhea is deserving of medical attention in this setting because it increases the workload of caregivers, who frequently have to wipe the affected child's chin (a mean of 73 times per day in one study), replace bibs (mean of 7 times per day), change clothing (often more than once a day), and run up to 25 loads of laundry per week [46]. Clothes, toys, books, and furniture can be regularly damaged, and facial skin can become excoriated and infected. Patient communication strategies also can become more limited due to frequent saliva-induced damage of electronic communication devices, computers, and audio equipment [46], as well as due to the reluctance of people to want to interact with a drooling child [8].

The submandibular glands account for approximately 60–70% of daily saliva production, and tend to secrete saliva at a steady rate throughout the day [8, 15]. It is the viscid saliva produced by the submandibular glands that accounts for the majority of drooling in neurologically devastated children. The saliva produced by the parotid glands is more serous in texture, and accounts for only about 20–25% of resting saliva, increasing its salivary output markedly during eating [8, 15]. The sublingual glands account for only about 5% of total daily saliva production [8].

When evaluating a neurologically impaired child with drooling, it has generally been recommended that a multidisciplinary team approach be taken, with evaluations from an otolaryngologist, speech pathologist, dentist, and pulmonologist, especially if the child is thought to be suffering from chronic or recurrent pulmonary infectious or inflammatory disease from salivary aspiration [8]. The initial evaluation should take into account position and control of head movement, nature of saliva (viscid or watery), tongue size and mobility, evaluation of swallowing function, and nasal, nasopharyngeal, and oropharyngeal obstruction. Correction of gingivitis, adenotonsillar hypertrophy, and other causes of upper airway obstruction should be pursued if feasible, and a head-back wheelchair may also help [8]. Salivary gland irradiation does reduce salivary flow, as evidenced by the xerostomia frequently seen in adults receiving radiation therapy for squamous cell carcinoma of the head and neck, but this modality is no longer recommended for children with sialorrhea due to the potential long-term risks of radiation exposure [40].

Oral Motor Therapy and Biofeedback Techniques

Oral motor training is typically performed by a speech-language pathologist who works with the patient over many sessions, and involves exercises that try to improve lip closure, jaw elevation, and tongue mobility [8]. During the initial intensive training period, drooling has been shown to dramatically and objectively improve in children with cerebral palsy; however, once training is stopped, the beneficial effects seems to gradually wear off over subsequent months [51]. Oral motor training was offered as the primary management option in only 18% of children presenting to a major multidisciplinary drooling center in Toronto, most likely reflecting the fact that such therapy is often either ineffective or difficult to sustain [8]. The new technology of VitalStim, in which pharyngeal muscles are electrically stimulated to try to improve the swallowing mechanism, also holds some promise [7].

Biofeedback therapy for chronic sialorrhea teaches children to swallow more frequently in response to an auditory stimulus. This technique, using an alarm linked to a timer, makes the act of swallowing a conscious one in those patients who are cognizant enough to participate. This type of therapy has been shown to lead to a significant decrease in drooling rates [25]. Drawbacks to this technique include the fact that it is time consuming, labor intensive, and requires highly motivated caregivers and children of adequate age and intelligence to participate. Long-term control of sialorrhea has unfortunately been difficult to achieve with this technique [8, 25].

Pharmacotherapy for Sialorrhea

Anticholinergic medication is the most commonly used pharmacotherapy for neurologically impaired children with chronic drooling. Since secretion of saliva from the salivary glands is controlled by the autonomic nervous system, anticholinergic agents are able to decrease salivation by blocking cholinergic muscarinic receptors, thus inhibiting salivary gland parasympathetic secretomotor innervation. However, the non-selective anticholinergic nature of these medications can lead to a variety of unwanted central and peripheral adverse effects, including constipation, urinary retention, blurred vision, and restlessness. Since most of the children treated would require pharmacotherapy for life, compliance difficulties frequently arise.

Systemic Pharmacotherapy

Glycopyrrolate is a quaternary ammonium compound structurally similar to atropine that is frequently used to control drooling in neurologically impaired children. In a survey of 41 caregivers of children with cerebral palsy, it was found that glycopyrrolate had been used in 37 of the patients, with significant improvement in drooling reported by 95% of the patients [2]. However, side effects such as dry mouth, thick secretions, urinary retention, and flushing were reported in 44% of patients, leading to discontinuation of the medication in nearly a third of the subjects.

In a placebo-controlled, double-blind, crossover dose-ranging study, 39 children with developmental disabilities and excessive drooling were randomized to receive either incrementally increasing doses of glycopyrrolate or placebo [33]. All children who completed the study demonstrated a significant improvement in drooling with glycopyrrolate when compared to placebo, in a dose-dependent fashion. However, adverse effects also occurred in a dose-dependent manner in 69% of those taking glycopyrrolate, leading 7 children (approximately 20%) to withdraw from the study. Side effects included behavioral changes such as restlessness and irritability, constipation, thick secretions, urinary retention, and facial flushing.

Transdermal scopolamine, another systemic anticholinergic medication, is also effective at reducing drooling. This medication, applied as a patch to the skin, allows drug delivery with a stable serum concentration over a 72-h period. In a double-blind, placebo-controlled crossover trial of 18 developmentally delayed children with drooling, the drug lead to a significant reduction of drooling from 24 to 72 h after the patch was applied, with drowsiness reported as the only side effect [4]. In another trial, 10 developmentally delayed children with excessive drooling were randomized in a double-blind, placebo-controlled trial to assess the efficacy and safety of transdermal scopolamine, and over half of the patients had a statistically significant reduction in drooling, with one third having cessation of drooling while wearing the patch [28]. However, like the other anticholinergic medications that have been tried, a variety of side effects have been reported with longer term use [23].

A recent report has noted that administration of modafinil, a psychostimulant used to treat conditions ranging from attention deficit hyperactivity disorder to narcolepsy, incidentally appeared to lead to complete cessation of drooling in two children with cerebral palsy. This remarkable result was presumed to be due to improvements in the muscular coordination of swallowing, and deserves further study [21].

Injectable Salivary Gland Pharmacotherapy (Botulinum Toxin A)

In an attempt to pharmacologically inhibit sialorrhea while minimizing the widespread side effects associated with systemic anticholinergic agents, the injection of botulinum toxin A into major salivary glands has begun to grow in popularity. Botulinum toxin A, a neurotoxin harvested from *Clostridium botulinum*, exerts its effect by inhibiting the release of presynaptic acetylcholine into the synaptic cleft [41]. Since the release of saliva from salivary glands is mediated by acetylcholine released from postganglionic parasympathetic nerve fibers within the salivary gland tissue, botulinum toxin A has been considered as a potential therapeutic option for drooling [41].

The effect of botulinum toxin A in children with severe drooling was first reported in 2002, with a 33% response rate noted with submandibular injections, and an 80% response rate with combined submandibular and parotid injections [44]. Studies of children with cerebral palsy and sialorrhea have shown that the majority of patients experience a reduction in drooling after botulinum toxin A is injected into the submandibular glands [22], or the parotid glands [18, 41], or both [44]. The response rate seems to be higher when submandibular glands are injected, which would be expected given the greater role submandibular secretory activity plays in baseline saliva production and drooling [23]. The beneficial effects on sialorrhea typically peak between 2 to 8 weeks after injection, after which they begin to wear off [23, 41]. Approximately 5–10 (up to 25) total units have been administered per gland, with injections usually occurring bilaterally, at two distinct sites per gland. In order to decrease the likelihood of erroneous needle placement with inadvertent paralysis of muscles involved with mastication and swallowing, ultrasound guidance of the needle has been recommended [18, 22], as has use of an electromyographic needle when injecting the parotid gland [41]. In children with cerebral palsy, the injections are typically performed under general anesthesia [22].

In a controlled clinical trial of children with cerebral palsy and severe drooling, botulinum toxin A injections into the submandibular glands led to a similar drooling response rate (49%) as cutaneous scopolamine application (53%), but 71% of patients receiving scopolamine experienced moderate to severe side effects, whereas patients injected with botulinum toxin A injections suffered only incidental, minor adverse side effects [23].

Although botulinum toxin A is not yet generally accepted as the first choice for controlling sialorrhea, it seems to have certain advantages over other pharmacologic options in children. The primary disadvantage appears to be the need for repeated injections, typically under general anesthesia.

Surgical Interventions for Sialorrhea

Surgical intervention targeting the major salivary glands ideally would be reserved for those neurologically impaired children who have failed at least 6 months of oral motor therapy, whose intellectual or physical disability is too severe for conservative treatment to be effective, and who are old enough (generally at least 6 years old) that no further maturation of swallowing function would be expected [8, 15].

The two general types of operations intended to help manage sialorrhea are those that try to decrease saliva production, and those that attempt to redirect the flow of saliva so that it may be swallowed more readily.

Procedures Designed to Redirect the Flow of Saliva

Relocation of the Parotid Duct

One of the earlier attempts to redirect saliva toward the oropharynx was described by Wilkie and Brody, who in 1977 reported their 10-year experience with relocation of the parotid duct into the tonsillar fossae, preceded by tonsillectomy and performed in conjunction with excision of the submandibular gland [48]. Although good control of sialorrhea was reported in 90% of patients, there was a high rate of complications (35% of cases), including wound breakdown, stenosis of the parotid duct, impaired oral hygiene with increased dental and gingival infections, and septic parotitis. This surgical strategy was generally abandoned by the mid 1980s due its morbidity [8].

Submandibular Duct Relocation

As it became increasingly understood that the submandibular glands were the main problem in sialorrhea, submandibular duct relocation emerged as one of the surgical procedures of choice for sialorrhea. With this procedure, an elliptical incision is made around the papilla of each submandibular duct, creating a mucosal island. The submandibular duct is dissected posteriorly, and the released papilla is threaded submucosally and sutured to the base of the tongue at an exit perforation [15]. Tonsillectomy is performed first, if indicated, based on tonsil size or chronic infection.

In 1989 and 1995, two major multidisciplinary centers for the treatment of drooling reported large series of the submandibular duct relocation technique for sialorrhea in neurologically disabled children [9, 47]. Drooling was reduced significantly in the majority of patients, and the high rate of complications seen with parotid duct rerouting was avoided. However, ranulas requiring intraoral sublingual gland excision occurred in 8–13% of patients [9, 47].

In 2001, clinicians working at the Drooling Control Clinic in Toronto reported that the addition of sublingual gland excision to the submandibular duct relocation procedure minimized the risk of postoperative ranula formation, while still maintaining the beneficial impact of the surgery on drooling [10]. This experience was also reproduced at the Saliva Control Clinic at the Royal Children's Hospital in Melbourne, Australia, where submandibular duct transposition combined with sublingual gland excision led to successful control of drooling in 66% of patients 5 years postoperatively, with no postoperative ranulae noted [15]. However, major complications still occurred in 10% of patients, including bleeding, tongue swelling with airway obstruction, submandibular abscess, lingual nerve injury, and aspiration pneumonia.

Procedures Designed to Decrease Salivary Flow

Tympanic Neurectomy

Tympanic neurectomy is a procedure in which the postganglionic parasympathetic nerve fibers providing secretomotor innervation to the parotid and submandibular glands are divided as they course through the middle ear. Through a standard tympanomeatal flap approach, division of the chorda tympani nerve (conveying secretomotor fibers to the submandibular and sublingual glands) and the tympanic plexus (containing similar fibers destined for the parotid glands) can be achieved. Since the 1970s, this procedure has been largely abandoned because, in addition to causing loss of taste, it has been reported that many patients resume their preoperative level of drooling within 6 months of surgery [8].

Bilateral Excision of the Submandibular Gland and Ligation of the Parotid Duct

Since 1984, bilateral excision of the submandibular gland, combined with ligation of the parotid duct, has been the treatment of choice for chronic sialorrhea at Children's Hospital in Cincinnati [43]. In a review of 93 children with chronic sialorrhea who underwent this procedure from 1988 to 1997, there were only 12 postoperative complications: xerostomia in 7 children, an increase in dental caries in 2 children, and one case each of wound hematoma, marked transient parotid gland swelling, and parotitis. With an average follow-up of 4.2 years, significant improvement in drooling was noted in 65% of patients, with cessation of drooling noted in 21%. This approach has also been the standard surgical approach for many years at Children's Hospital of Pittsburgh.

Bilateral Ligation of the Submandibular Duct and Ligation of the Parotid Duct

A recent report describing ligation of the submandibular duct also adds to the technique available for the management of drooling procedures [24]. The physiologic rationale behind the success of salivary duct ligation is believed to be functional atrophy of the affected gland [24]. Five children with cerebral palsy and recurrent pneumonitis due to aspirated saliva underwent bilateral submandibular and parotid duct ligation. Aside from a brief period of mild postoperative swelling, there were no adverse effects, and caregivers of every patient reported a substantial decrease in the amount of drooling, with no ranula formation and no xerostomia (median follow-up 13 months). One of the main beneficial features of this technique is the ease and rapidity with which it can be performed, although long-term results are not yet known.

Controversies Regarding Ligation of the Parotid Duct

For neurologically impaired children with problematic sialorrhea, it has been generally accepted that relocation of the parotid duct is fraught with complications, whereas parotidectomy is too aggressive an approach. Thus, transoral ligation of the parotid duct has emerged as the simplest and most feasible surgical option to pursue, should one choose to address the parotid gland surgically in this setting. However, vigorous debate exists regarding whether or not this procedure needs to be done at all, and as to what effect it may have on dental hygiene, xerostomia, and the thickness of oral secretions.

In one large series of neurologically impaired children with sialorrhea, unilateral ligation of the parotid duct (performed in conjunction with relocation of the submandibular duct) was blamed for complications such as thick, unmanageable saliva (46% of patients), xerostomia with oral crusting (32%), dysphagia (21%), and a high rate of dental caries [47]. Once ligation of the parotid duct was abandoned in favor of relocation of the submandibular duct with excision of the sublingual gland, the majority of these problems anecdotally resolved [15].

Aware that most problematic drooling arises from the submandibular glands, the Drooling Control Clinic in Toronto reserves ligation of the parotid duct only for those children in whom there is persistent watery sialorrhea after relocation of the submandibular duct with ligation of the parotid duct; this "back-up" procedure has only needed to be performed in approximately 3% of their patients [8].

However, bilateral parotid duct ligation in combination with bilateral excision of the submandibular gland has been the procedure of choice for chronic sialorrhea at Children's Hospital in Cincinnati for decades, with very low rates of xerostomia and dental caries [43]. Thus, the debate regarding whether or not to perform parotid duct ligation for sialorrhea, and under what circumstances, remains unresolved.

Controversies Regarding Excision of Submandibular Glands, Relocation and Ligation of the Duct

Those in favor of relocation of the submandibular ducts have argued that it is not logical to ligate the ducts of these major salivary glands, since the problem in children with cerebral palsy is usually not one of overproduction of saliva, but rather one of inability to direct saliva adequately from the mouth to the throat [15]. By relocating the submandibular ducts, physiologic saliva production is preserved, while reducing drooling, and reducing complications such as severe xerostomia, thick secretions, and dental caries [15].

Conversely, those who advocate surgical techniques that reduce saliva production (such as ligation of the submandibular duct or excision of the gland) argue that the increased posterior oropharyngeal salivary flow caused by submandibular duct relocation could increase the likelihood of contamination of the lower respiratory tract in children who, due to their neuromuscular swallowing disorders, may be prone to aspiration [43]. Advocates of major ductal ligation and gland excision presume that enough minor salivary gland saliva production persists to prevent xerostomia and dental caries in most patients undergoing these procedures [43].

Take Home Messages

- Most masses found within the salivary glands in the pediatric age group consist of either vascular anomalies or infectious intra- or perisalivary adenopathy, with glandular epithelial tumors being extremely rare.
- The rarity of salivary gland neoplasms in the pediatric age group should be taken into account during evaluation of the mass in the salivary gland, and the other more likely diagnoses in the differential must be considered and ruled out.
- In the absence of a true glandular neoplasm, parotidectomy and excision of the submandibular glands is rarely required for masses in the salivary glands, but many other less aggressive techniques, both surgical and pharmacologic, can be considered depending on the diagnosis.
- Problematic sialorrhea in neurologically impaired children can be managed with oral motor therapy, systemic anticholinergic medication, salivary gland injection with botulinum toxin A, relocation of the salivary ducts, ligation of the salivary duct, or excision of the glands; a multidisciplinary approach is advisable to help with this complex decision-making process.

References

1. Alqahtani A, Nguyen LT, Flageole H, et al. (1999) 25 years' experience with lymphangiomas in children. J Pediatr Surg 34:1164–1168
2. Bachrach SJ, Walter RS, Trzcinski K (1998) Use of glycopyrrolate and other anticholinegic medications for sialorrhea in children with cerebral palsy. Clin Pediatr (Phila) 37:485–590
3. Bentz BG, Hughes CA, Lüdemann JP, et al. (2000) Masses of the salivary gland region in children. Arch Otolaryngol Head Neck Surg 126:1435–1439
4. Brodtkorb E, Wyzocka-Bakowska MM, Lillevold PE, et al. (1988) Transdermal scopolamine in drooling. J Ment Defic Res 32:233–237

5. Camacho AE, Goodman ML, Eavey RD (1989) Pathologic correlation of the unknown solid parotid mass in children. Otolaryngol Head Neck Surg 101:566–571
6. Castro EB, Huvos AG, Strong EW, et al. (1972) Tumors of the major salivary glands in children. Cancer 29:312–317
7. Chetney R, Waro K (2004) A new home health approach to swallowing disorders. Home Health Nurse 22:703–707
8. Crysdale WS, The Management of Drooling. In: Bluestone CD, Stool SE, Alper CM, Arjmand EM, Casselbrant ML, Dohar JD, Yellon RF (2003) Pediatric Otolaryngology. Saunders Philadelphia 1138–1148
9. Crysdale WS, White A (1989) Submandibular duct relocation for drooling: a 10-year experience with 194 patients. Otolaryngol Head Neck Surg 101:87–92
10. Crysdale WS, Raveh E, McCann C, et al. (2001) Management of drooling in individuals with neurodisability: a surgical experience. Dev Med Child Neurol 43:379–383
11. Giglio MS, Landaeta M, Pinto ME (1997) Microbiology of recurrent parotitis. Pediatr Infect Dis J 16:386–390
12. Giguère CM, Bauman NM, Sato Y, et al. (2002) Treatment of lymphangiomas with OK-432 (picibanil) sclerotherapy. Arch Otolaryngol Head Neck Surg 128:1137–1144
13. Gondim LA, Zonta RF, Fortkamp E, et al. (2000) Otorhinolaryngological manifestations in children with human immunodeficiency virus infection. Int J Pediatr Otorhinolaryngol 54:97–102
14. Greene AK, Rogers GF, Mulliken JB (2004) Management of parotid hemangioma in 100 children. Plast Reconstr Surg 113:53–60
15. Greensmith AL, Johnstone BR, Reid SM, et al. (2005) Prospective analysis of the outcome of surgical management of drooling in the pediatric population: a 10-year experience. Plast Reconstr Surg 116:1233–1242
16. Gupta RK, Best J, MacMahon E (2005) Mumps and the UK epidemic 2005. BMJ 330:1132–1135
17. Hamoir M, Plouin-Gaudon I, Rombaux P, et al. (2001) Lymphatic malformations of the head and neck: a retrospective review and a support for staging. Head Neck 23:326–337
18. Hassin-Baer S, Scheuer E, Buchman AS, et al. (2005) Botulinum toxin injections for children with excessive drooling. J Child Neurol 20:120–123
19. Hockstein NG, Samadi DS, Gendron K, et al. (2004) Pediatric submandibular triangle masses: a fifteen-year experience. Head Neck 26:675–680
20. Houghton K, Malleson P, Cabral D, et al. (2005) Primary Sjögren's syndrome in children and adolescents: are proposed diagnostic criteria applicable? J Rheumatol 32:2225–2232
21. Hurst D, Cedrone N (2006) Modafinil for drooling in cerebral palsy. J Child Neurol 21:112–114
22. Jongerius PH, Joosten F, Hoogen FJA, et al. (2003) The treatment of drooling by ultrasound-guided intraglandular injections of botulinum toxin type A into the salivary glands. Laryngoscope 113:107–111
23. Jongerius PH, van den Hoogen FJ, van Limbeek J, et al. (2004) Effect of botulinum toxin in the treatment of drooling: a controlled clinical trial. Pediatrics 114:620–627
24. Klem C, Mair EA (1999) Four-duct ligation: a simple and effective treatment for chronic aspiration from sialorrhea. Arch Otolaryngol Head Neck Surg 125:796–800
25. Koheil R, Sochaniwskyj AE, Bablich K, et al. (1987) Biofeedback techniques and behaviour modification in the conservative remediation of drooling by children with cerebral palsy. Dev Med Child Neurol 29:19–26
26. Kono T, Sakurai H, Groff WF, et al. (2006) Comparison study of a traditional pulsed dye laser versus a long-pulsed dye laser in the treatment of early childhood hemangiomas. Lasers Surg Med 38:112–115
27. Krolls SO, Trodahl JN, Boyers RC (1972) Salivary gland lesions in children. A survey of 430 cases. Cancer 30:459–469
28. Lewis DW, Fontana C, Mehallick LK, et al. (1994) Transdermal scopolamine for reduction of drooling in developmentally delayed children. Dev Med Child Neurol 36:484–486
29. Mandel L, Abai S (2004) Diagnosing bulimia nervosa with parotid gland swelling. J Am Dent Assoc 135:613–616
30. Mandell DL (2000) Head and neck anomalies related to the branchial apparatus. Otolaryngol Clin North Am 33:1309–1332
31. Mandell DL, Wald ER, Michaels MG, et al. (2003) Management of nontuberculous mycobacterial cervical lymphadenitis. Arch Otolaryngol Head Neck Surg 129:341–344
32. Massei F, Gori L, Macchia P, et al. (2005) The expanded spectrum of bartonellosis in children. Infect Dis Clin North Am 19:691–711
33. Mier RJ, Bachrach SJ, Lakin RC, et al. (2000) Treatment of sialorrhea with glycopyrrolate: a double-blind, dose-ranging study. Arch Pediatr Adolesc Med 154:1214–1218
34. Ogata H, Ebihara S, Mukai K (1994) Salivary gland neoplasms in children. Jpn J Clin Oncol 24:88–93
35. Ogren FP, Huerter JV, Pearson PH, et al. (1987) Transient salivary gland hypertrophy in bulimics. Laryngoscope 97:951–953
36. Orvidas LJ, Kasperbauer JL, Lewis JE, et al. (2000) Pediatric parotid masses. Arch Otolaryngol Head Neck Surg 126:177–184

37. Ozen IO, Moralioglu S, Karabulut R, et al. (2005) Surgical treatment of cervicofacial cystic hygromas in children. ORL J Otorhinolaryngol Relat Spec 67:331–334
38. Rahbar R, Grimmer F, Vargas SO, et al. (2006) Mucoepidermoid carcinoma of the parotid gland in children. Arch Otolaryngol Head Neck Surg 132:375–380
39. Ricciardelli EJ, Richardson MA (1991) Cervicofacial cystic hygroma. Patterns of recurrence and management of the difficult case. Arch Otolaryngol Head Neck Surg 117:546–553
40. Robinson AC, Khoury GG, Robinson PM (1989) Role of irradiation in the suppression of parotid secretions. J Laryngol Otol 103:594–595
41. Savarese R, Diamond M, Elovic E, et al. (2004) Intraparotid injection of botulinum toxin A as a treatment to control sialorrhea in children with cerebral palsy. Am J Phys Med Rehabil 83:304–311
42. Spiegel R, Miron D, Sakran W, et al. (2004) Acute neonatal suppurative parotitis: case reports and review. Pediatr Infect Dis J 23:76–78
43. Stern Y, Feinmesser R, Collins M, et al. (2002) Bilateral submandibular gland excision with parotid duct ligation for treatment of sialorrhea in children. Arch Otolaryngol Head Neck Surg 128:801–803
44. Suskind DL, Tilton A (2002) Clinical study of botulinum-A toxin in the treatment of sialorrhea in children with cerebral palsy. Laryngoscope 112:73–81
45. Tahmassebi JF, Curzon ME (2003) Prevalence of drooling in children with cerebral palsy attending special schools. Dev Med Child Neurol 45:613–617
46. Van der Burg JJW, Jongerius PH, Van Hulst K, et al. (2006) Drooling in children with cerebral palsy: effect of salivary flow reduction on daily life and care. Dev Med Child Neurol 48:103–107
47. Webb K, Reddihough DS, Johnson H (1995) Long-term outcome of saliva-control surgery. Dev Med Child Neurol 37:755–762
48. Wilkie TF, Brody GS (1977) The surgical treatment of drooling. A ten-year review. Plast Reconstr Surg 59:791–797
49. Witman PM, Wagner AM, Scherer K, et al. (2006) Complications following pulsed dye laser treatment of superficial hemangiomas. Lasers Surg Med 38:116–123
50. Work WP (1972) Newer concepts of first branchial cleft defects. Laryngoscope 82:1581–1593
51. Yam WKL, Yang HLC, Abdullah V, et al. (2006) Management of drooling for children with neurological problems in Hong Kong. Brain Dev 28:24–29
52. Zhao YF, Jia Y, Chen XM, et al. (2004) Clinical review of 580 ranulas. Oral Surg Oral Med Oral Pathol Oral Radiol Endod 98:281–287

Chapter 14

Superficial Parotidectomy

14

Steven J. Wang and David W. Eisele

Contents

Core Features

- Indications
- Preoperative evaluation
- Surgical technique
- First branchial cleft anomaly excision
- Complications

Complications to Avoid

- Injury to the facial nerve
- Hemorrhage or hematoma
- Infection
- External otitis
- Skin-flap necrosis
- Intraoperative tumor rupture

Introduction

Superficial lobe parotidectomy describes removal of all or a portion of the parotid gland superficial to the facial nerve. The most common indications for this operative procedure are a neoplasm of the superficial lobe of the parotid gland, metastases to parotid lymph nodes from adjacent sites of skin cancer or melanoma, or from cancer of the external auditory meatus [1–4]. Another indication is access to the deep lobe of the gland or other structures deep to the facial nerve. Superficial parotidectomy may also be a component of first branchial cleft cyst resection or the management of chronic parotid sialadenitis [5–10]. Rarely, superficial parotidectomy is performed for cosmesis in cases of sialosis.

Preoperative Evaluation

A thorough history is obtained prior to consideration for surgery. Most patients with parotid neoplasms note a progressively enlarging asymptomatic mass. Pain can be associated with some neoplasms but is not a reliable indicator of malignancy. Symptoms of sensory loss, trismus, and facial weakness are worrisome for local tumor invasion by a malignant neoplasm [11–14]. The past medical history should include information regarding any prior cutaneous lesions or malignancies. In addition, the patient should be queried about any prior radiation exposure to the head and neck including dental radiographs. Smoking is associated with Warthin's tumor and, therefore, should be investigated [15–18]. This tumor can also occur bilaterally, thus any history of a prior parotid tumor should be elicited.

All patients should have a complete examination of the head and neck. Cranial nerve function should be examined and facial nerve function should be evaluated carefully. Facial nerve paralysis is usually an indication of nerve invasion by a malignant tumor. Facial weakness may be subtle and may involve only one branch or the entire facial nerve or facial muscle fasciculations may be noted. Fixation to the overlying skin, limited mobility of the mass, and associated cervical lymphadenopathy are other signs suggestive of malignancy.

Fine-needle aspiration biopsy (FNAB) is an accurate and useful investigation for the diagnosis of a parotid mass [19–21]. FNAB allows for improved patient selection for surgery since it can identify conditions such as reactive lymph nodes or cysts that might mimic parotid neoplasms clinically. The information gained by FNAB is useful for patient counseling, surgical timing and planning, and guiding the direction of preoperative consultation (see Chapter 8, Fine-needle Aspiration Biopsy).

Imaging studies are helpful to assess malignant neoplasms or neoplasms that are large, have diminished mobility, suspected local invasion or deep extension. In general, magnetic resonance imaging (MRI) is the preferred imaging study for parotid neoplasms (see Chapter 2, Imaging of the Salivary Glands).

Technique

Superficial parotidectomy is performed under general anesthesia. Long-term paralytic agents are avoided to allow for facial nerve monitoring. After the induction of general anesthesia, the endotracheal tube is positioned in the contralateral oral cavity and secured by tape on the contralateral face only. A modified Blair incision is planned in a preauricular crease coursing around the ear lobule and then into an upper neck crease (Fig. 14.1). An alternative incision is a modified face-lift incision. Methylene blue can be used to mark points along the proposed incision, which facilitates proper wound alignment and closure. The ipsilateral face is prepared with an antiseptic solution and the surgical field is draped with a transparent adhesive sterile drape to allow visualization of facial motion (Fig. 14.2). If electrophysiologic facial nerve monitoring is to be used intraoperatively, nerve electrodes are placed in the ipsilateral facial muscles and tested for electrical integrity.

The skin incision is made with a scalpel and carried down through the subcutaneous tissues and platysma muscle (Fig. 14.3). Care is taken to avoid division of the greater auricular nerve. An anterior flap is elevated superficial to the greater auricular nerve and the parotid fascia (Fig. 14.4). Elevation of a thick flap is desirable to reduce the occurrence of Frey's syndrome while carefully avoiding violation of any neoplasm at the surface of the gland. As the flap is elevated toward the anterior aspect of the gland, the peripheral branches of the facial nerve are carefully avoided. A posterior, inferior flap is also elevated to expose the tail of the parotid gland. After elevation, the flaps are retracted with silk sutures or self-retaining hooks.

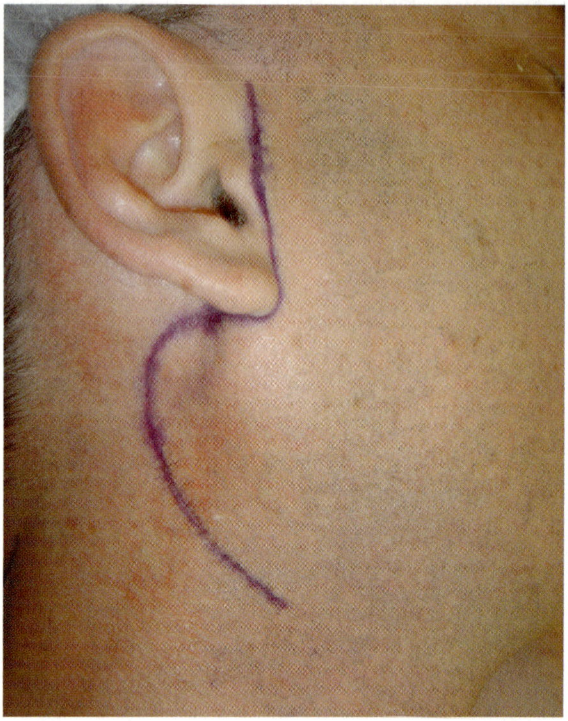

Fig. 14.1: Modified Blair incision marked

The tail of the parotid gland is dissected off of the sternocleidomastoid muscle by dissecting deep to the posterior branch of the greater auricular nerve, if preservation of this nerve is feasible based on tumor location. Next, the posterior belly of the digastric muscle is exposed with further elevation of the tail of the parotid gland (Fig. 14.5). The posterior belly of the digastric muscle serves as a landmark for the facial nerve. During elevation of the tail of the parotid, the integrity of the posterior facial vein also is preserved if possible. The facial nerve usually courses superficial to this vessel and division of this structure can contribute to increased venous bleeding during dissection of the gland. Occasionally some or all of the branches of the facial nerve will be found deep to the vein.

The preauricular space is opened by division of the attachments of the parotid gland to the cartilaginous external auditory canal with blunt and sharp dissection. This plane of dissection exposes the tragal cartilage pointer,

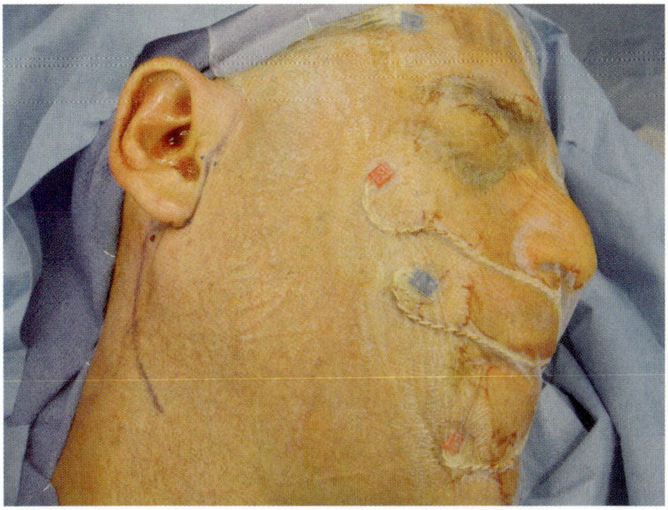

Fig. 14.2: Operative field draped. Electrodes for facial nerve monitoring are in position

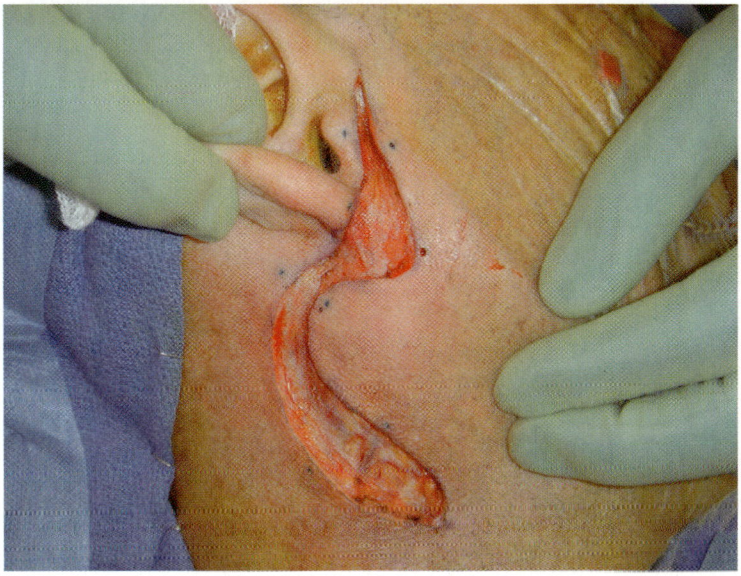

Fig. 14.3: Incision through skin and subcutaneous tissue. The greater auricular nerve is preserved

which serves as another landmark for the facial nerve. A wide plane of dissection from the zygoma to the digastric muscle is created to facilitate exposure of the facial nerve. Hemostasis is assured with bipolar electrocautery as indicated.

The gland is carefully retracted anteriorly. This exposes the operative field for identification of the facial nerve. Care must be taken to avoid pressure or traction injury of the facial nerve during retraction of the gland. The facial nerve is identified using anatomic landmarks, which include the posterior belly of the digastric muscle, the mastoid tip, the tragal cartilage pointer, and the tympanomastoid suture. If the proximal segment of the facial nerve is obscured, retrograde dissection of one or more of the peripheral facial nerve branches may be necessary to identify the main trunk. When necessary, the facial nerve can be identified in the mastoid bone by mastoidectomy and followed peripherally.

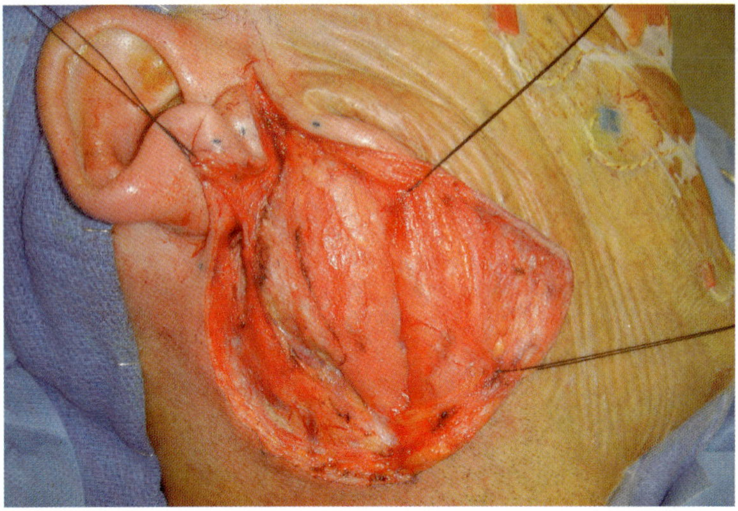

Fig. 14.4: Elevation of anterior flap

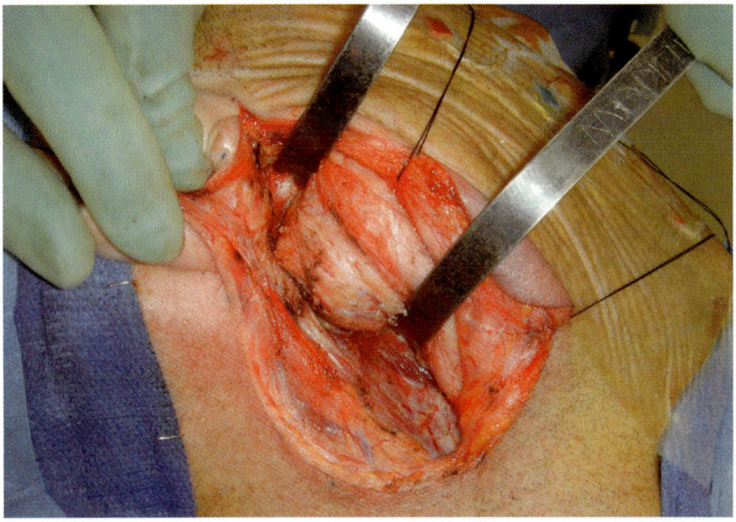

Fig. 14.5: Elevation of tail of parotid gland from sternocleidomastoid muscle and posterior belly of the digastric muscle with preservation of the posterior branch of the greater auricular nerve

Once the facial nerve is identified, the parotid gland superficial to the facial nerve is divided carefully, preserving the integrity of the nerve (Fig. 14.6). A McCabe dissector (an angled ratchetless dissecting clamp) is useful for dissection of the proximal facial nerve. The dissector is passed along the facial nerve, lifted, and then gently spread. The gland superficial to the exposed segment of the facial nerve is then carefully divided. The exact location of the facial nerve should always be determined prior to division of the gland tissue. Anatomic distortion by a neoplasm or operative manipulation must be considered. Various instruments are acceptable for the division of parotid gland tissue and include a standard scalpel, scissors, the Hemostatix scalpel, the harmonic scalpel, bipolar scissors, and the Ligasure Precise [22–24]. Any bleeding that occurs related to division of the gland is carefully controlled. Complete hemostasis is necessary to maintain a clear operative field relative to the facial nerve. The facial nerve is followed peripherally, the desired portion of the gland is dissected from successive facial nerve branches (Figs. 14.7, 14.8), and the specimen removed. In cases of previous parotid surgery or recurrent tumor, the usual dissection described above is not always possible. Retrograde dissection is an option and requires identifi-

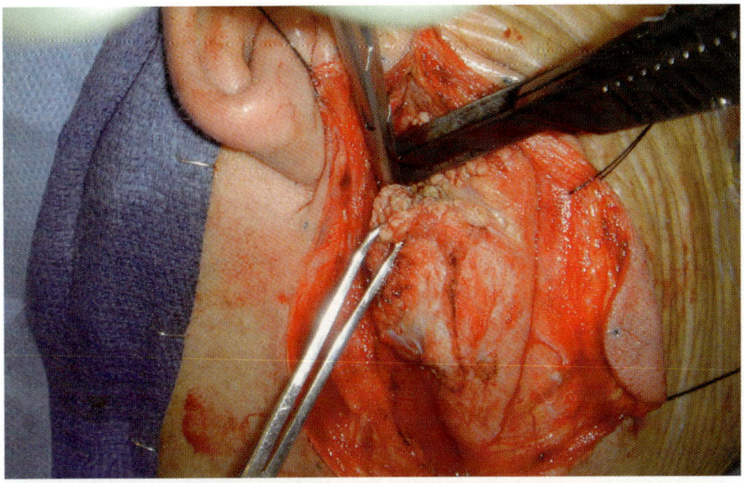

Fig. 14.6: Parotid gland divided superficial to the main trunk of the facial nerve

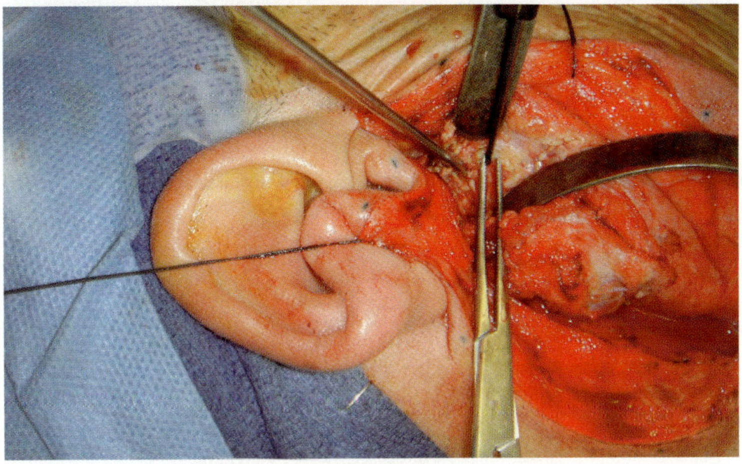

Fig. 14.7: Exposure of the buccal branch of the facial nerve

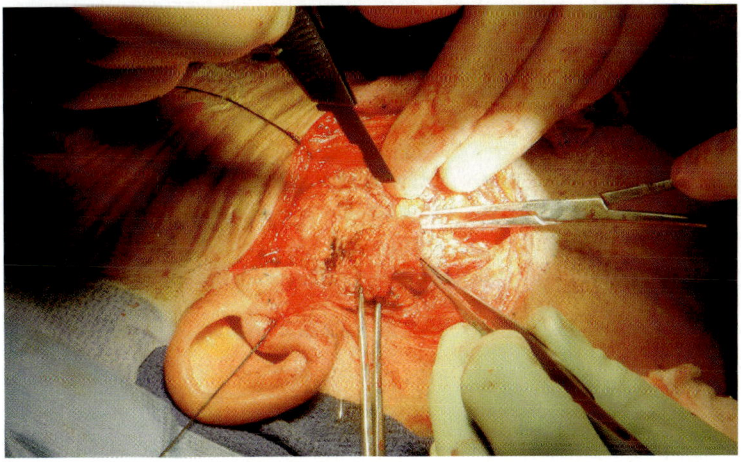

Fig. 14.8: Retrograde dissection of a peripheral facial nerve branch

cation of a peripheral branch and dissection of it proximally until the main trunk is identified.

The facial nerve is preserved except in cases when confirmed malignancy is found invading the nerve. In instances of facial nerve invasion by carcinoma, facial nerve resection is performed. Proximal and distal margins of the resected nerve are examined histologically by frozen section to ensure clear surgical margins. If the tumor involves the stylomastoid foramen, mastoidectomy is performed to identify the proximal facial nerve in the fallopian canal to achieve a clear margin. Immediate nerve reconstruction by a nerve interposition graft is usually indicated if facial nerve resection is performed. This topic is addressed in greater detail in Chapters 24, Facial Nerve Reconstruction, and 26, Reconstruction after Excision of Cancer of the Salivary Glands.

After the superficial portion of the gland is removed, the wound is carefully inspected and bleeding sites are controlled with bipolar electrocautery or ligatures (Figs. 14.9, 14.10). The integrity of the facial nerve is confirmed visually and by electrical stimulation of the main trunk of the facial nerve and all the peripheral branches. If any injured facial nerve branches are identified, they are repaired immediately using a microscopic repair technique.

A neck dissection is performed for clinically positive nodes. For the clinically negative neck, the first echelon nodes are inspected. Enlarged or suspicious nodes are examined and a neck dissection is performed if metastatic disease is confirmed by frozen section.

The wound is irrigated, realigned, and closed in layers over a closed-suction drain (Fig. 14.11). The drain is usually removed on the first postoperative day and the skin sutures are removed within one week.

Adjuvant radiation therapy is recommended for select malignancies including metastatic cutaneous squamous cell carcinoma, high-grade and advanced parotid malignancies, and other select malignancies.

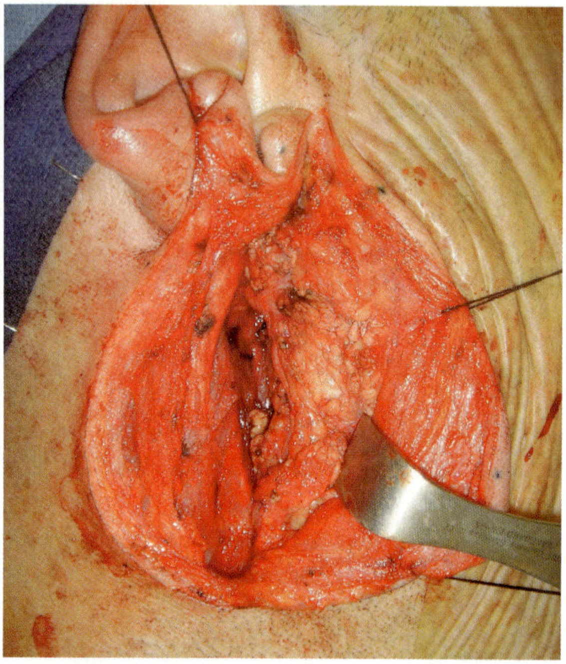

Fig. 14.9: Specimen removed with facial nerve integrity confirmed

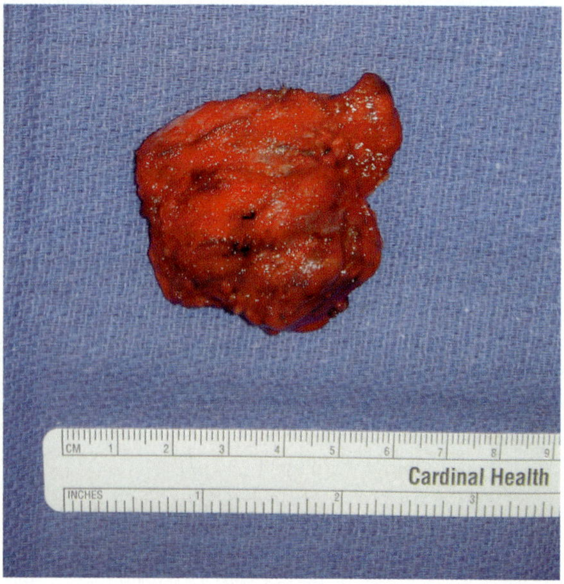

Fig. 14.10: Surgical specimen

First Branchial Cleft Anomaly Excision

First branchial cleft anomalies are uncommon developmental malformations that are anatomically in close proximity to the parotid gland and facial nerve [3–9, 25–27]. Thus, the management of these anomalies is described in this chapter. Anomalies of the first branchial cleft are thought to arise from embryologic development

14

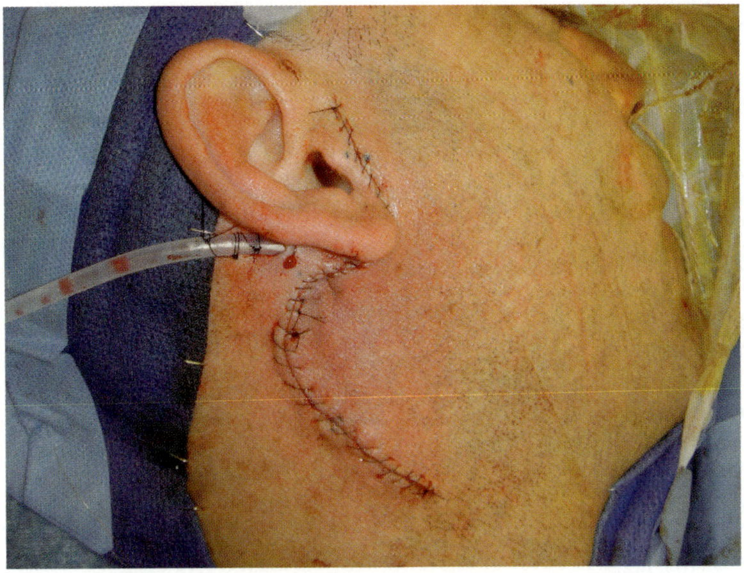

Fig. 14.11: Wound closed in layers over a closed suction drain

defects of the first branchial cleft and first branchial arch. They are rare, representing fewer than 10% of all branchial cleft anomalies [5].

A brief review of fetal embryologic development of the branchial arches is necessary to understand the proper management of first branchial cleft anomalies [25]. The six paired branchial arches are composed of ectodermal, mesodermal, and endodermal elements. Each arch is separated by a closing membrane, dividing the inner pharyngeal pouch from the outer branchial cleft, and contains muscle, skin, cartilage, and one cranial nerve. The facial nerve develops with the first branchial arch. The first branchial cleft persists as the external auditory canal, while the first pharyngeal pouch gives rise to the middle ear, mastoid antrum, and Eustachian tube. The parotid gland develops as an outward evagination of the gut endothelium and envelops the facial nerve. Thus, first branchial cleft anomalies may be intimately associated with the parotid gland and facial nerve.

First branchial cleft anomalies were classified by Work into two types [27]. Type I first branchial cleft anomalies represent a duplication anomaly of the membranous ear canal, while type II first branchial cleft anomalies are duplication anomalies of the membranous and cartilaginous ear canal. Type I first branchial cleft anomalies are often located close to the ear and parotid gland, while type II anomalies often present as a recurrent abscess in the neck. Clinical recognition of first branchial cleft anomalies, however, can be difficult. Suspicion of this diagnosis should be entertained in any patient with otorrhea in the absence of chronic otitis, with a cutaneous opening anterior to the sternocleidomastoid muscle in the suprahyoid neck, or with an isolated parotid cyst that fluctuates in size.

Because of frequent infections and misdiagnosis, appropriate treatment of first branchial cleft anomalies is often delayed. Definitive treatment requires complete surgical excision. The standard surgical approach involves wide exposure of the lesion with a parotidectomy with identification and protection of the facial nerve. This is particularly important in patients who have had recurrent infections or previous surgical procedures. Electrophysiologic monitoring of the facial nerve can be useful in these challenging cases [28]. The fistulous tract may be superficial to, deep to, or wrapped around the facial nerve. It is also crucial to excise any skin and cartilage surrounding the fistula near the external auditory canal, to ensure complete resection.

Complications

There are both early and late complications of superficial parotidectomy (Table 14.1). Facial nerve paresis or paralysis can occur as an early complication. Temporary facial nerve paralysis involving all or just one of the branches of the nerve occurs in 10–30% of superficial parotidectomies [29–33]. Permanent facial nerve paralysis occurs in less than 1% of superficial parotidectomies [32, 33]. The nerve at most risk for injury during superficial parotidectomy is the marginal mandibular branch of the facial nerve [31–33].

Excessive stimulation of the nerve with a battery-powered nerve stimulator may be responsible for a temporary facial nerve paresis. Temporary facial nerve paresis usually resolves from weeks to months postoperatively. Complete nerve transection can occur during surgery. Nerve transection requires immediate microsurgical repair.

Hemorrhage or hematoma is an uncommon early complication of superficial parotidectomy and is usually related to incomplete hemostasis during the procedure. Treatment consists of returning the patient to the operating room and, under general anesthesia, evacuation of the hematoma and surgical control of any identified bleeding vessels is carried out.

Infection is uncommon after superficial parotidectomy and is avoided by the use of aseptic techniques and careful handling of tissues. Perioperative antibiotics are not used. The rarity of infection is probably related to the rich vascular supply to the parotid region. Treatment of infection consists of appropriate antibiotics. Abscess formation is rare after superficial parotidectomy and requires surgical drainage and antibiotics.

External otitis can occur postoperatively and can be related to intraoperative blood collection in the external auditory canal. A petrolatum gauze pack placed in the external auditory canal can prevent blood entry during the procedure. Treatment of external otitis consists of cleaning the auditory canal and instillation of antibiotic ear drops.

Skin-flap necrosis is an uncommon complication. When it occurs it is usually located in the distal tip of the postauricular skin flap. Care must be taken to avoid compromise of the vascular supply to this portion of the skin flap. Smoking, prior radiation therapy, and diabetes mellitus may contribute to this complication due to impairment of the blood supply to the flap. Treatment of flap necrosis consists of conservative debridement of necrotic tissue and local wound care.

Mild trismus may occur following superficial parotidectomy and may be related to inflammation and fibrosis of the masseter muscle. This complication usually resolves with range of motion exercises of the jaw.

Table 14.1. Complications of superficial parotidectomy

Early complications	Late complications
Facial nerve paresis or paralysis	Frey's syndrome
Bleeding/hematoma	Hypertrophic scar or keloid
Infection	Recurrent tumor
Skin flap necrosis	Poor cosmesis
Salivary fistula/sialocele	Soft tissue deficit
Seroma	
External otitis	
Trismus	

Salivary fistula or sialocele can occur in approximately 10% of cases of superficial parotidectomy [34]. This problem is a result of leakage of saliva from remaining salivary gland tissue that collects beneath the flap or drains from the wound. This complication is usually mild and self-limited. Treatment of a sialocele consists of repeated needle aspirations. A salivary fistula is managed with local wound care. A chronic salivary fistula is rare following superficial parotidectomy.

Frey's syndrome or gustatory sweating is a relatively common long-term complication of superficial parotidectomy [35]. This complication is thought to be related to aberrant regeneration of nerve fibers from the postganglionic secretomotor parasympathetic innervation of the parotid gland to the severed postganglionic sympathetic fibers that supply the sweat glands of the skin of the face. As a result, sweating with or without dermal flushing occurs during salivary stimulation. If objective testing is performed, Frey's syndrome occurs in the majority of patients undergoing superficial parotidectomy. Only about 10% of patients, however, complain of symptomatic Frey's syndrome.

Most patients with Frey's syndrome do not seek therapy. Medical treatment of symptomatic Frey's syndrome includes topical application of antiperspirant, topical anticholinergics (1% glycopyrrolate), or injections of botulinum toxin (see Chapter 5, Treatment of Frey's Syndrome).

Take Home Messages

- Superficial parotidectomy is typically indicated for benign or malignant neoplasms of the parotid gland and metastases from adjacent skin cancers or external auditory canal tumors.
- Preoperative evaluation for superficial parotidectomy includes a complete history and thorough head and neck examination; fine-needle aspiration biopsy and MRI are often helpful.
- Knowledge of anatomy and meticulous surgical technique are essential.
- Facial nerve monitoring may facilitate safe, complete removal of parotid lesions, particularly in reoperations.
- First branchial cleft anomalies are often intimately associated with the facial nerve and parotid gland, and their complete excision with facial nerve preservation is necessary.
- Understanding potential complications that may be associated with superficial parotidectomy is necessary for appropriate postoperative management.

References

1. Guntinas-Lichius O, Klussmann JP, Wittekindt C, Stennert E Parotidectomy for benign parotid disease at a university teaching hospital: outcome of 963 operations. Laryngoscope 2006;116:534–540
2. O'Brien CJ Current management of benign parotid tumors – the role of limited superficial parotidectomy. Head Neck 2003;25:946–952
3. Leverstein H, van der Wal JE, Tiwari RM, van der Waal I, Snow GB. Surgical management of 246 previously untreated pleomorphic adenomas of the parotid gland. Br J Surg 1997;84:399–403
4. Lai SY, Weinstein GS, Chalian AA, Rosenthal DI, Weber RS. Parotidectomy in the treatment of aggressive cutaneous malignancies. Arch Otolaryngol Head Neck Surg 2002;128:521–526
5. Olsen KD, Maragos NE, Weiland LH. First branchial cleft anomalies. Laryngoscope 1980;90:423–436
6. Koltai PJ, Winkelmann PE. A first branchial cleft anomaly within the parotid gland. Otolaryngol Head Neck Surg 1980;88:44–48
7. Belenky WM, Medina JE. First branchial cleft anomalies. Laryngoscope 1980;90:28–39
8. McRae RG, Lee KJ, Goertzen E. First branchial cleft anomalies and the facial nerve. Otolaryngol Head Neck Surg 1983;91:197–202
9. Triglia JM, Nicollas R, Ducroz V, Koltai PJ, Garabedian EN. First branchial cleft anomalies: a study of 39 cases and a review of the literature. Arch Otolaryngol Head Neck Surg 1998;124:291–295
10. O'Brien CJ, Murrant NJ. Surgical management of chronic parotitis. Head Neck 1993;15:445–449
11. Conley J, Selfe RW. Occult neoplasms in facial paralysis. Laryngoscope 1981;91:205–210
12. Frankenthaler RA, Luna MA, Lee SS, Ang KK, Byers RM, Guillamondegui OM, Wolf P, Goepfert H. Prognostic variables in parotid gland cancer. Arch Otolaryngol Head Neck Surg 1991;117:1251–1256
13. Broderick JP, Auger RG, DeSanto LW. Facial paralysis and occult parotid cancer. A characteristic syndrome. Arch Otolaryngol Head Neck Surg 1988;114:195–197
14. Gurney TA, Eisele DW, Weinberg V, Shin E, Lee N. Adenoid cystic carcinoma of the major salivary glands treated with surgery and radiation. Laryngoscope 2005;115:1278–1282
15. de Ru JA, Plantinga RF, Majoor MH, van Benthem PP, Slootweg PJ, Peeters PH, Hordijk GJ. Warthin's tumour and smoking. B-ENT 2005;1:63–66
16. Yu GY, Liu XB, Li ZL, Peng X. Smoking and the development of Warthin's tumour of the parotid gland. Br J Oral Maxillofac Surg 1998;36:183–185
17. Gallo O, Bocciolini C. Warthin's tumour associated with autoimmune diseases and tobacco use. Acta Otolaryngol 1997;117:623–627
18. Yoo GH, Eisele DW, Askin FB, Driben JS, Johns ME. Warthin's tumor: a 40-year experience at The Johns Hopkins Hospital. Laryngoscope 1994;104:799–803
19. Weinberger MS, Rosenberg WW, Meurer WT, Robbins KT. Fine-needle aspiration of parotid gland lesions. Head Neck 1992;14:483–487
20. Cohen EG, Patel SG, Lin O, Boyle JO, Kraus DH, Singh B, Wong RJ, Shah JP, Shaha AR. Fine-needle aspiration biopsy of salivary gland lesions in a selected patient population. Arch Otolaryngol Head Neck Surg 2004;130:773–778
21. Alphs HH, Eisele DW, Westra WH. The role of fine needle aspiration in the evaluation of parotid masses. Curr Opin Otolaryngol Head Neck Surg 2006;14:62–66

22. Eisele DW. The Shaw hemostatic scalpel in parotid surgery. Arch Otolaryngol Head Neck Surg 1999;125:119
23. Jackson LL, Gourin CG, Thomas DS, Porubsky ES, Klippert FN, Terris DJ. Use of the harmonic scalpel in superficial and total parotidectomy for benign and malignant disease. Laryngoscope 2005;115(6):1070–1073
24. Ussmueller JO, Jaehne M, Neumann BG. The use of diathermy scissors in parotid gland surgery. Arch Otolaryngol Head Neck Surg 2004;130(2):187–189
25. Nofsinger YC, Tom LW, LaRossa D, Wetmore RF, Handler SD. Periauricular cysts and sinuses. Laryngoscope 1997;107:883–887
26. Sichel JY, Halperin D, Dano I, Dangoor E. Clinical update on type II first branchial cleft cysts. Laryngoscope 1998;108:1524–1527
27. Work WP. Newer concept of first branchial cleft defects. Laryngoscope 1972;82:1581–1592
28. Isaacson G, Martin WH. First branchial cleft cyst excision with electrophysiological facial nerve localization. Arch Otolaryngol Head Neck Surg 2000;126:513–516
29. Bron LP, O'Brien CJ. Facial nerve function after parotidectomy. Arch Otolaryngol Head Neck Surg 1997;123:1091–1096
30. Gaillard C, Perie S, Susini B, St Guily JL. Facial nerve dysfunction after parotidectomy: the role of local factors. Laryngoscope 2005;115:287–291
31. Reilly J, Myssiorek D. Facial nerve stimulation and post parotidectomy facial paresis. Otolaryngol Head Neck Surg 2003;128:530–533
32. Witt RL. Facial nerve function after partial superficial parotidectomy: An 11-year review (1987–1997). Otolaryngol Head Neck Surg 1999;121:210–213
33. Dulguerov P, Marchal F, Lehmann W. Postparotidectomy facial nerve paralysis: possible etiologic factors and results with routine facial nerve monitoring. Laryngoscope 1999;109:754–762
34. Wax M, Tarshis L. Post-parotidectomy fistula. J Otolaryngol 1991;20:10–13
35. Eisele DW. Simple method for the assessment of Frey's syndrome. Laryngoscope 1992;102:583–584

Chapter 15

Total Parotidectomy

15

Eric J. Moore and Kerry D. Olsen

Contents

Core Features

- Total parotidectomy is a spectrum of operations based on anatomy and on tumor extent.
- The surgeon applies knowledge of embryology, anatomy, tumor pathology and behavior, and tumor extent to individualize the operation to the patient.
- The deep parotid gland contains lymphatic nodes that must be adequately managed in malignant tumors.
- Adequate management of the deep parotid gland requires control of the intraglandular external carotid artery and its branches.

Complications to Avoid

- The surgeon should not embark on parotidectomy without the availability of frozen-section pathologic review.
- The surgeon should not embark on parotidectomy without the capability to perform total parotidectomy, neck dissection, and extended operation.
- The surgeon should not be reassured that a parotid mass is benign solely on the basis of fine-needle aspiration.
- The surgeon should be prepared to address facial nerve deficits at the time of the initial operation.

"... it follows from the complex relations of the parotid gland that its entire removal as a surgical procedure is an anatomic impossibility."

Sir Frederic Treves, 1901

Introduction

The first reference to removing the parotid gland with identification and preservation of the facial nerve was by Carwardine in 1907 [8]. In 1916, Sistrunk described 112 cases of parotidectomy with preservation of the facial nerve [3]. Like many operations performed today, the procedure languished in relative obscurity until advances in anesthesia and hemostasis and the modifications of talented practitioners advanced it to the prominent position that it holds in the armamentarium of the modern head and neck surgeon. Experience gained during the past half century of parotid surgery at Mayo Clinic by surgeons such as Oliver H. Beahrs, Lawrence W. DeSanto, and Kerry D. Olsen, continually performing 75–100 parotid operations a year, serves as the foundation for this chapter. The outcomes of the operation have shown a need for flexibility and the ability to individualize the approach and the procedure to a particular patient and tumor. This chapter discusses definitions, indications, preoperative evaluation, procedural technique, and postoperative care with an emphasis on the need for an experienced surgeon to have a flexible approach to parotid conditions. The interested student who studies and rigorously applies these techniques will realize the exhilaration that accompanies a well-designed and executed parotid operation.

Parotidectomy is one of the most challenging of all operations facing the head and neck surgeon. The tumors requiring treatment are usually benign, but if left to observation they can lead to disfiguring facial masses or malignant degeneration. Meticulous removal of the tumor with inclusion of surrounding normal glandular tissue is necessary to prevent recurrence. The operation requires careful dissection and preservation of the facial nerve trunk and its peripheral branches because both the surgeon and the patient usually expect a high level of facial function postoperatively. Tumors of the parotid gland are uncommon, but the histologic variety, variability of tumor site in relationship to the facial nerve, and complexity of different operative maneuvers to achieve tumor eradication require experience and expertise on the part of the surgeon. Some tumors may require only simple excision with partial parotidectomy, whereas other tumors may require radical excision with sacrifice of the facial nerve, lymph node dissection, or resection of surrounding structures. Finally, preoperative evaluation with clinical examination, imaging, and even cytologic examination often cannot adequately prepare the surgeon for the situation in the operating theater. Sound decision-making based on adequate experience must be practiced intraoperatively to achieve a successful outcome. All of these facets of parotidectomy make it one of the most interesting and formidable in the job description of an oncologic surgeon—casual operators need not apply.

The surgeon must rely on detailed anatomic knowledge of the parotid gland and its relationship to surrounding structures, particularly neural and vascular, to perform the operation safely. The pertinent relationships are presented in the anatomy section of this chapter, but the surgeon who wants to minimize operative complications in this area must master the anatomy through careful study of anatomic texts and the practice of anatomic dissection. The varieties of tissue thickness, neural and vascular structural heterogeneity, and variability of tumor relationships to surrounding structures are too vast to present pictorially. The surgeon will spend a career mastering this complexity, and technique improves with further performance of the task. Still, several anatomic points are worth presenting more than once: (1) the anatomy of the facial nerve trunk as it exits the stylomastoid foramen and enters the parotid gland is very constant; (2) the separation of the parotid gland into a superficial and deep portion divided by the facial nerve is a surgical, and not an embryologic, distinction, and thus the tumors that present in these regions and their relationship to lymphatic structures are not different; and (3) roughly 80% of the parotid gland (and 80% of the 15–20 intraglandular lymph nodes) lies superficial to the facial nerve, and 20%

of the gland and its lymphatics lie in the deep portion medial to the nerve.

What constitutes a total parotidectomy? This question deserves some attention because of the variability in techniques and philosophies of different surgeons. In general, total parotidectomy connotes the removal of both the superficial portion of the gland and the entire deep gland beneath the facial nerve. In extreme cases, the operation also may entail removal of the peripheral facial nerve and even surrounding muscle, bone, and skin. In practice, the more extensive version of the operation is rarely indicated. When performed, it is usually in the treatment of advanced malignancies. More commonly, the surgeon finds the need to perform a subtotal parotidectomy by removing the superficial gland and a portion of the gland deep to the facial nerve. The surgeon performing parotid surgery must possess the skill and knowledge to perform the various forms of total parotidectomy, thereby adequately removing disease while avoiding unnecessary morbidity.

When does a surgeon need to contemplate total parotidectomy? Surgeons who perform parotidectomy also need thorough knowledge regarding clinical behavior of the various pathologic lesions that can arise in the major salivary glands. Benign tumors, such as pleomorphic adenomas, oncocytomas, and Warthin's tumors, usually necessitate only subtotal removal of the gland with preservation of the facial nerve. Benign tumors that arise in the deep lobe often require initial elevation or removal of the superficial lobe followed by mobilization of the facial nerve before subtotal removal of the deep portion of the gland. Occasionally the surgeon may not be able to determine the deep lobe origin of the tumor before mobilization of the superficial gland. Operative exploration may show the need for removal of the deep lobe in tumors that arise in the midpoint of the parotid adjacent to the facial nerve. The inexperienced operator may omit the possibility of total gland removal and facial nerve mobilization during the preoperative consent process for a patient with a seemingly innocuous parotid mass. Some multifocal tumors, despite benign behavior, may require total parotidectomy to ensure complete removal. Parapharyngeal tumors may require superficial and deep parotid removal if they are dumbbell-shaped tumors that pass through the stylomandibular tunnel, or they may require only deep lobe removal if they are confined to the parapharyngeal space.

Malignant tumors of the parotid gland often require total removal of the gland. The exception is low-grade tumors with a low risk of nodal metastasis. All malignant tumors that arise in the deep gland and any tumor with confirmed metastasis to the parotid gland require total parotidectomy for adequate removal. High-grade tumors arising in the superficial gland warrant total parotidectomy to ensure adequate treatment of the parotid lymph nodes. Tumors that spread outside the parotid gland or involve the facial nerve usually warrant total parotidectomy. Because of the complexity of tumor presentation and behavior, the parotid surgeon benefits from considerable familiarity with the behavior of the many types of parotid tumors, both benign and malignant. The surgeon also needs to understand how histologic grade can influence tumor behavior and consequently dictate the extent of surgery necessary for adequate extirpation. Obviously the availability of a competent pathologist who has equally detailed familiarity with the evaluation and diagnosis of salivary gland conditions is essential for adequate surgical treatment of parotid tumors. If the surgeon cannot work closely and efficiently in the operating room with a skilled frozen-section pathologist, then that surgeon should question the ability to perform competent surgical care of the patient with a parotid mass.

Background Information

Embryology

The major salivary glands develop by the ingrowth of oral epithelium into the underlying mesenchyme [7]. In the case of the parotid gland, the ectoderm grows backward across the masseter muscle and is against the developing external ear structures. Although the embryologic development of the facial nerve was a source of some controversy for more than a century, it is now known that the facial nerve migrates anteriorly and becomes surrounded by the developing gland. The gland then insinuates into the spaces around the mandible, temporal bone, and surrounding muscles. The clinical implication of this embryologic development is that the histologic features of the superficial and deep portions of the gland are identical. Despite being the first of the major salivary glands to initiate development, the parotid gland is the last to become encapsulated by fascia. The clinical implication of late encapsulation is incorporation of a variable but substantial number of lymph nodes within the parenchyma of the parotid gland, in both the superficial and the deep lobes. Fascial structures also interdigitate between the superficial and deep lobes of the gland and around the intraglandular facial nerve.

Surgical Anatomy

The adult parotid gland occupies a region in front of the ear, varying in width from 3.4 to 5.8 cm. It weighs between 14 and 28 g [5]. It is irregular and variable in shape, and it has been described as having four surfaces: superficial, deep, anterior, and posterior [1]. The posterior surface overlaps and is grooved by its contact with the sternocleidomastoid muscle, mastoid process, and external auditory meatus. This inferior variability in size and shape has the clinical implication that any infra-auricular mass should be assumed to have an origin in the parotid gland until proved otherwise with imaging or surgical exploration. Many inexperienced practitioners have inadvertently incised this area with the intent of "excisional" biopsy, only to find themselves within the parenchyma of the gland dealing with an unexpected parotid neoplasm.

The deep surface of the gland is molded against the medial wall of the musculoskeletal recess formed by the mastoid process, external acoustic meatus, head of the mandible, and ascending ramus of the mandible. These surrounding structures have surgical importance. The medial wall of the bony recess is the styloid process and, deeper, the transverse process of the atlas. The medial bony recess is incomplete, but helping to fill it are the posterior belly of the digastric muscle and the styloid musculature. These muscles, particularly the digastric muscle and stylohyoid muscle, indent the deep surface of the gland and are easily seen during complete parotidectomy. Anteriorly, the ramus of the mandible and the masseter muscle contact the deep portion of the parotid. The bulk of the pterygoid muscles in the infratemporal fossa is not visualized during total parotidectomy, but the insertion of the lateral pterygoid at the temporomandibular joint is related to the deep portion of the gland that extends deep to the posterior border of the mandible. The stylomandibular ligament unites the styloid process to the mandibular ramus. Together with the ascending ramus of the mandible and the skull base, it forms the stylomandibular tunnel described by Patey and Thackray [11]. Tumors from the retromandibular portion of the parotid gland may pass through the stylomandibular tunnel and thus extend to the prestyloid portion of the parapharyngeal space.

Related Fascia

The superficial layer of the deep cervical fascia splits to invest the parotid gland and then fuses superiorly with the periosteum of the zygoma. Over the lateral surface of the gland, this fascia is often termed the parotid fascia, and it serves as an excellent barrier above which a tissue flap containing the superficial fascia and subcutaneous fat can be raised. The parotid fascia sends numerous septae passing among the lobules of glandular tissue. Anterior to the gland, the fascia continues to invest the masseter muscle. The deep fascia of the medial gland is thinner, is continuous with the fascia of the styloid muscles, and continues downward to form a portion of the stylomandibular ligament before fusing with the fascia of the digastric muscle and periosteum of the angle of the mandible.

Vascular Anatomy

The variability of the venous system in and around the parotid gland makes it difficult for the surgeon to understand many clinically useful relationships. Two important relationships bear mention: (1) the superficial temporal and internal maxillary veins fuse within the gland to form the posterior facial vein, which generally splits as it exits the gland into a posterior (retromandibular) branch that drains into the external jugular vein and an anterior branch that drains into the common facial vein and then into the internal jugular vein, and (2) the veins generally lie deep to the facial nerve within the gland, the cervical branch of the facial nerve usually passing over the posterior facial vein and the marginal nerve passing over the anterior facial vein.

The external carotid artery and its terminal branches are intimately connected to the parotid gland. Unlike the posterior facial vein, which runs superficial to the digastric and stylohyoid muscles, the external carotid artery runs deep to these muscles before curving upward and entering that portion of the gland molded inward by the styloid process. The branches of the external carotid artery are commonly divided as anterior, posterior, ascending, and terminal, but the branches involved in total parotidectomy are best considered in terms of the relationship of their origin proximal or distal to the digastric muscle. The superior thyroid, lingual, and ascending pharyngeal arteries originate proximal to the digastric muscle, and generally are not encountered during parotidectomy.

The occipital and facial arteries originate at the inferior border of the digastric muscle. The occipital artery runs posteriorly under the digastric muscle, grooves the mastoid near the insertion of this muscle, and runs away from the parotid bed. The facial artery ascends deep to the digastric muscle and curves back over the stylohyoid muscle before passing between the submandibular gland and mandible. The artery crosses over the mandible at the anterior border of the masseter muscle.

The remaining distal branches of the carotid artery are more intimately related to the parotid gland. The posterior auricular artery originates near the superior border of the digastric muscle and runs backward between the mastoid process and external auditory meatus. It sometimes is encountered in the dissection of the facial nerve trunk, but it does not run in the glandular tissue. The internal maxillary artery and superficial temporal arteries originate from the intraglandular portion of the external carotid artery. The internal maxillary artery runs deep to the ascending ramus of the mandible to lie deep or superficial to the lateral pterygoid muscle. The superficial temporal artery grooves the deep surface of the gland and runs upward between the tragus and temporomandibular joint. It gives off the transverse facial artery, which runs anteriorly over the mandibular ramus toward the masseter muscle.

The internal jugular vein passes deep to the operative field during total parotidectomy. It is rarely encountered, except in the removal of tumors that extend to the parapharyngeal space. The internal jugular vein leaves the skull base medial and posterior to the styloid process and descends immediately on the anterior surface of the transverse process of C1. It runs deep to the digastric and styloid muscles.

The internal carotid artery ascends vertically on the anteromedial surface of the internal jugular vein. It also is rarely encountered during complete parotidectomy, being confined to the poststyloid portion of the parapharyngeal space. The exception is tortuous turns in the superior cervical internal carotid artery, which can sometimes bring the artery far more lateral than the surgeon might expect.

Lymphatic Anatomy

The parotid gland contains a rich and intricate system of both afferent and efferent lymphatics. The afferent lymphatic channels draining into lymph nodes on the superficial surface of the gland serve as the principal collecting system for the frontotemporal scalp, upper face, lacrimal gland, and external ear. The afferent lymphatic channels draining to lymph nodes on the deep surface of the gland drain the palate, nasopharynx, auditory canal, and middle ear.

The efferent channels drain to both the superficial and the deep cervical lymphatic systems. The average adult parotid gland contains 15–20 intraglandular lymph nodes [12]. In the past there has been some controversy over the density of deep glandular lymph nodes and the necessity of doing total parotidectomy for lymphatic metastasis. However, the current understanding of embryologic formation of the superficial and deep portions from a singular gland anlage, coupled with the dense interconnection of lymphatics between the glandular and paraglandular lymphatics and superficial and deep portions of the gland, argue for total parotidectomy in these situations. The adult deep lobe parotid gland contains lymph nodes 75% of the time, and the average number of nodes in the deep gland is 2.3 [4].

Neural Anatomy

Although the anatomic variability of the facial nerve and detailed descriptions of the percentages of different branching patterns have contributed to the body of knowledge surrounding parotid surgery, the surgeon should be aware of the constancy of the position of the main trunk of the facial nerve [1]. The facial nerve exits the stylomandibular foramen, which lies at the base of the styloid process at the end of the tympanomastoid fissure. After leaving the foramen, the main trunk of the facial nerve gives off branches to the postauricular muscles and posterior belly of the digastric muscle, and then it curves anteriorly. These branches may have to be divided during mobilization of the nerve in the performance of total parotidectomy. The facial nerve then becomes embedded in parotid tissue and usually runs superficial to the posterior facial vein (often in contact with it) and lateral to the external carotid artery. Occasionally, some of the branches of the facial nerve run deep to the facial vein.

To identify the facial nerve trunk, the surgeon can utilize the spatial relationships mentioned, but none of these structures is actually visible during mobilization of the gland. The structures that are most useful for identification of the facial nerve early in parotidectomy are the posterior belly of the digastric muscle, cartilaginous tragal pointer, and mastoid tip. A finger tip placed on the lateral surface of the mastoid process will direct the surgeon to the proper plane and zone of dissection to identify the facial nerve trunk. Every parotid surgeon has encountered that moment of uncertainty when dissecting through a thick parotid gland before encountering the facial trunk, but one must remember that in a plane along the anterior surface of the mastoid tip no vital structure exists between the fingertip and the trunk of the seventh nerve. It exists as a singular white structure that is 2–3 mm in diameter at this location [1]. In the case of deep lobe tumors, the main trunk of the facial nerve may be more lateral, and it may be encountered sooner than expected. In children, the main trunk may not be as deep as expected.

The major division of the facial nerve, the pes anserinus, is located within 1.3 cm of the stylomastoid foramen [3]. The nerve divides into an upper temporofacial division and a lower cervicofacial division. Anastomotic branches occur commonly between the upper division nerves, rarely between the mandibular branch and other branches, and never between the branches of the cervicofacial division. Considerable controversy exists about the relationship of the facial nerve and the surrounding parotid parenchyma. The controversy has significance from two separate clinical aspects, namely, (1) what can be done surgically, and (2) what should be done oncologically.

From the standpoint of surgical technique, a definite plane of dissection can be developed along the facial nerve. This is commonly the technique used in removal of tumors of the superficial portion of the parotid gland. From an oncologic standpoint, the parotid gland is a unilobar, multilobular structure. The intimate continuity of ducts and parenchymal connections that traverse the plane of the facial nerve makes separation of the gland along this plane a surgical, and arbitrary, separation when dealing with invasive neoplasms.

The greater auricular nerve crosses over the sternocleidomastoid muscle and divides into multiple branches below the external ear. The anterior branch sends sensory fibers to the ear lobe as well as the skin and fascia over the parotid gland. Posterior branches of the greater auricular nerve may be preserved during parotidectomy for benign disease.

The auriculotemporal nerve, a branch of the fifth cranial nerve, passes in the superior deep portion of the gland as it leaves the infratemporal fossa. It gives sensory fibers and postganglionic parasympathetic fibers from the otic ganglion to the parotid gland.

Parotid Duct

The parotid duct is formed at the anterior border of the gland as smaller tributaries from within the gland converge. An "accessory" lobe of the parotid gland may be loosely connected to the main body of the gland or completely separate from it and lie adjacent to the duct. Variations in the distribution of the tributaries have limited surgical significance.

Definitions and Indications

Superficial Parotidectomy

Superficial parotidectomy entails removal of the lateral portion of the parotid gland with preservation of the facial nerve. It is the standard operation for masses that arise in the portion of the parotid gland lateral to the facial nerve, particularly when the histopathologic nature of the mass has not been confirmed. Superficial parotidectomy is adequate treatment for benign tumors of the superficial parotid gland, such as pleomorphic adenoma, and for localized, well-encapsulated malignant tumors of low histologic grade which arise in the lateral lobe of the parotid gland. High recurrence rates following operation for pleomorphic adenoma have been attributed to inadequate surgical excision, and superficial parotidectomy should be the standard operative procedure in the armamentarium of the parotid surgeon [9]. Some surgeons advocate partial or subtotal parotidectomy for tumors that arise in the lateral parotid tail. The surgeon entertaining the decision to perform subtotal superficial parotidectomy needs to be confident in both the histologic nature of the mass and the encapsulation and localized nature of the tumor. If either of these issues is in question, a formal superficial parotidectomy should be performed. The goal of removal of a benign parotid tumor is complete removal with a cuff of normal parotid tissue around the tumor and preservation of the facial nerve. No parotid tumor should be removed by excisional biopsy without clear visualization of the branches of the facial nerve.

Deep Parotidectomy

To understand deep parotidectomy, the components of the deep gland need to be conceptualized. From a surgical dissection view, the deep parotid consists of three main parts (again, contiguous): (1) the portion of the gland between cranial nerve VII and over the masseter muscle, (2) the gland deep to cranial nerve VII between the mandible and the mastoid/external auditory canal (greatest volume), and (3) the retromandibular gland that extends to or into the parapharyngeal space. The surgeon may individualize the extent of resection to involve some or all of these portions on the basis of the pathologic findings and presentation of the tumor. The major operations involving the deep parotid may include superficial parotidectomy combined with partial deep lobe parotidectomy, superficial parotidectomy with total deep lobe parotidectomy with or without resection of cranial nerve VII, isolated deep parotidectomy, deep lobe parotidectomy with parapharyngeal space extension, and extended total parotidectomy usually with resection of cranial nerve VII. These operations are described separately below, and illustrative cases are used to highlight typical indications.

Superficial Parotidectomy with Partial Deep Lobe Resection

This operation is commonly performed for benign tumors of the central deep parotid gland, such as pleomorphic adenoma involving the gland deep to the facial nerve. The surgeon may not always be able to predict the relationship of the tumor to the peripheral nerve from preoperative examination or imaging, and the decision to resect the deep gland may evolve during the operation after dissection of the superficial gland. This operation also may be performed for low-grade malignancies of the superficial gland for which the surgeon wants to include a portion of the deep gland to ensure an adequate margin of resection. Rarely, this operation is performed in patients with refractory chronic sialadenitis in an effort to remove all chronically infected gland and prevent postoperative sialocele. The operation also may be used for patients with mucosa-associated lymphoid tissue (MALT) lymphoma of the parotid gland in the absence of other signs of lymphoma. This situation should be expected in patients with rheumatoid arthritis or Sjögren's syndrome who have development of nodular enlargement of the parotid gland.

Case Example 1

A 37-year-old dental hygienist was referred from her primary physician with a 2-year history of a right-sided 2.5-cm infra-auricular mass. She came with a computed tomogram that showed a 2.5-cm mass within the parenchyma of the inferior parotid gland. The mass was nontender, and she had no adenopathy, skin changes, or facial nerve paresis. She had done extensive research on parotid gland conditions, and she was intensely concerned with the aesthetic outcome of any surgical intervention. She underwent preoperative examination and discussion, and intraoperative exploration progressed with exposure of the parotid gland, identification of the facial nerve, and mobilization of the superficial lobe of the parotid gland. As the operation progressed, it became obvious that the mass was deep to the facial nerve trunk and cervicomandibular division. The main trunk was draped over the main portion of the mass in the deep parotid gland. The superficial lobe was removed, the facial nerve trunk and peripheral branches were mobilized, and the deep gland between the mandible and mastoid and a portion of the gland over the masseter were removed in continuity with the mass. Frozen-section pathologic findings confirmed pleomorphic adenoma arising within the deep gland. The parotid defect was reconstructed with an abdominal dermal fat graft to mask the perimandibular defect.

Superficial Parotidectomy with Total Deep Lobe Resection

Total removal of the superficial and deep parotid gland should be performed for malignant neoplasms with confirmed or suspected metastasis to the parotid lymph nodes, including the following situations: (1) metastasis to a superficial parotid node from a primary parotid tumor or an extraparotid malignancy, (2) any parotid malignancy that indicates metastasis by involvement of cervical lymph nodes, and (3) any high-grade parotid malignancy with a high risk of metastasis. Total parotidectomy also is performed for primary parotid malignancies originating in the deep lobe and for primary malignancies that extend outside the parotid gland. The operation also is performed for multifocal tumors, such as oncocytomas, to ensure complete removal. The operation may involve sparing or sacrifice of the facial nerve branches or trunk depending on tumor extent to the nerve.

Case Example 2

A 45-year-old man was referred for treatment of a biopsy-proven malignant melanoma 1.3 mm in greatest depth centered over the temporal skin in the supra-auricular area. Preoperative positron emission tomography showed a fluorodeoxyglucose-avid 1.2-cm node in the superficial parotid gland. The patient underwent wide local excision of the temporal melanoma and superficial and deep parotidectomy with facial nerve preservation and upper neck dissection. Frozen and permanent pathologic findings included 2 of 6 neck nodes in the superficial parotid gland positive for metastatic melanoma, 1 of 3 nodes in the deep parotid glands positive for melanoma, and 1 of 25 neck nodes positive for melanoma. The patient was treated with postoperative radiation and followed for the possibility of locoregional or distant recurrence.

Isolated Deep Parotidectomy

Isolated removal of the deep parotid gland is most often performed for benign tumors of the inferior parotid gland deep to the facial nerve. This operation can be used for "dumbbell" tumors of the deep parotid gland that enter the parapharyngeal space through the stylomandibular tunnel. During this operation, the superficial gland is mobilized to aid in identification of the facial nerve, but it is not removed if not involved with tumor.

Case Example 3

A 37-year-old woman was involved in a motor vehicle accident and examined for superficial wounds in the emergency department. On physical examination, she had fullness of her soft palate and tonsillar asymmetry. Magnetic resonance imaging showed a 3.5-cm mass in the prestyloid parapharyngeal space with a small cuff of tissue contiguous with the deep parotid gland. She had no other head or neck abnormalities. She underwent surgical exploration with a cervicoparotid approach, mobilization of the inferior parotid gland, and identification of the facial trunk and inferior nerve division. Blunt finger dissection was used to mobilize the mass from the parapharyngeal space and deliver it into the neck, with care taken to avoid rupturing the capsule of the mass against the styloid process. The mass was sent for pathologic review with a cuff of inferior deep parotid tissue. Histopathologic results confirmed the presence of encapsulated pleomorphic adenoma. The patient was discharged from the hospital after overnight observation and was free of evidence of recurrent disease at 4 years postoperatively.

Extended Total Parotidectomy

Removal of the superficial and deep parotid gland also may be extended to involve adjacent structures such as the overlying skin, the underlying mandible, the temporal bone and external auditory canal, or the deep musculature of the parapharyngeal space. These extensions are dictated by tumor growth and behavior. Patients with extensive parotid malignancies must be counseled regarding the possibility of extended resections and the resulting functional and cosmetic morbidity. The head and neck surgeon may need to anticipate the extent of defect and incorporate plans for reconstruction into the overall surgical design.

Case Example 4

A 63-year-old attorney presented with a mass in the left parotid gland, jaw pain, and upper facial weakness of 4 weeks' duration. He had a history of removal of a squamous cell carcinoma from the ipsilateral forehead skin 18 months earlier. On physical examination, a fixed 3.5-cm mass was present in the superior parotid gland. The patient also had trismus and House grade 2/6 ipsilateral upper facial nerve dysfunction. Imaging disclosed an enhancing mass present in the parotid gland with central necrosis and extension to the mandibular ramus, temporalis muscle, and pterygoid musculature. He underwent surgical excision with total parotidectomy, including facial nerve sacrifice, partial mandibulectomy, and resection of the overlying skin, ear canal, lateral temporal bone, and surrounding musculature. Pathologic findings included metastatic squamous cell carcinoma to 5 of 12 intraparotid nodes and 6 of 48 ipsilateral neck nodes. He underwent reconstruction with fibular free tissue transfer, cervicofacial rotation flap, and sural nerve interposition graft to the facial nerve defect. The patient underwent postoperative radiation therapy. Distant metastasis developed 2.5 years after therapy was completed.

Evaluation of the Patient

Evaluation of the patient with a parotid mass should always start with a history concentrating on tumor presentation. Factors such as slow versus rapid growth, pain, facial paresis or paralysis, and overlying skin changes or associated lymphadenopathy can be informative in the distinction between benign and malignant lesions. Risk factors for malignancy such as prior radiation exposure and tobacco abuse should be sought, and inquiry should be made into previous diagnostic and therapeutic forays. The evaluation should review possible coagulation disorders, medical conditions, medications, dietary supplements, and allergies that could affect general anesthesia. The physician should inquire about a history of recurrent or chronic infections or inflammation of the parotid gland. With ready access to electronic medical information, today's patients are often partially or thoroughly informed as to the pathophysiology and treatment of parotid masses. Time spent during the history to explore patients' concerns and preconceived notions regarding their parotid mass can serve to relieve anxiety and foster realistic expectations.

After the history is obtained, a careful examination of the head and neck should concentrate on the preauricular and malar skin. The external auditory canal and tympanic membrane should be examined. Ipsilateral and contralateral facial nerve function should be evaluated with a standardized grading system. Generally, patients with intact facial nerve function can retain their facial nerve, even in the setting of malignancy, but patients with impaired facial nerve function usually have significant invasion of the nerve. During palpation of the gland and mass, the key factors to assess are size, consistency, mobility, and location. Intraoral examination should investigate the palate and lateral pharynx for asymmetry suggesting parapharyngeal extension. The neck is then palpated to assess for lymphadenopathy.

The role of imaging in parotidectomy is controversial. Imaging is not necessary for the evaluation of a patient with an easily identifiable mass in the parotid gland with benign characteristics on history and physical examination. Imaging begins to add clinically useful information when, after the physical examination, the surgeon is uncertain about the presence or extent of the lesion. It also is useful when the surgeon suspects extension outside the parotid gland. Parotid masses extending deep to the mandible into the parapharyngeal space should always be imaged preoperatively. Magnetic resonance imaging with gadolinium usually provides the greatest amount of information regarding tumor consistency, extent, and relationship to surrounding gland and other structures. Computed tomography with contrast may be added or substituted to gain information regarding tumor relationship to adjacent bony or vascular structures. The role of positron emission tomography is growing in the evaluation of malignant tumors with potential metastasis (see Chapter 2, Imaging of the Salivary Glands).

Fine-needle aspiration for the evaluation of parotid masses is also controversial. The literature reports variable accuracy when it is used for parotid masses, and the experience of the cytopathologist can greatly influence the results [13]. Fine-needle aspiration rarely alters the decision for the treatment of parotid masses. It may have use for evaluation of a patient with a parotid mass who is of poor health or reluctant to undergo surgical removal of the mass. For a patient with an obvious malignancy, it may help characterize the type of malignancy, which may be useful for pretreatment counseling (see Chapter 8, Fine-needle Aspiration Biopsy).

Preoperative Discussion

After the complete evaluation, the surgeon should thoroughly discuss the assessment, treatment plan, and goals of operation with the patient. This plan should be individualized to the patient and the tumor characteristics. The discussion includes an assessment of benign versus malignant tumor behavior. Even when the diagnosis is based on the findings of fine-needle aspiration, the surgeon should prepare the patient for an alteration of the diagnosis based on intraoperative findings and frozen-section analysis. The treatment plan must be designed around safe and complete tumor extirpation, avoidance of piecemeal removal, appropriate management of cervical lymphatics, facial nerve preservation if oncologically sound, and appropriate rehabilitation measures. All patients undergoing parotid surgery should be counseled regarding placement of the incision and postoperative scar, expected cosmetic defect, expected postoperative function and time to full recovery, possibility of the need for adjunctive radiation therapy for high-grade malignant tumors, and postoperative sequelae such as paresthesias and gustatory sweating. All patients undergoing parotidectomy should be counseled regarding the possibility of postoperative facial paresis or paralysis. This point becomes especially salient in patients undergoing total parotidectomy, particularly the elderly. Older patients have both slower and more incomplete recovery of facial function after manipulation of the nerve to the degree necessary for complete parotidectomy. If the facial nerve is involved with tumor, as evidenced on examination or imaging, the patient should be counseled regarding nerve sacrifice and rehabilitation.

Reconstruction of the functional and cosmetic deficits resulting from the operation should be discussed with the patient, including, as appropriate, the possible need for nerve grafting, the donor site incisions, and morbidity. Superficial parotidectomy results in mild to moderate facial contour asymmetry, and total parotidectomy results in a significant depression in the preauricular and inframandibular areas. The surgeon can attempt to minimize contour irregularity in removal of benign deep parotid masses by preservation of the superficial lobe. The patient should be counseled regarding the possibility of parotid bed reconstruction with autologous material (such as dermal fat graft) or artificial material.

Sometimes a patient has previously had partial parotid surgery for a tumor that requires total parotidectomy for adequate management. Often this situation results when the permanent pathologic findings show a malignant high-grade lesion and the preoperative or intraoperative histopathologic findings indicated a benign or low-grade lesion. Our advice in these situations is to complete the treatment that would have been recommended and performed if the surgeon had had the correct information at the outset. This advice often involves reentering a previously operated field, carefully identifying and mobilizing the facial nerve, removing the remainder of the parotid gland, and performing a neck dissection. This can be a difficult dissection, and the patient should be counseled regarding the possible need for facial nerve monitoring, facial nerve injury, and need for facial reanimation and nerve reconstruction procedures. Following sound principles of management is still preferable to observation in the face of uncertainty regarding adequate tumor removal.

The necessity for thorough preoperative counseling when this operation is to be performed cannot be overestimated, and a carefully planned and executed operation can still result in a dissatisfied surgeon and patient if the patient has not been counseled about appropriate expectations after the operation.

Surgical Technique

Preparation

Before entering the operating theater, the surgeon should arrange for a pathologist to provide reliable frozen-section review of the tissue. This approach will save many patients the cost, time, and morbidity of returning for further surgical resection for an undiagnosed malignancy. A quality assurance system should be in place to ensure the correct patient and site of surgery. Appropriate imaging studies should be thoroughly reviewed and visible during the operation. The risk of bleeding is low, and typing and cross-matching for blood transfusion are not needed during the operation. Antibiotics are not routinely administered unless there are preoperative signs of infection. The operation is performed with the patient under general endotracheal anesthesia, and the endotracheal tube is positioned and taped to the oral commissure and cheek opposite to the lesion. The patient is placed in a 45° reverse-Trendelenburg position or lounge-chair position with the head higher than the heart. The head is turned to the opposite side of the lesion, and the neck is extended by placement of a rolled sheet under the shoulders. The patient is prepared by sterile scrub and draped so that the ear, lateral corner of the ipsilateral eye, ipsilateral oral commissure, and entire ipsilateral neck are visible in the field. If facial nerve monitoring is to be used, the nerve monitor is placed in the orbicularis oris and orbicularis oculi muscles to ensure upper and lower division monitoring. The surgeon stands on the side of the patient ipsilateral to the gland to be dissected, the assistant stands at the head and opposite the surgeon, and the scrub technician stands on the side of the surgeon.

Incisions and Flap Elevation

The incision site is marked with a surgical marker. The incision begins in the preauricular crease at the superior root of the helix and curves gently below the lobule, and then turns anteriorly to run horizontally in a skin crease approximately two finger widths below the angle of the mandible (Fig. 15.1). This limb of the incision should be oriented so that it could be extended into an incision that will accommodate dissection of the neck. The incision should not extend far posteriorly into the thin skin below the lobule over the mastoid tip. This skin will become ischemic in patients who use tobacco or have diabetes, and the surgeon will risk development of skin flap loss.

In patients who are particularly concerned with scar camouflage, the incision can be placed in the retrotragal area to hide the scar better. If the surgeon performs this type of incision, the incision line should lie just inside the anterior edge of the tragus and the dissection of the skin over the tragus should be very thin, in the immediate subcutaneous plane to avoid elevation of the tragal

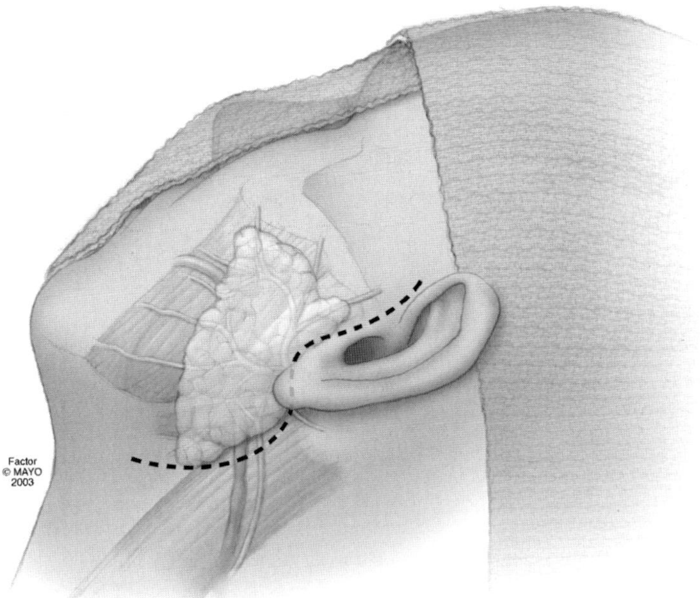

Fig. 15.1: Parotid incision. (From Olsen [10]. Used with permission of Mayo Foundation for Medical Education and Research)

perichondrium. The inferior incision also can be curved around the lobule and up onto the posterior conchal cartilage and back into the hairline. This incision is similar to the incision used in rhytidectomy, and its use can allow the surgeon to totally hide the incisional sequelae of parotidectomy. Although the exposure offered with this incision can allow full mobilization of the parotid gland, it is more difficult to incorporate neck dissection into the operation with this exposure. For this reason, postauricular incisions should be used only when the surgeon is convinced that the patient has benign disease.

The surgeon may crosshatch the incision lines superficially with a no. 10 or 15 blade to assist in precise realignment during closure. The incision is then made from superior to inferior through the skin into the subcutaneous tissue with the scalpel. Double skin hooks are placed into the facial flap, and the flap is raised for 1 cm with the blade. The assistant places firm upward retraction on the skin flap with the hooks, and back-traction is applied on the skin with a sponge by the surgeon or a second assistant. The surgeon should raise the flap immediately over the parotid fascia, which is recognizable as a white fibrous layer deep to the subcutaneous fat and superficial musculoaponeurotic system layer. Care should be taken not to enter a superficial tumor or the substance of the gland during flap elevation. Flap elevation continues with Jones scissors spread open perpendicularly along the parotid fascia; the scissors opens tunnels along the parotid gland which are then connected with blunt and sharp dissection over the parotid fascia (Fig. 15.2). In this way, the filamentous cutaneous ligaments that anchor the skin to the deep facial structures are divided, and small vessels are coagulated with bipolar cauterization. Flap elevation in this fashion can be carried to the anterior edge of the parotid gland. At this point, tissues are no longer cut, and the surgeon only bluntly spreads the tissue beyond the edge of the parotid gland. Spreading should occur in the same perpendicular orientation of the scissors tips, with the long axis of the scissors oriented parallel to the branches of the facial nerve. Dissection should continue anteriorly over the fascia of the masseter muscle. Branches of the facial nerve may be seen coursing toward the mid face just deep to this fascia. At the periphery, the parotid duct should not be looked for or isolated during this portion of the operation. Doing so could put the buccal branches of the facial nerve that accompany this duct at risk.

Skin hooks should next be placed on the inferior and posterior edges of the skin flap beneath the lobule. The anterior edge of the sternocleidomastoid muscle is identified, and the greater auricular nerve and external jugular vein, located just anterior to the nerve, are identi-

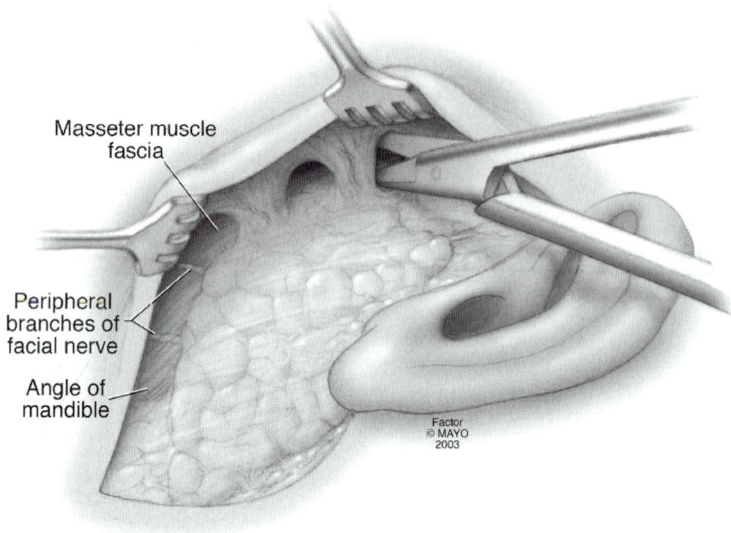

Fig. 15.2: Separation of the facial flap from the parotid gland. (From Olsen [10]. Used with permission of Mayo Foundation for Medical Education and Research)

fied. The greater auricular nerve and its branches are the largest component of the upper surgical plexus [10]. The nerve divides into mastoid, auricular, and facial branches, and the posterior branches can be preserved in some operations. The greater auricular nerve should be followed distally beyond its branch point before division. It then can be divided at its branches and reflected inferiorly, thereby allowing for the potential for nerve grafting from the facial nerve trunk to distal branches if the facial nerve has to be sacrificed. If possible, the external jugular vein should not be divided. After elevation of the skin flaps, the skin is secured with elastic hook retraction or self-retaining retractors to allow for adequate visualization of the entire field.

Deeper Dissection

The parotid gland is next separated from the anterior sternocleidomastoid muscle by sharp dissection. The gland is secured with Kocher clamps along its inferior border away from any tumor and retracted superomedially to assist in dissection. The gland also is separated bluntly from the tragal cartilage by spreading with Jones scissors parallel to the plane of the cartilage down to the level of the tragal cartilaginous pointer. A small bridge of tissue is divided to permit contiguous exposure of the entire anterior border of the sternocleidomastoid muscle and the tragal pointer. Several veins in this tissue require bipolar cauterization. A finger placed to the depth of the cartilaginous canal can allow palpation of the bony canal, the mastoid tip, and the tympanomastoid suture line.

After the parotid gland has been completely separated from the sternocleidomastoid muscle and the tragus, the posterior belly of the digastric muscle should be identified. The search for this muscle should not be too low in the surgical field, thereby putting the internal jugular vein or accessory nerve at unnecessary risk. Another common error is to search for the muscle too anterior in the field, thereby putting the marginal branch of the facial nerve at risk. The mastoid tip and the posterior border of the angle of the mandible serve as landmarks for the posterior digastric muscle. Once the muscle belly is identified immediately deep to the angle of the mandible, the remainder of the parotid gland is freed with blunt dissection. The surgeon is advised to trade the Jones scissors for a curved clamp at this point and to use this instrument for the remainder of the dissection as a means to resist the temptation to cut tissue until the facial nerve is clearly identified and mobilized. At this point, this dissection should have allowed for generous exposure of the entire inferior surface of the parotid gland, the posterior belly of the digastric muscle, and the mastoid tip and tragal cartilage. Some of the musculature that makes up the bed of the deep parotid gland may also be seen. The surgeon may visualize the stylohyoid muscle; the stylopharyngeus and styloglossus muscles are more superior and not seen yet. Near the angle of the mandible between the

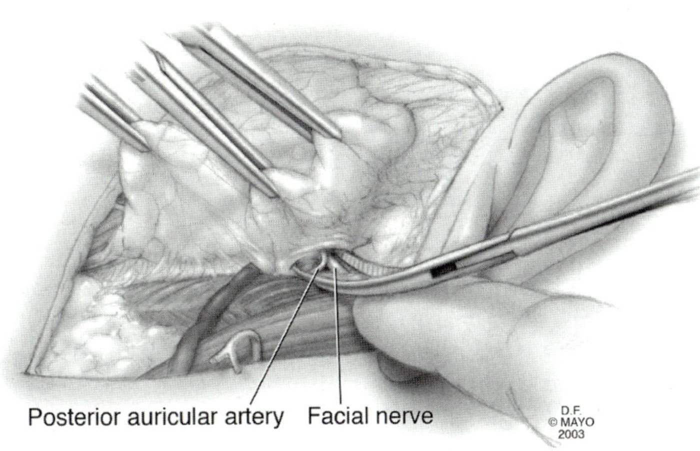

Fig. 15.3: Identification of the facial nerve. (From Olsen [10]. Used with permission of Mayo Foundation for Medical Education and Research)

stylohyoid and stylopharyngeus muscles, the external carotid artery enters the deep portion of the parotid gland. Hemostasis should be achieved with bipolar cauterization. Only when the field is widely exposed on a broad front and meticulous hemostasis has been achieved should the surgeon begin to expose the main trunk of the facial nerve.

Facial Nerve Mobilization

Kocher clamps are repositioned along the posterior parotid gland to provide adequate countertraction (Fig. 15.3). The assistant, in addition to providing traction, should also watch the patient's face to report movement as "twitching" of the facial musculature, which indicates stimulation of the facial nerve. The main trunk of the facial nerve exits the stylomastoid foramen immediately posterior to the styloid process. The styloid process is rarely felt during superficial parotidectomy. The nerve gives off branches to the posterior belly of the digastric muscle and postauricular muscles before it turns anterolaterally and enters the parotid gland just anterior to the border where the digastric muscle inserts into the mastoid. Tumors may thin the nerve or displace the trunk, but the position where the nerve enters the gland is constant.

Placing a finger on the mastoid tip, the surgeon uses the position of the cartilaginous tragal pointer and superior edge of the digastric muscle to identify the position of the facial nerve. It may be helpful to identify deeper structures such as the styloid process or tympanomastoid suture line to aid in nerve identification though these structures are not in view during this portion of the dissection. A small curved clamp is oriented perpendicular to the anticipated direction of the facial trunk to elevate tissues layer by layer. Scissors are never used for dissection down to the nerve, and no tissue is cut in this area until the nerve is seen. The tissue will separate with blunt dissection and traction before the nerve will tear, and this technique will prevent the surgeon from ever inadvertently cutting the facial nerve. Blunt dissection proceeds posterior to anterior until the surgeon identifies the nerve as a white cord 2–3 mm wide. The nerve is striking once it is identified, and it will not be confused with other structures in the vicinity. Further mobilization is performed by separating gland from the nerve, proceeding anteriorly; often the assistant will notice some twitching of the face during this separation (Fig. 15.4). The surgeon should dissect distally along the nerve to identify the pes and confirm that the main trunk has been identified proximal to any significant branches. By increasing upward retraction on the gland, the assistant can reduce any bleeding that may obscure the field. The only troublesome vessel in this area is the posterior auricular artery.

The posterior auricular artery travels posteriorly along the digastric muscle after it arises from the external carotid artery or, more rarely, the occipital artery. It usually lies inferior to the facial nerve trunk, but it may overlie it before sending branches to the mastoid and external auditory canal. The artery should not be divided until the facial nerve is identified. After identification of the trunk and during mobilization of the inferior parotid gland, the artery is ligated to prevent later hemorrhage.

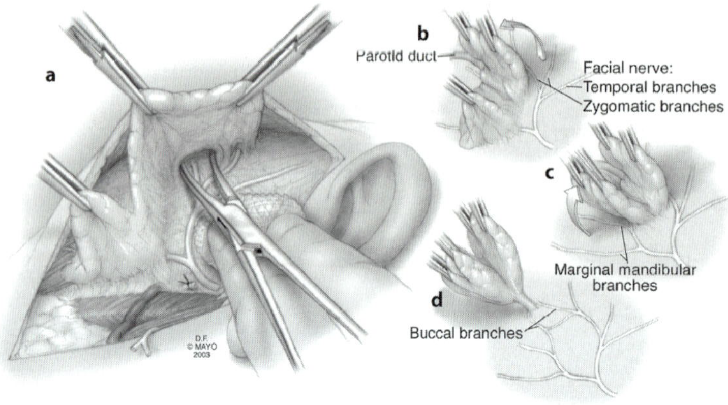

Fig. 15.4: Dissecting the facial nerve from the superficial gland. (From Olsen [10]. Used with permission of Mayo Foundation for Medical Education and Research)

Removal of the Superficial Gland

Traction on the gland should be in an upward direction; often the assistant retracts the gland anteriorly to enable the assistant to see the procedure, and the surgeon may have to redirect the retraction repetitively to ensure efficient direction of pull. The surgeon chooses either a superior division or an inferior division to work along initially. Often it is helpful to work away from the majority of the tumor to mobilize as much of the gland as possible before working along the less forgiving portion of the gland. The gland is separated at its edge, the temporal or marginal branches being followed to the periphery. The thickest fascia is encountered posterosuperiorly; this must be divided sharply or the surgeon will make tunnels into the gland along the nerve, and the procedure will slow to a crawl. Posteriorly, the surgeon will encounter branches of the superficial temporal vein, and these veins can be cauterized with bipolar cautery or ligated depending on their size.

Inferiorly, the surgeon will encounter the posterior facial vein, which is crossed by the inferior branches of the facial nerve. The marginal branch usually passes directly anterior to this vein and the anterior facial vein. The cervical branch may be superficial or deep or have branches on both sides of this vein. The vein should be carefully ligated after identification and preservation of these branches. Troublesome bleeding during dissection usually can be controlled by traction on the Kocher clamps by the assistant and by countertraction applied with a sponge on the gland by the surgeon. Obvious bleeding vessels can be cauterized with bipolar cautery. Vessels directly adjacent to the nerve branches should not be cauterized until the superficial lobe is completely mobilized.

After following a nerve branch to its peripheral emergence from the parotid gland, the surgeon returns to a proximal position along that nerve and searches for another branch to follow. In this manner the dissection progresses from posterior to anterior and either superiorly or inferiorly until the superficial gland has been completely separated from the facial nerve and the deep parotid gland. At this point, the surgeon should have a clear impression of the relationship of the tumor to the facial nerve, superficial gland, deep gland, and surrounding structures. It may be necessary to dissect along the tumor capsule to separate it from the deep gland and facial nerve. Careful retraction and meticulous dissection can prevent rupture of the tumor capsule, which is often pivotal in the prevention of recurrence. If the facial nerve is adherent to the tumor, the surgeon may elect to perform a biopsy of the nerve based on what is known about the histopathologic nature of the main tumor.

The gland is now left attached to only the parotid duct. The surgeon inspects this area to ensure that no buccal branches are adherent to the duct. The duct is divided and ligated, and the specimen is sent for examination by the pathologist. The wound should now be irrigated and the field inspected for bleeding vessels, which are ligated. The surgeon may need to wait for frozen-section pathologic results to make a decision about proceeding with total parotidectomy or closing. This time can be spent inspecting the wound, achieving meticulous hemostasis, and palpating the deep gland and neck to assess adequate tumor removal and lymphadenopathy. This is also an excellent time to review anatomic relationships and teach parotid anatomy and tumor pathology to assistants and surgeons in training.

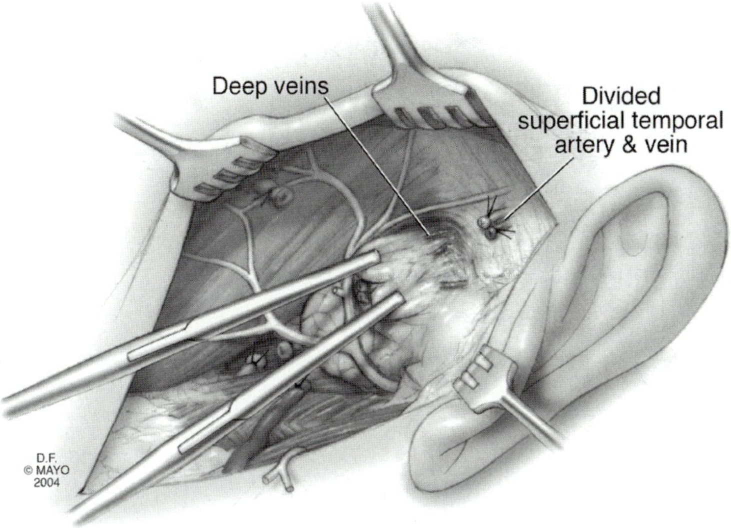

Fig. 15.5: Mobilization of the deep parotid gland and gaining of vascular control. (Used with permission of Mayo Foundation for Medical Education and Research)

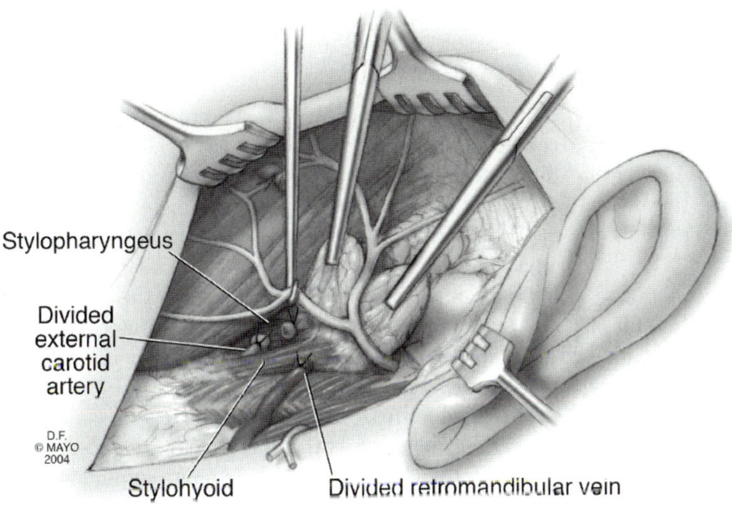

Fig. 15.6: Division of the carotid artery and posterior facial vein. (Used with permission of Mayo Foundation for Medical Education and Research)

Deep Parotidectomy

The essence of deep parotidectomy is vascular control. Once the surgeon has made the decision to perform deep parotid gland removal, the intraglandular segments of the external carotid artery and deep veins are ligated and divided (Fig. 15.5). The superficial temporal artery and vein are ligated at the superior periphery of the gland. Often the surgeon must ligate several branches in this area, because the vessels may branch at the periphery of the gland. The external carotid artery is isolated superior to the digastric muscle before it enters the inferior surface of the gland. The surgeon may need to divide the digastric and stylohyoid musculature to gain adequate access. In some elderly patients, the artery is tortuous in this area, and care should be taken to visualize branches off the artery, or to clearly identify the internal carotid artery and differentiate it from the external carotid artery, before ligation of the external carotid vessel. The posterior facial vein is divided and ligated if this step has not already been performed (Fig. 15.6). The transverse facial artery is divided at the superior anterior periphery of the gland. The only

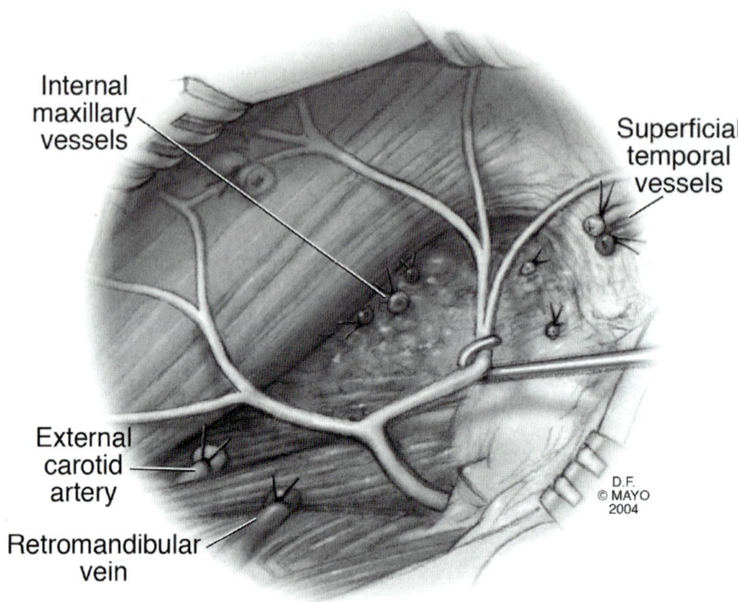

Fig. 15.7: Removal of the deep gland by mobilization of the facial nerve. (Used with permission of Mayo Foundation for Medical Education and Research)

significant vascular structures remaining at this point are the internal maxillary artery and venous tributaries to the pterygoid musculature located at the posterior border of the masseter muscle and mandibular ramus. These vessels are managed later in the procedure after mobilization of the deep gland for better exposure.

After control of the intraglandular vessels is obtained, the facial nerve trunk and branches are mobilized off of the underlying tumor. This step is best performed with a combination of blunt and sharp dissection with the nerve directly in view and gently retracted by the assistant with a nerve hook (Fig. 15.7). After complete mobilization of the nerve, the gland can be bluntly dissected from the deep bed with retraction and separation of the fascial attachments with a small curved clamp. The gland is separated from the temporomandibular joint, bony ear canal, condyle of the mandible, and styloglossus and stylopharyngeus muscles.

Now the deep venous tributaries that enter the pterygoid musculature can be cauterized or ligated and divided. The internal maxillary artery and adjacent veins will be encountered at the posterior mandibular ramus and need to be ligated and divided. The gland is now easily mobilized from superior to inferior and delivered from beneath the facial nerve trunk and inferior facial nerve division into the neck. The deep portion of the gland adjacent to the parapharyngeal space is mobilized with blunt dissection. If necessary for access, the stylomandibular ligament can be mobilized anteriorly to further open the stylomandibular tunnel. Portions of the tumor or gland that enter this area can be mobilized with finger dissection.

The gland is completely freed from attachment to any adjacent structures and sent for frozen-section pathologic examination. Small vessels around the deep gland adjacent to the mastoid and trunk can be cauterized using the bipolar forceps. The wound is irrigated, and meticulous hemostasis is achieved. If necessary, the incision can be extended for neck dissection at this time.

At the conclusion of the operation, a suction drain is placed in the wound through a separate stab incision in the postauricular skin and sewn into place. The wound is closed with interrupted absorbable sutures of 4-0 poliglecaprone 25 in the deep dermis and platysma and 5-0 absorbable sutures in the subcuticular skin. A conforming dressing or antibiotic ointment can be applied, and the patient is awakened and extubated.

Total Parotidectomy with Facial Nerve Sacrifice

In general, if facial nerve function is normal preoperatively, even in patients with malignancy, then the nerve can be preserved with careful dissection of the tumor off the nerve sheath. If the nerve is paretic or fully paralyzed preoperatively, then it is involved with tumor and is normally resected during tumor resection. Nerve that is clearly invaded by high-grade malignant tumor should be resected with the specimen to negative proximal and distal margins. This may necessitate sacrificing peripheral branches, divisions, or even the main trunk of the facial nerve. Intraoperatively, a nerve that is infiltrated with tumor will appear swollen and usually darker than the normal glistening white appearance of normal facial nerve. A biopsy of a questionably involved peripheral nerve branch can be performed intraoperatively, but biopsy of the nerve will result in paresis or paralysis. Once a decision has been made to resect a nerve that is embedded in or infiltrated by tumor, the surgeon should check the proximal and distal nerve margins repetitively until they are both cleared, as evidenced on frozen-section pathologic examination. This may necessitate following the nerve into the mastoid bone by performing mastoidectomy to access the vertical or horizontal section of the proximal facial nerve.

After negative proximal and distal facial nerve margins are obtained, the nerve is reconstructed with primary neurorraphy or grafting. Mastoidectomy and nerve mobilization may be necessary to attain proper length of the facial nerve for tension-free anastomosis. Appropriate grafts include the ipsilateral greater auricular nerve if it is not involved with tumor or an ipsilateral sural nerve graft. The graft should be harvested with meticulous technique, freshened, and approximated without tension or redundancy with minimal use of well-placed 9-0 nylon sutures. If the proximal facial nerve is not suitable for grafting, peripheral branches can be grafted to the ipsilateral hypoglossal nerve by placement of an interpositional jump graft to preserve facial tone.

The surgeon may elect to perform additional procedures after resection of the facial nerve. The upper eyelid may be managed by placement of a gold-weight or temporary lateral tarsorrhaphy, the brow may be elevated with direct browlift, and the lower lid may be suspended with lateral canthoplasty and lid shortening. These maneuvers become more essential in elderly patients with skin laxity because of the potential for early problems with ectropion and corneal exposure, which develop much more readily than in younger patients with tighter skin tone [6]. Management of the lower face with suspension may be performed primarily or secondarily based on the surgeon's and the patient's expectations for facial nerve recovery. The surgeon should be cautious in performing temporalis transfer after total parotidectomy performed as previously described, because the deep and superficial temporalis vasculature has been compromised by division of the external carotid contributions.

Resection of Adjacent Structures and Reconstruction

The operation may be extended to involve resection of adjacent structures that are involved with tumor. It may include lateral or subtotal temporal bone resection, partial mandibular resection, resection of the overlying skin, resection of portions or all of the auditory canal, and resection of surrounding musculature. The surgeon should be guided by the extent of gross tumor and the frozen-section results. The surgeon should not be limited by inexperience, less than thorough knowledge of adjacent anatomy, or concerns with the potential for reconstruction. The goal after embarking on this operation for malignancy is total tumor removal with negative margins. The preoperative work-up should have assessed the resectability of the tumor. Patients with extensive parotid malignancies should be cared for only in an operating theater that possesses technically adept and competent teams supplying necessary skills in frozen-section pathology. The team should possess the capability to perform full tumor extirpation at the parotid bed, skull base, temporal bone, and neck. The team should also be competent with reconstruction use of locoregional flaps and microvascular reconstruction. If these capabilities are not available in one center at one setting, then the patient deserves referral to a more experienced team. At no time should the surgeon subject the patient to the fallacy that near total tumor removal is adequate treatment and that additional adjuvant chemotherapy or radiation will "mop up" the remaining positive margins.

After complete removal of the parotid gland, the patient is left with a significant cosmetic defect. If the operation included resection of the facial nerve or adjacent structures, the patient may be left with a significant cosmetic or functional defect. Reconstruction of these defects depends on the patient's desires, age, additional treatment plans, and expected outcomes and on many other factors. In short, it is highly individualized to the patient. The preoperative discussion should have explored these options in depth to fully guide the surgeon at the time of the operation. We often divide the resection and the reconstruction into separate but intimately coordinated teams. Among the many benefits of this approach is the concept that the resecting surgeon is not influenced subconsciously to minimize the operation because of concerns with the feasibility of reconstructing the defect.

Options for reconstruction include primary closure, dermal fat grafting, muscle transposition with locoregional flaps of the sternocleidomastoid or pectoralis muscles, and microvascular cutaneous, musculocutaneous, and innervated muscular flaps. Again, the reconstruction will be guided by the functional and aesthetic goals of the surgeon and patient. The details of these reconstructions are discussed elsewhere in this book (see Chapter 26, Reconstruction after Excision of Cancer of the Salivary Glands).

Postoperative Care

Hospitalization and Wound Care

After total parotidectomy with nerve preservation, patients are admitted to the hospital for overnight observation. Undetected and expanding hematoma can cause airway compromise that can be life-threatening. If a dressing has been applied, it is removed the next morning, the wound is inspected, and the patient can be discharged with instructions in wound care, bathing, and activity. Patients are instructed to watch the wound for redness, swelling, or drainage that indicates the presence of infection, seroma, or hematoma.

Young patients may have minimal to moderate facial paresis (House grade 2–3) after total parotidectomy. Older patients will generally have more significant paresis after the operation, and it will usually take longer (3–6 months) to recover fully. Facial paresis may actually worsen during the first 2 days after the operation because of neurapraxia. During recovery, adequate eye care is essential to prevent exposure-related ophthalmologic complications. Patients are instructed to lubricate the eye with an ophthalmic ointment before sleeping, and they should be instructed to use moisturizing drops frequently during the day. This prophylaxis should be continued until full eye closure is achieved. A moisture chamber may be helpful for some patients. For patients without adequate Bell phenomenon or who lack dexterity or mental faculty to adequately assess and self-treat dryness of the eye, consideration should be given to more aggressive eye care such as temporary tarsorrhaphy and regular ophthalmologic examination.

Patients are instructed that they will experience numbness of the auricle, particularly around the lobule. The numbness will be most noticeable in patients with pierced ears. It will improve for up to a year after the operation, but the inferior lobule usually remains anesthetic. The depression around the ear improves slightly with time, but it will persist in patients with total parotidectomy, and it will be more severe with greater removal of surrounding tissue. Patients are instructed to move their head and neck after the operation, and they are given instructions on shoulder exercises if a neck dissection has been performed. Counseling is given on "first-bite" pain which consists of pain on initiating chewing. Patients are instructed to chew gum for physiotherapy. The pain usually resolves completely with time.

Long-term Care and Expectations

Frey's syndrome (gustatory sweating) results when the postganglionic parasympathetic nerve fibers of the parotid gland aberrantly reinnervate the sweat glands in the skin. This develops 6–12 months postoperatively, and it is present in all patients. Patients may not volunteer its presence until questioned, or they may complain of "leaking saliva" from the incision when eating. Management may range from reassurance and explanation, which are more readily accepted when a patient has been counseled preoperatively, to application of clear antiperspirants to anticholinergic therapy and botulinum toxin application to interpositional grafting. Rarely are aggressive treatments necessary, because the potential complications of infection, seroma, and nerve injury rarely are justified by the severity of the symptoms (see Chapter 5, Treatment of Frey's Syndrome).

Few patients have sialocele develop after total parotidectomy; the incidence decreases as the majority to all of the gland is removed. If it develops, it can be managed by needle aspiration and a pressure dressing. Rarely, insertion of a Penrose or suction drain, compression dressing, and a short course of anticholinergic therapy may be necessary.

Patients are referred for adjuvant therapy as indicated by tumor histology and extent. Indications for radiotherapy postoperatively include high-grade tumors with perineural invasion, nodal extent to multiple nodes, extracapsular nodal extension, and close margins with a high chance of tumor recurrence [14].

Adequate follow-up for patients who undergo parotidectomy for malignancy entails regular 3-month examinations for 2 years followed by 6-month examinations for 3 years and thereafter yearly follow-up. This schedule can be modified according to the pathologic findings and suspicion of recurrence by the surgeon. Some parotid tumors, such as mucoepidermoid carcinoma, have a very low chance of recurrence after adequate removal, whereas others, such as adenoid cystic carcinoma, may recur years after wide resection [2]. Regular imaging with serial magnetic resonance imaging or positron emission tomography can aid in the detection of recurrence when meaningful intervention is still possible. Patients may be hesitant to come for follow-up because of fear, denial, or inappropriate confidence of cure, and the surgeon should be thorough and assure the patient of the importance of this part of the treatment.

Finally, patients should be reassured that the healing after total parotidectomy takes months rather than days. Discomfort, cosmetic deficits, and functional deficits generally improve for up to 2 years postoperatively. Patients who have had both proper treatment and preparation for the sequelae of total parotidectomy will return regularly and have disease-free survival and improvement that will satisfy both the patient and the surgeon.

Take Home Messages

- Total parotidectomy is a spectrum of operations from straightforward to complex.
- The surgeon performing total parotidectomy should possess detailed knowledge of parotid and periparotid anatomy, experience in parotid surgery and facial nerve surgery, and thorough knowledge of the behavior of benign and malignant parotid tumors.
- The surgeon individualizes the operation to the tumor and the patient.
- The parotid gland is separated artificially by the surgeon into a large portion superficial to the facial nerve and a smaller portion deep to the nerve.
- Both portions of the parotid gland can develop benign and malignant tumors and contain lymph nodes.
- Cancer with the potential to metastasize to lymphatics in the parotid gland should be managed by total parotidectomy.
- Thorough preoperative work-up and discussion build rapport and confidence between the surgeon and patient.
- Fine-needle aspiration is rarely necessary or completely accurate preoperatively.
- Frozen-section pathologic examination is essential for decision making during parotidectomy.
- If the facial nerve functions normally preoperatively, it generally should be preserved.
- If the facial nerve is dysfunctional preoperatively or infiltrated by tumor intraoperatively, it should be resected to achieve negative margins.
- The key to total parotidectomy is adequate control of the intraglandular external carotid artery and deep veins.
- Total parotidectomy results in a defect that may require reconstruction.

References

1. Beahrs OH, Adson MA (1958) The surgical anatomy and technic of parotidectomy. Am J Surg 95:885–896
2. Boahene DKO, Olsen KD, Lewis JE, et al. (2004) Mucoepidermoid carcinoma of the parotid gland: the Mayo Clinic experience. Arch Otolaryngol Head Neck Surg 130:849–856
3. Davis RA, Anson BJ, Budinger JM, et al. (1956) Surgical anatomy of the facial nerve and parotid gland based upon a study of 350 cervicofacial halves. Surg Gynecol Obstet 102:385–412
4. Garatea-Crelgo J, Gay-Escoda C, Bermejo B, et al. (1993) Morphological study of the parotid lymph nodes. J Craniomaxillofac Surg 21:207–209
5. Gray H (1966) Anatomy of the human body, 28th edn. Lea & Febiger, Philadelphia

6. Guntinas-Lichius O, Gabriel B, Peter Klussmann J (2006) Risk of facial palsy and severe Frey's syndrome after conservative parotidectomy for benign disease: analysis of 610 operations. Acta Otolaryngol 126:1104–1109
7. Johns ME (1977) The salivary glands: anatomy and embryology. Otolaryngol Clin North Am 10:261–271
8. Kidd HA (1950) Complete excision of the parotid gland with preservation of the facial nerve. Br Med J 1:989–991
9. Krolls SO, Boyers RC (1972) Mixed tumors of salivary glands: long-term follow-up. Cancer 30:276–281
10. Olsen KD (2004) Superficial parotidectomy. Oper Tech Gen Surg 6:102–114
11. Patey DH, Thackray AC (1957) The pathological anatomy and treatment of parotid tumours with retropharyngeal extension (dumb-bell tumours); with a report of 4 personal cases. Br J Surg 44:352–358
12. Pisani P, Ramponi A, Pia F (1996) The deep parotid lymph nodes: an anatomical and oncological study. J Laryngol Otol 110:148–150
13. Zbaren P, Nuyens M, Loosli H, et al. (2004) Diagnostic accuracy of fine-needle aspiration cytology and frozen section in primary parotid carcinoma. Cancer 100:1876–1883
14. Zbaren P, Nuyens M, Caversaccio M, et al. (2006) Postoperative radiation therapy for T1 and T2 primary parotid carcinoma: is it useful? Otolaryngol Head Neck Surg 135:140–143

Chapter 16

Recurrent Pleomorphic Adenoma

16

Patrick J. Bradley

Contents

Core Features

- Causes of recurrence
- Clinical presentations
- Assessment of risk for recurrence
- Options for treatment
- Management of the facial nerve
- Results of treatment of the parotid gland
- Risks of Malignant Transformation
- Role of radiation therapy
- Recurrent submandibular gland pleomorphic adenoma
- Recurrent minor salivary gland pleomorphic adenoma
- Conclusion

Complications to Avoid

- In primary surgery, attention to surgical technique, avoidance of tumor manipulation, and adequate exposure will reduce the likelihood of recurrence of pleomorphic adenoma.
- When recurrence is suspected, review the histology from previous surgery and confirm accurately the persistence or recurrence of the pleomorphic adenoma.
- Revision surgery usually reveals a tumor more extensive than was evaluated both clinically and by imaging.

- If complete excision is unlikely with or without preservation of neurological structures then referral to a specialist center is warranted.

Introduction

The treatment of choice for salivary gland neoplasms, both benign and malignant, is surgery with preservation of vascular and neurological structures. This assumes, of course, that the patient is willing to undergo the proposed surgery and that their comorbidities do not contraindicate surgery. The aim of salivary gland tumor surgery is complete excision, with as safe of a margin of normal tissue that is feasible and oncologically appropriate.

Recurrent tumor following surgery or any treatment usually presents as a recurrent swelling at the primary site, with or without local symptoms: a mass or multiple masses, pain, ulcer, facial palsy, dyspnea, diplopia, or dysphonia depending upon whether the primary site is of major or minor salivary gland origin. Tumors of salivary gland origin may recur in sites distant from the primary site, and may present singly or in combination with such as cervical nodal involvement or distant metastases to lung, bone, and brain. The recurrence may present months or years following treatment, and hence 5-year survival figures for tumors of salivary gland origin are generally meaningless unless data include patients followed up and observed for more than 15–20 years [5, 11]. Unfortunately in the current climate of nationalized care in the UK, the cost and time for this protracted follow-up has dissuaded some specialists from providing prolonged surveillance.

Pleomorphic Adenoma

The most common benign tumor of salivary gland origin is the pleomorphic adenoma (80%) and presents at all sites in the head and neck, as salivary gland tissue is distributed widely. The most frequent site is the parotid gland (Fig. 16.1), followed by the submandibular gland and the minor salivary glands, particularly in the oral cavity. Pleomorphic adenomas are usually solitary lesions, although synchronous or metachronous involvement of two or more major glands can occur [25] (Fig. 16.2). Pleomorphic adenomas may also be found in combination with other salivary gland tumors, most commonly Warthin's tumor [15, 74]. Pleomorphic adenoma may develop in patients from a wide range of ages but are most commonly diagnosed in patients between the ages of 30 and 50 years; they are uncommon in the first two decades of life, although they have been reported [8].

The usual clinical presentation is of a painless, slowly growing, firm mass when diagnosed in all sites of the head and neck. The tumor is usually surrounded by a fibrous capsule of varying thickness with a clear demarcation between the tumor and the adjacent salivary tissue. Morphological diversity is the hallmark of pleomorphic adenoma, and few other tumors of salivary gland origin manifest such a wide spectrum. All tumors demonstrate combinations of gland-like epithelium and mesenchymal-like tissue, but the proportions of each vary widely. Pleomorphic adenomas are categorized into four types: principally myxoid; myxoid and cellular components present in equal proportions; predominantly cellular; and extreme cellular [74]. Pleomorphic adenomas arising in the oral and pharyngeal minor salivary glands demonstrate the same histological features as those in the major glands. Pleomorphic adenomas arising in the minor salivary gland generally present as well-circumscribed, smooth, firm masses, most commonly located on the palate, upper lip, and buccal mucosa [75], but also present in the nasal cavity, oropharynx, and larynx. Because most pleomorphic adenomas arising in minor salivary glands are removed when they are less than 2.0 cm, surface bosselation is uncommon; it is seen frequently when tumors are bigger than 3 cm. A fibrous capsule is not often apparent, but the tumor is clearly demarcated from the surrounding tissues.

The management of a primary pleomorphic adenoma is complete surgical excision with preservation of local neurological structures wherever its location in the head and neck. Accurate assessment by computed tomography (CT) or magnetic resonance imaging (MRI) and the judicious use of fine-needle aspiration cytology (FNAC) provide important information which is used in formulating a plan of management. In the parotid gland this implies that the surgical goal should be to achieve tumor clearance within the confines imposed by the facial nerve [26]. The tumor capsule and margins can be violated by any surgical procedure, which makes this form of surgery of the parotid gland precise, and the technique used is of paramount importance for successful tumor surgery [6, 28].

It has been reported [33] that the use of cell proliferation fraction measurements by flow cytometry as a biological parameter for the prediction of recurrence in pleomorphic adenomas should be considered. The authors stated that tumors of a larger size showed a higher

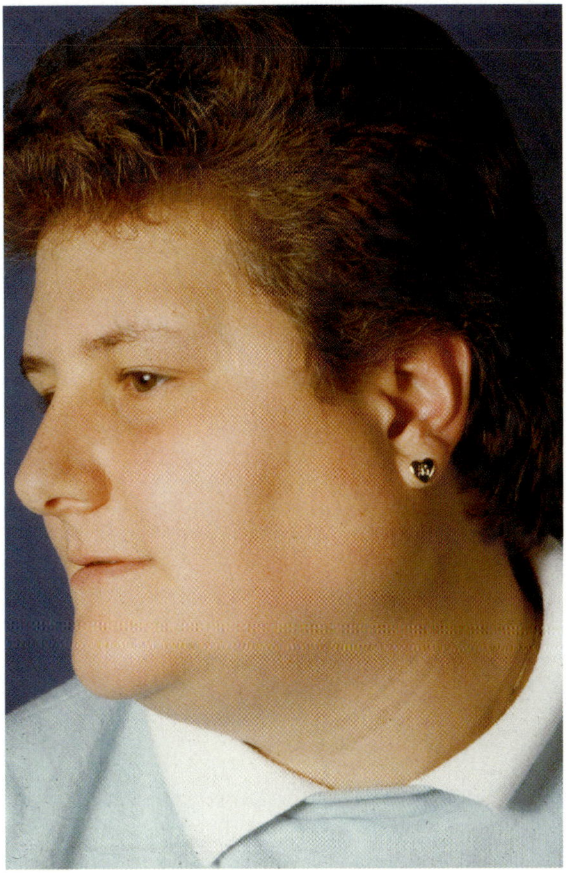

Fig. 16.1: Young nurse with large pleomorphic adenoma of the parotid gland

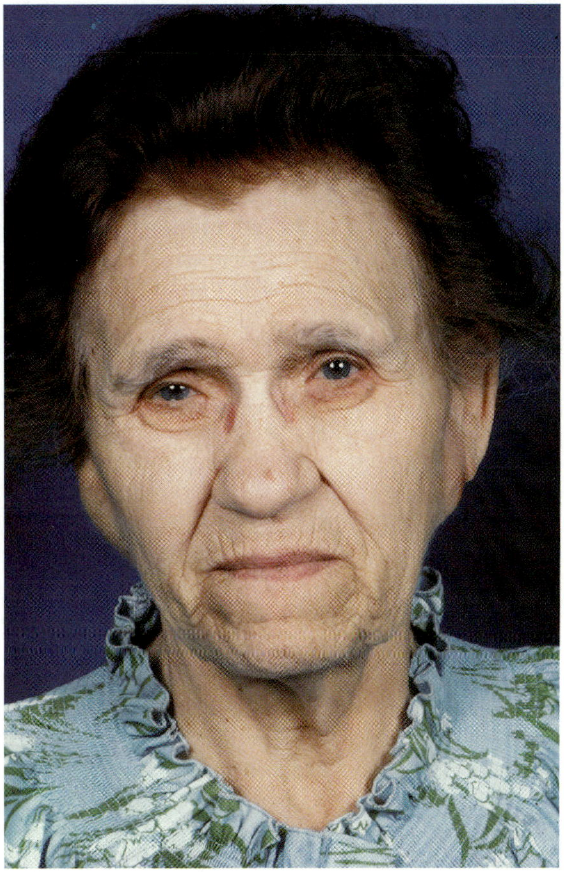

Fig. 16.2: Elderly woman with pleomorphic adenoma of both parotid glands

percentage of cells in the S-phase fraction and probably a greater tendency for recurrence. The incidence of recurrence following surgery varies depending on the surgical technique used, the experience of the surgeons, the duration of patient's follow-up, and clinical honesty. Whatever the series and its duration of patient follow-up, a recurrence rate of less than 1% is considered acceptable.

Causes of Recurrence

Multicentricity

Pleomorphic adenomas are unifocal disease in the major salivary glands; surgeons and pathologists no longer support this theory.

The Bare Area

The tumor capsule may vary in thickness from very thin (a few cells) to very thick; this variation may occur on the surface of the same tumor [68, 76]. Because many pleomorphic adenomas have a nodular surface, there is always the possibility of a nodule attached by a narrow stalk becoming separated from the main tumor mass thus giving rise to a recurrence. Pseudopodia (microscopic finger-like formations of tumor tissue which extends beyond the main mass of tumor) are a significant risk factor for local recurrence of benign pleomorphic adenomas [12, 29]. This is referred to as "capsule penetration" which occurs earlier and is more common in the bosselation process [37]. In capsular perforation, the tumor cells perforate the capsule and lie adjacent to the normal parotid tissue. Subcapsular splitting may be no more than a dehiscence resulting from perioperative handling, and the presence of blood within the split would support this hypothesis. Another publication [46] confirmed that no tumor has a smooth surface, and all tumors have a "bare area." The bare area is not always exposed to the facial nerve and may occur at any location along the tumor surface. The surgeon should carry out a wide local excision with the tumor contained within as much normal tissue as is possible. The bare area or deep surface of the tumor can lie against the cartilaginous external auditory meatus, styloid process, facial nerve, or masseter muscle.

Tumor Rupture

Rupture of the tumor, because of overzealous traction, instrument compression, rough handling, or poor surgical technique, with spillage into the surgical wound are factors which have been thought to predispose to recurrence. The interior of a pleomorphic adenoma is usually soft and gelatinous, and it is these myxoid and friable cellular tumors that are at highest risk for rupture [46]. It has been suggested that the recurrence of pleomorphic adenoma cannot be fully explained by the characteristics of the tumor itself, but the cause of recurrence can usually be laid at the door of the surgeon, and his or her technique [27]. Recent reports suggest that there is no correlation between tumor capsule rupture and recurrence in pleomorphic adenoma [10, 29, 53]. However, this evidence does not fully explain the most frequent finding of multiple nodules (Fig. 16.3a–c) rather than solitary, isolated recurrences. These observations suggest that rupture of the capsule of the tumor and spillage of tumor cells are still the most likely factors contributing to recurrence of tumor. Long-term follow-up, even annual follow-up by mail, may give a more accurate picture of tumor-free disease survival, than hoping that patients who develop a recurrence will come back and consult with their original surgeon.

Extension of Tumor into Other Areas

Extension of tumor into other areas which may go unrecognized at the time of surgery has been cited [42, 62]. For instance, the tumor may become wedged between the mastoid process and the body of the mandible.

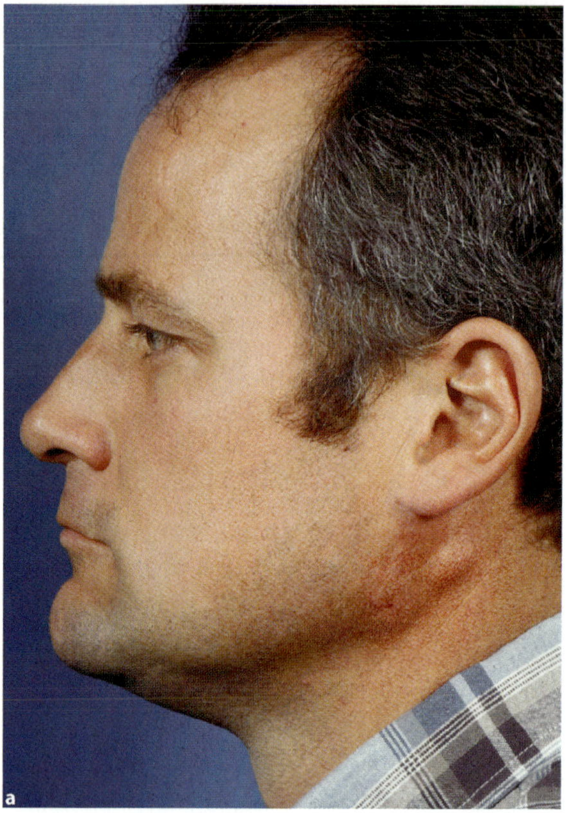

Fig. 16.3a–c: **a** Patient with recurrent pleomorphic adenoma of the tail of the parotid gland. A formal parotidectomy was not done in this case. **b–c** *see next page*

Misdiagnosis

Many clinicians still believe that a small mass in the preauricular area is more likely to be a lymph node or a sebaceous cyst than a pleomorphic adenoma. This belief results in an incisional biopsy or a local enucleation, followed by the discovery days later that the lesion was actually a pleomorphic adenoma. The clinician often elects to follow a "watch and wait" policy, and the recurrence becomes evident years later.

Enucleation

Local excision or "enucleation" was a practice recommended in the 1970s and 1980s as primary treatment

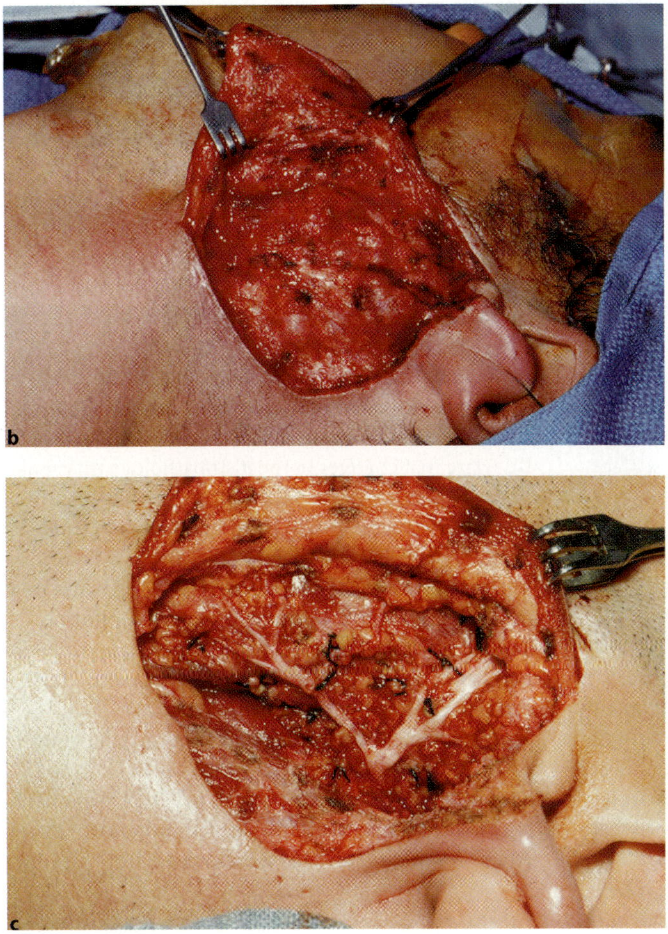

Fig. 16.3b–c: *(continued)* **b** With the flap elevated, multiple nodules of recurrent pleomorphic adenoma became apparent. **c** A total parotidectomy was carried out with preservation of the facial nerve

of pleomorphic adenoma in the parotid gland followed by postoperative radiotherapy [16, 17]. These procedures fell out of favor many years ago but advocates are resurgent again, suggesting that in "expert hands" using extracapsular dissection benign tumors can be removed safely by techniques much less invasive than a formal parotidectomy [47, 49]. However, a recurrence rate of 2% has been associated with this procedure. Other authors, reviewing the literature, continue to discourage minimal margin surgery in the parotid gland [58, 61, 69, 78]. Unfortunately the capsule surrounding the benign pleomorphic adenoma is at best a pseudocapsule that allows for bits of satellite tumors to be left behind at enucleation surgery or allows spillage during handling or manipulation during surgery, possibilities that have been discussed by many authors [2, 13, 45]. If the tumor has been enucleated with obvious rupture or documented spillage, then the proper course of treatment is a formal parotidectomy or excision of the submandibular gland.

Implantation of Tumor Cells

Implantation of tumor cells may take place along the tract of a suction drain or at the point of egress from the skin in cases of tumor rupture. Recurrences tend to be found within the surgical scar or on either side of it, marking the entry and exit points of the suture needle [42]. Soiling and contamination of instruments and gloves from an unrecognized microrupture may also give rise to recurrence.

Preoperative Biopsy

Preoperative biopsy or intraoperative sampling of the tumor may lead to soiling of the surrounding tissues and create a potential risk of recurrence. A survey of 34 internationally recognized head and neck oncologists concluded that the routine use of FNAC does not alter the treatment of a discreet mass in the parotid [48].

Poorly Designed Incisions

The incision may be poorly designed, most often in parotid surgery, usually too small limiting complete exposure of the tumor mass, and as a consequence, the surgeon may cut across the posterior border or outer surface of the tumor when the flap is being raised [70].

The Clinical Course of Recurrent Pleomorphic Adenoma

The patient with a recurrent pleomorphic adenoma usually presents with a mass and a history of parotid or submandibular surgery done some years previously. In the parotid gland there is frequently evidence of a formal parotidectomy with a large scar or a smaller scar in the preauricular area suggesting local surgery, most commonly involving the lower pole of parotid. In the submandibular gland the mass or masses may be small or extremely large. If a minor salivary gland pleomorphic adenoma has been shelled out, the patient will usually be able to relate the story.

16

Recurrences are best classified clinically as uninodular or solitary isolated lump or multinodular or with multiple nodules extending above and below the scar. Areas of multiple nodules and islands of tumor are more common in parotid and submandibular recurrences than they are in the case of intraoral tumors of minor salivary gland origin. In one series [42], the authors reported 63.2% recurrences of multinodular tumors in their series of recurrent parotid tumors. Solitary and multinodular recurrences account for 47–67%, depending on the referral pattern [42, 60]. The palpable single nodule is almost always discovered at microscopy to be a small cluster of grapes (nodules) lacking even the most rudimentary capsule.

The time interval between the first operation and presentation with recurrence varies. Few tumors recur within the first 12 months and most recurrences present between 5 and 7 years [21, 42]. Assessment of recurrent disease must include CT and/or MRI and probably ultrasound. Tumors of minor salivary glands require fastidious assessment in a three-dimensional manner by imaging before biopsy. FNAC analysis is mandatory to ensure that the tumor presenting is still a pleomorphic adenoma, as errors initially may have occurred or pathological changes may have developed in the interval between original surgery and the current presentation.

Assessment of a Recurrent Pleomorphic Adenoma of the Parotid Gland

- The pathological recurrence will be much bigger and more extensive than clinically suspected [69].
- Be aware that changes in the histopathology may make decision making more difficult.
- The revision surgery will be difficult and time consuming.
- The risk of trauma to the facial nerve is high and may be difficult to identify even with nerve monitoring.
- The facial nerve if traumatized may never recover normal function, and even may be permanently paralyzed.
- The skin may need to be replaced if recurrences invade or are adherent to the skin.
- Should the patient have had prior adjuvant radiotherapy or further recurrences, further surgery if offered will be more difficult than anticipated.

Options for the Management of Recurrent Pleomorphic Adenoma of Major Salivary Gland Origin

The best policy to prevent recurrence of pleomorphic adenoma of the salivary gland is excisional biopsy of the tumor with maximal safe margin. Functional neurological preservation is the ultimate goal [79].

Treatment of the recurrent tumor is be determined by the age and physical health of the patient, the number of pervious operations, and the anatomical extent of the recurrence. The preoperative assessment must be thorough, with radiological imaging and biopsy. Available options include:

- No treatment: The elderly and infirmed; very small tumors to palpation only, or an isolated recurrence (all must be confirmed as benign on FNAC); enormous tumors with complex anatomical involvement in an elderly patient.

Local excision of a solitary recurrence including the overlying scar (rarely feasible).

Parotid location: Superficial parotidectomy and facial nerve dissection—the recently enucleated tumor of small size and limited to the superficial lobe in which there has been no attempt to locate the facial nerve [36, 39].

Parotid location: Total parotidectomy with facial nerve dissection and preservation; the overlying scar is excised in continuity [36].

Parotid location: Total parotidectomy with resection of the involved nerve and immediate nerve graft with or without replacement of overlying skin.

Submandibular gland location: Supraomohyoid neck dissection with or without partial mandibulectomy, with or without removal of cranial nerve, and excision of the floor of the mouth may be necessary if tumor is massive or adherent [4].

Major or minor gland location: en bloc resection of the involved tissues with reconstruction by a pedicled or free tissue transfer with or without bone replacement and prosthesis [14, 54].

Any of these surgical procedures followed by radiotherapy [14, 40].

Possible use of radiotherapy alone after FNAC confirmation of pleomorphic adenoma, with full patient and family consent.

The Facial Nerve

The treatment of recurrent pleomorphic adenoma has added controversy about its management and more so when tumor and/or scar are confluent with the facial nerve. Radical excision with sacrifice if the facial nerve has been advocated but morbidity is naturally high. Even if the nerve is grafted a House-Brackman grade III is as good a result as one gets [22, 23, 38, 72]. A number of authors express reservations about forfeiting neural integrity in the presence of benign disease and recommend parotidectomy with dissection and preservation of the facial nerve [52, 54, 60]. Facial nerve paralysis after the first operation for recurrent pleomorphic adenoma is reported to be approximately 15%. In practice, the risk to the facial nerve depends on the extent of previous surgery, whether the facial nerve was paralyzed previously but recovered, and the resultant scarring; dense scarring is more likely to predispose to nerve injury. There is a greater risk of permanent nerve damage with each ensuing operation (30% chance of permanent nerve injury after three operations).

The likelihood of a temporary facial nerve weakness for 6 months was 27% at the first operation, 14% after the second, and rose to 33% at the third attempt. The likelihood of permanent paralysis rose from 27% after the first surgery to 29% at the second surgery [21].

A retrospective series of 35 patients treated surgically for first recurrence of a pleomorphic adenoma of the parotid gland were seen over a 15-year period, with a minimum follow-up of 7 years. Locoregional control was 77%, and malignant transformation was 5.7% [44].

In a series of 126 patients from the Mayo Clinic [60], rates of tumor recurrence after one operation were 32.3%, 7.1% after two operations, and 1.6% after three. After all procedures, partial facial nerve paralysis was recorded in 13.5% of patients and total paralysis was recorded in 5.5% of patients. Facial nerve injury is more likely if the tumor is deep, is in multiple sites, or if extensive scar tissue is present. In 24 patients who had had multiple operations, the rate of facial nerve paralysis was 53% (38% temporary and 15% permanent).

In another series of 42 patients [38], all patients had multinodular, non-tender recurrent nodules following one to four prior surgical procedures, and 6 patients had been treated with radiotherapy. In 30 patients the facial nerve was preserved. Ten patients had House-Brackmann Facial Nerve Grading grade I–II, 14 patients had grade III–IV, and 6 patients had grade V–VI. In the 12 patients who had the facial nerve sacrificed, the facial nerve function was grade III–IV in 5 and grade V–VI in 7.

The use of loupes and the operating microscope have greatly helped with minimizing permanent paralysis of the facial nerve after revision surgery for recurrent pleomorphic adenoma. The use of continuous facial nerve monitoring has also greatly minimized trauma to the facial nerve that has already been operated upon [19, 56]. When facial nerve monitoring is used during surgery for recurrent pleomorphic adenoma of the parotid gland, the facial nerve deficit can be reduced and the recovery of the facial nerve is faster [43, 80].

Results of Treating Recurrent Pleomorphic Adenoma of the Parotid Gland

Myssiorek et al. [52] reported that only 67% of patients with recurrent tumors ultimately achieved tumor-free status after surgery. Although initial recurrence of pleomorphic adenoma can occur as long as 20 years following the first surgery, most subsequent recurrences are known to develop within 2–5 years [16, 21]. In the parotid gland, recurrence deep to the facial nerve, which would include recurrences in the parapharyngeal space, are less likely to be controlled by further surgery than recurrences lateral to the nerve [11]. Patients with more than one recurrence were significantly younger than patients who have had only one recurrence [36]. Once a patient has a second recurrence the tumor appears to become more aggressive. Subsequent recurrences are more likely and appear more quickly than the initial recurrence [21], and the likelihood of histological malignant degeneration is also greater [16, 38, 60].

Risks of Malignant Transformation

The risk of malignant transformation of recurrent pleomorphic adenoma is said to increase with time. In the literature, this incidence has varied from less than 10% to as much as 40% [39]. In a series, 2:36 (6.9%) patients treated for multiple recurrences developed malignant disease [32]. In another series 2:40 (5%) patients in similar circumstance developed carcinoma ex-pleomorphic adenoma and died of disseminated metastases to the lung and bone [38]. The literature warns that patients with recurrent pleomorphic adenoma require thorough investigation and biopsy to confirm the true nature of the persistent clinical benign disease to exclude malignant change, prior to recommencing treatment [60]. Also it must be remembered that patients who have been treated with radiotherapy for recurrent pleomorphic adenoma also continue to have a risk of malignancy [3, 64].

Factors associated with a higher change of malignant transformation in pleomorphic adenoma of the parotid gland [60] (Fig. 16.4a, b) were age greater than 40 years at initial treatment, male sex, nodules greater than 2 cm in diameter, tumors of the deep lobe [32], solitary nodules, more frequent recurrences (more than 4) [41], and having had more than one previous operation. Malignant tumors were reported in 9 (7.1%) patients. An appraisal of adenocarcinoma ex-pleomorphic adenoma or carcinosarcoma confirms that there is a malignant change in both the epithelial and mesenchymal elements [24, 57].

The enigma of the metastasizing pleomorphic adenoma needs to be considered. It seems to be associated with incomplete surgery or enucleation, leading to multiple recurrences that appear to be a prerequisite for the development of distant metastasis [31]. The evidence is overwhelming that this is associated with persistent disease at the following sites: 95% associated with the parotid gland, followed by the submandibular gland (4%) and the minor salivary glands (1%). This should be considered a low-grade malignancy but has lethal potential and can be associated with a fatal outcome [7]. In a virtual case series, 42 patients [55] had sufficient data to analyze. The mean presentation-to-metastasis latency was 16 years. Bone (45%) was the most common site for metastases, followed by the head and neck (43%) and lung (36%). There was significant morbidity and mortality from distant metastases with 5-year disease-specific and disease-free survival of 58% and 50%, respectively.

The Role of Radiotherapy

The role of radiotherapy remains controversial in the management of primary or recurrent pleomorphic adenoma [36, 39,53]. Radiotherapy should be considered if there has been tumor spillage or residual tumor following reoperation [30, 32]. Some surgeons have not treated with radiotherapy for first-time recurrence [39] because of its ineffectiveness in preventing further recurrences as well as concerns about subsequent morbidity [11, 17]. The risk for patients who have had radiotherapy for recurrent or incompletely excised pleomorphic adenoma is well documented and should be discussed with each patient and his or her relatives before treatment is recommended for a benign tumor [66].

In another series of patients, a decision was made not to sacrifice the facial nerve in 17/21 patients and performed instead a subtotal excision of recurrent pleomorphic adenoma followed by postoperative radiotherapy. Sixteen of the 17 patients (94%) remained free of clinical recurrence, with an average follow-up of 5.9 years [65]. The dose of radiotherapy ranged from 50 to 67 Gy (average 50.5 Gy). A report is awaited to learn of the long-term follow-up of this group of patients.

There is no study to date that compares surgery alone versus surgery with radiotherapy for treatment of these recurrent tumors [64]. The recurrence rate after the first operation was 15% in this series. Subanalysis of multinodular and uninodular recurrent tumors showed that patients with multinodular disease are particularly at risk when treated by surgery alone. The use of postoperative radiotherapy demonstrated an advantage only in patients

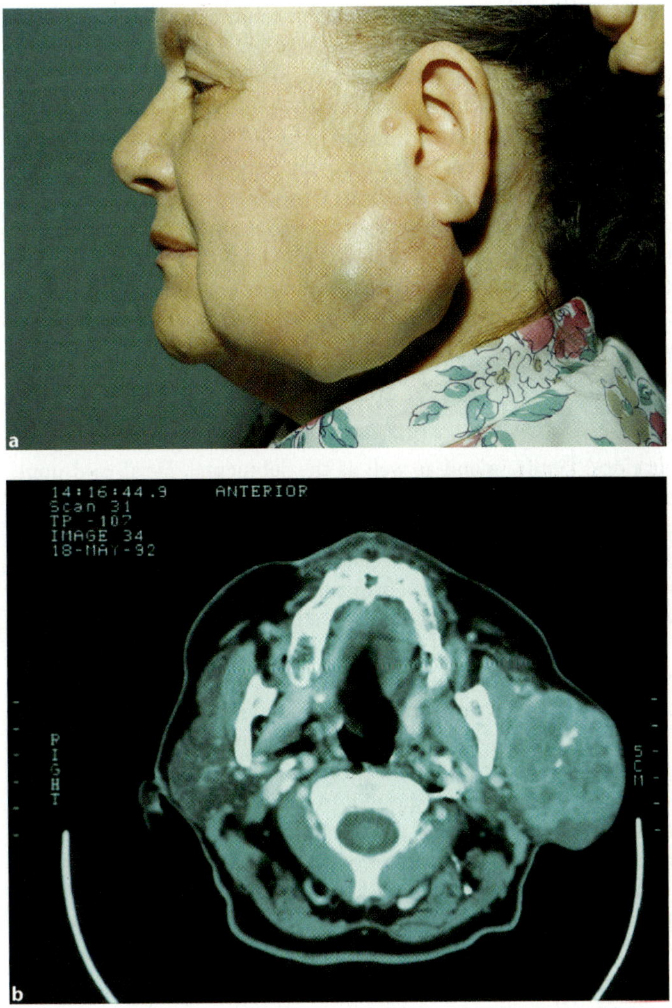

Fig. 16.4: **a** A 65-year-old patient with a 20-year history of a 7×5 cm mass in the parotid gland with a recent history of rapid increase in size and pain. Parotidectomy revealed carcinoma ex-pleomorphic adenoma. The patient was treated with adjunctive postoperative radiotherapy, had local and regional control, but died of distant metastasis within two years. **b** CT scan of same patient with carcinoma ex-pleomorphic adenoma

with multinodular recurrences [64]. None of the patients who received postoperative radiotherapy had local failure, although this difference was not statistically significant [11]. It is to be recommended that certain patients who have undergone surgery and who had ominous clinical and pathological presentations should receive postoperative radiotherapy [11].

In a large series (187 patients) from the Christie Hospital, Manchester, UK [3], all had pleomorphic adenomas of the parotid gland treated by surgery and postoperative radiotherapy by one of two techniques. Until 1976, needle implant was used, to a dose of 60 Gy, and after that time, external beam radiotherapy using megavoltage linear accelerators using an inclined plane to avoid the eyes was used. The tumor dose was 50 Gy in 15–16 fractions. This treatment followed surgery for incomplete excision or tumor spillage. The median age was 46 years, with half of the patients (87/187) having had ages between 40 and 60 years. Median follow-up for all patients was 14 years. A total of 115 patients had radiotherapy after their first operation, with a recurrence rate of 0.9% (1 of 115); of the 115 cases there were two cases of radionecrosis (one major and one minor), one case of facial palsy, one case of Frey's syndrome, and one case of salivary fistula. Seventy-two patients had radiotherapy delayed until one or more recurrences had been surgically treated. Nine of these patients (12.5%) developed yet another recurrence after radiotherapy. There were two cases of radionecrosis (one major), four cases of facial palsy (three were complete), 16 cases of Frey's syndrome, and one case of malignant change.

Recurrence after radiotherapy continued after 20 years of follow-up. It is recommended that patients having unsatisfactory surgery due to spillage at surgery or residual tumor left behind should have radiotherapy immediately, rather than delaying treatment until local recurrence occurs, because of the increased morbidity and the higher complication incidence of yet further recurrences. A similar treatment plan [40] has been recommended at Princess Margaret Hospital, Toronto with treatment to 45 Gy in 20 fractions over 4 weeks, using an ipsilateral technique encompassing the parotid bed. Using this approach, the authors report the long-term control of tumor to be in excess of 90%.

The use of neutron radiotherapy has been recommended for the management of recurrent pleomorphic adenoma of the parotid gland [9, 18]. The indications included gross residual disease and multirecurrent multinodular disease. The actuarial 15-year locoregional control was 76% for patients with gross residual disease versus 100% for those with microscopic disease [18]. The use of neutron therapy may be considered an alternative to further surgery when patients present with more than two recurrences, with a functioning facial nerve, and with a tumor less than 5 cm as there is less likely resultant damage to the facial nerve.

16

The long-term risks of radiotherapy as well as neutron therapy in the head and neck include osteosarcoma of the mandible, malignant fibrous histiocytoma, synovial fistula of the temporomandibular joint, and osteonecrosis of the temporal bone [59, 71].

Recurrent Pleomorphic Adenoma of the Submandibular Gland

It is estimated that 8% of all pleomorphic adenomas presenting in the head and neck arise in the submandibular gland and the fact that the condition is rare is reflected in the paucity of any large series of patients [1, 20, 35, 50, 63, 77]. Recurrent tumors, however, are often multifocal and difficult to re-excise completely, hence more likely to further relapse if followed up for long enough [1]. Surgical excision, by means of an extracapsular gland excision, is the mainstay primary treatment to be recommended for all clinically suspected neoplasms of the submandibular gland [1, 63, 77], not only malignant lesions but also in benign neoplasms, and more extensive resections are recommended for any subsequent recurrent pleomorphic adenoma of the submandibular gland [50, 67]. Another school of thought, however, suggests that the initial procedure for all submandibular masses should be a regional dissection of the submandibular triangle, including the entire gland as well as the submental, facial, and upper cervical lymph nodes [4, 50, 67, 77]. This ensures a definitive operation for benign lesions, avoiding the risks of tumor spillage associated with a more limited excision, and removes the primary echelon of lymph nodes at risk of metastasis if the pathology in fact turns out to be malignant [77].

The propensity of pleomorphic adenoma to recur is well documented, and although most recurrences will be evident within 5 years, a significant proportion of tumors will occur 10 or more years after treatment [67]. Pathological factors thought to contribute to tumor recurrence include tumor multicentricity and microscopic tumor capsule penetration by finger-like formations. However, one of the major risk factors for recurrence of pleomorphic adenoma is related to the adequacy and technique of surgical excision. The ideal method of excision is to remove the submandibular gland with the tumor with a margin of normal tissue, thereby reducing the risk of recurrence, as no marginal areas of tissue are left behind and no spilling of tumor cells will have occurred from breaches of the tumor capsule. Other surgical factors implicated in recurrence include intraoperative tumor rupture, misdiagnosis, and surgical implantation of tumor cells [73]. The evidence suggests that recurrent pleomorphic adenoma of the submandibular gland requires a more major excision of the submandibular triangle tissue than previously undertaken, and to ensure that a wide area is excised to encompass the multifocal disease. A selective neck dissection (supraomohyoid neck dissection) clearing levels Ib, IIa, and III should also be undertaken [51].

Recurrent Pleomorphic Adenoma of the Minor Salivary Glands

The most common site for pleomorphic adenoma is in the oral cavity, and the majority are located in the palate. Recurrent pleomorphic adenomas of the palate are usually larger than the initial tumor and are best re-biopsied and imaged before undertaking any revision surgery. The imaging of recurrent tumor is similar to that seen with a malignant process, so a change from the original pleomorphic adenoma must be excluded before proceeding with treatment. Other areas in the oral cavity where pleomorphic adenomas tend to recur commonly are the buccal mucosa and the upper lip. Wide excision should ensure that such recurrences are controlled; most of the recurrent pleomorphic adenomas arising in the oral cavity are unifocal and are suitable for further surgery. Surgeons should be aware of the possibility of malignant change in recurrent intraoral pleomorphic adenoma [34].

Conclusion

Recurrent pleomorphic adenoma is being encountered much less frequently now because the correct primary surgical procedure of complete excision of the tumor is being performed initially. The persisting major factor associated with tumor recurrence is poor surgical technique rather than tumor biology. Management of recurrent pleomorphic adenoma is currently further surgery, aiming at complete local excision with preservation of neurological structures, with consideration to adding adjunctive radiotherapy postoperatively. The use of radiotherapy currently should be reserved for patients who refuse surgery if there is likelihood that the facial nerve would need to be excised and the resultant paralysis would be unacceptable in an adjunctive setting following resection of a carcinoma ex-pleomorphic adenoma. There remains, however the persistent risk of malignant degeneration in patients who have pleomorphic adenoma of salivary gland origin. Repeated recurrences, whether the patient has had adjunctive radiotherapy or not, carry a life-long risk of malignant degeneration which may result in a fatal outcome.

Take Home Messages

- A recurrence rate in surgery for pleomorphic adenoma of >1% is considered acceptable.
- Presentation is by a painless, slow-growing mass.
- Recurrences may present 15–20 years after initial surgery.
- Beware of change in histopathology—review the original and perform FNAC prior to commencing further treatment.
- Recurrences are most commonly due to poor surgical technique.
- If further surgery is offered then functional neurological preservation is the ultimate goal.
- There remains a risk of further recurrence even after apparent successful revision surgery.
- External beam and neutron radiotherapy may be an alternative treatment offered to some selected patients
- Frequent or persistent pleomorphic adenoma recurrences may proceed to the metastasizing pleomorphic adenoma with a potential fatal outcome.

References

1. Alves FA, Perez DEC, Almeida OP, et al. (2002) Pleomorphic adenoma of the submandibular gland. Arch Otolaryngol Head Neck Surg 128:1400–1403
2. Armitstead PR, Smiddy FG, Frank HG (1979) Simple enucleation and radiotherapy in the treatment of pleomorphic adenoma of the parotid gland. Br J Surg 66:716–717
3. Barton J, Slevin NJ, Gleaves EN (1992) Radiotherapy for pleomorphic adenoma of the parotid gland. Int J Radiat Oncol Biol Phys 22:925–928
4. Bradley PJ (1999) Submandibular gland and minor salivary gland neoplasms. Curr Opin Otolaryngol Head Neck Surg 7:72–78
5. Bradley PJ (2001) Recurrent salivary gland pleomorphic adenoma: etiology, management, and results. Curr Opin Otolaryngol Head Neck Surg 9:100–109
6. Bradley PJ (2004) Editorial overview. Pleomorphic salivary adenoma of the parotid gland: which operation to perform? Curr Opin Otolaryngol Head Neck Surg 12:69–70
7. Bradley PJ (2005) Metastasizing pleomorphic salivary adenoma should now be considered a low-grade malignancy with a lethal potential. Curr Opin Otolaryngol Head Neck Surg 13:123–126
8. Bradley PJ, McClelland L, Metha D (2006) Paediatric salivary gland epithelial neoplasms. ORL J Otorhinolaryngol Relat Spec 69:137–145
9. Buchholz TA, Laramore GE, Griffin TW (1992) Fast neutron radiation for recurrent pleomorphic adenoma of the parotid gland. Am J Clin Oncol 15:441–115
10. Buchman G, Stringer SP, Mendenhall WM (1994) Pleomorphic adenoma: effect of tumor spill and inadequate resection on tumor recurrence. Laryngoscope 104:1231–1234
11. Carew JF, Spiro RH, Singh B, et al. (1999) Treatment of recurrent pleomorphic adenoma of the parotid gland. Otolaryngol Head Neck Surg 121:539–542
12. Chen RL, Wang CM, Wen YM (2004) Study of the relative factors of the biological behaviour of pleomorphic adenoma of parotid. Zhonghua Kou Qiang Yi Xue Za Zhi 39:277–279
13. Clairmont AA, Richardson GS, Hanna DC (1977) The pseudocapsule of pleomorphic adenoma (benign mixed tumors). Am J Surg 134:242–243
14. Commins DJ, Roberts D, Fisher C, et al. (1995) Seeding of a parotid pleomorphic adenoma. J Laryngol Otol 109:671–673
15. Curry JL, Petruzzelli GJ, McClatchey KD, et al. (2002) Synchronous benign and malignant salivary gland tumors in ipsilateral glands: a report of two cases and a review of literature. Head Neck 24:302–306
16. Dawson AK (1989) Radiation therapy in recurrent pleomorphic adenoma of the parotid gland. Int J Radiat Oncol Biol Phys 16:819–821
17. Dawson AK, Orr LA (1985) Long-term results of local excision and radiotherapy in pleomorphic adenoma of the parotid gland. Int J Radiat Oncol Biol Phys 11:451–455
18. Douglas JG, Einck J, Austin-Seymour M, et al. (2001) Neutron radiotherapy for recurrent pleomorphic adenomas of major salivary glands. Head Neck 23:1037–1042
19. Dulguerov P, Marchal F, Lehmann W (1999) Post parotidectomy facial nerve paralysis: possible aetiological factors and results with routine facial nerve monitoring. Laryngoscope 109:754–762
20. Erol B, Ozer N, Unlu G, et al. (1997) A massive pleomorphic adenoma of the submandibular salivary gland. J Oral Maxillofac Surg 55:1011–1014
21. Fee WE Jr, Goffinet DR, Calcaterra TC (1987) Recurrent mixed tumors of the parotid gland: results of surgical therapy. Laryngoscope 88:265–273
22. Fleming WB (1987) Recurrent pleomorphic adenoma of the parotid gland. Aust N Z J Surg 57:173–176
23. Glas AS, Vermey A, Hollema H, et al. (2001) Surgical treatment of recurrent pleomorphic adenoma of the parotid gland: a clinical analysis of 52 patients. Head Neck 23:311–316
24. Gnepp DR (1993) Malignant mixed tumors of the salivary glands: a review. Pathol Ann 28:279–328
25. Gnepp DR, Schroeder W, Heffner D (1989) Synchronous tumors arising in a single major salivary gland. Cancer 63:1219–1224
26. Graham SM, McCullach TM, Funk GF, et al. (1999) Recurrent benign parotid tumors: the lesson not learnt yet [comment]. Aust N Z Surg 69:531
27. Hancock BD (1999) Clinically benign parotid tumors: local dissection as an alternative to superficial parotidectomy in selected cases. Ann R Coll Surg Engl 81:299–301
28. Helmus C, Myssiorek D, Shemem LJ (1999) Clinical challenges in otolaryngology: conservation vs superficial parotidectomy for benign lesions of the parotid tail. Arch Otolaryngol Head Neck Surg 125:1164–1167
29. Hendrikisson HH, Westrin KM, Carlsoo B, et al. (1998) Recurrent primary pleomorphic adenomas of salivary origin. Cancer 82:617–620
30. Hodge CW, Morris CG, Werning JW, et al. (2005) Role of radiotherapy for pleomorphic adenoma. Am J Clin Oncol 28:148–151
31. Hoorweg JJ, Hilgers FJM, Keus RB, et al. (1998) Metastasizing pleomorphic adenoma: a report of three cases. Eur J Surg Oncol 24:452–455

32. Jackson SR, Roland NJ, Clarke RW, et al. (1993) Recurrent pleomorphic adenoma. J Laryngol Otol 103:546–549
33. Junquera L, Alonso D, Sampedro A, et al. (1999) Pleomorphic adenoma of the salivary glands: prospective clinicopathologic and flow cytometric study. Head Neck 21:652–656
34. Karatzanis AD, Drivas EI, Giannikaki ES, et al. (2005) Malignant myoepithelioma arising from recurrent pleomorphic adenoma of the soft palate. Auris Nasus Larynx 32:435–437
35. Laskawi R, Ellies M, Arglebe C, et al. (1995) Surgical management of benign tumors of the submandibular gland: a follow-up study. J Oral Maxillofac Surg 53:506–508
36. Laskawi R, Schott T, Schroder M (1998) Recurrent pleomorphic adenoma of the parotid gland: clinician evaluation and long-term follow up. Br J Oral Maxillofac Surg 36:48–51
37. Lawson HH (1989) Capsular penetration and perforation in pleomorphic adenoma of the parotid salivary gland. Br J Surg 76:594–596
38. Leonetti JP, Marzo SJ, Petruzzelli GJ, et al. (2005) Recurrent pleomorphic adenoma of the parotid gland. Otolaryngol Head Neck Surg 133:319–322
39. Leverstein H, Tiwari RM, Snow GB, et al. (1997) The surgical management of recurrent or residual pleomorphic adenoma of the parotid gland: analysis and results of 40 patients. Eur Arch Otorhinolaryngol 254:313–317
40. Liu F-F, Rotstein L, Davison AJ, et al. (1995) Benign parotid adenomas: a review of the Princess Margaret Hospital Experience. Head Neck 17:177–183
41. Mann W, Beck C, Karatay MC (1985) Recurrent benign tumors of the parotid gland and their tendency for becoming malignant. Laryngol Rhinol Otol (Stuttg) 64:133–135
42. Maran AGD, MacKenzie IJ, Stanley RE (1984) Recurrent pleomorphic adenoma of the parotid gland. Arch Otolaryngol 110:167–171
43. Makeieff M, Venail F, Cartier C, et al. (2005) Continuous facial nerve monitoring during pleomorphic adenoma recurrence surgery. Laryngoscope 115:1310–1314
44. Maxwell EL, Hall FT, Freeman JL (2004) Recurrent pleomorphic adenoma of the parotid gland. J Otolaryngol 33:181–184
45. McEvedy BV, Ross WM (1976) The treatment of mixed parotid tumors by enucleation and radiotherapy. Br J Surg 63:341–342
46. McGregor AD, Burgoyne M, Tan KC (1988) Recurrent pleomorphic adenoma salivary adenoma: the relevance of age at first presentation. Br J Plast Surg 41:177–181
47. McGurk M (2004) Benign parotid tumors. BMJ 329:1299–1300
48. McGurk M, Hussain K (1997) Role of fine needle aspiration cytology in the management of the discrete parotid lump. Ann R Coll Surg Engl 79:198–202
49. McGurk M, Thomas BL, Renehan AG (2003) Extracapsular dissection for clinically benign parotid lumps: reduced morbidity without oncological compromise. Br J Cancer 89:1610–1613
50. Munir N, Bradley PJ (2007) Pleomorphic adenoma of the submandibular gland: what form of surgical management should be undertaken? Eur Arch Otorhinolaryngol Head Neck Surg (in press)
51. Munir N, Bradley PJ (2007) Diagnosis and management of neoplastic lesions of the submandibular triangle. Oral Oncol (in press)
52. Myssiorek D, Ruah GB, Hybels RL (1990) Recurrent pleomorphic adenomas of the parotid gland. Head Neck 12:332–336
53. Natvig K, Soberg R (1994) Relationship of intraoperative rupture of pleomorphic adenoma to recurrence: an 11–25 year follow up study. Head Neck 16:213–217
54. Niparko JK, Beauchamp ML, Krause CJ, et al. (1986) Surgical treatment of recurrent pleomorphic adenoma of the parotid gland. Arch Otolaryngol Head Neck Surg 112:1180–1184
55. Nouraei SAR, Fergusin MS, Clarke PM, et al. (2006) Metastasizing pleomorphic salivary adenoma. Arch Otolaryngol Head Neck Surg 132:788–793
56. Olsen KD, Daube JR (1994) Intra-operative monitoring of the facial nerve: an aid in the management of parotid gland pleomorphic adenomas. Laryngoscope 104:232–239
57. Olsen KD, Lewis JE (2001) Carcinoma ex-pleomorphic adenoma: a clinicopathologic review. Head Neck 23:705–712
58. Paris J, Facon F, Chrestian MA, et al. (2003) Recurrences of pleomorphic adenomas of the parotid: changing attitudes. Rev Laryngol Otol Rhinol (Bord) 124:229–234
59. Patel SG, See ACH, Williamson PA, et al. (1999) Radiation induced sarcoma of the head and neck. Head Neck 21:346–349
60. Phillips PP, Olsen KD (1995) Recurrent pleomorphic adenoma of the parotid gland: report of 126 cases and a review of the literature. Ann Otol Rhinol Laryngol 104:100–104
61. Piekarski J, Nejc D, Szymczak W, et al. (2004) Results of extracapsular dissection of pleomorphic adenoma of parotid gland. J Oral MaxilloFac Surg 62:1198–1202
62. Rabinov CR, Canalis RF, Alavi S, et al. (1997) Recurrent pleomorphic adenoma of the parotid gland involving the osseous external auditory canal. Ann Otol Rhinol Laryngol 106:589–593

63. Rapidis AD, Stavrianos S, Lagogiannia G, et al. (2004) Tumors of the submandibular gland: clinicopathologic analysis of 23 patients. J Oral Maxillofac Surg 62:1203–1208
64. Renehan A, Gleaves EN, McGurk M (1996) An analysis of the treatment of 114 patients with recurrent pleomorphic adenoma of the parotid gland. Am J Surg 172:710–714
65. Samson MJ, Metson R, Wang CC, et al. (1991) Preservation of the facial nerve in the management of recurrent pleomorphic adenomas of the parotid gland. Laryngoscope 101:1060–1062
66. Schot LJ, Hilgers FJM, Keus RB, et al. (1992) Late effects of radiotherapy on hearing. Eur Arch Otorhinolaryngol 249:305–308
67. Spiro JD, Spiro RH (1994) Submandibular gland tumors. In: Shockley WW (ed) The Neck: Diagnosis and Surgery. Mosby, St Louis, pp 295–306
68. Stennert E, Guntinas-Lichius O, Klaussmann JP, et al. (2001) Histopathology of pleomorphic adenoma in the parotid gland: a prospective unselected series of 100 cases. Laryngoscope 111:2195–2200
69. Stennert E, Wittekindt C, Klaussmann JP, et al. (2004) Recurrent pleomorphic adenoma of the parotid gland: a prospective histological and immunohistochemical study. Laryngoscope 114:158–163
70. Touquet R, McKenzie IJ, Carrouth JAS (1990) Management of the parotid pleomorphic adenoma: the problem of exposing tumor tissue at operation: the logical pursuit of treatment policies. Br J Oral Maxillofac Surg 28:404–408
71. van der Laan BFAM, Baris G, Gregor RT, et al. (1995) Radiation induced tumors of the head and neck. J Laryngol Otol 109:346–349
72. Vaughan ED, Richardson D (1993) Facial nerve reconstruction following ablative parotid surgery. Br J Oral Maxillofac Surg 31:274–280
73. Wai-Hei E, Tsang WM, Tse GMK (2003) Mucoepidermoid carcinoma ex-pleomorphic adenoma of the submandibular gland. Am J Otolaryngol 24:253–257
74. Waldron CA (1991) Mixed tumor (pleomorphic adenoma) and myoepithelioma. In: Ellis GL, Auclair PL, Gnepp DR (eds) Surgical Pathology of the Salivary Glands. Saunders, Philadelphia, pp 165–186
75. Waldron CA, El-Mofty S, Gnepp DR (1988) Tumors of the intraoral minor salivary glands. Oral Surg Oral Med Oral Pathol 66:323–333
76. Webb AJ, Eveson JW (2001) Pleomorphic adenomas of the major salivary glands: a study of the capsule form in relation to surgical management. Clin Otolaryngol 26:134–142
77. Weber RS, Byers RM, Petit B, et al. (1990) Submandibular gland tumors. Arch Otolaryngol Head Neck Surg 116:1055–1060
78. Witt RL (2002) The significance of the margin in parotid surgery for pleomorphic adenoma. Laryngoscope 112:2141–2154
79. Yugueros P, Goellner JR, Petty PM, et al. (1998) Treating recurrence of parotid pleomorphic adenoma. Ann Plast Surg 40:573–576
80. Zabren P, Tschumi I, Nuyens M, et al. (2005) Recurrent pleomorphic adenoma of the parotid gland. Am J Surg 189:203–207

Chapter 17

Management of the Mass in the Buccal Space

Rohan R. Walvekar and Eugene N. Myers

17

Contents

Core Features

- To provide a concept of the three-dimensional anatomy of the buccal space.
- To describe the clinical presentation and specific features of buccal space tumors.
- To discuss the advantages, disadvantages, and rationale for various surgical approaches to the tumors of the buccal space.

Complications to Avoid

- Excellent exposure of the mass and buccal branches of the facial nerve will help to avoid damage to the facial nerve.
- Damage to Stensen's duct with resultant sialocele can be avoided by using the external approach.

Introduction

The mass in the substance of the cheek, also known as the "buccal space" presents a diagnostic and therapeutic challenge. A mass appearing in the buccal space usually suggests a tumor arising in the buccal space or the accessory lobe of the parotid gland. These tumors are unusual and present in a unique fashion. The diagnosis of these lesions is often difficult to make. A detailed clinical examination and imaging studies are helpful in defining the location and extent of these tumors. However, the definitive diagnosis of a mass in the buccal space is obtained by excision of the mass and histopathological evaluation. A variety of benign and malignant lesions may arise within the buccal space. Some more commonly occurring lesions include benign and malignant tumors of salivary gland origin, lymphoma, lipomas (see Fig. 17.1), and metastasis from a distant site. There are many reports describing various masses in the buccal space and several surgical approaches have been described in the literature [10, 18–20, 25, 26, 29, 34, 40]. Table 17.1 lists lesions reported within the buccal space [1–6, 8, 10, 14–16, 21–23, 26–28, 32, 33, 35–40]. The surgical management of these tumors is challenging because the operative technique must provide good exposure, prevent damage to the facial nerve and Stensen's duct, and have a good cosmetic result.

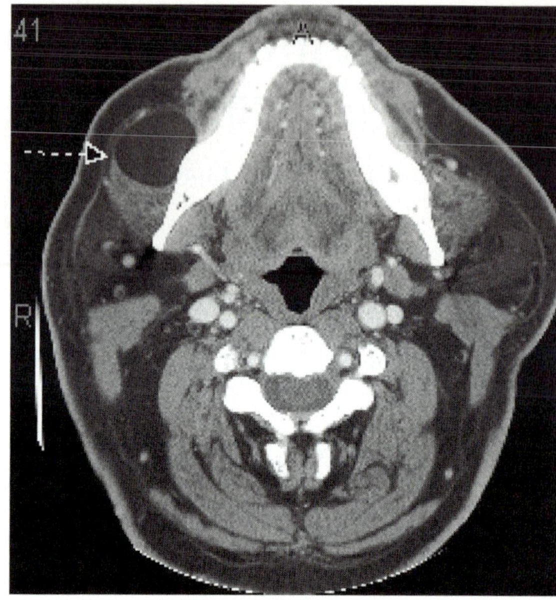

Fig. 17.1: Lipoma of the buccal space

Anatomy of the Buccal Space

The head and neck surgeon must have an understanding of the three-dimensional anatomy of the buccal space, in order to provide safe surgical therapy [10, 34]. Madorsky and Allison mention that the buccal space was first described in 1935 by Coller and Yglesias, and Kostrubala in 1945 further subdivided the masticator space into temporal, infratemporal, retrozygomatic, and buccal, describing the extent of these spaces [25]. Kostrubala described the buccal space as being a fascial space in the mid-cheek, anterior to the masticator space and anterior to and separate from the parotid gland [18]. Figure 17.2 is a schematic illustration of the buccal space and its contents. The anatomical boundaries of the buccal space include the buccinator muscle medially with its overlying fascia, extending superiorly to the zygoma and inferiorly to the mandible [10]. The anterolateral wall of the buccal space is formed laterally by the skin and superficial layer of the deep cervical fascia and medially by the muscles of facial expression [15]. The anterior limit of the buccal space is defined by the orbicularis oris muscle [10]. The posterior wall of the buccal space is formed by the masseter muscle, mandible, lateral and medial pterygoid muscles, and the parotid gland. The buccal space frequently communicates posteriorly with the masseteric space through deficiencies in the parotidomasseteric fascia [15]. There are no true superior or inferior boundaries to the buccal space, however, these are formed as the superficial layer of the deep cervical fascia attaches to the periosteum of the zygomatic arch and mandible, respectively [10, 15].

Most of the buccal space is filled with adipose tissue that has been termed the "buccal fat pad" and lymph nodes. The buccal fat pad has also been described as "Bichat's fat pad" or the "suctorial fat pad" and has been studied in great detail by Gaughran in 1957 [25]. The buccal fat pad with its extensions can serve as a conduit for the spread of infections or tumors originating in the oral cavity or parotid gland [10, 15]. Other important contents of the buccal space include the parotid duct (Stensen's duct), as it passes anteriorly from the gland to pierce the buccinator muscle opposite the second maxillary molar. The duct separates the buccal space into two equal-sized anterior and posterior compartments. Moving laterally, the anterior facial vein, the facial artery, and the lymphatic channels are encountered. Even more laterally, the branches of the facial nerve can be located as they pierce the medial surface of several muscles of facial expression which form the deep portion of the lateral wall, such as the risorius, zygomaticus major, and levator labii superioris along with their fascia [10].

Superficial Musculoaponeurotic System (SMAS)

The SMAS was first described by Mitz and Peyronie in 1976 [29]. The SMAS is thought to be a fibrous degeneration of the platysma, or a distinct fibromuscular layer

Table 17.1. Lesions reported in the buccal space

Glandular	Vascular	Lymph node	Connective	Muscular	Inflammatory	Neural	Miscellaneous
Accessory parotid or aberrant salivary gland tumors	Hylanized thrombus[a]	Calcified node	Fibromatosis	Myositis ossificans	Abscess formation	Neurofibroma	Foreign body granuloma e.g., paraffinoma [15]
Mixed tumors (benign[a] and malignant)	False aneurysm	Benign reactive node	Lipoma	Masseteric hypertrophy	Bacterial abscess	Neuroma	Kimura disease [15]
Mucoepidermoid carcinoma (low- and high-grade)	Hemangioma	Lymphoma[a]	Liposarcoma		Aspergilloma		
Acinic cell carcinoma	Recurrent juvenile nasopharyngeal angiofibroma [3]	Lymphosarcoma	Spindle cell lipoma[a]		Sarcoidosis[a]		
Adenoid cystic carcinoma		Metastatic nodal involvement	Fibroma		Polymorphic low-grade adenocarcinoma [21]		
Carcinoma ex-pleomorphic adenoma		Lymphangioma	Fibrosarcoma		Tuberculous granuloma and adenoid cystic carcinoma presenting as a single buccal space mass [22]		
Metastatic clear cell carcinoma			Solitary fibrous tumor [5]		Clear cell carcinoma metastatic from kidney		
Chronic sialadenitis[a]			Rhabdomyosarcoma				

[a] Identifies the diagnoses of 10 patients treated between 1975 and 1985

Table 17.1. *(continued)* Lesions reported in the buccal space

Glandular	Vascular	Lymph node	Connective	Muscular	Inflammatory	Neural	Miscellaneous
Oncocytoma[a]			Pseudoherniation of buccal fat pad [27]				
Papillary cystadenoma lymphomatosum			Nodular fasciitis[a]				
Sebaceous adenoma[a]			Alveolar soft-part sarcoma of the head neck [16]				
Parotid duct tumor or calculus							
Minor salivary gland calculus							

[a] Identifies the diagnoses of 10 patients treated between 1975 and 1985

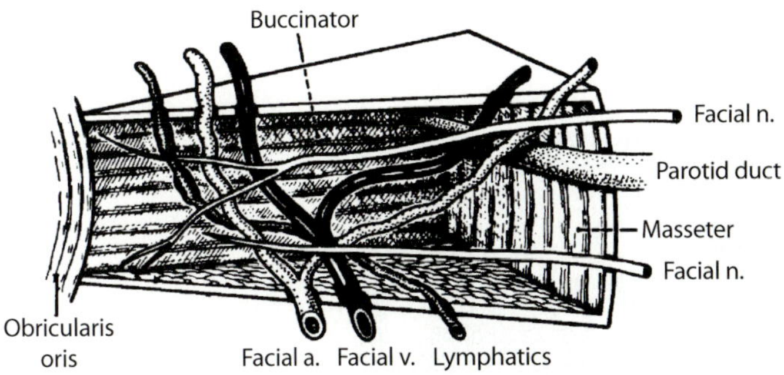

Fig. 17.2: Schematic illustration in oblique lateral view of left buccal space and its contents [10]. [Reprinted with permission from: Rodgers GK and Myers EN (1988) Surgical management of the mass in the buccal space. Laryngoscope 98:749–53]

composed of platysma muscle and parotid fascia, or an extension of the cervical fascia. There are several other explanations of the origins of the SMAS. The SMAS splits the subcutaneous layer in the face into a superficial layer that contains tenuous fat lobes interspersed with fibrous septa that insert into the dermis and a deeper layer which extends to the facial muscles and contains fat which is more abundant and less organized due to the absence of fibrous septation [7]. The SMAS is lateral to the facial nerve and the facial vessels. It is thicker over the parotid gland and is thinner in the mid-cheek area. It reinforces the contour of the face, and identification and repair of this layer is essential to minimize facial deformity following surgery for tumors in the buccal space [25].

Accessory Lobe of the Parotid Gland

One of the important differential diagnoses of a mass presenting in the mid-cheek area is the accessory lobe of the parotid gland. The accessory lobe of the parotid gland is an island of salivary gland tissue found anterior to and separate from the main parotid gland. Anterior processes or extension of the main parotid gland are not considered to be accessory parotid tissue [17]. Frommer, in cadaver studies, demonstrated that the accessory lobe of the parotid gland is found in approximately 21% of the population [9]. The accessory lobe is found along the line of the Stensen's duct in the soft parts of the cheek and is usually separated from it by an average of 6 mm [24, 31]. As a result a mass arising in the accessory parotid tissue presents in the central one third of a line drawn from the middle of the tragus to a point midway between the ala of the nose and the vermillion border of the upper lip, about a fingerbreadth below the zygomatic arch [31, 32]. The accessory lobe of the parotid gland drains through one or more ducts into the nearby Stensen's duct, and is usually closely related to the buccal space and zygomatic branches of the facial nerve [31]. The normal size of an accessory lobe of the parotid gland, when present, is described to be "pea-sized" or "lima bean-sized" varying from 0.5 to 2.5 cm in diameter, and is spheroidal in shape, firm in consistency, and separate from the overlying skin [14, 31].

One to eight percent of all parotid neoplasms arise within the accessory lobe of the parotid gland. The rate of malignancy has been reported to be from 26% to 50% [24]. The histology, variety, and distribution of neoplasms within the accessory lobe of the parotid gland are similar to those occurring within the main parotid gland. As with the main parotid gland, pleomorphic adenoma is the most common benign tumor. Most malignant tumors of the accessory lobe of the parotid gland are cancers of salivary gland origin. There are, however, a few reports of metastases to this site from primary tumors in the head and neck or distant sites [11, 17]. We recently encountered a case of metastasis of a renal cell carcinoma to the accessory lobe of the parotid gland (Fig. 17.3).

Preoperative Evaluation

Clinical Presentation and Physical Examination

A mass within the substance of the cheek poses a diagnostic problem. It may arise from any of the several types of tissues present in the buccal space. A detailed history, clinical examination, and imaging studies may suggest a specific etiology, however, the final diagnosis of buccal space masses is often elusive and must be confirmed by surgical removal and histopathological evaluation [10]. An accurate history and physical examination helps to

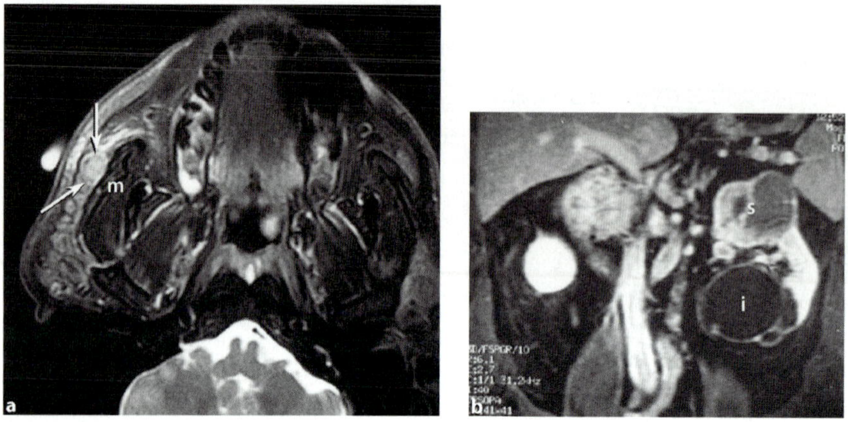

Fig. 17.3: **a** T2-weighted axial MRI through the parotid gland demonstrates a round 10-mm mass (*arrows*) overlying the masseter muscle (*m*). The mass has signal intensity slightly higher than the adjacent gland, but not high enough to be definitive for pleomorphic adenoma. This proved to be renal cell carcinoma metastatic to the accessory lobe. **b** Sagittal postcontrast spoiled-gradient MRI of the abdomen with T1 weighting shows two distinct masses in the left kidney. The superior mass (*s*) has cystic and solid components. The inferior mass (*i*) is predominantly cystic and has extensive septations

localize the site of the lesion as originating in the buccal space. Buccal space masses present in a unique fashion. The lesions in the buccal space are readily apparent because they are easily palpated just beneath the buccal mucosa or the skin of the cheek (see Fig. 17.4) [13]. The typical history encountered in patients with a mass in the buccal space is that of a slowly growing painless mass in the cheek, which disturbs the facial symmetry. These lesions are typically nontender and can be best assessed by a bimanual examination. They are not always well circumscribed and are often ill-defined merging with the adjacent buccal fat pad [10]. The mass may lie closer to the oral mucosa and the patient may be able to feel the intraoral mass with the tongue. When the mass presents in the oral cavity, the patients are often seen initially by their dentist or an oromaxillofacial surgeon. Skin involvement, facial nerve paralysis, Stensen's duct obstruction, and pain often all suggest indications of a malignant tumor within the buccal space, as benign tumors almost never produce pressure or obstructive symptoms [10].

17

Imaging

Imaging studies can provide valuable information that can help to limit the differential diagnosis of a mass in the buccal space. Kurabayashi et al. evaluated the computed tomography (CT) features of a buccal space mass in 53 patients [20]. CT images were assessed for the number, location, internal architecture, and margin of the lesions and their relation to the surrounding structures. Their series included 44 tumors (33 benign and 11 malignant) and 9 masses which were not tumors. The criteria used to diagnose malignant tumors included, ill-defined margins, violation of fascial planes, and aggressive bone destruction. CT was useful in demonstrating the presence and location of the masses in the buccal space, and sometimes aided in the differential diagnosis. However, the study concluded that CT had a limited value in differentiating malignant from benign lesions. Only 7 out of 11 malignant tumor were correctly identified (sensitivity 64%) [20].

Kurabayashi et al. also studied 30 patients with benign and malignant lesions in the buccal space using magnetic resonance imaging (MRI) [19]. The authors evaluated the MRI characteristics of lesions in the buccal space. They concluded that MRI was useful in demonstrating the extent of lesions in the buccal space because of its excellent soft tissue contrast, however, the sensitivity of predicting malignancy was very poor (29%). This was especially true for malignant tumors of minor salivary gland origin, which were typically seen as well-defined masses without infiltration into surrounding structures on MRI [19]. Table 17.2 lists the CT and MRI characteristics of tumors encountered commonly in the buccal space [15, 19, 20].

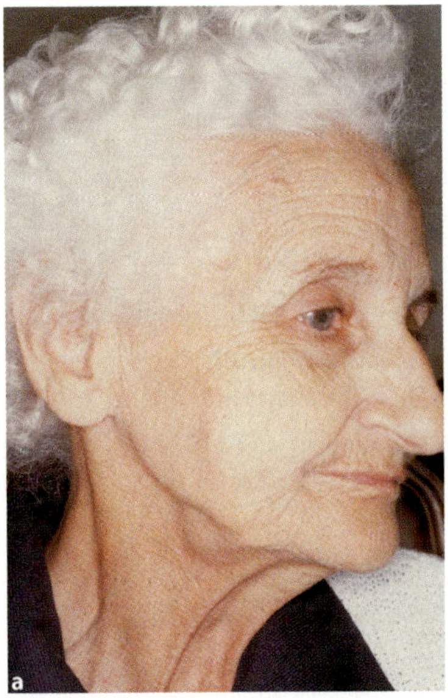

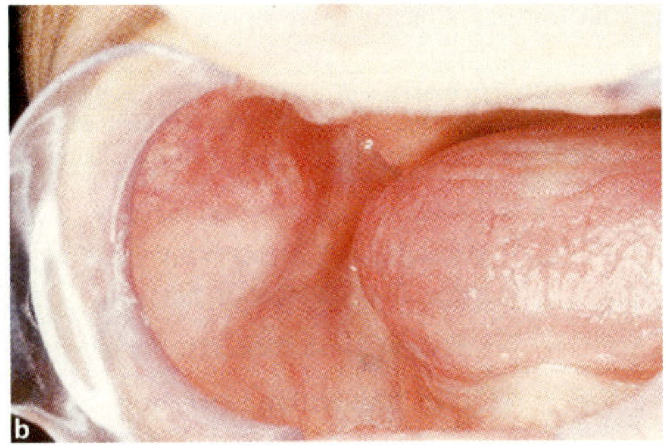

Fig. 17.4: **a** External view of a right buccal space mass. **b** Internal view. Note the intraoral bulge produced by the mass. [Reprinted with permission from: Rodgers GK and Myers EN (1988) Surgical management of the mass in the buccal space. Laryngoscope 98:749–53]

Positron emission tomography (PET) as well as PET-CT can also be useful in defining the location of the lesions and in forming the differential diagnosis. PET-CT scanning can also add valuable information that may alter management. Gomes et al. reported a case of high-grade mucoepidermoid carcinoma of the accessory lobe of the parotid gland in which the CT and MRI did not show any abnormality other than the primary lesion. However, an 18F-fluorodeoxyglucose (FDG) PET-CT scan showed multiple distant metastases. In view of this finding, curative treatment was deferred and the patient was offered palliation only [12].

Fine-needle Aspiration Biopsy (FNAB)

Fine-needle aspiration biopsy provides a valuable tool in the evaluation of a mid-cheek mass [24]. Johnson and Spiro [14] studied 23 patients having a mass in the mid-cheek arising from the accessory parotid gland. Aspiration biopsy was done in 8 patients, yielding the diagnosis in 7. They concluded that FNAB can be useful in selected cases of buccal space masses, however the authors did not routinely employ the use of FNAB in such cases. FNAB does have certain disadvantages, such as possible facial nerve damage, introduction of infection, hemorrhage, tumor spillage, and possible scarring of tissue planes around the facial nerve, which increases the chances of facial nerve paresis during surgical excision. These complications can be minimized by using image guidance for this procedure. However, since FNAB does not alter the management of these lesions, we do not advocate routine FNAB as a routine diagnostic tool in the evaluation of buccal space masses.

Surgical Approaches to the Buccal Space Masses

Several surgical approaches to the buccal space have been described (Fig. 17.5, Table 17.3) [10].

Internal or Intraoral Approach

The approach used most commonly is a direct intraoral, transmucosal incision with dissection and removal of the mass. This approach is appealing because the bulging of the tumor into the intraoral area appears to lend itself to easy excision and of course eliminates a skin incision with its inevitable scar. The transoral approach has several advantages, such as it limiting the area of dissection and hence the potential area of tumor implantation. It is quicker owing to lesser dissections. A transmucosal

Table 17.2. Characteristic radiographic features of buccal space lesions

Tumor type	CT findings	MRI findings
Accessory parotid tissue	• Identified better by CT • Location: separate from main parotid gland, lateral to the masseter along its anterior margin	
Hemangiomas	• Adjacent to buccinator • Phleboliths are characteristic	• Homogenous internal architecture • Higher signal intensity on T2-weighted images • Enhancement with contrast is a typical feature
Vascular malformations:		
• Venous malformations	• Presence of phleboliths	• Discrete areas of high signal intensity representing venous lakes
• Arteriovenous malformations		• Serpiginous flow voids
• Lymphatic malformations	• Smooth, irregular • Adjacent to the buccinator muscle	• Cystic and septated lesions with fluid-fluid levels
Infection and inflammatory lesions	• Inflammatory changes in the fat planes • Abscess appears as a single or multiloculated low-density area with peripheral rim enhancement	• Edema within surrounding fat • Rim enhancement
Tumors of minor salivary gland origin[a]:		
• Benign: pleomorphic adenoma[b]	• Smooth margins	• Rounded appearance • Low signal intensity on T1-weighted images • High signal intensity on T2-weighted images
• Malignant: adenoid cystic carcinoma[c]	• Invasion of surrounding tissue suggests malignant tumor	• Tumors with high signal intensity on T2-weighted images—better prognosis • Tumors with low/intermediate intensity on T2-weighted images—poor prognosis • Invasion of surrounding tissues—poor prognosis
Rhabdomyosarcoma	• Appear as muscle density masses • Show soft tissue and bone infiltration	• Signal intensity is greater that muscle on T2-weighted images • Bone destruction is characteristic

[a] CT/MRIhave limited value in differentiating malignant versus benign tumors—small malignant salivary gland tumors may have a sharp margin mimicking a benign tumor

[b] Pleomorphic adenoma is the most common benign salivary gland tumor

[c] Adenoid cystic carcinomas form 25% of malignant minor salivary gland tumors

Table 17.2. *(continued)* Characteristic radiographic features of buccal space lesions

Tumor type	CT findings	MRI findings
Neurofibroma		• Low intensity signal on T1-weighted images, high intensity on T2-weighted images • Single neurofibroma: target sign—peripheral hyperintensity with central hypointensity
Lipoma	• Internal architecture shows fat density	• T1/T2-weighted signal intensity in high/high
Metastatic lymph node	• Well-circumscribed mass with rim enhancement and central low attenuation	• High signal intensity on T2-weighted images

[a] CT/MRIhave limited value in differentiating malignant versus benign tumors—small malignant salivary gland tumors may have a sharp margin mimicking a benign tumor
[b] Pleomorphic adenoma is the most common benign salivary gland tumor
[c] Adenoid cystic carcinomas form 25% of malignant minor salivary gland tumors

Table 17.3. Surgical approaches to the buccal space

Internal/intraoral approach External approaches:
• Direct approach • Paranasal approach • Preauricular approach • Submandibular approach • Preauricular-suborbital approach • Extended parotid-submandibular approach • Rhytidectomy approach

incision eliminates the complications associated with raising skin flaps, such as flap necrosis. The intraoral approach, however, does not provide adequate exposure to the branches of the facial nerve, which is at greater risk while using this approach, especially since branches of the facial nerve are always closely associated with or actually incorporated into the capsule on the lateral aspect of the tumor, which cannot be visualized well through the intraoral approach. Stensen's duct is also closely associated with these tumors, which increases the risk of injury to the duct and sialocele. Transoral excision may only be suitable for an oral submucosal lesion located medial to the buccinator muscle [10, 25].

External Approaches

The transcutaneous direct external approach has similar advantages to the transoral approach. However, the transcutaneous incision leaves a highly visible scar and the limited exposure makes it difficult to use local tissue to fill any resultant depressed areas [25].

The preauricular approach provides access to superficial tumors that are located posteriorly in the buccal space while the submandibular approach provides access to the lower buccal space. The paranasal approach with its extensions provides excellent exposure but does not permit identification and dissection of the facial nerve. The preauricular-suborbital approach leaves a visible scar along the upper limb of the incision [25].

Essentially most other external approaches described in the literature are suboptimal as they also provide limited exposure for tumor removal or do not allow identification and dissection of the facial nerve.

We have designed the extended parotid-submandibular incision specifically for use in the removal of tumors of the buccal space because it provides excellent exposure and minimizes the risk of complications, such as injury to Stensen's duct or the facial nerve during excision of these tumors [10, 34]. We have found that this technique also provides an excellent cosmetic result. Patients are counseled that the buccal branch of the facial nerve will be dis-

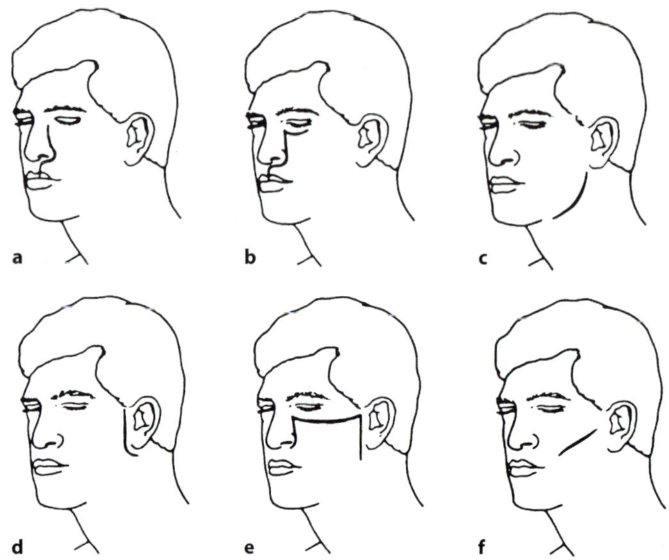

Fig. 17.5: Approaches to the buccal space. **a** Paranasal. **b** Paranasal with suborbital extension. **c** Submandibular. **d** Preauricular. **e** Suborbital-preauricular. **f** Direct cutaneous. [Reprinted with permission from: Rodgers GK and Myers EN (1988) Surgical management of the mass in the buccal space. Laryngoscope 98:749–53]

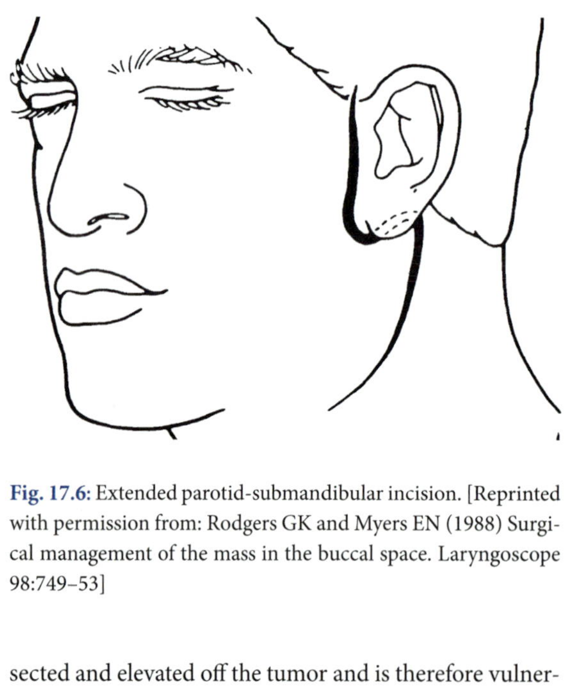

Fig. 17.6: Extended parotid-submandibular incision. [Reprinted with permission from: Rodgers GK and Myers EN (1988) Surgical management of the mass in the buccal space. Laryngoscope 98:749–53]

sected and elevated off the tumor and is therefore vulnerable to intraoperative injury and postoperative weakness from dissection and stretching of the nerve. The use of intraoperative facial nerve stimulators facilitates the accurate identification of the facial nerve and its branches. The rhytidectomy approach also has advantages similar to the parotid-submandibular approach. The latter leaves a scar in the neck, which normally can be masked in the horizontal skin folds. In our experience, this has proved to be a very effective technique providing excellent masking of the cervical limb of the incision. Though the rhytidectomy incision avoids the neck scar it does not allow access for cervical lymphadenectomy if required [25]. We recommend the extended parotid-submandibular approach and the rhytidectomy approach for management of the buccal space tumors. These two procedures and associated complications are described here.

Extended Parotid-Submandibular Incision

The incision is a modification of the standard parotidectomy incision (Fig. 17.6). Extension of the preauricular incision somewhat superiorly and extension of the cervical incision into a skin crease in the submandibular space allows for wide undermining of the flap, which is necessary in order to gain exposure anterior to the parotid gland to expose the tumor. It is not necessary to carry out a formal parotidectomy or to identify the facial nerve at the stylomastoid foramen because the tumor is located anterior to the anterior border of the parotid gland therefore only the buccal branches of the nerve are anatomically associated with these tumors.

The skin flap is elevated anterior to the anterior border of the parotid gland where the mass begins to be encountered. Further evaluation of the flap provides exposure of the entire mass. The location of the buccal branches of the facial nerve is easily identified, usually during blunt dissection of the mass, and confirmed with a facial nerve stimulator (Fig. 17.7a–d). Stensen's duct may also be identified during this phase of the dissection. Dissection of the branches of the nerves somewhat anterior and posterior to the mass itself will allow undermining and mobilizing the nerve. A small nerve retractor is then used to retract the branches of the nerve away from the mass. The nerves once dissected may be marked with arterial loops. The mass itself may be made more prominent and easier to dissect by inserting a sponge into the oral cavity adjacent to the buccal mucosa. The mass is then removed by sharp and blunt dissection. After removal of the mass, the nerves are returned to their normal anatomical position. Removal of the tumor leaves a noticeable defect in the facial contour, which is eliminated by approximating the superficial musculoaponeurotic system (SMAS).

Hemostasis is obtained, the wound is irrigated, and a Hemovac drain is inserted under the skin flap and brought

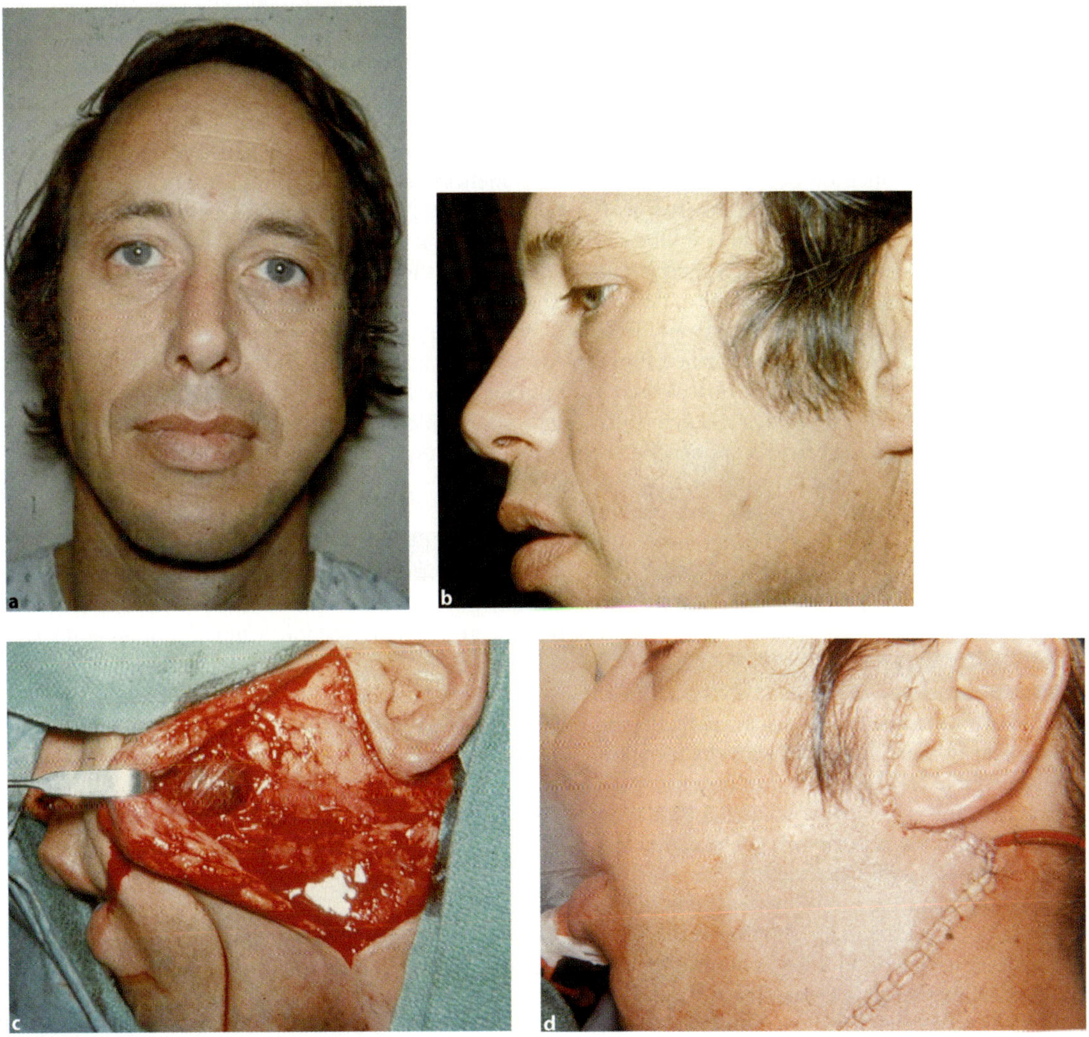

Fig. 17.7: **a** Left cheek mass (frontal view). **b** Left cheek mass (lateral view). **c** Surgical exposure of a buccal space tumor demonstrating the facial nerve branches adherent to the lateral aspect of the mass (*black arrow*). **d** Postoperative picture showing the closure of the standard extended parotid-submandibular incision

out through the skin 1 cm posterior to the incision. The skin flap is closed with subcutaneous chromic sutures and then continuous closure with 6-0 fast absorbing catgut suture. Steri-Strips and a pressure dressing are applied. The patient is allowed to recover from anesthesia. Within 24 h the drainage has usually stopped, the pressure dressing and the drain are removed, and the patient is discharged. The Steri-Strips and sutures are removed within 5–7 days.

Rhytidectomy Approach

Mitz and Peyronie, in 1976, described the rhytidectomy approach and how this technique allows for reconstruction of the contour defect associated with tumor extirpation using the SMAS interposition [29]. The incision employed in these cases is the one used for cosmetic rhytidectomy (Fig. 17.8). The incision begins at the temple and continues in a preauricular crease, and then is posttragal. The incision is carried inferior to the ear lobe and up to the level of the posterior auricularis muscle and posteriorly into the hairline. The skin is undermined anterior to the tumor, mobilized, and retracted away from the tumor. The tumor is then excised as described above. After removal of the tumor, the SMAS is closed directly to give sufficient support to the cheek to avoid deformity. Rotation of a flap of SMAS has been recommended for defects that are too large for direct closure or advancement closure. This technique distributes the volume defect over a wider area and makes the depression of a gradual transition, and therefore less noticeable [25].

Complications

Complications of the extended parotid-submandibular approach are similar to those associated with rhytidectomy and are listed in Table 17.4 [34]. The most common perioperative complication is hematoma occurring with a frequency of 1–15%. This was also the only complication that we had in our series of buccal space tumors. The incidence of large hematomas requiring surgical intervention ranges from 1.9% to 3.6%. Other important complications include injury to the facial nerve and to the parotid gland or the parotid duct which may result in facial asymmetry and parotid pseudocysts (sialocele) or parotid fistulas [30]. Care must be taken in undermining the superior aspect of the flap because the zygomatic branch of the upper division of the facial nerve is superficial in this area and the branch could be injured with resultant facial nerve paralysis.

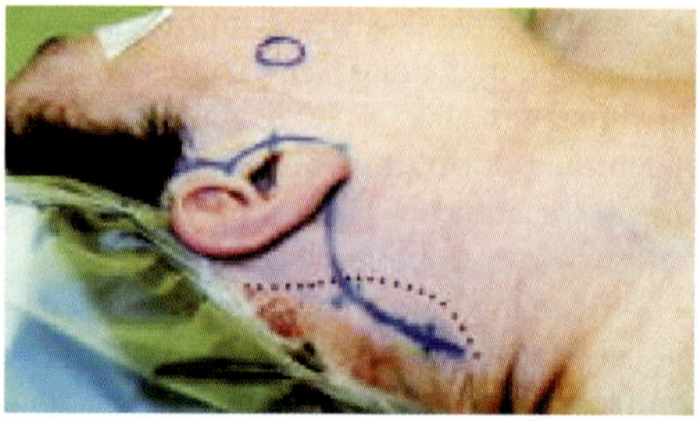

Fig. 17.8: Standard rhytidectomy incision (*blue line*) and hairline (*dotted line*). [Reprinted with permission from: Lin DT, Coppit GL, Burkey BB, and Netterville JL (2004) Tumors of the accessory lobe of the parotid gland: a 10-year experience. Laryngoscope 114:1652-5]

Complications can be minimized by excellent exposure, meticulous dissection, and identification of important structures, which is exactly why we use the parotid-submandibular approach, which is a systematic surgical approach for the management tumors in the buccal space. The experience of caring for a patient who had a mass previously removed through an incision in the buccal mucosa, sustaining injury to the facial nerve and developing a sialocele in the buccal space due to inadvertent injury to Stensen's duct, was the incentive to design the extended parotid-submandibular incision.

Conclusions

Tumors arising in the buccal space are rare tumors that present in a unique fashion. Clinical examination and

Table 17.4. Complications associated with extended parotid-submandibular approach/rhytidectomy approach

Hematoma
Nerve injury: facial nerve, greater auricular nerve
Necrosis of skin flap
Hair loss
Infection
Parotid injury: salivary fistula, sialocele
Contour deformity
Pigmentary changes in the skin
Keloid/scar formation

radiological correlation provide valuable information regarding the location and extent of these tumors. FNAB may provide additional information in certain cases. However, the only way to characterize these tumors is by excision and pathological evaluation. Surgery is both diagnostic as well as therapeutic in this situation. The parotid-submandibular is a systematic, versatile, and cosmetically acceptable approach that provides excellent exposure to the buccal space and allows identification of the facial nerve branches.

Take Home Messages

- Surgical management and treatment planning through a rigorous evaluation including imaging studies and FNAB. In patients suspected to have a malignant tumor, PET-CT may provide valuable information that could alter the treatment plan.
- Educating the patient regarding postoperative appearance and possible complications is critical. Evaluate the patient's needs as to cosmetic appearance. The modified parotid incision leaves a visible scar so for the female patient a rhytidectomy approach should be considered, whereas the incision in the male patient is usually hidden in the beard line hair and is acceptable.
- Undermine in the plane between the subcutaneous tissue and the SMAS.
- Begin to look for the branches of the buccal branch of the facial nerve once the soft tissues have been undermined to the anterior border of the parotid gland.
- Identify the branches of the facial nerve using the nerve stimulator and dissect them off the tumor.
- Retract the branches of the nerve away from the tumor in order to excise it without nerve injury.
- Closing the SMAS either primarily or with a flap will prevent an unsightly depression in the cheek.

References

1. Allan JH, Finch LD, Chippendale I (1969) Sialolithiasis of the minor salivary glands. Oral Surg Oral Med Oral Pathol 27:780–785
2. Barnard JD (1975) Primary clinical manifestation of bronchial carcinoma as a buccal metastasis. Br Dent J 138:174–176
3. Berger SB, Chaloupka JC, Putman CM, Citardi MJ, Lamb T, Sasaki CL (1996) Hypervascular tumor of the buccal space in an adult as a late recurrence of juvenile angiofibroma. AJNR Am J Neuroradiol 17:1384–1387
4. Calhoun NR (1963) Lipoma of the buccal space. Report of a case. Oral Surg Oral Med Oral Pathol 16:246–249
5. Dunfee BL, Sakai O, Spiegel JH, Pistey R (2005) Solitary fibrous tumor of the buccal space. AJNR Am J Neuroradiol 26:2114–2116
6. Ewbank RL, Mitchell DF (1964) Hyalinized thrombi of the cheek: report of case. J Oral Surg Anesth Hosp Dent Serv 22:456–459
7. Ferreira LM, Hochman B, Locali RF, Rosa-Oliveira LM (2006) A stratigraphic approach to the superficial musculoaponeurotic system and its anatomic correlation with the superficial fascia. Aesthetic Plast Surg 30:549–552
8. Fritz GW, Petti NA, Abitbol A, Thelmo WL (1980) Extranodal malignant histiocytic lymphoma of the cheek: report of case. J Oral Surg, 38(3):200–202
9. Frommer J (1977) The human accessory parotid gland: its incidence, nature, and significance. Oral Surg Oral Med Oral Pathol 43:671–676
10. Gallia L, Rood SR, Myers EN (1981) Management of buccal space masses. Otolaryngol Head Neck Surg 89:221–225
11. Goldberg JA, Georgiade GS (1990) Accessory parotid glands as a site of metastases from outside the head and neck: case report. Head Neck 12:421–425
12. Gomes M, Pepe G, Bomanji J, Al-Salihi O, Du Y, Gacinovic S, Ell P (2006) High-grade mucoepidermoid carcinoma of the accessory parotid gland with distant metastases identified by 18F-FDG PET-CT. Pediatr Blood Cancer
13. Harnesberger HR (1995) The masticator space. In: Harnsberger HR (ed) Handbook of Head and Neck Imaging. Mosby Year Book, St Louis, pp 46–59
14. Johnson FE, Spiro RH (1979) Tumors arising in accessory parotid tissue. Am J Surg 138:576–578
15. Kim HC, Han MH, Moon MH, Kim JH, Kim IO, Chang KH (2005) CT and MR imaging of the buccal space: normal anatomy and abnormalities. Korean J Radiol 6:22–30
16. Kim HS, Lee HK, Weon YC, Kim HJ (2005) Alveolar soft-part sarcoma of the head and neck: clinical and imaging features in five cases. AJNR Am J Neuroradiol 26:1331–1335

17. Klotz DA, Coniglio JU (2000) Prudent management of the mid-cheek mass: revisiting the accessory parotid gland tumor. Laryngoscope 110:1627–1632
18. Kostrubala JG (1945) Potential anatomical spaces in the face. Am J Surg 68:28
19. Kurabayashi T, Ida M, Tetsumura A, Ohbayashi N, Yasumoto M, Sasaki T (2002) MR imaging of benign and malignant lesions in the buccal space. Dentomaxillofac Radiol 31:344–349
20. Kurabayashi T, Ida M, Yoshino N, Sasaki T, Kishi T, Kusama M (1997) Computed tomography in the diagnosis of buccal space masses. Dentomaxillofac Radiol 26:347–353
21. Kwong MD, Bert RJ (1999) Neuroradiology case of the day. Polymorphous low-grade adenocarcinoma of a minor salivary gland in the right buccal space. AJR Am J Roentgenol 173:805, 808–809
22. Landa LE, Kathju S, Nepomuceno-Perez MC, Gordon C, Sotereanos GC (2002) Tuberculous granuloma and adenoid cystic carcinoma presenting as a single buccal space mass. J Craniofac Surg 13:533–537
23. Larsson A, Svartz K (1976) Nodular fascitis in the oral cavity. Int J Oral Surg 5:122–127
24. Lin DT, Coppit GL, Burkey BB, Netterville JL (2004) Tumors of the accessory lobe of the parotid gland: a 10-year experience. Laryngoscope 114:1652–1655
25. Madorsky SJ, Allison GR (1999) Management of buccal space tumors by rhytidectomy approach with superficial musculoaponeurotic system reconstruction. Am J Otolaryngol 20:51–55
26. Maguire CP, Horton CE, Pickrell KL (1955) Tumors of the cheek; observations on etiology, differential diagnosis, and methods of surgical approach. AMA Arch Surg 71:869–906
27. Matarasso A (1997) Pseudoherniation of the buccal fat pad: a new clinical syndrome. Plast Reconstr Surg 100:723–730; discussion 731–736
28. Merchant NE (1972) Cavernous haemangioma of the cheek. Dent Pract Dent Rec 22:436
29. Mitz V, Peyronie M (1976) The superficial musculo-aponeurotic system (SMAS) in the parotid and cheek area. Plast Reconstr Surg 58:80–88
30. Moyer JS, Baker SR (2005) Complications of rhytidectomy. Facial Plast Surg Clin North Am 13:469–478
31. Perzik SL, White IL (1966) Surgical management of preauricular tumors of the accessory parotid apparatus. Am J Surg 112:498–503
32. Polayes IM, Rankow RM (1979) Cysts, masses, and tumors of the accessory parotid gland. Plast Reconstr Surg 64:17–23
33. Robbins JP, Fitz-Hugh GS, Constable WC (1971) Involvement of the buccinator node in facial malignancy. Arch Otolaryngol 94:356–358
34. Rodgers GK, Myers EN (1988) Surgical management of the mass in the buccal space. Laryngoscope 98:749–753
35. Rodriguez V, Bardwil JM, Bodey GP (1971) Primary aspergilloma cured with amphotericin B. South Med J 64:396–398
36. Smith JF (1967) Nodular fasciitis of the buccal pad. Arch Otolaryngol 86:217–218
37. Tate RJ (1971) Unusual facial abscess. Report of a case. Br Dent J 131:504
38. Tomizawa M, Nakajima T, Fukushima M (1979) False aneurysm of the cheek: report of two cases. J Oral Surg 37:515–518
39. Trester PH, Markovitch E, Zambito RF, Stratigos GT (1969) Myositis ossificans, circumscripta and progressiva, with surgical correction of the masseter muscle: report of two cases. J Oral Surg 27:201–205
40. Weaver DF (1964) Tumors of the cheek. Arch Otolaryngol 79:229–238

Chapter 18

Management of the Mass in the Prestyloid Parapharyngeal Space

18

Rohan R. Walvekar and Eugene N. Myers

Contents

Core Features

- To provide a concept of the three-dimensional anatomy of the prestyloid parapharyngeal space (PPS).
- To present the various options for preoperative evaluation of PPS masses.
- To discuss the surgical approaches to the prestyloid PPS and their applications.

Complications to Avoid

- Injury to the facial nerve can be minimized by accurate preoperative planning using CT scanning and by meticulous dissection of the main trunk and its branches.
- Gustatory sweating (Frey's syndrome) can be avoided by preserving the superficial lobe of the parotid gland and returning it to its anatomical position after excision of a deep lobe parotid tumor.

Introduction

The management of the patient with a tumor of the PPS is a challenging task. The PPS is a complex anatomical region due to its three-dimensional shape, deep location, and its intricate surroundings [10]. The PPS is a difficult region to examine, and thus presents a number of technical challenges for diagnosis and surgical management of these tumors. In fact surgery of the PPS is a relatively recent activity in our field, as the PPS with its components has only been characterized since the introduction of the computed tomography (CT) scan [20].

Anatomy

The PPS has been described as being an inverted triangle with its base at the base of the skull and apex at the hyoid bone (see Fig. 18.1). The lateral wall of the PPS is the pterygoid muscles and the ascending ramus of the mandible [13]. The medial boundary is the pharyngobasilar fascia and the superior constrictor muscle [8]. The posterior limit of the PPS consists of the cervical spine and the adjacent deep muscles of the neck. The anterior boundary is formed by the medial pterygoid muscle [7, 10]. The apex of the PPS is the submandibular triangle to the level of the hyoid bone. Two sides of the PPS are bone, i.e., the skull base superiorly and the mandible laterally. As a result, the tumors of the prestyloid PPS spread along the path of least resistance, which is the anterior, medial, and inferior direction. These tumors displace the pharyngeal wall and the tonsil and often present as a submucosal mass in the pharynx.

The prestyloid PPS is a potential space within the PPS. The fascia of the tensor veli palatini extends from the styloid process to the skull base dividing the PPS into the prestyloid and poststyloid compartments [13] (Fig. 18.2). The prestyloid PPS contains the pterygoid muscles, the retromandibular portion of the deep lobe of the parotid gland, the internal maxillary artery, the lingual nerve, and the inferior dental nerves. It also contains adipose tissue, minor nerves, vessels, and lymphatics [7]. Though the fascia itself cannot be visualized on imaging, CT and/or magnetic resonance imaging (MRI) can accurately classify tumors of the PPS as being in the prestyloid or poststyloid compartment [8]. This information is vital in identifying the tissue of origin of the tumors within the PPS and in developing a differential diagnosis and plan for further management.

Tumors may develop from the various types of tissue present within this anatomical space. The origin of tumors in the PPS, whether prestyloid or poststyloid, is important in their differential diagnosis and management. The clinical correlation of imaging studies and surgical findings has provided information which allows the clinician to predict the tumor type from the imaging studies with a high degree of accuracy. The key anatomical landmarks for this differentiation are the prestyloid fat, the medial pterygoid muscle, the carotid artery, the posterior edge of the mandible, and the styloid process. Of these the carotid artery and the styloid process are the most important landmarks for the clinician.

Tumors of the prestyloid PPS are usually of salivary gland origin, usually arising from the deep lobe of the parotid gland. Most of these tumors are pleomorphic adenomas which arise from the deep lobe of the parotid gland (see Fig. 18.3a, b) but can also arise less frequently, de novo in the prestyloid PPS. An enhanced CT scan or MRI will clearly demonstrate extension of deep lobe tumors of the parotid gland through the stylomandibular tunnel, extending medially and displacing the parapharyngeal structures (see Fig. 18.4a, b). The demonstration of a fat plane between the deep lobe of the parotid gland and the tumor is indicative of tumor originating de novo in the PPS, most commonly from the extraparotid minor salivary glands. The lack of visualization of this plane indicates a tumor originating in the deep parotid lobe or invading it [9]. High resolution images of the MRI are superior to the CT scan to make such a differentiation [10].

A wide variety of benign and malignant tumors can occur in the PPS (see Table 18.1). About 80% of PPS masses are benign, while 20% are malignant [5]. The primary radiological differential diagnosis for a tumor originating in the prestyloid PPS is a deep lobe parotid tumor and or a neurilemoma (arising from the lingual nerve, inferior alveolar nerve, or auriculotemporal nerve). Although a mass in the prestyloid PPS is more likely to be of salivary gland origin, it is extremely difficult to differentiate it radiologically from a neurilemoma and hence the possibility of a neurilemoma must be taken into consideration in the differential diagnosis. Cancers arising in other sites such as thyroid [6], nasopharynx [24], and maxilla [22], with metastasis to the prestyloid PPS have been described. Raut et al. reported a case of metastatic carcinoma of the breast which presented as a deep lobe parotid tumor in the PPS 15 years after the primary presentation [17].

Clinical Presentation

Tumors of the PPS may be present for several years prior to clinical presentation. They often have to grow to at least 2.5–3.0 cm before they are detected [20]. Carrau et al. found that 20% of masses were also found incidentally [3]. Such incidental findings are not surprising with the routine use of imaging for diagnostic purposes today. The

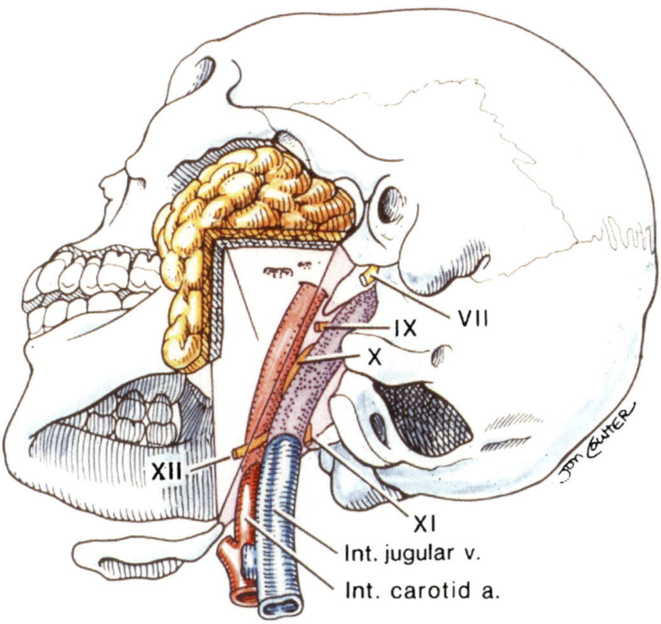

Fig. 18.1: Parapharyngeal space: an inverted triangle with base at skull base and apex at the hyoid bone. [Reprinted with permission from: Carrau RL, Myers EN, and Johnson JT (1990) Management of tumors arising in the parapharyngeal space. Laryngoscope 100:583–9]

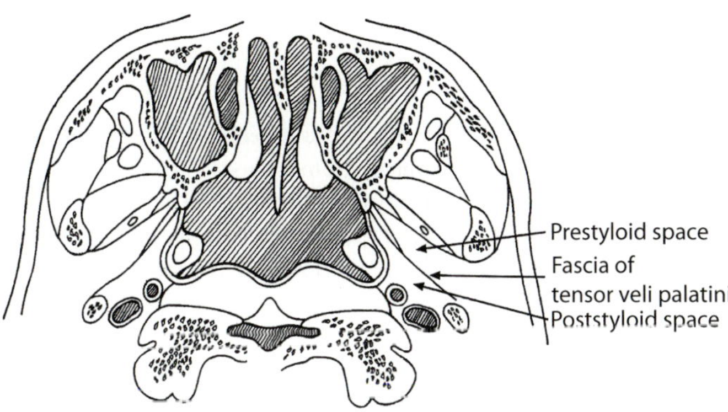

Fig. 18.2: Parapharyngeal space: anatomical boundaries. [Reprinted with permission from: Johnson JT (1997) Parapharyngeal space. In: Myers EN (ed) Operative Otolaryngology: Head and Neck Surgery. Saunders, Philadelphia]

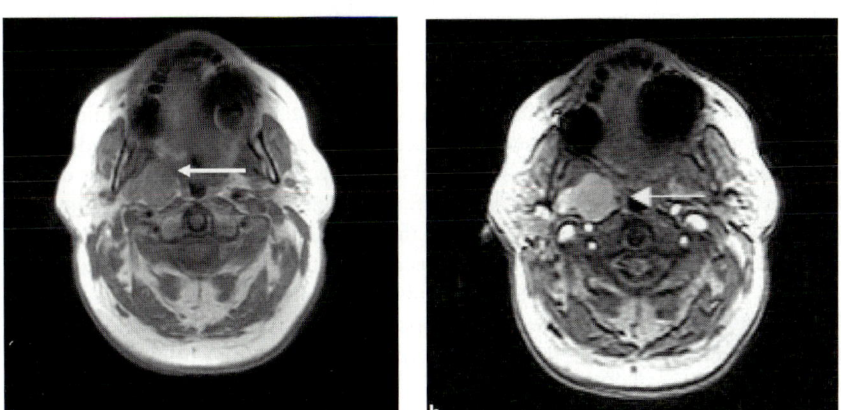

Fig. 18.3: **a** T1-weighted MRI image of a pleomorphic adenoma involving the prestyloid PPS. **b** T2-weighted MRI image of a pleomorphic adenoma originating the prestyloid PPS

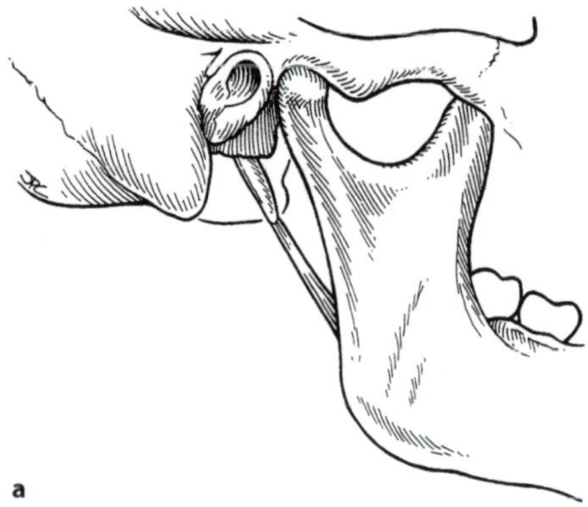

a

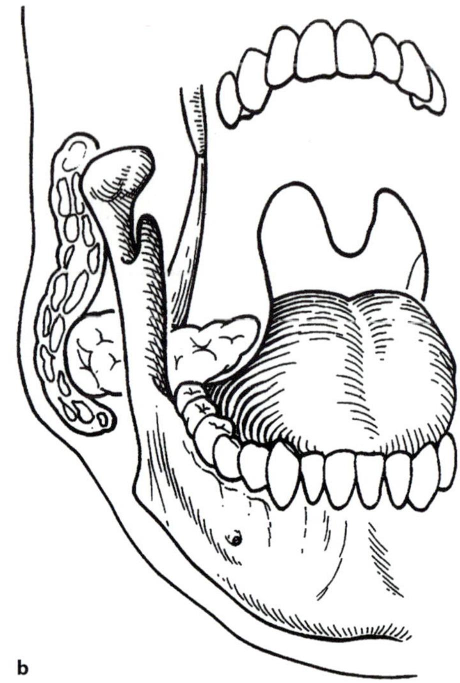

b

Fig. 18.4: **a** Styloid process and its relationship to the mandible forming the stylomandibular tunnel with the stylomandibular ligament as the inferior boundary. [Reprinted with permission from: Johnson JT (1997) Prestyloid parapharyngeal space. In: Myers EN (ed) Operative Otolaryngology: Head and Neck Surgery. Saunders, Philadelphia] **b** Deep lobe tumors of the parotid gland passing through the stylomandibular tunnel, often presenting as an oropharyngeal mass [Reprinted with permission from: Johnson JT (1997) Prestyloid parapharyngeal space. In: Myers EN (ed) Operative Otolaryngology: Head and Neck Surgery. Saunders, Philadelphia]

most commonly encountered presentation of a neoplasm involving the prestyloid PPS is an asymptomatic submucosal mass in the lateral wall of the oropharynx with or without a mass in the parotid gland or the neck (see Table 18.2) (Fig. 18.5). Expansion of these tumors may interfere with the proper fit of an upper denture and on occasion may become symptomatic based on the large size, producing interference with breathing and swallowing. In a retrospective study of 166 PPS tumors, about 25% of patients did not report any symptoms at the time of diagnosis [5]. The presence of a mass in the parotid gland is often associated with the mass in the oral cavity. The presence of pain or neuropathy should direct the clinician to suspect a primary or metastatic cancer. In addition to the clinical signs and symptoms, a detailed examination of the head and neck, which would include an examination of the cranial nerves, and bimanual palpation allows the clinician to formulate a clinical impression of the extent of the tumor.

Preoperative Evaluation

Patients being evaluated for a tumor in the prestyloid PPS should undergo a thorough history and physical examination. Tumors of the head and neck, and poststyloid PPS masses such as paragangliomas should be ruled out. Certain aspects of the physical examination, such as indirect laryngoscopy or fiberoptic laryngoscopy, should be performed to evaluate the motion of the vocal cords.

Imaging

The distinction between tumors of the prestyloid and poststyloid space may be made radiologically based on a clear understanding of anatomy in this region. Som et al. [20], developed a CT protocol to provide a preoperative diagnosis accurately in 88% of PPS tumors. There were ten large tumors in their study of 104 cases which could not be diagnosed initially but the CT scan helped to limit the differential diagnosis in the ten cases. In our department, CT scan with contrast has been used almost exclusively with the exception of certain patients in whom there is a suspicion of intracranial extension who benefit from MRI studies. The prestyloid PPS has a significant fat content which is easily displaced and deformed, and it has high signal intensity on T1-weighted images (see Fig. 18.6) [10]. The posterior displacement of the carotid artery and internal jugular vein on MRI is suggestive of a

Table 18.1. Tumors of the PPS removed at the Department of Otolaryngology, University of Pittsburgh

Histology	Number of tumors
Paraganglioma	69
Pleomorphic adenoma	32
Squamous cell carcinoma	10
Neurilemoma	7
Salivary duct carcinoma	3
Sarcoma	3
Schwannoma	3
Adenocarcinoma	2
Adenoid cystic carcinoma	2
Carcinoma ex pleomorphic adenoma	2
Lipoma	2
Lymphangioma	2
Lymphoma	2
Meningioma	2
Hemangioma	1
Hemangiopericytoma	1
Leiomyosarcoma	1
Liposarcoma	1
Lymphoepithelial carcinoma	1
Mucoepidermoid carcinoma	1
Myoepithelioma	1
Neurofibroma	1
Oncocytic papillary cystadenoma	1
Thyroid carcinoma	1
Warthin's tumor	1

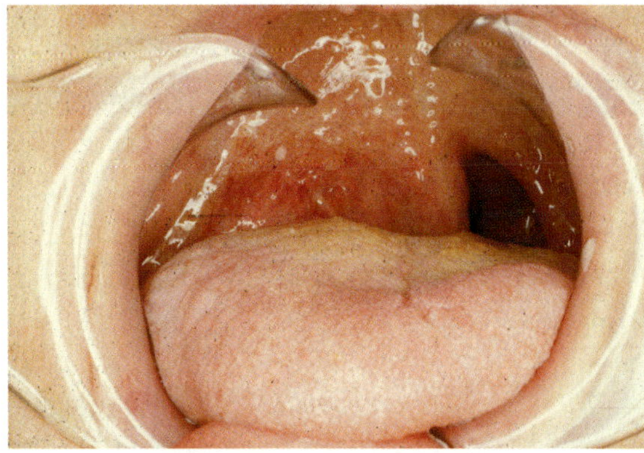

Fig. 18.5: Prestyloid PPS tumor presenting as an intraoral mass. [Reprinted with permission from: Johnson JT (1997) Prestyloid parapharyngeal space. In: Myers EN (ed) Operative Otolaryngology: Head and Neck Surgery. Saunders, Philadelphia]

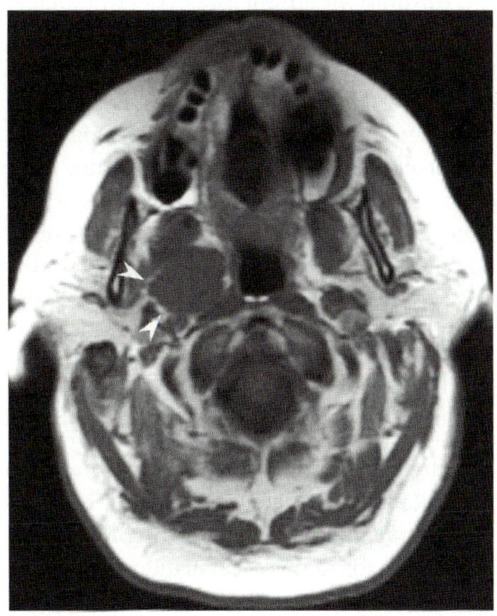

Fig. 18.6: Axial unenhanced T1-weighted image through the PPS demonstrates a 3-cm parapharyngeal mass separated from the deep lobe of the parotid by an intact fat plane (*arrowheads*). This mass, which displaces the fat plane medially, was excised and shown to be a pleomorphic adenoma

Table 18.2. Clinical presentation of prestyloid PPS tumors

Symptoms		Signs
Asymptomatic	→	Normal examination (incidentaloma)
Lump in the neck	→	Mass in the neck/parotid region
Difficulty swallowing or breathing	→	Intraoral mass
Asymmetry of the face	→	Facial paresis or palsy
Hearing loss or otalgia	→	Serous otitis media
Others		
Pain		Trismus
Globus sensation		

prestyloid PPS tumor. Dynamic MRI and magnetic resonance angiography (MRA) are additional tools that can provide supportive evidence for vascular tumors originating in the region.

The distinction between prestyloid and poststyloid space tumors is the most important aspect of radiological evaluation. Clinical correlation along with imaging can help to clearly define what type of tumor the patient has and provides us with a very clear plan of management based on location and histology. In most cases, this clinicoradiological correlation can serve as a substitute for a biopsy.

Recently other types of imaging studies have emerged. In a recent study, a three-dimensional (3D) digital reconstruction of the prestyloid PPS was performed with the help of two-dimensional MRI data and thin cadaveric sections of the PPS. The digitalized 3D model could clearly demonstrate the spatial relationship of various structures in the PPS. In the prestyloid PPS, besides the pharyngeal vein, the ascending pharyngeal artery with its branches and the submandibular nerve could be clearly demonstrated. Such 3D reconstructed images of the MRI would provide important data for radiological diagnosis, surgical planning, and radiotherapy. Positron emission tomography (PET) and PET with CT may also help to diagnose and monitor tumors of the PPS. The PET scan has been shown to have the ability to reflect tumor growth in pleomorphic adenomas, which are the most common tumors found in the prestyloid PPS [12]. In the same way as F-DOPA-PET with CT does seem to improve the diagnostic accuracy of paragangliomas in the PPS [1, 2], an image fusion of the PET and CT may help to improve diagnostic accuracy and anatomical definition of the prestyloid PPS lesions.

18

Tumors of the deep lobe of the parotid gland can be differentiated from those arising de novo in the prestyloid PPS by the presence of a fat plane between the deep lobe of the parotid gland and the tumor. This is a very important point in planning the surgical approach for these tumors, since the tumors independent of the parotid gland may be removed through a cervical approach whereas tumors arising in the deep lobe of the parotid gland with extension into the PPS must be approached through a parotid-submandibular approach with dissection of the facial nerve off the deep lobe in order to avoid injury to the facial nerve.

Fine-needle Aspiration Biopsy (FNAB)

Fine-needle aspiration biopsy may contribute to preoperative histopathological evaluation of prestyloid PPS tumors. Palpable tumors can be easily aspirated; however more deeply seated tumors may need accurate fine-needle aspiration with ultrasound or CT guidance [13]. The current literature on histopathology of prestyloid PPS tumors is based on the study of surgical specimens, with much less emphasis on FNAB or incisional biopsies. This may have been due to the fact that regardless of preoperative histological findings, most tumors will require excision. Secondly, there is a theoretical possibility of hemorrhage, infection, and tumor seeding with FNAB creating a bias against performing FNAB for diagnostic purposes. More recent reports have shown these beliefs to be unfounded [14]. Wilson et al. reported no instances of tumor seeding after diagnostic aspiration [23]. With respect to hemorrhage, the aspiration of a carotid body tumor, which is not a tumor found in the prestyloid PPS, seems to be the only contraindication to FNAB. A recent review of PPS tumors has shown that FNAB for PPS tumors has an accuracy, sensitivity, and specificity of 94%, 86%, and 100%, respectively [14].

Fine-needle aspiration biopsy may be especially helpful in patients suspected of harboring malignant tumors. Clinical findings such as pain, nerve involvement, rapid growth, and fixation, with radiological evidence of bone involvement are suggestive of a malignant tumor. In these cases, an FNAB may be helpful to confirm the clinical suspicion and provide valuable information for treatment planning and counseling the patient and family preoperatively. It does seem reasonable to assume that FNAB of prestyloid PPS tumors can be done safely under image guidance, if necessary, to help in treatment planning. However, traditionally we have not advocated FNAB prior to surgical resection since in most cases it does alter the plan of management.

Surgical Approaches to Tumors of the Prestyloid Parapharyngeal Space

There are a variety of surgical approaches which may be used for the management of tumors of the PPS (see Table 18.3). The traditional approaches to the prestyloid PPS are the transcervical or transcervical-transparotid approaches, either of which may be augmented with a mandibulotomy [5, 21]. Other than PPS extensions of deep lobe parotid tumors, most PPS masses can be excised by the transcervical technique alone.

Transoral/Transoral-Transcervical Approach

Transoral excision has been advocated for neoplasms arising in the prestyloid PPS especially when the tumors are limited to the prestyloid PPS and cannot be felt in the neck or parotid gland. A pure transoral approach provides several advantages. It is the most direct approach to the tumors of the prestyloid PPS, which may bulge into the oropharynx or lateral pharyngeal wall. Exposure of the tumor requires less surgery, and careful dissection will prevent damage to important adjacent structures, including the facial nerve [7]. Disadvantages of this approach include incomplete exposure and lack of proximal control of the internal carotid artery. Transoral excision alone has also been criticized for an associated increased risk of bleeding, tumor spillage, and increased rate of recurrence [5]. In our opinion, lack of adequate exposure deprives the surgeon of the opportunity to identify the closely related neurovascular structures or Stensen's duct, which can increase the risk of injury to these structures. Transoral excision may also compromise the wound through contamination by oral secretions or seed the tumor into the mucosa of the palate.

Table 18.3. Surgical approaches used in surgery of the prestyloid PPS

Surgical approaches
• Transoral
• Transoral-transcervical
• Transcervical
• Transcervical-transparotid
• Mandibulotomy

For these reasons we do not advocate transoral/ transmucosal biopsies or partial removal. In addition to contaminating the mucosa, scarring increases the difficulty of subsequent removal. In cases where prior biopsy has been done, a combined transoral-transcervical approach would ensure complete and safe resection. In case of a recurrence, the scar from the previous transoral surgery should be removed at the time of the transcervical revision surgery.

Transcervical/Submandibular Approach

The prestyloid PPS is ideally approached using the transcervical submandibular technique (see Fig. 18.7). The skin incision is made in the major transverse skin crease in the neck. A facelift incision may also be used. This is carried down through the subcutaneous tissue and platysma muscle. The mandibular branch of the facial nerve must be identified and preserved. Identification of the anterior border of the sternocleidomastoid muscle facilitates identification of the posterior belly of the digastric muscle. The submandibular gland is then dissected free of the surrounding tissues. The facial artery is identified deep to the posterior belly of the digastric muscle and is clamped, transected, and doubly ligated with silk suture. The submandibular gland is then mobilized anteriorly where it is pedicled on the submaxillary ganglion and Warthin's duct

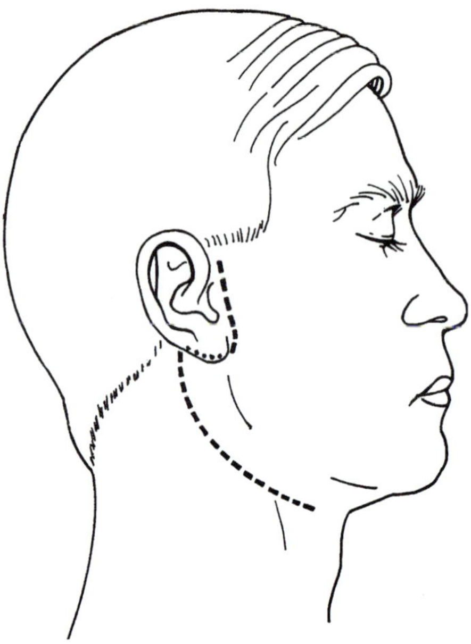

Fig. 18.7: Transcervical approach. [Reprinted with permission from: Johnson JT (1997) Prestyloid parapharyngeal space. In: Myers EN (ed) Operative Otolaryngology: Head and Neck Surgery. Saunders, Philadelphia]

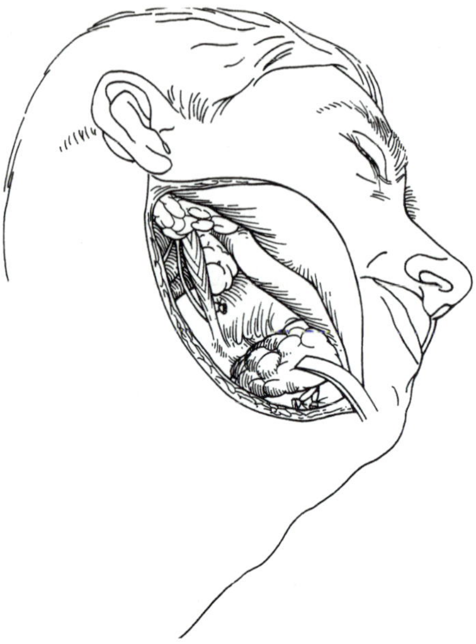

Fig. 18.8: Mobilization and anterior retraction of the submandibular gland to gain access to the parapharyngeal space. [Reprinted with permission from: Johnson JT (1997) Prestyloid parapharyngeal space. In: Myers EN (ed) Operative Otolaryngology: Head and Neck Surgery. Saunders, Philadelphia]

(see Fig. 18.8). It is not necessary to remove the submandibular gland as has been reported by Malone et al. [11], but it is important to retract it anteriorly since this exposure provides direct access to the apex of the prestyloid PPS. Once the gland has been mobilized the tumor is identified and using sharp and blunt dissection the tumor is separated from surrounding tissues (see Fig. 18.9). There are some specific maneuvers that can increase exposure at this stage of dissection. A stylomandibular release and anterior dislocation of the mandible can increase exposure by 50%. Subsequently, the styloid process, styloid musculature, and posterior belly of the digastric muscle can be removed for additional exposure [5, 16].

Tumors in the prestyloid PPS are usually pleomorphic adenoma which does not invade the surrounding soft tissue. However, to prevent recurrence every effort should be made to preserve the capsule of the tumor. A suction drain is placed in the depths of the wound and brought out just posterior to the skin incision in order to collapse the dead space. The wound is then meticulously closed and a dressing applied.

Transcervical-Transparotid Approach

The majority of tumors of the prestyloid PPS require formal identification and preservation of the main trunk of the facial nerve. We advocate the parotid-submandibular approach for prestyloid PPS tumors which arise from the deep lobe of the parotid gland. Other authors have also recommended the transcervical-transparotid approach for all deep lobe parotid tumors [15, 19]. The potential injury to the facial nerve from tumors that either arise from the deep lobe of the parotid or are adherent to it are the most important reasons for this approach which allows adequate exposure and early identification of the facial nerve.

An extended parotid-submandibular incision includes a modified Blair incision in the preauricular skin crease, carried around the earlobe and then extended into the neck in a prominent horizontal skin crease to the level of the submandibular gland (Fig. 18.10). The submandibular gland is then mobilized by ligating the facial artery and displacing the gland anteriorly. The skin

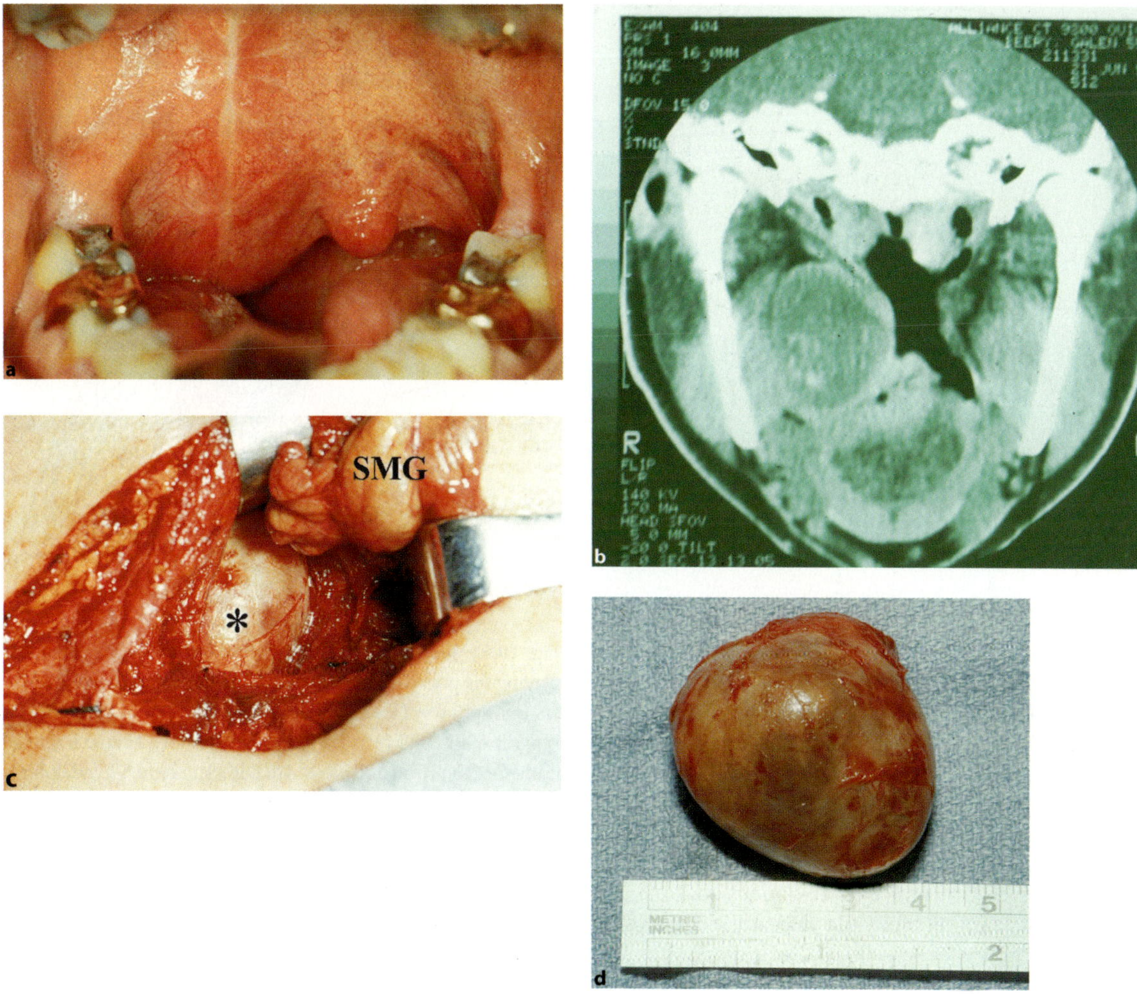

Fig. 18.9: **a** A prestyloid PPS tumor presenting as an intraoral submucosal mass. [Reprinted with permission from: Myers EN, Johnson JT, Curtin HD (2003) Tumors of the parapharyngeal space. In: Myers EN, Suen JY, Myers JN, Hanna EH (eds) Cancer of the Head and Neck, 4th edn. Saunders, Philadelphia] **b** A coronal CT scan showing the mass occupying the prestyloid PPS displacing the lateral oropharyngeal wall medially. [Reprinted with permission from: Myers EN, Johnson JT, Curtin HD (2003) Tumors of the parapharyngeal space. In: Myers EN, Suen JY, Myers JN, Hanna EH (eds) Cancer of the Head and Neck, 4th edn. Saunders, Philadelphia] **c** The mass (*asterisk*) is exposed through a transcervical incision displacing the submandibular gland anteriorly (*SMG*). **d** Specimen of the prestyloid PPS tumor showing the smooth surface of the mass which facilitates mobilization by blunt dissection

flaps are raised as in a parotidectomy, and the main trunk of the facial nerve is identified by using the landmarks of the anterior border of the sternocleidomastoid, the mastoid tip, and the cartilaginous external auditory meatus. The main trunk of the facial nerve is identified and the divisions of the facial nerve are exposed (Fig. 18.11). In doing this, the superficial lobe is dissected from the facial nerve, pedicled anteriorly and preserved. Tumors of the deep lobe of the parotid gland which involve the prestyloid PPS will most often lie just beneath the branches of the facial nerve. The branches of the facial nerve are dissected free of the capsule of the tumor and the nerve

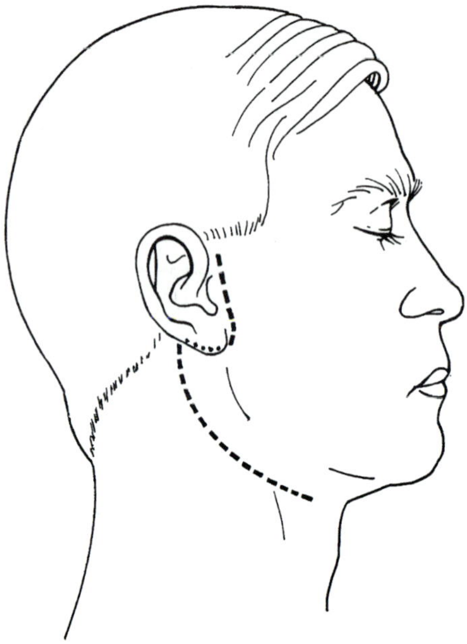

Fig. 18.10: Incision for the transcervical-transparotid approach. [Reprinted with permission from: Johnson JT (1997) Prestyloid parapharyngeal space. In: Myers EN (ed) Operative Otolaryngology: Head and Neck Surgery. Saunders, Philadelphia]

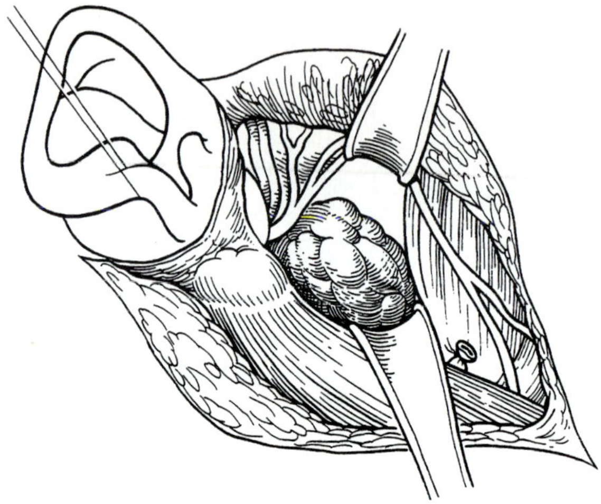

Fig. 18.11: Identification and dissection of the facial nerve displaying the pes anserinus. [Reprinted with permission from: Myers EN, Johnson JT, Curtin HD (2003) Tumors of the parapharyngeal space. In: Myers EN, Suen JY, Myers JN, Hanna EH (eds) Cancer of the Head and Neck, 4th edn. Saunders, Philadelphia]

is mobilized. The deep lobe tumor is then delivered through this exposure in a three-dimensional manner with a combination of blunt and sharp dissection. Blunt finger dissection is often sufficient for extraparotid salivary gland tumors of the prestyloid PPS. The maneuvers used to increase exposure for the transcervical approach such as a stylomandibular tenotomy and anterior retraction of the mandible can also be employed to increase exposure if needed. At the end of the procedure, after hemostasis is obtained and the wound irrigated, the superficial lobe of the parotid gland is replaced in its anatomical position in order to ensure that the contour of the face is preserved. The wound is then closed in layers over a suction drain.

Mandibulotomy Approach

The mandibulotomy approach is usually reserved for tumors of the poststyloid PPS. Such a midline or anterior mandibulotomy may be helpful to increase exposure for lesions in the superior PPS, tumors larger than 8 cm, tumors encasing the internal carotid artery, and malignant tumors invading the skull base or vertebral bodies. This approach has limited utility for the management of prestyloid PPS tumors. In our opinion, most prestyloid PPS tumors can be managed satisfactorily with a transcervical approach and its modifications with the exception of deep lobe parotid tumors, which can be safely approached via a transcervical-transparotid approach. An interesting new approach described by Teng et al. [21] described a subcutaneous mandibulotomy which the authors feel affords excellent access to the PPS without the lip-split, chin-split, and floor of mouth incisions which are a part of the usual midline mandibulotomy. They propose the approach for tumors which are inaccessible through the transcervical approach yet do not require a full midline mandibulotomy for a safe and complete removal.

Complications

Complications of the surgery could be either sequelae expected from the operation (e.g., if a cranial nerve is

Table 18.4. Complications of PPS surgery

Complication	Causative factor
Facial nerve weakness	Traction injury to the facial nerve
First bite syndrome	Parotid "sympathectomy"
Trismus/temporomandibular joint pain	Dislocation of the temporomandibular joint during mandibular swing
Tongue weakness	Hypoglossal nerve injury
Hematoma	Inadequate hemostasis, slippage of ligature especially from the facial artery
Seroma	

resected for oncological reasons) or unexpected complications such as facial nerve damage and the first bite syndrome which are the most frequent complications of surgery for prestyloid PPS tumors [5] (Table 18.4).

Damage to the Facial Nerve

The most common complication of dissection of the prestyloid PPS relates to the facial nerve. If the tumor is separated from the deep lobe of the parotid by a distinct fat plane, removal of tumor completely without injury to the nerve can be expected. If, however, the tumor is a PPS extension of a deep lobe parotid tumor, then it is possible that injury to the facial nerve, either from inaccurate dissection or traction on the nerve, may occur. Traction injuries to the facial nerve can be expected to recover within 3 months [5].

Proper eye care is essential for patients with facial nerve injury. In the immediate postoperative period a moisture chamber is used. Patients who are expected to have a prolonged recovery from facial paralysis benefit from insertion of a gold weight into the upper eyelid. In cases where excision of the facial nerve is necessary, options for rehabilitation of facial function include an immediate reconstruction with an interposition nerve graft (greater auricular nerve) or a temporalis muscle sling to reanimate the oral commissure [9] (refer to Chapter 24, Facial Nerve Reconstruction, and Chapter 26, Reconstruction after Excision of Cancer of the Salivary Glands, for further details on facial nerve rehabilitation and reconstruction).

First Bite Syndrome

The "first bite syndrome" may occur in patients with dissection of prestyloid PPS tumors. It is characterized by a pain in the parotid region immediately after the first bite of each meal, which lasts for a few seconds, improves with each bite, and is at its worst with the first meal of the day. Symptoms are usually mild but can be severe enough to hinder a patient's quality of life and ability to eat. This syndrome is commonly seen when parotid tissue is left behind after deep lobe parotid surgery via the transcervical-transparotid approach, accompanied by an interruption of sympathetic supply to the parotid either due to a injury to the cervical sympathetic chain or due to a selective sympathetic denervation accompanying an external carotid artery ligation. This concept of a parotid "sympathectomy" has been proposed by Chiu et al. [4]. In the authors' experience, current treatment options have not been effective. Medical treatment is symptomatic with nonsteroidal anti-inflammatory medications or carbamazepine. If medical treatment fails, tympanic neurectomy may provide relief in some patients [4].

Conclusion

The management of prestyloid PPS masses is surgical. A detailed preoperative evaluation will help define the location, type, and the extent of the tumor. In most cases a complete resection of the tumor is possible via the transcervical approach. For tumor originating in the deep parotid lobe, facial nerve identification and dissection should be performed to prevent inadvertent injury to the facial nerve.

Take Home Messages

- Tumors in the prestyloid PPS are usually of salivary gland origin.
- Modern imaging techniques permit the surgeon to formulate a plan of management without a preoperative biopsy.
- Image-guided fine-needle aspiration can be considered for tumor limited to the prestyloid PPS, particularly if malignancy is suspected.
- A transcervical approach with its modifications will provide adequate exposure for a complete resection in most cases if the mass is not a PPS extension of a tumor of the deep lobe of the parotid gland.
- Excision of a tumor in the deep lobe of the parotid gland with extension to the PPS requires that the branches of the facial nerve be identified and mobilized off the tumor.
- Transoral incisional biopsy of a tumor of the PPS may result in contamination of the mucosa and make eventual transcervical resection more difficult.

References

1. Baysal BE, Myers EN (2002) Etiopathogenesis and clinical presentation of carotid body tumors. Microsc Res Tech 59:256–261
2. Brink I, et al. (2005) Imaging of pheochromocytoma and paraganglioma. Fam Cancer 4:61–68
3. Carrau RL, Myers EN, Johnson JT (1990) Management of tumors arising in the parapharyngeal space. Laryngoscope 100:583–539
4. Chiu AG, et al. (2002) First bite syndrome: a complication of surgery involving the parapharyngeal space. Head Neck 24:996–999
5. Cohen SM, Burkey BB, Netterville JL (2005) Surgical management of parapharyngeal space masses. Head Neck 27:669–675
6. Desuter G, et al. (2004) Parapharyngeal metastases from thyroid cancer. Eur J Surg Oncol 30: 80–84
7. Goodwin WJ Jr, Chandler JR (1988) Transoral excision of lateral parapharyngeal space tumors presenting intraorally. Laryngoscope 98:266–269
8. Hamza A, et al. (1997) Neurilemmomas of the parapharyngeal space. Arch Otolaryngol Head Neck Surg 123:622–626
9. Khafif A, et al. (2005) Surgical management of parapharyngeal space tumors: a 10-year review. Otolaryngol Head Neck Surg 132:401–406
10. Li QY, et al. (2004) The pre-styloid compartment of the parapharyngeal space: a three-dimensional digitized model based on the Chinese Visible Human. Surg Radiol Anat 26:411–416
11. Malone JP, Agrawal A, Schuller DE (2001) Safety and efficacy of transcervical resection of parapharyngeal space neoplasms. Ann Otol Rhinol Laryngol 110:1093–1098
12. Matsuda M, et al. (1998) Positron emission tomographic imaging of pleomorphic adenoma in the parotid gland. Acta Otolaryngol Suppl 538:214–220
13. Myers EN, Johnson JT, Curtin HD (2003) Tumors of the parapharyngeal space. In: Myers EN, et al. (eds) Cancer of the Head and Neck. Saunders, Philadelphia, pp 511–530
14. Oliai BR, et al. (2005) Parapharyngeal space tumors: a cytopathological study of 24 cases on fine-needle aspiration cytology. Diag Cytopathol 32:11–15
15. Olsen KD (1994) Tumors and surgery of the parapharyngeal space. Laryngoscope 104(suppl 63):1–28
16. Orabi AA, Riad MA, O'Regan MB (2002) Stylomandibular tenotomy in the transcervical removal of large benign parapharyngeal tumours. Br J Oral Maxillofac Surg 40:313–316
17. Raut V, et al. (2001) Metastatic breast carcinoma in the parapharyngeal space. J Laryngol Otol 115:750–752
18. Raut V, et al. (2001) Metastatic breast carcinoma in the parapharyngeal space. J Laryngol Otol 115:750–2
19. Som PM, Biller HF, Lawson W (1981) Tumors of the parapharyngeal space: preoperative evaluation, diagnosis and surgical approaches. Ann Otol Rhinol Laryngol Suppl 90:3–15
20. Som PM, et al. (1984) Parapharyngeal space masses: an updated protocol based upon 104 cases. Radiology 153:149–156

21. Teng MS, et al. (2003) Subcutaneous mandibulotomy: a new surgical access for large tumors of the parapharyngeal space. Laryngoscope 113:1893–1897
22. Umeda M, et al. (2002) Metastasis of maxillary carcinoma to the parapharyngeal space: rationale and technique for concomitant en bloc parapharyngeal dissection. J Oral Maxillofac Surg 60:408–413
23. Wilson JA, et al. (1987) Fine needle aspiration biopsy and the otolaryngologist. J Laryngol Otol 101:595–600
24. Xiao GL, Gao L, Xu GZ (2002) Prognostic influence of parapharyngeal space involvement in nasopharyngeal carcinoma. Int J Radiat Oncol Biol 52:957–963

Chapter 19

Vascular Lesions of Salivary Glands

19

Lisa Buckmiller, Brendan C. Stack Jr, and James Y. Suen

Contents

Core Features

- Vascular lesions can involve major and minor salivary glands.
- An understanding of the correct diagnosis of a vascular lesion is key to its adequate management.
- All vascular lesions are not hemangiomas and all do not spontaneously regress.

Complications to Avoid

- Misdiagnosis of vascular lesions.
- Misunderstanding of the natural history of hemangiomas, venous malformations lymphatic malformations, and arteriovenous malformations.

Introduction

The most common vascular anomalies of the salivary glands are congenital. They do not arise from salivary gland tissue but may involve it intimately. When these vascular anomalies are treated surgically, the involved salivary glands frequently must be removed. In the parotid gland, the facial nerve is at risk and should be preserved when possible.

The parotid is the salivary gland most commonly involved. Hemangiomas and vascular malformations are common in the face and frequently involve the parotid gland. The submandibular gland can be involved by vascular malformations, as can the minor salivary glands. In the latter, a lymphatic malformation may be confused with a ranula in the floor of mouth.

The goals of treatment for vascular lesions depend upon the type and extent of the lesion. Hemangiomas eventually regress during childhood whereas vascular malformations continue to grow or expand throughout life unless they are treated and controlled. Arteriovenous malformations are destructive and life threatening and must be surgically resected; however, the goal of treatment for venous and lymphatic malformations may be to control the disease rather than to cure it.

It is crucial to understand the classification of these lesions for proper diagnosis and to formulate a plan of management.

Classification

One of the greatest advances in the understanding and treatment of congenital vascular lesions, regardless of their location, is their correct classification. Classification allows for an orderly understanding of various groups of vascular lesions which leads to a correct diagnosis and therefore appropriate management. A major reason for problematic management of these lesions in the past has been a lack of understanding of the nature of these lesions by most primary care providers to whom these patients initially present. Many patients have had an incorrect diagnosis, uninformed medical opinions, and even inappropriate treatments because of a lack of understanding of these lesions in general, and their classification in particular. The key to understanding vascular lesions is: knowledge of their natural history, understanding of the vessel of origin/etiology, and which therapy is most appropriate for a given type of lesion. The therapeutic approach can differ significantly depending on the diagnosis.

The understanding of vascular lesions was revolutionized by the biologic classification proposed in 1982 by Mulliken and Glowacki [1] (Table 19.1). The basic paradigm is that congenital vascular lesions can be subdivided into two groups, malformations and hemangiomas. Vascular malformations are present at birth, but some can be difficult to recognize initially due to their small size or hidden location. Malformations have a natural history which distinguishes them from hemangiomas and is often an initial point of misinformation provided to patients and their families. Vascular malformations are not proliferative, they grow with their host and they never involute spontaneously. It is important that parents should not be told that these lesions will disappear.

Hemangiomas are considered by many practitioners to be the classic pediatric vascular lesion. As a result, they are overdiagnosed, and this misinformation results in inappropriate or delayed management. Hemangiomas are not usually present at birth but may have a pink, purple, or hypopigmented area which predicts its position. They usually become clinically apparent in the early postnatal period and they proliferate (grow faster than their host) in the first year of life. The pathologic hallmark of these lesions is increased endothelial growth. These lesions share many cellular markers with placental tissue and are now thought to represent a placental metastasis from the mother to child [2]. These lesions spontaneously begin to regress between 1 and 2 years of age. Involution may require 6–12 years. Those that regress more quickly tend to leave less fibrofatty tissue than those that persist longer.

Waner and Suen have further refined the classification system of Mulliken and Glowacki by further subcategorizing vascular malformations based on their vessel of origin (Table 19.1) [3].

Table 19.1. Classification of vascular lesions (modified from Mulliken [1])

Hemangiomas
Vascular malformations
Venous
Capillary (port-wine stains)
Lymphatic (cystic hygromas, lymphangiomas)
Arteriovenous
Mixed
Venous-lymphatic
Venous venular

Source: Waner M, Suen JY (eds) (1999) Hemangiomas and Vascular Malformations of the Head and Neck. New York: Wiley-Liss, Tables 1.1, 1.3–1.5

Diagnosis

Proper classification of vascular lesions is the first goal in the management of these patients. A diagnosis is generated through thorough history taking, physical examination, imaging studies, and postoperative pathology results. Imaging is the principal modality for characterization of extent of the lesion. Imaging, although frequently characteristic of certain lesions, cannot always provide a definitive diagnosis. For example, cases of venous and lymphatic lesions may not be distinguished from each other by magnetic resonance imaging (MRI). Imaging is, therefore, not a substitute for an understanding of the presentation and natural history of these lesions.

The principal imaging modality that delineates vascular lesions and helps the surgeon arrive at the proper diagnosis is MRI. MRI provides the greatest contrast between vascular lesions and surrounding soft tissue. MRI can delineate lesions that extend beyond the capabilities of ultrasound. Imaging can also be used as part of treatment in cases of primary sclerotherapy or as part of a surgical plan which might include preoperative sclerotherapy or embolization. Arteriography is typically reserved for diagnosis and embolization of arteriovenous malformations.

Hemangiomas

Hemangiomas are congenital vascular tumors comprised of proliferative capillary tissues that are related to placenta. This astonishing observation was realized within the last decade, when it was discovered that hemangiomas share tissue markers with placenta [2]. Specifically, the tissue marker GLUT1 is now used routinely to distinguish hemangiomas from all other types of vascular anomalies. Hemangiomas frequently occur in the parotid gland, where they present a particular treatment challenge. These lesions are usually not clearly apparent at birth but may present with an overlying pinkish stain or hypopigmented area. They undergo a rapid proliferative phase and can greatly increase in volume, much to the distress of both parents and physician (Fig. 19.1). Hemangiomas will continue to proliferate over the next 10–14 months and then undergo a variable involution phase, in which the lesion will soften, frequently shrink, and be replaced by fibrofatty tissue. Diagnosis of deep lesions can be aided by MRI which is the diagnostic modality of choice, but if there is superficial involvement MRI is usually not necessary [4]. In the past, medical professionals have advised that no treatment is indicated for these lesions since they "all go away." However, hemangiomas can leave a very disfiguring residual in a large percentage of patients, and may take years to involute. This frequently requires some type of intervention to allow a more normal appearance. In many cases, the residual fibrofatty tissue, overlying stretched and scarred skin, and a continued mass deformity needs to be addressed. Other indications for surgical intervention include complications such as loss of vision, ulceration of the skin, and cartilage destruction.

Various modalities for the treatment of hemangiomas exist and specific treatment regimens need to be individualized for each patient.

Observation

Observation remains an option in the treatment of hemangiomas, however, this should be reserved only for small lesions that are unlikely to leave unsightly residua such as bulky fibrofatty tissue and skin redundancy. Since it is difficult to predict the extent of growth of a given hemangioma or the likelihood of complete involution, intervention to potentially avoid the need for future extensive surgery is advised. In many cases, the growth of the hemangioma or its appearance can be controlled by other means.

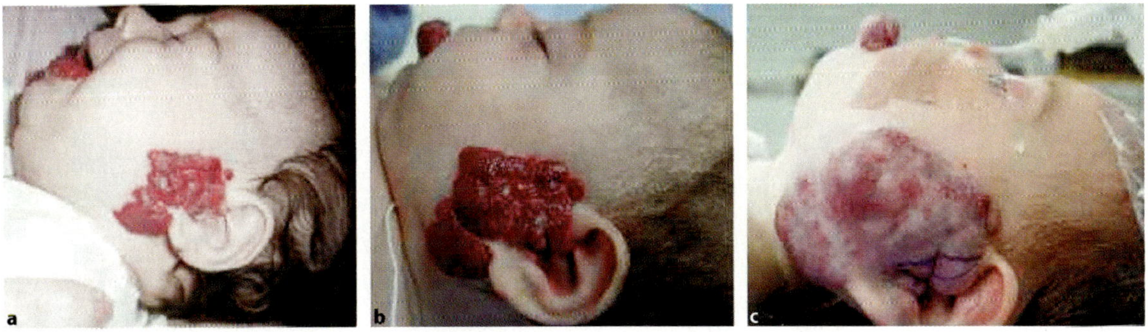

Fig. 19.1a–c: Progressive proliferation of parotid (beard distribution) hemangiomas

Medical Management

Steroid therapy has long been the mainstay of treatment of hemangiomas. However caution must be used with systemic steroid use in children in order to minimize long-term side effects, such as growth disturbance and hormonal imbalances. Oral steroids such as prednisone in high doses, 2–6 mg/kg per day, have been shown to slow, and in many cases reverse the growth of hemangiomas [5–7]. This is usually short-lived since, in our experience, most patients who have been on long-term use of oral steroids have problems with rebound growth upon cessation of the steroids, which then leads to an observation period hopeful for involution.

Intralesional injection of steroid is gaining favor for some patients. The objective is to deliver high-dose steroids to the areas involved with the hemangioma while minimizing potential systemic side effects. A combination of long- and short-acting steroids is usually chosen. We prefer triamcinolone 40 mg/cc and betamethasone 6 mg/cc in a 1:1 ratio. Usually softening of the hemangioma as well as cessation of growth and actual shrinkage of the lesion can be seen in 48–72 h. It is common for the hemangioma to begin proliferating again in the following weeks to months and injections are repeated at 8- to 12-week intervals (Fig. 19.2). Steroid injection has proven to be a useful modality to control growth during the proliferative phase; however it does not eliminate the need for further intervention in every case [8, 9].

Other medical interventions for hemangiomas warrant mentioning, including vincristine and interferon. Vincristine is useful in several situations. We use vincristine as a first-line treatment in patients who have high output cardiac failure, in extensive but surgically inaccessible lesions such as hemangiomas of the liver, or in cases where the hemangioma is otherwise life- or organ-threatening such as in ocular hemangiomas where the patient is at risk for blindness. The drawbacks to such treatment are the need for catheter placement and close monitoring of immune and electrolyte status while the patient is receiving chemotherapy. Vincristine has proven very effective in these cases, however several courses of treatment are usually necessary. Interferon is only recommended in life-threatening cases that have failed other treatment modalities, due to the substantial risk of irreversible spastic diplegia when given to young patients.

Laser Therapy

Hemangiomas involving the superficial tissues can be treated with pulsed dye laser. Lasers can be useful to speed the lightening of the skin during involution or in treating overlying skin ulceration caused by the rapid growth of the hemangioma. The exact mechanism for skin breakdown is unclear but is theorized to be due to a form of vascular steal phenomenon (Fig. 19.2). Flash pump dye laser, 585–595 nm, is very useful in treating ulcerations, greatly lessening healing time. Wound care is very important and includes application of Silvadine cream, which also prevents localized infection.

Surgery

Decisions on timing of surgery for hemangiomas remains controversial, however it is imperative to treat these children early enough to allow them to have as normal an appearance as possible when entering school [8, 10–12]. After about 1 year of age, hemangiomas be-

19

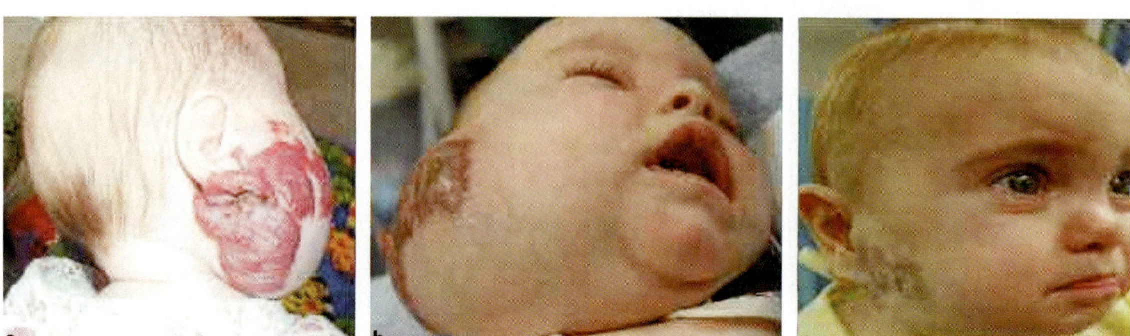

Fig. 19.2: Patient with large parotid hemangiomas before (**a**, **b**) and after three steroid injections (**c**)

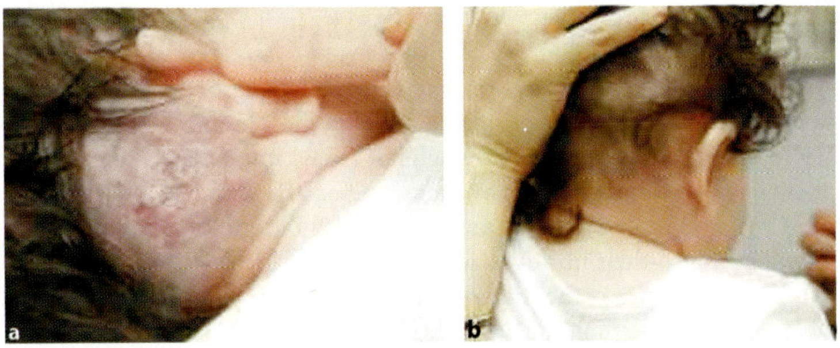

Fig. 19.3: Congenital hemangioma at birth (**a**) and at 6 months of age (**b**)

gin a variable involution rate, with some lesions disappearing in several months and others remaining large with very little change. Parents should be advised of this variability and it is usually recommended that removal of hemangiomas involving the parotid be delayed to assess for adequate involution. If the hemangioma remains large at the age of approximately 3–4 years, then surgical removal is indicated to provide the child with facial symmetry. Surgery can be difficult and frequently involves substantial blood loss and a risk to the facial nerve. The nerve frequently is surrounded by hemangioma and dissection can be difficult. Waiting for initial involution can improve ease of dissection due to fewer vessels and more fibrofatty tissue, although this is not true in all cases. The goal of surgery is not necessarily to remove all of the hemangioma but to create symmetry and eliminate bulk. Since hemangiomas will never reproliferate, the remaining hemangioma acts as a fibrofatty filler and causes no future problems. Usually a superficial parotidectomy is sufficient to accomplish these goals, and further dissection of the nerve is unnecessary. Time should be given to allow for recovery of any nerve apraxia prior to entry to school.

Frequently, enough of the hemangioma will involute to obviate the need for extensive surgery with nerve dissection. In many cases, redundant scarred skin can be resected without formal identification of the facial nerve as long as superficial planes are respected.

Other Hemangiomas

Although rare, two other types of hemangiomas need to be mentioned. These are termed congenital hemangiomas in the literature but this term can be misleading since all hemangiomas are technically congenital. These two other types of hemangiomas that differ from the more common infantile hemangioma, is the rapidly involuting congenital hemangioma (RICH), and the other is the non-involuting congenital hemangioma (NICH). These are lesions which are fully formed at birth and do not undergo a rapid growth phase during the first year of life like infantile hemangiomas. They also differ from the more common hemangiomas in that they are GLUT1 negative, and this can aid in their diagnosis [12]. They can be classified as either rapidly involuting or non-involuting depending on their history. The rapidly involuting hemangiomas will frequently be quite large at birth but the mass completely disappears within several months. Usually, residual scarring of the skin with atrophy of the subcutaneous tissues is all that remains (Fig. 19.3). The non-involuting congenital hemangioma will undergo little change and may require removal at some time to improve appearance. These two lesions appear very similar at birth and only time will tell if the lesion will undergo involution.

Kasabach-Merritt Syndrome

Traditionally, it was thought that Kasabach-Merritt syndrome was caused by hemangiomas, however, it has been shown that the lesion is actually kaposiform hemangioendothelioma (KHE). Kasabach-Merritt is defined by platelet trapping, ecchymosis, high output cardiac failure, and can be associated with a high mortality rate. KHE lesions tend to be very firm, have less distinct borders and appear purplish in color. These lesions can occur anywhere, including the salivary glands. KHE can be diagnosed on the basis of history, it is usually present at birth with rapid growth thereafter, or by laboratory studies, a fall in platelet count or a biopsy. Treatment consists of high-dose steroids, vincristine, and possibly surgical excision once the lesion and the patient are stable and depending on the location of the lesion. These lesions can involve multiple and/or diffuse sites.

Vascular Malformations

One of the greatest advances in the understanding and treatment of congenital vascular lesions, wherever their location, is their correct classification. The key to understanding vascular lesions is: knowledge of their natural history, understanding of the vessel of origin/etiology, and which therapy is most appropriate for a given type of lesion.

Venular Malformations

Venular malformations are commonly termed port-wine stains (PWS) or classified as capillary malformations. Venular malformations have, as their name implies, low flow, postcapillary vessels of origin (Table 19.1). This group is distinct, however, from simply lesions of dilated veins (venous malformations, see below). Venular lesions arise from the small venules just distal to the capillary beds, usually highly regulated resistance vessels which manage capillary perfusion. Although these lesions can involve facial skin which overlies major salivary glands, these lesions do not extend into these glands (Fig. 19.4). Minor salivary glands are involved when venular lesions are located on mucosa. Treatment for these lesions includes laser photocoagulation with non-contact YAG or pulse dye (PDL) lasers [13–20]. Redundant tissue resulting from these lesions may be excised for cosmetic and functional reasons.

Venous Malformations

Venous malformations are lesions of grouped ectatic veins. They are considered to be low flow lesions. They are present at birth, although not always immediately recognized, and progress by increasing ectasia with age. Veins within these lesions may reach a 10-fold greater diameter than their normal size. Phleboliths, palpable calcified thrombi, are pathognomonic of this lesion, if present. Clinical presentation is variable due to size, location (internal versus external), and vertical location within the layers of the soft tissue. The deeper the lesion, the less overlying purple/blue discoloration would be expected. Some lesions are so deep that they have no overlying color changes and are diagnosed by their mass effect, ability to compress with refilling, and their imaging characteristics (Fig. 19.5).

Venous lesions grow over the life of the patient, but the velocity of growth can be variable. Predictable periods of rapid expansion include: puberty, use of oral contraceptives, pregnancy, or trauma. They can present as an isolated lesion or as multiple foci of apparently discontinuous lesions, or diffuse areas of involvement. It is not uncommon when a patient presents with a single venous lesions for others to be discovered during physical examination, flexible laryngoscopy, or upon review of imaging studies. MRI scans can identify and delineate areas involved by venous lesions and these scans are necessary for treatment planning should intervention be elected (Fig. 19.6). Sites of predilection of venous lesions within the head and neck include: buccal mucosa, tongue, oral

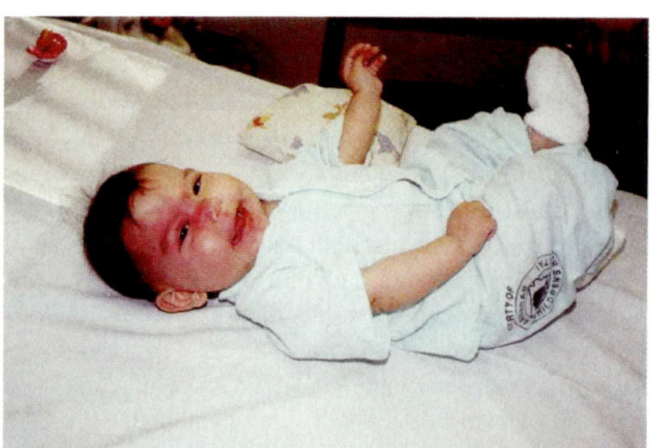

Fig. 19.4: Infant with port-wine stain over right face including parotid/preauricular area

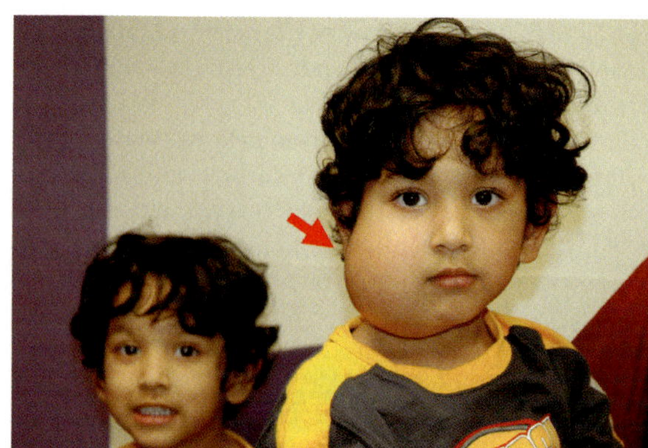

Fig. 19.5: Identical twins with child in foreground with a large right-sided facial venous malformation involving the parotid gland

19

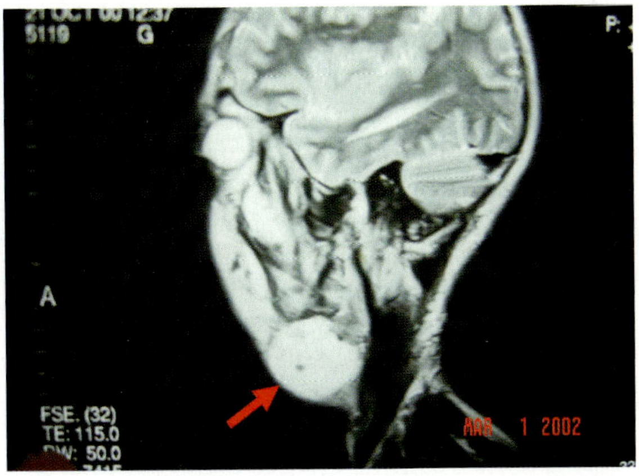

Fig. 19.6: Patient with venous malformation of submaxillary-parotid area which was consolidated with a phlebolith in the center. It was totally resectable. *Arrow* points to consolidated lesion

commissure, buccal space, parotid, and the soft tissue of the neck. Venous malformations frequently involve muscle groups. Major and minor salivary gland infiltration is commonly seen.

Treatment of venous malformations of the head and neck may be accomplished by multiple modalities. The decision to treat these lesions is based on their location, symptoms, and presence of functional impairment, aesthetic considerations, and the interest of the patients. Conservative treatment may be all that is required for lesions that result in no functional impairment. This can be done by having the patient sleep with the head of the bed elevated and minimizing excessive strenuous activity. Surface disfiguration and discoloration by smaller lesions may be managed by non-contact YAG laser treatments [21]. These treatments are limited to superficial obliteration of veins. Often this technique is applied to areas of mucosal involvement such as to the oral cavity, tongue, pharynx, or larynx. When lesions are treated endoscopically, one should start with the deepest (most distal to the point of endoscope insertion) lesion first. This prevents contact with the treated mucosa by retractors or the laryngoscope which may result in hemorrhage. YAG laser treatment shrinks the venous malformation away from overlying mucosa. The mucosa heals well with minimal scaring because of a lack of melanin. Interstitial placement of laser fibers can allow for internal laser treatment of venous malformations [22].

Sclerotherapy is an option to control the expansion of venous malformations [23]. This is particularly useful in areas where surgical access is difficult or risky, such as diffuse involvement of the tongue or face. Sclerotherapy treatments using ethanol throughout the lesion can promote thrombosis and shrinkage of the lesion. Multiple treatments are usually required, however, and it is important that the patient and family are aware of this. It is also useful preoperatively, to lessen intraoperative blood loss and facilitate dissection. Alcohol sclerotherapy should be performed by experienced interventional radiologists because complications and even death may occur.

Lesions that are localized and symptomatic can be resected. This is not a procedure for the inexperienced surgeon but is feasible when certain surgical principles are applied. Alternatively, image-directed sclerotherapy can be used to manage these lesions.

Lymphatic Malformations

Lymphatic malformations are slow flow malformations consisting of ectatic lymph channels and can be classified as focal or diffuse depending on the extent of the lesion as well as microcystic versus macrocystic which can be determined on MRI. Microcystic lesions contain cystic spaces that are less than 2 cm in diameter and present a much greater challenge to treat and cure than their macrocystic (cysts >2 cm) counterparts (Fig. 19.7). Many malformations are actually a combination of micro- and macrocystic, with pure composition of one or the other being rare. Lymphatic malformations are frequently quite large at birth and may result in airway problems. They can often be diagnosed on prenatal ultrasound. Multiple terms have been used in the past to label these lesions including cystic hygroma and lymphangioma. To eliminate confusion in diagnosis, these terms should be avoided.

Lymphatic malformations tend to be quite extensive with the parotid and submandibular areas frequently being involved. They are commonly bilateral in these extensive cervicofacial lymphatic malformations and present a great challenge in management for both physician as well as caregivers. The initial primary concern is the patient's airway. Infants with extensive disease usually will undergo tracheotomy to help maintain the airway from compression by the mass as well as from expected periods of swelling that are typical in areas involved with malformation.

The natural history of these lesions is they usually present at birth and they tend to grow slowly through-

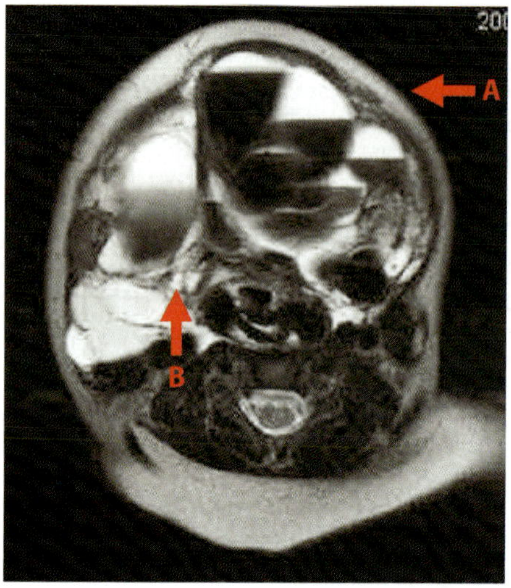

Fig. 19.7: MRI lymphatic malformation demonstrating both micro- (*vertical arrow*) and macrocysts (*horizontal arrow*) as well as fluid/fluid levels

out the patient's lifetime. The lesions never involute or proliferate, but grow by slow expansion of the ectatic vessels and they are exacerbated by infection, trauma and hormonal changes. Spontaneous regression has been reported in the literature, but this is rare, and in many instances these reports lack long-term follow-up. Parents or patients may report increased swelling with infection, due to the increased immune system activity and lymph flow during these times; the tissue surrounding the malformation may also become intermittently infected itself. It is important to treat infections which cause flare-up of the malformation with antibiotics and steroids to help control the expansion of the lesion and prevent irreversible growth. Hormonal control of these lesions has long been suspected, since puberty, pregnancy, and use of oral contraceptives can all greatly exacerbate these lesions.

Treatment of lymphatic malformations of the parotid will usually involve treating a more extensive cervicofacial malformation as well (Fig. 19.8). Intervention becomes necessary to preserve functions such as swallowing and speaking (i.e., tongue), as well as to correct or limit deformity (i.e., enlarged parotid/submaxillary area). Conservative management is one method of slowing the progress of extensive lesions and can be helpful in managing swelling after procedures. These include elevation of the head of the bed to limit expansion pressure on the walls of the malformation, and intermittent steroid and/or antibiotic treatments are also used for flare-up swelling. It is important that when a pulse of high-dose steroids is prescribed that proton pump inhibitors or a H2 blocker be prescribed as well.

Two main methods of treatment for lymphatic malformations of the salivary gland are surgery and sclerotherapy. Many factors go into the decision to use one of the two of these methods or a combination of both. Focal

19

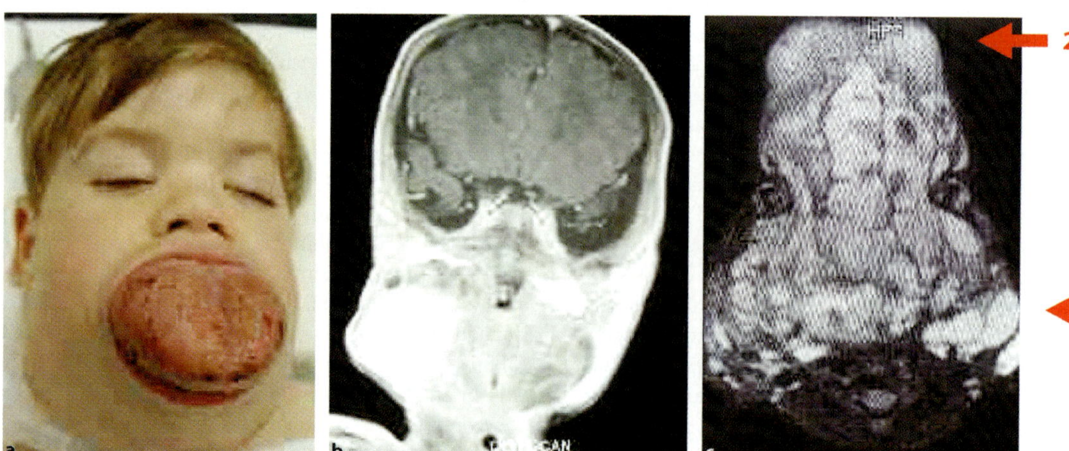

Fig. 19.8: Patient with extensive cervicofacial lymphatic malformation and macroglossia (**a**), with MRI (**b, c**) showing micro (*1*) and macrocystic (*2*) areas

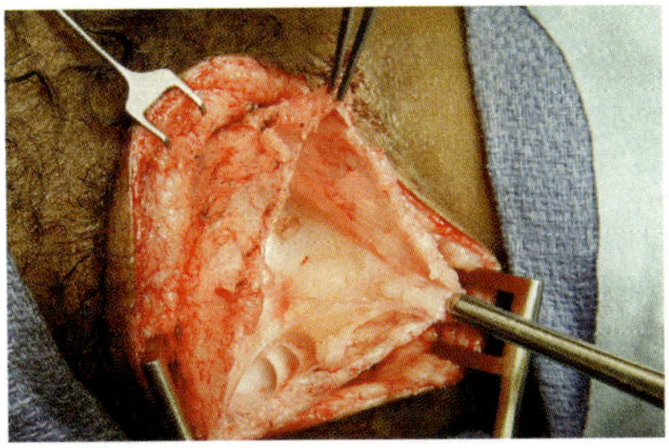

Fig. 19.9: Intraoperative view of large macrocystic lymphatic malformation

lesions, which are frequently macrocystic, are the easiest to treat with cure rates for both surgery as well as sclerotherapy being very high (Fig. 19.9). This is likely due to the ease of removing the entire lesion surgically due to the less diffuse nature of the malformation, and similarly, interventional radiologists are able to access the entire abnormal area to adequately inject all macrocystic sacs of the malformation which allows inflammation to promote scarring and decrease the potential for re-expansion.

Sclerotherapy is useful in treating macrocystic lesions only; however this may include the macrocystic areas of a mixed lesion and can be especially useful to treat areas that are less surgically accessible. Sclerotherapy is not useful in treating microcystic malformations. Sclerotherapy may need to be repeated but in these smaller focal lesions, cure is possible.

There are many sclerosing agents used today, and a complete discussion of these is beyond the scope of this chapter, however, OK432 as a sclerosant, has shown promising results in clinical trials here in the USA and is being considered for Food and Drug Administration (FDA) approval. Other agents include alcohol, doxycycline, and bleomycin, all of which carry their own risks. In the area of the parotid gland, with the considerations of the facial nerve, if the malformation is predominantly macrocystic, a series of sclerotherapy injections may adequately shrink and control the lesion, thus eliminating or postponing the need for extensive surgery with extensive facial nerve dissection. Whenever malformation is left in the tissues, as with sclerotherapy treatments and frequently with surgery especially on diffuse microcystic malformations, there is always a chance of re-growth of the lesion. Exacerbating factors such as infection or pregnancy should be discussed extensively with the patients so they have a realistic idea of what their treatment may involve.

Surgery has become the mainstay of treatment for lymphatic malformations of the salivary glands when the lesions are focal but have failed to be controlled by sclerotherapy or when the lesions are diffuse and have microcystic components (Fig. 19.10). This surgery can be very time consuming and a good surgical plan is imperative. In removal of the parotid components of the malformation, it is better to remove as much of the malformation as possible without putting vital structures at undue risk. The more malformation left behind, the quicker its recurrence. Therefore, total parotidectomy as well as removal of non-vital structures should be done carefully, thus leaving a soft tissue defect that can frequently be filled in with autologous fat graft from the abdomen or cadaveric dermis. Surgery can be very difficult due to the web-like appearance of the malformation which usually envelopes all vital structures requiring tedious dissection.

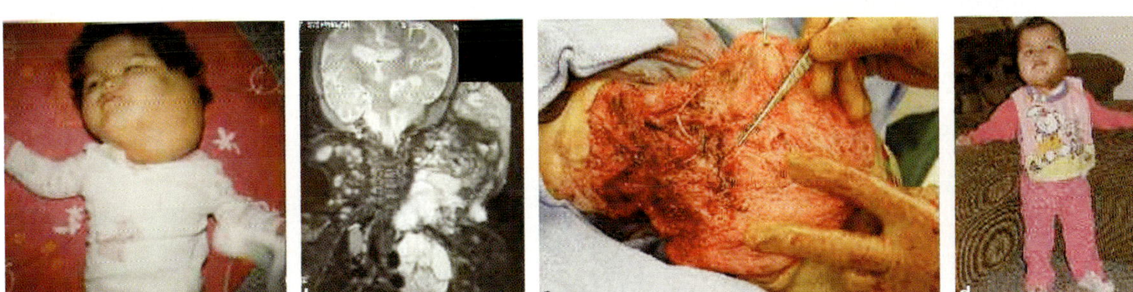

Fig. 19.10: Patient with large cervicofacial/thoracic lymphatic malformation, before surgery (**a**), preoperative MRI (**b**), intraoperative view after debulking (**c**), and postoperative (**d**)

When operating on a previously operated patient or one who has had many infections/sclerotherapy, formation of extremely dense scar tissue is the norm and should be anticipated during surgical planning. With patience, the scar-encased nerves/structures can be freed and the majority of the malformation removed (Fig. 19.10). In extensive lesions, involving all cervicofacial compartments, patients/parents need to be counseled about the near impossibility of complete cure. In many patients, it is impossible to remove all of the diseased tissue without causing unacceptable cosmetic and functional deformity and, therefore, small areas of malformation may be left. When this occurs, we frequently employ intraoperative sclerotherapy with doxycyclinesoaked Gelfoam to help scar these areas down so that this will be less of a problem later.

Postoperative care is important including placement of large-bore drains, IV steroids, and elevation of the head of the bed. Early removal of drains should be particularly discouraged due to the leaky nature of remaining lymphatic channels which can take several weeks to slow down. Early drain removal will result in fluid accumulation which will either need to be treated by drain replacement or doxycycline injections to seal the skin flap into place.

Although lymphatic malformations can present a unique challenge to the surgeon, the care of these patients is important and gratifying. A significant improvement in the quality of life of these patients can be made, as seen in this patient who could not sit up on her own prior to surgery due to the bulk of her malformation. After surgery, she was able to sit upright (Fig. 19.10). Another patient who presented with a large parotid lymphatic malformation as a young adult benefited from its removal prior to her marriage and childbearing [24, 25] (Fig. 19.11).

Arteriovenous Fistula

Arteriovenous (AV) fistulas should not be confused with AV malformations. Fistulas are acquired and usually are the result of trauma. An AV fistula can occur in or around the parotid gland and involve the superficial temporal ar-

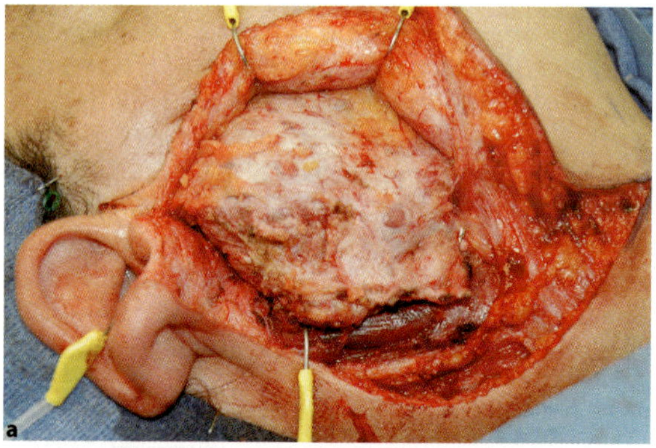

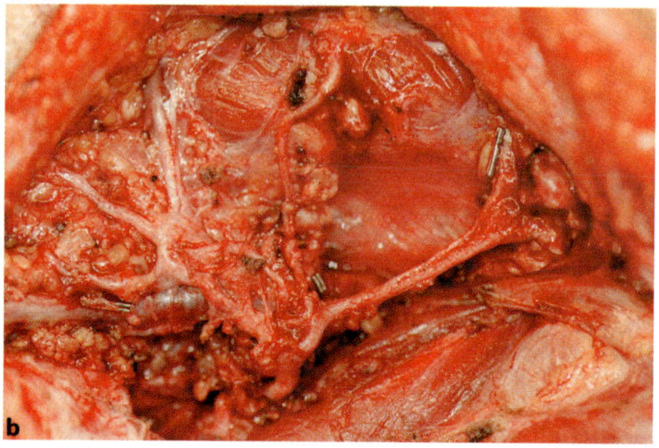

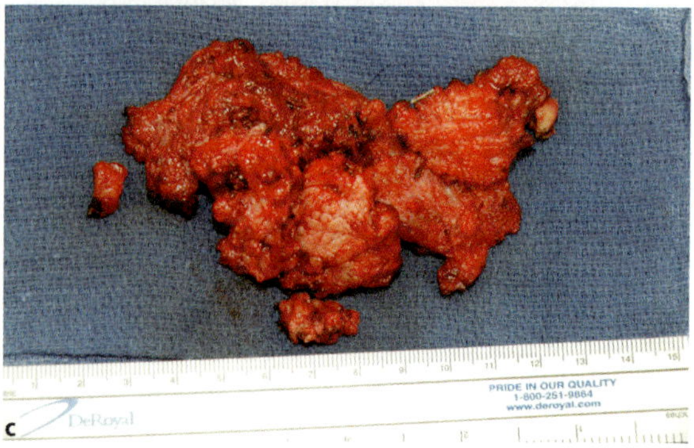

Fig. 19.11: This figure demonstrates the exposed right parotid gland completely replaced by lymphatic malformation (**a**), the facial nerve after total parotidectomy (**b**), and the excised specimen (**c**)

tery and vein. There is usually a history of trauma with a pulsatile fullness around the parotid gland a few months after the injury. Treatment is surgical resection to remove the fistulous tracts and a partial or superficial parotidectomy to gain access. With good interventional radiology availability, embolization can be an alternative treatment.

Arteriovenous Malformations

Arteriovenous malformations (AVM) frequently involve the major and minor salivary glands. They are usually present at birth but may not be obvious until several years later. Most manifest themselves before the age of 20 years old. AVM are affected by hormonal changes and commonly enlarge significantly at the beginning of puberty and especially with pregnancy. As they expand, they are invasive and destructive to all involved tissue. Bleeding is a common problem. Hypertrophy of involved and adjacent tissue will occur so that bone and soft tissue enlargement is seen. The AVM will infiltrate the major and minor salivary glands so that they are intimately involved.

Diagnosis is based on the history of a progressive vascular lesion in the face, tongue, or neck. It is common to see a vascular blush on the skin or mucosal surface similar to a port-wine stain. The patient may report a noticeable pulsation or bleeding from the mucosa (usually gingival) or where skin is involved. The involved tissues are hypertrophied and vascularity is usually obvious. Occasionally there is atrophy of the skin indicating a "steal" syndrome.

Imaging is important to assess the extent of disease and for diagnosis. MRI, magnetic resonance angiography (MRA), or arteriogram are the best imaging studies. On MRI the involved areas will reveal a hyperintense lesion with many flow voids scattered throughout (Fig. 19.12). MRA will demonstrate a very vascular lesion.

An arteriogram will demonstrate a rapid filling lesion with extravasation of dye in the lesion (nidus) and rapid filling veins draining it (Fig. 19.13). The nidus is where the AV shunting occurs and is the abnormal area. The imaging studies help to diagnose the AVM and identify the feeder vessels but do not usually delineate the extent of the disease. Catheterization is also necessary for embolization when indicated.

The treatment of AVM involving the salivary glands is usually embolization and/or surgical resection. Embolization can be via arteriogram or direct puncture technique. Embolization is usually a temporary treatment and

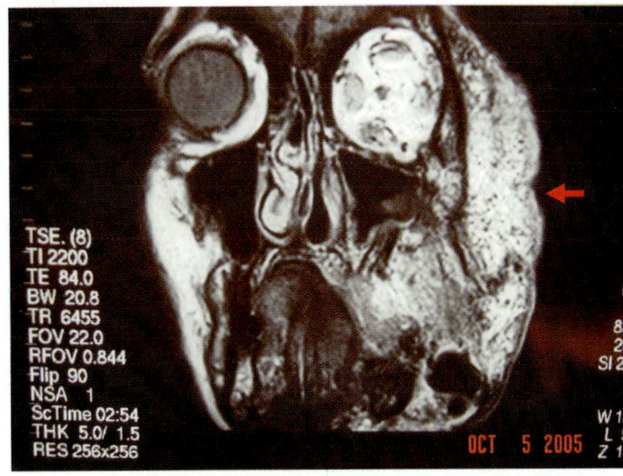

Fig. 19.12: A typical MRI of an arteriovenous malformation of the left face

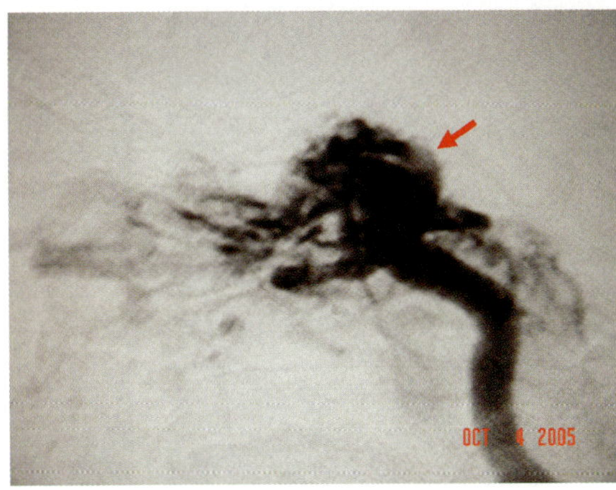

Fig. 19.13: An angiogram demonstrating the nidus (*arrow*) of an arteriovenous malformation

if major feeder vessels are embolized, new or collateral flow develops quickly and can make it more difficult to treat. Using alcohol injections may be potentially curable but requires multiple injections and carries possible devastating complications, such as death in a small percent of cases (<1%).

Surgery can be performed but the entire AVM must be removed. There are many feeder arteries and draining veins which may not be part of the nidus and do not necessarily have to be resected. When the parotid gland is involved or the face where peripheral branches of the facial nerve are involved, the nerve must be identified and dissected out early and preserved. This is what makes surgical resection so difficult. If the muscles of facial expression are involved they usually must also be removed, rendering the facial nerve non-functional (Fig. 19.14).

When the submandibular or sublingual glands are involved, they can be removed but the adjacent major nerves must be identified and preserved if possible. Minor salivary glands can be involved with mucosa and can usually be resected with the involved mucosa. Laser treatment of the skin or mucosa is rarely effective for AVM involving those areas.

Radical ablative procedures are commonly necessary with large AVM of the face. The facial nerve or the recipient facial muscles may be removed necessitating major reconstructive procedures, such as nerve grafts or microvascular free flaps [26] (Figs. 19.14, 19.15). Wound breakdown is common after resection of large AVM and occurs in the first few days postoperative resulting in further surgery. This occurs in spite of the remaining well-vascularized tissue.

Summary

Hemangiomas and vascular malformations frequently involve the major and minor salivary glands. Hemangiomas can be treated with several modalities. During involution, surgery may be indicated and is relatively safe. Vascular malformations will continue to grow by expansion and

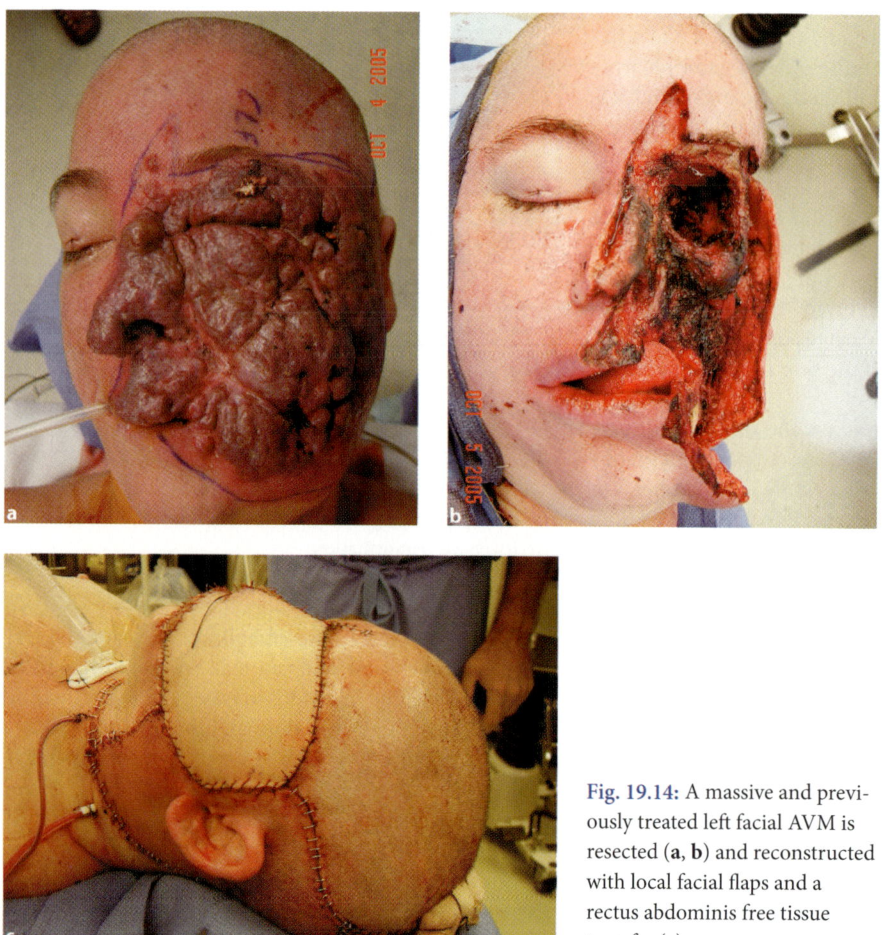

Fig. 19.14: A massive and previously treated left facial AVM is resected (**a**, **b**) and reconstructed with local facial flaps and a rectus abdominis free tissue transfer (**c**)

recruitment of adjacent tissues and usually require intervention. Many venous and lymphatic malformations are not curable and the goal should be to control symptoms with sclerotherapy, lasers and/or surgery.

Arteriovenous malformations are very destructive and can be life threatening. They must be treated as early as possible and complete removal or control should be the goal. Sclerotherapy and embolization may be useful but are rarely curative. Complete surgical resection is necessary and may require extensive ablation and reconstruction.

Salivary glands involved by these vascular lesions is uncommon but presents a major dilemma. Understanding the classification and natural history is crucial to their management.

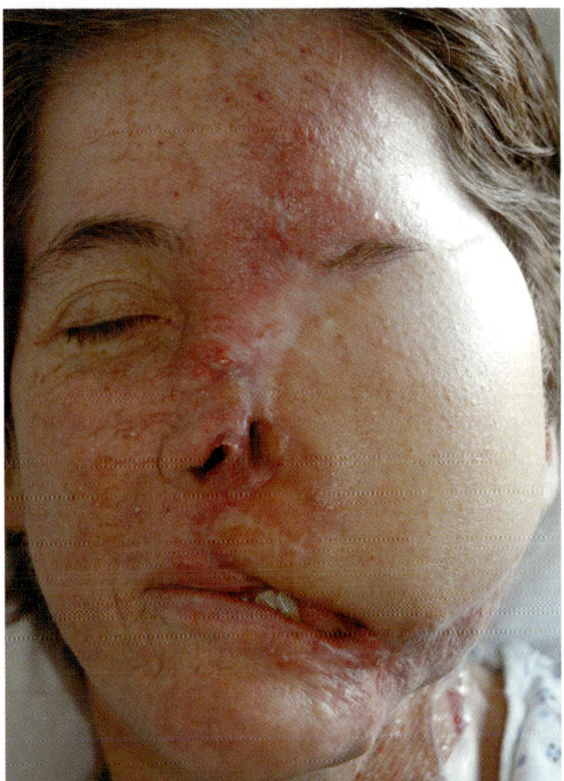

Fig. 19.15: Six months postresection of massive left facial AVM

Take Home Messages

- Congenital vascular lesions are classified as either hemangiomas or vascular malformations.
- Proper diagnosis of vascular lesions is crucial to prescribe the most appropriate treatment, whether medical or surgical.
- Vascular malformations do not regress and will require surgical resection to treat functional and cosmetic impairments.
- Venous and lymphatic malformations can be controlled with sclerotherapy, laser phototherapy, and/or surgery; the goal may be control of symptoms produced by the lesions when they are extensive.
- Arteriovenous malformations are progressive, life-threatening, and need aggressive treatment; treatment should include complete surgical resection but may also include sclerotherapy and embolization.

References

1. Mulliken JB, Glowacki J (1982) Hemangiomas and vascular malformations in infants and children. A classification based on endothelial characteristics. Plast Reconstr Surg 69:412
2. North PE, Waner M, Mizeracki A, Mrak RE, Nicholas R, Kincannon J, Suen JY, Mihm MC Jr (2001) A unique microvascular phenotype shared by juvenile hemangiomas and human placenta. Arch Dermatol 137:559–570
3. Waner M, Suen JY (eds) (1999) Hemangiomas and vascular malfomations of the head and neck. New York: Wiley-Liss
4. Andronikou S, McHugh K, Jadwat S, Linward J (2003) MRI features of bilateral parotid haemangiomas of infancy. Eur Radiol 13:711–716
5. Bennett M, Fleischer A, Chamlin S, Frieden I (2001) Oral Corticosteroid Use is Effective for Cutneous Hemangiomas. Arch Dermatol 137:1208–1213

6. Blei F, Isakoff M, Deb G (1997) The Response of Parotid Hemangiomas to the Use of Systemic Interferon Alfa-2a or Corticosteroids. Arch Otolaryngol 123:841–844
7. Hasan Q, Tan S, Gush J, Peters S, Davis P (2000) Steroid Therapy of a Proliferating Hemangioma: Histochemical and Molecular Changes. Pediatrics 105:117–120
8. Buckmiller L (2004) Update on hemangiomas and vascular malformations. Curr Opin Otolaryngol 12:476–487
9. Chen M, Yeong E, Horng S (2000) Intralesional Corticosteroid Therapy in Proliferating Head and Neck Hemangiomas: A Review of 155 cases. J Pediatr Surg 35:420–423
10. Greene A, Rogers G, Mulliken J (2004) Management of Parotid Hemangiomas in 100 Children. Plast Reconstr Surg 113:53–60
11. Greene A, Rogers G, Mulliken J (2005) Management of Parotid Hemangioma. Plast Reconstr Surg 116:676–677
12. North PE, Waner M, James CA, Mizeracki A, Frieden IJ, Mihm MC (2001) Congenital Nonprogressive Hemangioma: a distinct clinicopathologic entity unlike infantile hemangioma. Arch Dermatol 137:1607–1620
13. Reinisch J, Kim R, Harshbarger R, Meara J (2004) Surgical Management of Parotid Hemangioma. Plast Reconstr Surg 113:1940–1948
14. Selim MM, Kelly KM, Nelson JS, Wendelschafer-Crabb G, Kennedy WR, Zelickson BD (2004) Confocal microscopy study of nerves and blood vessels in untreated and treated port wine stains: preliminary observations. Dermatol Surg 30:892–897
15. Edstrom DW, Hedblad MA, Ros AM (2002) Flashlamp pulsed dye laser and argon-pumped dye laser in the treatment of port-wine stains: a clinical and histological comparison. Br J Dermatol 146:285–289
16. Ho WS, Ying SY, Chan PC, Chan HH (2004) Treatment of port wine stains with intense pulsed light: a prospective study. Dermatol Surg 30:887–890; Discussion 890–891
17. Troilius A, Svendsen G, Ljunggren B (2000) Ultrasound investigation of port wine stains. Acta Derm Venereol 80:196–199
18. Lorenz S, Scherer K, Wimmershoff MB, Landthaler M, Hohenleutner U (2003) Variable pulse frequency-doubled Nd:YAG laser versus flashlamp-pumped pulsed dye laser in the treatment of port wine stains. Acta Derm Venereol 83:210–213
19. Orten S, Waner M, Flock S, Roberson P, Kincannon J (1996) Port-wine stains: An assessment of 5 years of treatment. Arch Otolaryngol Head Neck Surg 122:1174
20. Smoller BR, Rosen S (1996) Port-wine stains: a disease of altered neural modulation of blood vessels. Arch Dermatol 122:177
21. Suen JY, Waner M (1989) Treatment of oral cavity vascular malformations using the neodymium:YAG laser. Arch Otolaryngol Head Neck Surg 115:1329–1333
22. Werner JA, Lippert BM, Gottschlich S, Folz BJ, Fleiner B, Hoeft S, Rudert H (1998) Ultrasound-guided interstitial Nd: YAG laser treatment of voluminous hemangiomas and vascular malformations in 92 patients. Laryngoscope 108:463–470
23. De Lorimier A (1995) Sclerotherapy of venous malformations. J Pediatr Surg 30:188–194
24. Harsha WJ, Perkins JA, Lewis CW, Mianning SC (2005) Pediatric admissions and procedures for lymphatic malformations in the United States: 1997 and 2000. Lymphat Res Biol 3:58–65
25. Lee BB (2005) New approaches to the treatment of congenital vascular malformations (CVMs): a single centre experience. Eur J Vasc Endovasc Surg 30:184–197
26. Cho SK, Do YS, Shin SW, Kim DI, Kim YW, Park KB, Kim EJ, Ahn HJ, Choo SW, Choo IW (2006) Arteriovenous malformations of the body and extremities: analysis of therapeutic outcomes and approaches according to a modified angiographic classification. J Endovasc Ther 13:527–538

Chapter 20

Tumors of Minor Salivary Gland Origin

20

Patrick J. Bradley

Contents

Core Features

- Anatomy
- Presentation
- Diagnostic strategy
- Staging
- Histology – general/specific:
  - Polymorphous low-grade adenocarcinoma
  - Adenoid cystic carcinoma
  - Mucoepidermoid carcinoma
- Prognostic factors
- Treatment approaches
- Results of treatment
- Tumors by specific site:
  - Oral cavity
  - Palate
  - Oropharynx
  - Nose/paranasal sinuses
  - Nasopharynx
  - Larynx

Complications to Avoid

- Failure to consider a diagnosis of tumor of salivary gland origin in every painless, non-ulcerative submucosal swelling in the clinical head and neck area may lead to misdiagnosis and mismanagement of the patient.
- Perform an incisional biopsy/punch biopsy prior to imaging or commencing treatment.
- Thorough imaging studies provide valuable information in planning management of these tumors whether benign or malignant.
- Failure to achieve clear surgical margins predisposes to local recurrence.
- Consider postoperative radiotherapy within 6 weeks, after definitive surgery, to minimize the risk of persistence/recurrence when a malignant disease demonstrates histopathological features associated with a poor prognosis.

Introduction

An estimation of the incidence of salivary gland neoplasms in the population, is that for every 100 tumors of the parotid gland, there are likely to be 10 of the submandibular gland, one of the sublingual gland, and 10 of the minor salivary glands. The probability of a malignant diagnosis is less than 25% in patients with a tumor of the parotid gland, about 50% in those with a tumor of the submandibular gland, more than 80% in those patients with a tumor of minor salivary gland origin, and virtually 100% in those few with a tumor of the sublingual gland [59]. The current incidence of a benign tumor of salivary gland origin is difficult to be certain about, as this disease is not registered, but is estimated to be 60–80/million population per year. For malignant salivary tumors in the USA, it is 10/1 million population per year and in the UK is 0.6/1 million population per year [8].

Tumors of the minor salivary glands account for 10–15% of all salivary gland neoplasms [68]. Because of the limited volume clinician experience regarding the natural history, prognostic factors, and recommending the best treatment modality is scarce, making prospective evaluation of these disease aspects almost impossible [26, 33, 53, 62]. Data still arise from case reports and retrospective analysis, which report treatment results and prognostic factors for overall survival, disease-specific survival (DSS), or tumor recurrence [31, 38, 47, 60, 61]. It has been proposed by the author that the apparent rarity of salivary gland tumors in these sites reflects either errors of histological diagnosis, or classification of these tumors by site (oral cavity or larynx) rather than by salivary gland tumors [8]. Another factor which has been reported is the difficulty associated with salivary gland neoplasms and more so with minor salivary gland malignancy with a re-classification rate of up to 29%, which has resulted from the introduction of a new histological classification system [67, 68].

Anatomy

Minor salivary glands, estimated to number 450–1,000, are widely distributed in the head and neck area [19]. The majority (70–90%) are located in the oral cavity and oropharynx, including the lateral margins of the tongue, the lips and the buccal mucosa, palate, glossopharyngeal area, and the retromolar trigone. The remainder are located in the nose, paranasal sinuses, pharynx, and the larynx. The minor salivary glands have been classified according to their anatomical location. These salivary glands, as compared with the major salivary glands, are more numerous and have a reduced volume and size of tissue, an abbreviated ductal system, and a paucity of capsular tissue. Overall, they contribute about 8–10% of the volume of unstimulated and stimulated whole saliva.

Presentation

The signs and symptoms of tumors associated with minor salivary glands vary relative to their diverse anatomical sites. The majority of patients are aged 60 years or older. Many of the larger series had reported a gender distribution of 66% women, and may be explained by referral bias [68]. The most frequent site of origin is the oral cavity and oropharynx, and within the oral cavity most tumors develop in the region of the hard palate because this is the area with the highest density of glands. The majority of patients present with a painless non-ulcerative, submucosal swelling. The mucosal layer is adherent to the mass and a small ulcer may be present. Other sites within the head and neck have a tendency to present clinically with obstructive symptoms of the nose, ear by Eustachian tube obstruction, and larynx and pharynx by hoarseness, altered voice, or dyspnea. It has been reported that up to 26% of patients present with local pain [12, 68]. Pain or numbness warrants investigation by magnetic resonance imaging (MRI) to rule out nerve invasion [69]. More than 15% of patients at presentation will have cervical lymph node metastases [38, 47].

Diagnostic Strategy

Physical examination and awareness that a clinically "benign" submucosal swelling any place in the head and neck may be a tumor of salivary gland origin and that statistically the pathology of that tumor is more likely to be malignant rather than benign, is the most important clinical information that will improve accurate diagnosis, and allow for a rational plan of management. Currently, imaging using computed tomography (CT) and/or MRI may help with the delineation of the tumor, the accurate staging of the disease, and for the correct planning of a surgical approach. The use of fine-needle aspiration cytology (FNAC) in tumors of minor salivary gland origin may be helpful in correctly classifying the tumor as benign or malignant, however the use of incisional biopsy or punch biopsy may reveal a better and more representative specimen, thus revealing the correct histological type. Complete excision should be avoided as it is likely that the margins will be close or positive, and that orientation of these incomplete margins will not be possible at the time of pathological analysis, and will result in anger by the patient and increased frustration for the clinicians in the subsequent planning of surgical salvage.

Staging

There is no TNM staging system for cancer of the minor salivary gland origin. It is agreed, however, that these tumors, when diagnosed as malignant should be staged as per the TNM system for each site as in squamous cell carcinoma of the head and neck [61, 68].

Histology

Tumors of salivary gland origin of all types have been reported in the majority of minor salivary gland sites. These include both the common benign and the malignant types. The proportions of benign to malignant vary greatly and range from 20–50% benign to 50–80% malignant. The series with the higher percentage of malignant disease may be a result from "harvesting effect," with the majority of clinicians treating benign diseases and referring malignant cases to the larger academic institutes [28, 59]. Tumors of minor salivary gland origin are more common in women with a ratio ranging from 1.2:1 to 1.9:1. Some series suggest that there is a higher incidence of tumors of minor salivary gland origin in blacks than whites in the South African population [27], as well as in Ugandans [13].

Benign tumors of minor salivary gland origin are most frequently pleomorphic adenoma and have been located in areas as diverse as tongue [66], posterior tongue [22], nasal cavity and septum [65] (Fig. 20.1a, b), larynx [55], and trachea [5]. The most common site for pleomorphic adenoma is the hard palate, followed by the upper lip. Some of these pleomorphic adenomas can become massive with malignant degeneration before presentation [7] and young children may also present with pleomorphic adenoma [46], the majority of which are located in the region of the hard palate. Canalicular adenoma has a predilection for the upper lip [23]. Other benign neoplasms of salivary gland origin that have been reported in the oral cavity include basal cell adenoma [38].

The most frequently encountered malignant tumors of minor salivary gland origin are adenoid cystic carcinoma (32–69%) and mucoepidermoid carcinoma (15–35%), with acinic cell carcinoma, polymorphous adenocarcinoma, myoepithelial carcinoma, and carcinoma ex-pleomorphic adenoma seen less frequently [31]. There remains an area of controversy concerning the grading of salivary gland malignancy, more so with minor salivary glands because of inter-observer error, and a policy of treating all grades of minor salivary gland malignant disease similarly with postoperative radiotherapy [61, 68], except for low-grade polymorphous adenocarcinoma.

Specific Histopathology

Polymorphous low-grade adenocarcinoma (PLGA) (Fig. 20.2) needs to be differentiated from other types of adenocarcinoma because of differing biological behaviors. PLGA generally has a better prognosis than other types of adenocarcinoma [6, 11, 14]. Histologically, the cells are described as cuboid or columnar with oval or elongated basophilic nuclei, and the cytoplasm is scanty. The cytoplasm may appear eosinophilic or basophilic, and mitotic figures are infrequent. Because of its variable microscopic appearance, PLGA may be mistaken for monomorphic or pleomorphic adenoma, or occasionally

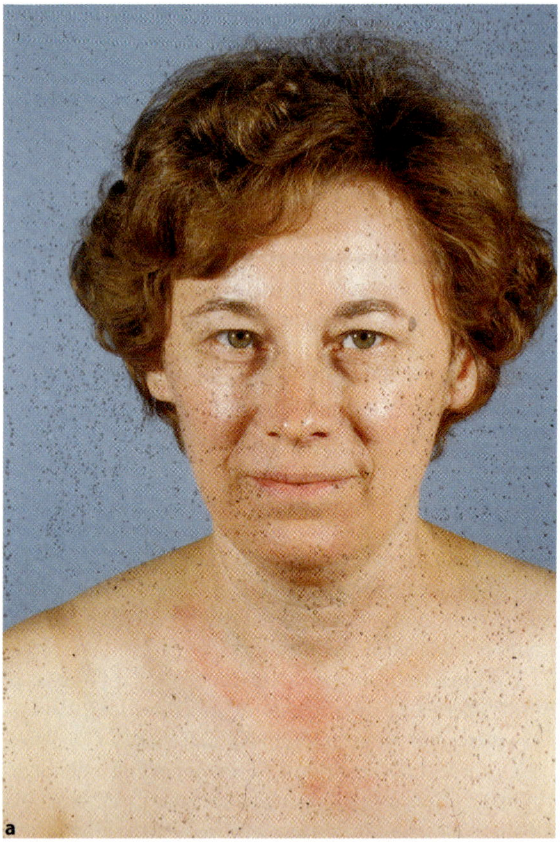
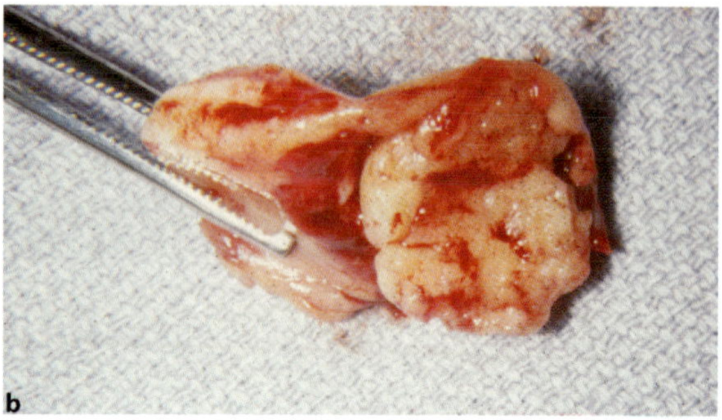

Fig. 20.1: **a** Patient with left lateral rhinotomy for pleomorphic adenoma of the septum. **b** Pleomorphic adenoma of septum completely excised

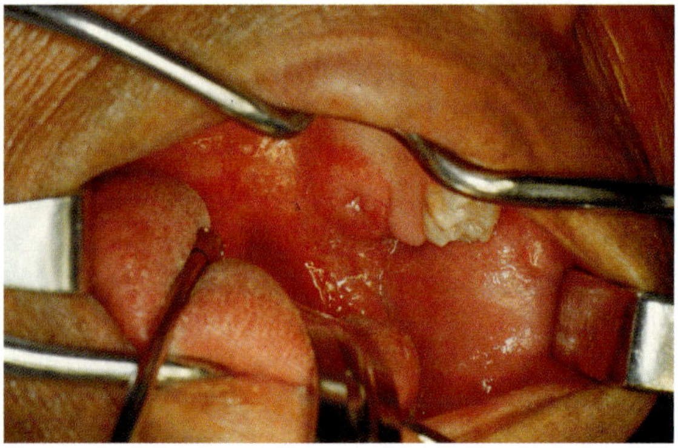

Fig. 20.2: Polymorphous low-grade adenocarcinoma of the hard palate

adenoid cystic carcinoma due to the presence of perineural invasion. There has been reported a case of PLGA presenting as a cervical lymph node metastasis from a primary located in the soft palate [49]. In another review, the authors emphasize the occasional malignant nature of pleomorphic adenoma—whether these carcinomas should now be correctly diagnosis as PLGA has not been settled [66].

Adenoid cystic carcinoma (ACC) is the most common malignancy of minor salivary gland origin (60%). ACC of the minor salivary glands occurs most frequently in the oral cavity (palate) followed by the paranasal sinuses (14–17%). The tumor is often very advanced at the time of diagnosis, and complete excision is limited by the large size (with perineural extension involving the skull base) and the proximity of the tumor to important neural and vascular structures. The clinical behavior of ACC is a paradox. First, the tumor grows slowly, but its clinical course is relentless and progressive. Second, operative interventions are usually feasible, but multiple local recurrences are the rule. Third, metastatic spread to regional lymph nodes is uncommon, but distant spread to the lungs and bones is frequent. And fourth, 5-year survival rates are optimistically high, but 10- and 20-year survival rates are dismally low [71].

A unique feature of ACC is the propensity for perineural invasion, even in early-stage tumors (Fig. 20.3). These tumors can be graded according to Szanto et al. [64] as cribriform or tubular (grade I), less than 30% solid (grade II), or greater than 30% solid (grade III). In patients treated similarly by whatever modalities, the cribriform and tubular variants of ACC demonstrated no difference in the rate of distant metastases and overall survival. The cribriform variant demonstrated a significantly worse prognosis in terms of local recurrence rates. The patients who had a solid histological pattern of ACC appear to have an overall worse prognosis in terms of distant metastases and long-term survival [42]. ACC of the minor salivary glands should be treated by radical local excision and postoperative radiotherapy [9]. Patients who receive postoperative radiation therapy have an improved outcome with radical surgery compared with biopsy alone [51]. The role of neutron therapy in the management of advanced or recurrent ACC shows promising results but is not commonly available [16, 17, 25, 52]. Chemotherapy currently is seeking a role in the management of advanced and metastatic cancer of salivary gland origin. There is a need for biomarkers that will allow for better identification of the risk of distant dissemination to make this approach cost effective [59].

Mucoepidermoid carcinoma (MEC) is the most frequent malignant tumor arising from intraoral minor sali-

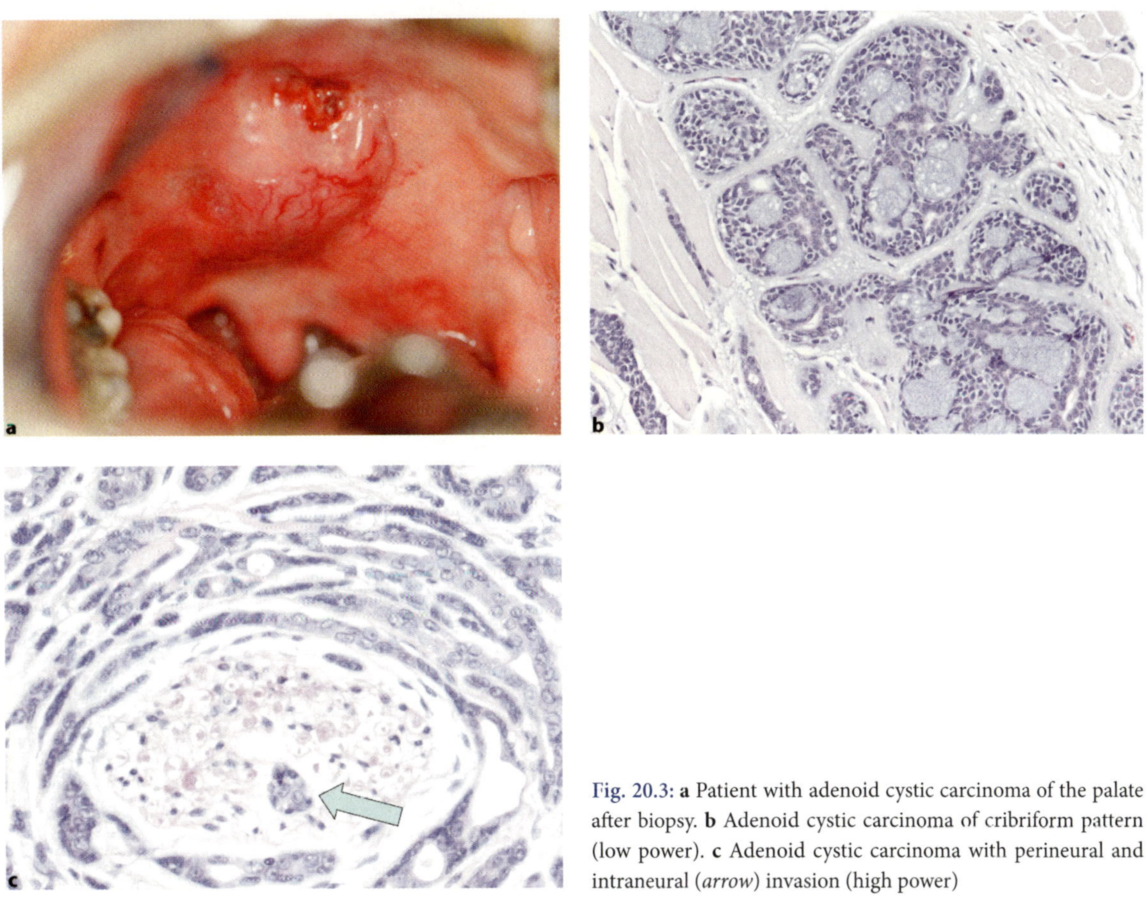

Fig. 20.3: **a** Patient with adenoid cystic carcinoma of the palate after biopsy. **b** Adenoid cystic carcinoma of cribriform pattern (low power). **c** Adenoid cystic carcinoma with perineural and intraneural (*arrow*) invasion (high power)

vary glands, representing about 36–59% of all malignant intraoral salivary gland tumors [40] (Fig. 20.4). The prognosis of MEC is mainly influenced by the clinical stage and histological grade [3]. Patients who have tumors of low-grade malignancy and with early clinical stage disease at presentation have a better prognosis than patients with high-grade tumors or with advanced clinical stage. Investigation of a series of 27 patients collected over a period of 40 years were analyzed for clinicopathological and immunohistological features [40], and the results showed a reduced survival was associated with: male gender, regional metastases, high-grade of malignancy, strong expression of proliferating cell nuclear factor (PCNA), and weak expression of c-erbB-2 gene (a gene with an important role in the development, differentiation, and mitogenic signaling in normal cells).

Prognostic Factors

Tumor stage, histology, and grade of malignancy are the most important predictors for survival [60]. These are independent variables and all are able to influence treatment outcome, although stage seems to be more important than grading [2, 47]. In adenoid cystic carcinoma the prognostic factors associated with poor prognosis are perineural invasion, positive margins and solid histological features [20, 30].

Treatment

The standard treatment of resectable tumors of minor salivary gland origin—benign and malignant—is surgi-

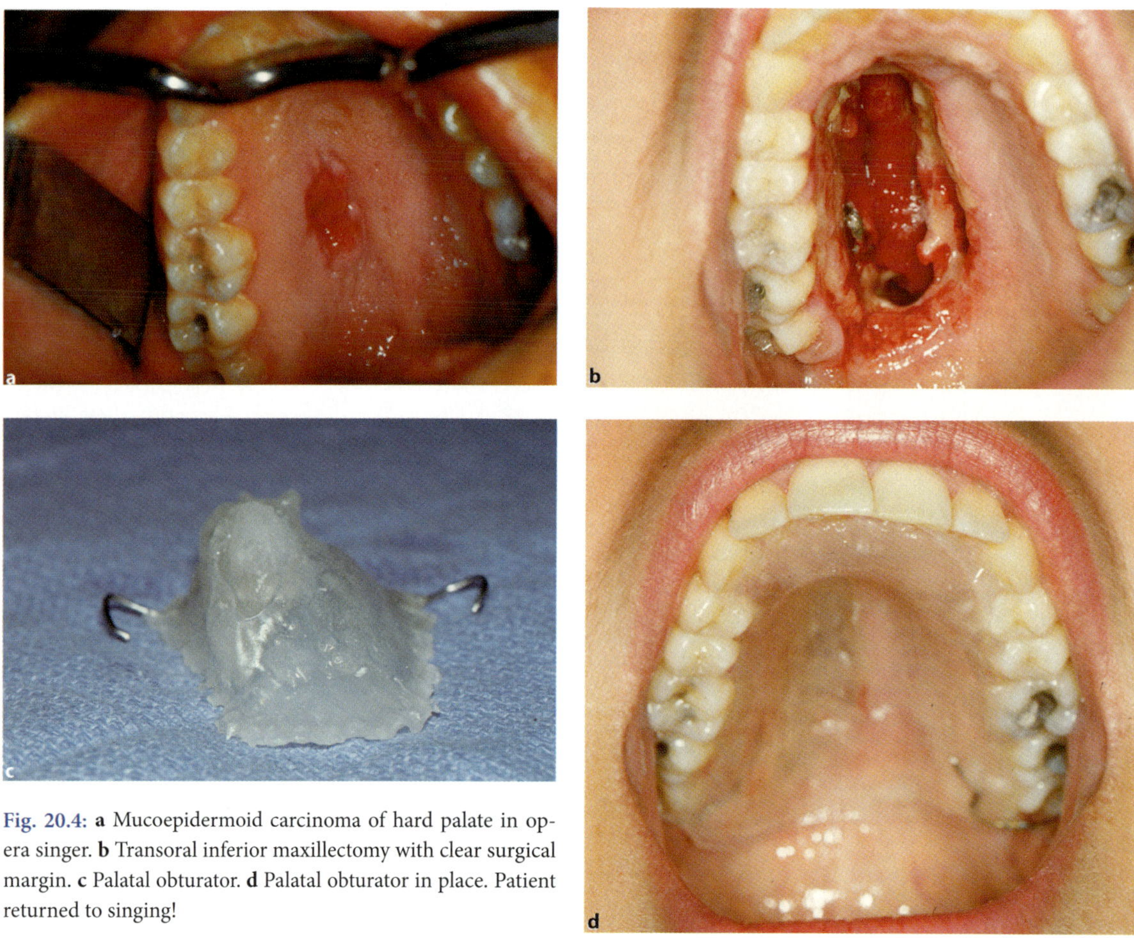

Fig. 20.4: **a** Mucoepidermoid carcinoma of hard palate in opera singer. **b** Transoral inferior maxillectomy with clear surgical margin. **c** Palatal obturator. **d** Palatal obturator in place. Patient returned to singing!

cal excision. Currently, the indications for treatment of the neck is to do a neck dissection only when there are demonstrable metastases present (clinical or imaging), or when the neck is being surgically entered as an approach to the primary tumor. Postoperative radiotherapy is recommended in selected patients, most commonly those patients with adenoid cystic carcinoma [29, 35]. Primary radiotherapy is indicated for patients who refuse surgery or who have an inoperable/unresectable tumor [37]. The role of neutron radiotherapy is indicated, when available, for unresectable or inoperable locoregional cancer [18].

The role of chemotherapy remains controversial and should be selected for individual patients, such as in a palliative situation for relief of symptoms when the cancer is unresectable or recurrent after treatment, for patients not amenable to radiotherapy, and for patients with distant metastatic cancer.

Results of Treatment

In a review of 55 patients treated in Amsterdam [68] over a 22-year period to 1995 and followed up till 1998, the majority (76%) had malignant tumors located in the oral cavity including hard palate (7%), base of the tongue (11%), as well as soft palate (7%), nasopharynx (4%), and maxillary sinus (2%). The most common cancer encountered was adenoid cystic carcinoma (22/55), followed by mucoepidermoid, adenocarcinoma and others in 9/55, respectively, acinic cell 3/55, and malignant mixed and undifferentiated one each. The overall 5- and 10-year survival rates were 66% [standard error (SE): 7%] and 57% (SE: 7%), respectively. The 5- and 10-year disease-specific survival rates were 76% (SE: 6%) and 74% (SE: 6%), respectively. All patients had their treatment individualized: 19 underwent surgical excision alone, 20 patients received a combination of surgery and radiotherapy without chemotherapy, 1 patient received intra-arterial chemotherapy (5FU) prior to surgery, not followed by radiotherapy. In 2 patients, the combination surgery-radiotherapy was preceded by intra-arterial chemotherapy (5FU) in the context of a clinical trial. One patient was judged inoperable by another institution and received radiotherapy there, but subsequently was operated upon and irradiated with neutrons. Palliative treatment for inoperable patients ($n = 8$) consisted of isolated radiotherapy ($n = 2$), isolated chemotherapy ($n = 1$), and a combination of chemoradiotherapy ($n = 5$). Four patients were not treated. The reasons were advanced age and extended disease ($n = 3$) and a coexistent extended esophageal carcinoma ($n = 1$).

The percentage of patients remaining free of tumor recurrence for 5 years from the day of therapy was 63% (SE: 7%), and the percentage of patients remaining free of tumor recurrence for 10 years was 60% (SE: 7%). There was total tumor control after the first treatment in 34 patients (62%). Eventually locoregional control was achieved in 42 of 55 patients (76%). Distant metastases occurred in 8 initially M0 patients (14.5%) treated originally with curative intent after a median period of 19 months. Distant metastases were first observed in the lungs ($n = 4$), in the skeleton ($n = 3$), and in multiple sites ($n = 1$). Univariate analysis was associated with 5-year survival stage I – 84%, stage II – 73%, stage III – 60%, and stage IV – 29% patients (trend log rank test: $P = 0.0006$). In summary, there is a significant difference in survival rates according to: advanced stage disease, N stage at presentation, bone metastasis, tumor histology, sex, and whether clear surgical margins have been achieved at surgery.

Tumors by Specific Site

Tumors Located in the Oral Cavity

The majority of patients seen have an age range of 45–60 years for benign salivary tumors and a median age of 40–55 years for malignant salivary tumors [39, 69]. About 10% present in children in their early teens [28].

The most common complaint was a painless swelling in the mouth (60%), with symptoms having been present for more than 12 months. The most common sites for tumors of minor salivary gland origin are the palate, buccal mucosa, and upper lip, which accounts for more than 75% of cases. The palate is the most common site for all tumors of minor salivary gland origin (55%) and more than (60%) of these are malignant [28]. The most common sites for malignant tumors of minor salivary gland origin are the palate, buccal mucosa, maxilla, and retromolar trigone.

The majority (80%) of the cancers histopathologically are mucoepidermoid carcinoma or adenoid cystic carcinoma, with other lesions less common: adenocarcinoma, polymorphous low-grade adenocarcinoma, salivary duct carcinoma, and acinic cell carcinoma. Patients with mucoepidermoid carcinoma generally present at an early stage compared to patients with adenoid cystic carcinoma, which is in an advanced stage when diagnosed.

Less than 10% of patients present with palpable cervical lymph adenopathy and these patients should undergo treatment. Controversy persists concerning the role of elective neck dissections, and currently the indication for elective neck dissection in many centers is clinical or radiological presence of significant or positive cervical adenopathy.

The treatment of all benign tumors is wide surgical excision, which may require an obturator or tissue reconstruction depending on the location of the primary tumor. A wide local excision and composite repair with or without neck dissections is required for cancer of minor salivary gland origin.

Tumors Located in the Palate

In one large series of 149 patients seen over a 46-year period at the MD Anderson Cancer Center in Houston, Texas, USA, malignant tumors were found in 116 patients (78%) and benign lesions in 33 patients (22%) [4]. The most common benign tumor was pleomorphic adenoma 30 (20%), while the most frequent malignant tumor was adenoid cystic carcinoma 43 (29%), followed by terminal duct adenocarcinoma 28 (19%), mucoepidermoid 24 (16%), adenocarcinoma 6 (4%), myoepithelioma 6 (4%), and others. Of the malignant tumors, 60 (52%) occurred on the hard palate alone, with the remaining arising from the soft palate or junction between hard and soft palate.

Local invasion as assessed radiologically or at the time of surgery included bone invasion, 36 (31%) malignant and 2 (6%) benign tumors, followed by sinonasal cavity invasion, 36 (31%) by malignant and 4 (11%) by benign disease. Also invaded by the malignant tumors were the pterygoid muscles 5%, nasopharynx 3%, and intracranial extension 3%. Histopathologically there was evidence of perineural invasion in 41 (35%) of the malignant tumors. Of the 116 patients with malignancy, 112 (97%) were staged N0, and 4 (3%) had clinical evidence of cervical lymph node metastasis.

The treatment of the benign tumors was surgical excision, but one patient had positive margins and received adjunctive postoperative radiotherapy; none recurred. Patients with malignant cancer had decreased survival ($P < 0.05$) and on multivariate analysis showed high-grade tumors, tumor size greater than or equal to 3.0 cm, and margin status (both positive margins and positive initial but final negative margins). In this series there was no significant difference between the patients treated with surgery alone and those treated with surgery plus postoperative radiotherapy. Histological types found to be associated with primary tumor recurrence include: adenoid cystic carcinoma (30%), mucoepidermoid carcinoma (8%), and terminal duct carcinoma (4%). The 2-, 5-, and 10-year disease-specific survival rates for patients with malignant cancer were 96%, 87%, and 80%, respectively. Overall survival rates at 2, 5, and 10 years were 93%, 79%, and 67%, respectively. This overall good survival reflects the tendency that cancers with less aggressive nature occur in the palate, or it may indicate an earlier-stage presentation and easier treatment course.

One of the findings that should be highlighted by this series is the importance of complete excision of the cancer with an adequate margin of normal tissue on the initial attempt, because subsequent attempts at complete excision are far more difficult to achieve technically (Fig. 20.5). The other lesson is that patients who have a cancer with high-grade histology and perineural invasion had a statistically significant improvement in locoregional control with postoperative radiotherapy, although no statistically significant improvement in survival was seen, though admittedly the power of analysis was small.

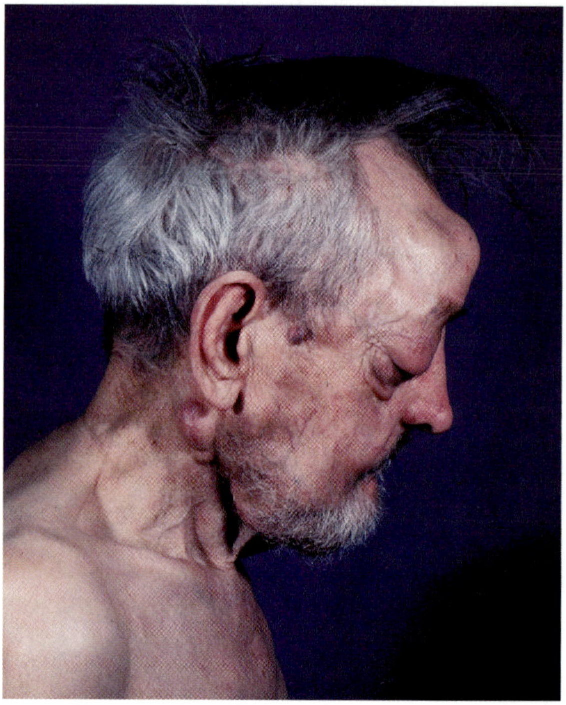

Fig. 20.5: Patient with inadequately excised malignant mixed tumor of hard palate with metastases to neck and frontal bone

Tumors Located in the Oropharynx

There are few series reporting on tumors of salivary gland origin of the oropharynx, especially the base of tongue [15, 32, 42] (Fig. 20.6). The majority are malignant with symptoms of tongue swelling, throat pain, and the presence of a mass in the neck being the most common presentation. The mean age is mid 50 years, with average duration of symptoms more than 9 months before diagnosis. The most frequent malignant tumor is adenoid cys-

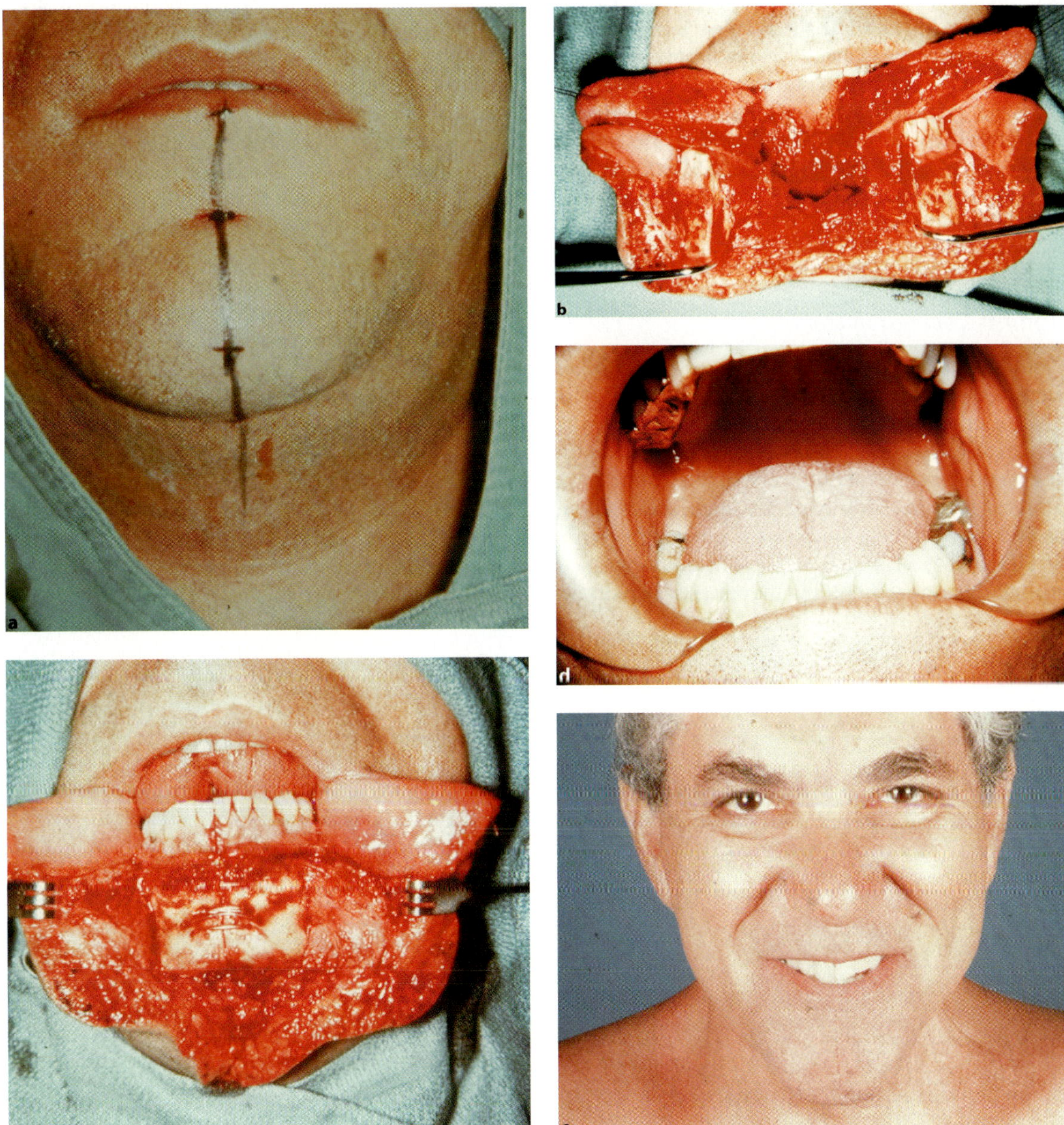

Fig. 20.6: **a** Patient with adenocarcinoma of the base of the tongue. **b** Labiomandibuloglossotomy and excision of the base of the tongue. **c** Tongue and mandible have been reapproximated. **d** Normal appearance of tongue postoperatively. **e** Patient completely healed with good cosmetic and functional result

tic carcinoma and mucoepidermoid carcinoma, followed by adenocarcinoma.

Treatment as for all salivary gland tumors is surgery, but suitability for such treatment is dependent upon the size of the tumor, site, presence of cervical lymph node metastases, patients' comorbidities, and patient preference. Should the patients be treated surgically then it is recommended that all but the smallest totally excised cancer be treated by adjunctive radiotherapy. In another series [45] of 14 patients, all of whom had adenoid cystic carcinoma, the authors conclude that this tumor is difficult to eradicate by surgical excision alone. The authors further emphasized the need for wide local excision with adequate surgical margins since local recurrence correlated with positive margins.

Tumors Located in the Nose and Paranasal Sinuses

Adenoid cystic carcinoma is the most frequent cancer of minor salivary gland origin found in the nasal cavity and paranasal sinuses. These tumors usually present with the common symptoms of nasal obstruction, rhinorrhea, pain, and epistaxis. Identifying the single site of origin can be difficult, as these tumors are frequently very large, and the radiological findings are those of any malignancy, especially bone destruction and the presence of a soft tissue mass [24, 34, 44, 54]. It has been considered that adenoid cystic carcinoma of the nasal cavity and paranasal sinuses has a worse prognosis than in any other area of the head and neck [24, 51] (Fig. 20.7). There is a propensity for frequent local recurrences and early perineural spread and hematogenous spread, with as many as 50% presenting with distant metastases. The incidence of recurrence is lower in those patients receiving more radical primary surgery, with or without postoperative radiotherapy [51, 58], but the choice between conservation and radical management may not alter prognosis. Indeed some authors suggested that "it is doubtful is any patients are cured of this disease" [24]. However, recent advancements in surgery [48, 50, 63] and radiotherapy [36, 57] have allowed many patients who would have previously been deemed inoperable to undergo local radical surgery with postoperative radiotherapy, or gamma knife for persistence or recurrence, with an anticipated better quality of life than achieved previously (Fig. 20.8).

Tumors Located in the Nasopharynx

In a review article of cancer of salivary gland origin of the nasopharynx [56], the authors comment that less than 100 cases have been reported. The most common histological types were adenoid cystic carcinoma (94%) and mucoepidermoid carcinoma (6%). Cancer of the na-

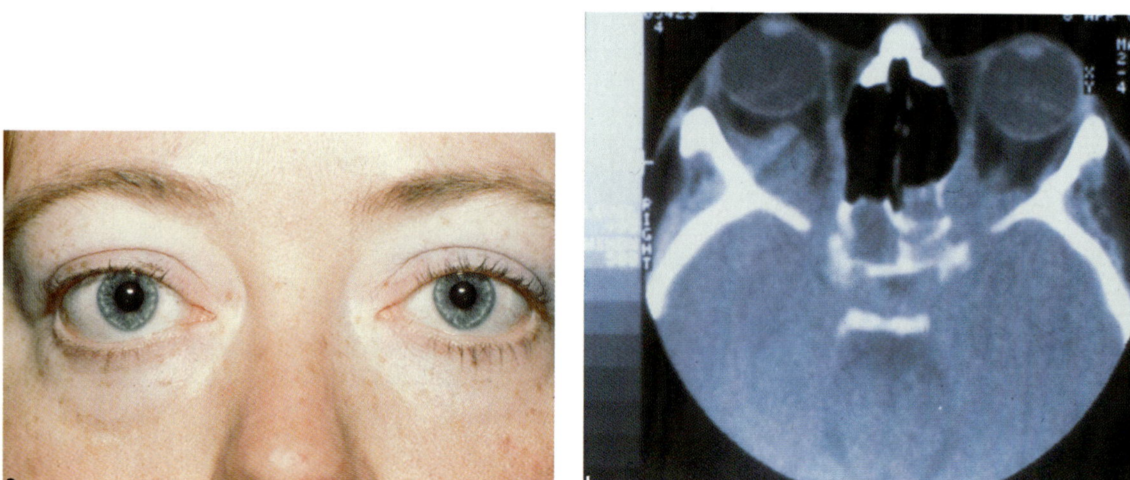

Fig. 20.7: **a** Young woman with bilateral proptosis. **b** CT scan of same patient demonstrating primary tumor in sphenoid sinus with bilateral invasion of orbits. Biopsy revealed adenoid cystic carcinoma. Patient was treated with radiation therapy which resulted in a long remission

20

sopharynx typically presents at an advanced stage, often with invasion of the skull base, intracranial extension, and involvement of cranial nerves. It is only recently with advances in surgical techniques that it is possible to treat cancer in this anatomical site, in a manner similar to cancer of salivary gland origin in other sites, by primary surgery with or without radiotherapy.

The patients seen tend to be younger, compared to patients with other types of cancers of the head and neck, with a median age of 46 years. As this is a "silent area" for tumors, there is a significant delay, with a mean lag time of 20 months from the onset of symptoms to diagnosis. The majority of patients present with sinonasal symptoms: nasal obstruction, headaches/facial pain, recurrent "sinusitis," epistaxis and posterior rhinorrhea, cranial nerve neuropathy including isolated involvement of branches of the trigeminal nerve, oculomotor nerve, abducens nerve and optic nerve, or otological findings

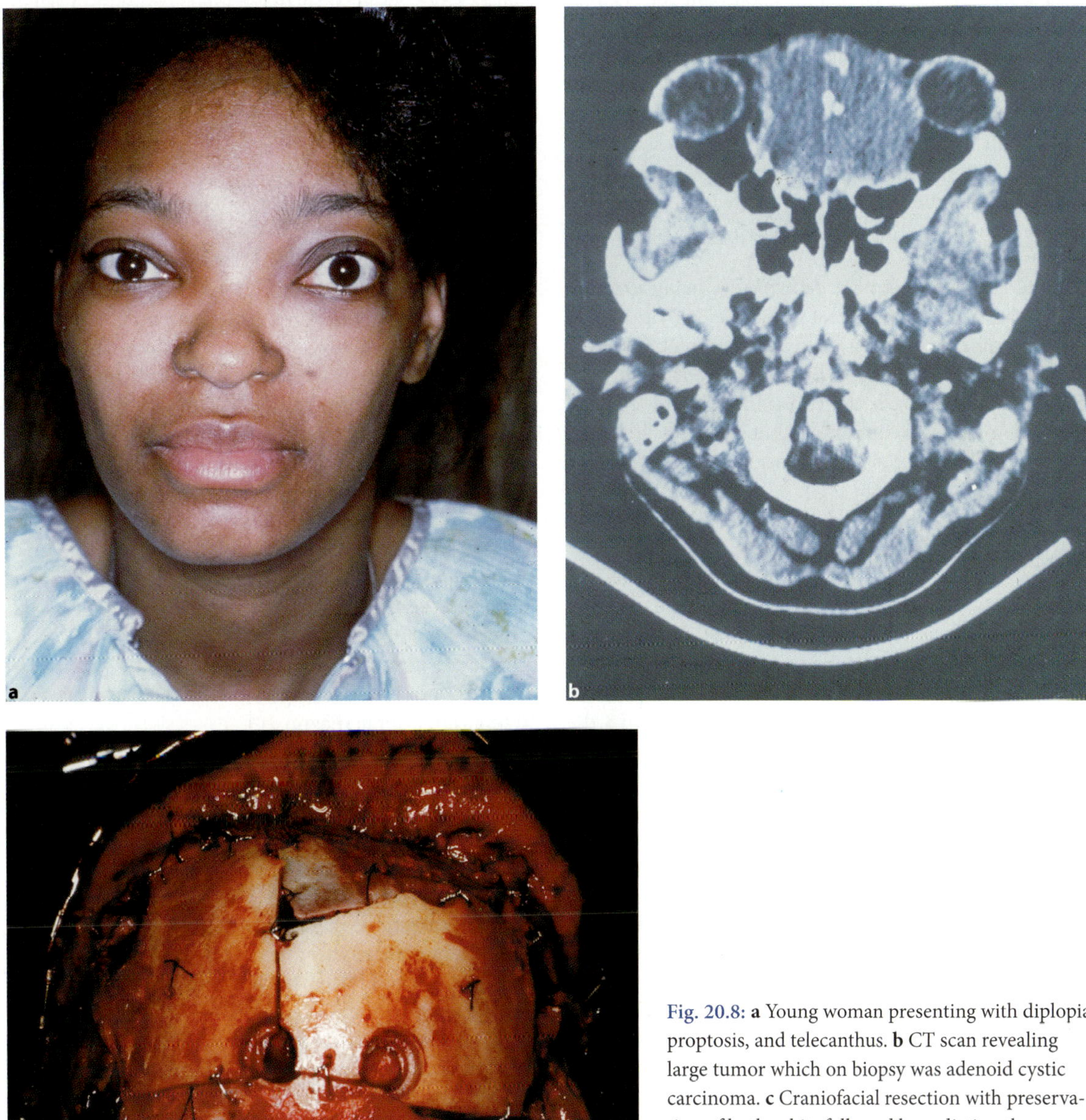

Fig. 20.8: **a** Young woman presenting with diplopia, proptosis, and telecanthus. **b** CT scan revealing large tumor which on biopsy was adenoid cystic carcinoma. **c** Craniofacial resection with preservation of both orbits followed by radiation therapy

including aural fullness, hearing loss, otorrhea, tinnitus, and vertigo.

The surgical approach used in this report was the lateral infratemporal middle fossa approach, but other approaches have been used including subfrontal, lateral rhinotomy, transoral palatal, and transoral maxillary. This type of surgery may involve transposing or resecting the carotid artery, excision and grafting of dura, and dissection of cancer from the cavernous sinus. Repair of the defect can involve repair of the dura using temporalis fascia or pericranial patches, and lateral skull defects were repaired by using a vascularized flap such as a temporalis flap, a free rectus abdominis muscle graft, a free gastro-omental graft, or a latissimus dorsi muscle flap. Adjuvant radiotherapy either neutrons or photons is preferred postoperatively if it has not been used previously. In this series, disease-specific survival was 67% at 5 years and 48% at 10 years for the overall group, with a worse survival in high-grade tumors of 31% at 5 years versus 78% for low-grade tumors [56].

An alternative treatment described is using external beam photon radiation to treat adenoid cystic carcinoma of the nasopharynx [70, 72], and reported 5- and 10-year survival rates of 78% and 49.5%, respectively, with a local control rate of 45.5% at 5 years. The authors reported a low rate of early complications but there was a risk of treatment-related complications in long-term survivors.

Tumors Located in the Larynx

In the larynx, minor salivary gland tumors are rare and are reported to comprise less than 1% of all tumors of the larynx. These tumors arise from submucosal glands, which are located most prevalently in the subglottis, but are also located in the supraglottis mostly found in the aryepiglottic folds, and the distal inferior aspect of the epiglottis [1, 41]. These tumors also have been reported in the floor of the ventricle and the undersurface of the anterior commissure [21].

Both benign and malignant tumors have been reported in the literature. The most common benign tumor is the pleomorphic adenoma; approximately 30 cases have been reported. These tumors are most frequently located in the supraglottis, the base of the epiglottis, and the posterior commissure [55].

The most frequent malignant tumor reported is the adenoid cystic carcinoma and is most frequently located in the subglottis [21]. More than 80 cases of mucoepidermoid carcinoma have been reported in the larynx [10]. The majority of cancers arising from salivary gland origin are advanced when diagnosed (stage III/IV) which reflects the submucosal growth and large size at the time of presentation. Other histological types of tumors may present with minimal symptoms of hoarseness, globus sensation, or dyspnea due to the size of the tumor.

Surgical excision is the preferred treatment. For benign tumors, such as pleomorphic adenoma, the treatment will depend on the size and location of the tumor. Conservation surgery, such as a pharyngotomy, laryngofissure, or transoral laser surgery, has been reported to be successfully used. Recurrence depends upon the adequacy of local excision, and most patients who recur will do so within 18 months. Long-term follow-up is recommended, as risk of recurrence may remain life long for such patients [43].

When the tumor has been proven malignant the indication for partial laryngeal surgery may be indicated on very few and very selected cases, since if the margins are positive then the retention of a functioning organ will not be achieved or worse yet, recurrence may result in the patient's death. The use of adjuvant postoperative radiotherapy should be considered in all patients and certainly must be considered in the presence of unfavorable prognostic factors—cartilage invasion, perineural, perivascular involvement [21].

Patients may also present with cervical lymph node metastases, including adenoid cystic carcinoma, and all patients should be clinically and radiologically staged, and the presence of nodal enlargement should always be treated at the time of surgery. Patients who fail partial surgery should be offered a total laryngectomy when appropriate. Sadly patients may develop distant metastases, most commonly in the lungs, which can occur more than 10 years after initial diagnosis.

Conclusion

Tumors of minor salivary gland origin are uncommon, and medical practitioners over a lifetime are unlikely to gain expertise in the management of this uncommon disease, except perhaps those tumors located in the oral cavity. The more away from the lips one moves in the head and neck region the more likely is that the tumor being treated is malignant. Pleomorphic adenoma remains the most common benign neoplasm and treatment is with local excision with a safe margin. Malignant tumors may present in a benign manner, with symptoms of a mass lesion, obstruction of a functioning organ, or pain. Biopsy is mandatory when a patient presents and is diagnosed with a non-ulcerated swelling, so that the true nature of the neoplasm can be appreciated prior to investigation and recommending management. Surgery is the treatment of choice, followed by radiotherapy when adverse pathology parameters are present. Local symptom relief can be anticipated in the short term, but long-term cure must be guarded. The most common malignant tumor encountered is the adenoid cystic carcinoma, which has a good short-term outcome, with evidence of distant metastases resulting in death should the patient live more than 10–15 years. Other histopathological types of malignant tumors are all potentially curable by surgery with or without postoperative radiotherapy, with anticipated long-term tumor-free survival.

Take Home Messages

- Tumors of minor salivary gland origin are uncommon and have been reported in all anatomical sites of the head and neck.
- Tumors of minor salivary gland origin are more likely to be histologically malignant than benign.
- Clinical presentation is most commonly a "benign," non-ulcerative, submucosal swelling.
- Incisional or punch biopsy should be performed prior to planning radiological imaging and/or definitive treatment.
- Complete surgical excision is the preferred treatment.
- Should the tumor be malignant and have poor prognostic histopathological parameters, then elective postoperative radiotherapy should be recommended.
- Patients with inoperable tumors or patients who refuse surgical excision should be offered radiotherapy, external beam or neutron radiotherapy.

References

1. Alavi S, Namazie A, Calcaterra TC, Blackwell KE (1999) Glandular Carcinoma of the Larynx; The UCLA Experience. Ann Otol Rhinol Laryngol 108:485–489
2. Anderson JN, Beenken SW, Crowe R, et al. (1995) Prognostic Factors in Minor Salivary Gland Cancer. Head Neck 17:480–486
3. Auclair PL, Goode RK, Ellis GL (1992) Mucoepidermoid Carcinoma of Intraoral Salivary Glands. Cancer 69:2012–2030
4. Beckhardt RN, Weber RS, Zane R, et al. (1995) Minor Salivary Gland Tumors of the Palate: Clinical and Pathologic Correlates of Outcome. Laryngoscope 105:1155–1160
5. Bizal JC, Righal SK, Kesler KA (1997) Pleomorphic Adenoma of the Trachea. Otolaryngol Head Neck Surg 116: 139–140
6. Blachaert RH, Ord RA (1998) Polymorphous Low-Grade Adenocarcinoma of the Sublingual Gland. Int J Oral Maxillofac Surg 27:115–117
7. Boneu F, Gonzalez-Lagunas J, Huguet P, et al. (1998) Massive Malignant Pleomorphic Adenoma of the Palate. J Oral Maxillofac Surg 56:91–96
8. Bradley PJ (1999) Submandibular Gland and Minor Salivary Gland Neoplasms. Curr Opin Otolaryngol Head Neck Surg 7:72–78
9. Bradley PJ (2004) Adenoid Cystic Carcinoma of the Head and Neck: A Review. Curr Opin Otolaryngol Head Neck Surg 12:127–130
10. Calis AB, Coskun BU, Seven H, et al. (2006) Laryngeal Mucoepidermoid Carcinoma: Report of 2 cases. Auris Nasus Larynx 33:211–214
11. Castle JT, Thompson LDR, Frommelt RA, et al. (1999) Polymorphous Low-Grade Adenocarcinoma. Cancer 86:207–219
12. Chou C, Zhu G, Luo M, et al. (1996) Carcinoma of the Minor Salivary Glands: results of surgery and combined therapy. J Oral Maxillofac Surg 54:448–453
13. Davies JNP, Dodge OG, Burkitt DP, et al. (1964) Salivary Gland Tumors in Uganda. Cancer 17:1310–1313
14. de Diego JL, Bernaldez R, Prim MP, et al. (1996) Polymorphous low-grade adenocarcinoma of the tongue. J Laryngol Otol 110:700–703
15. De Vries A, Johnson JT, Myers EN, et al. (1987) Base of Tongue Salivary Gland Tumors. Head Neck Surg 9:329–331
16. Douglas JG, Laramore GE, Austin-Seymour M, et al. (1996) Neutron radiotherapy for adenoid cystic carcinoma of minor salivary glands. Int J Radiat Oncol Biol Phys 36:87–93

17. Douglas JG, Laramore GE, Austin-Seymour M (2000) Treatment of Locally Advanced Adenoid Cystic Carcinoma of the Head and Neck with Neutron Radiotherapy. Int J Radiat Oncol Biol Phys 46:551–557
18. Douglas JG, Koh W-J, Austin-Seymour M, et al. (2003) Treatment of Salivary Gland Neoplasms with Fast Neutron Radiotherapy. Arch Otolaryngol Head Neck Surg 129:944–948
19. Ellis GL, Auclair PL (1996) The normal salivary glands. In Ellis GL, Auclair PL, Atlas of tumor pathology; tumors of the salivary glands. Third Series, Seventeenth fascicle. Washington D.C. Armed Forces Institute of Pathology, pp 1–23
20. Fordice J, Kershaw C, El-Naggar A, et al. (1999) Adenoid Cystic Carcinoma of the Head and Neck. Arch Otolaryngol Head Neck Surg 125:149–152
21. Ganly I, Patel SG, Coleman M, et al. (2006) Malignant Minor Salivary Gland Tumors of the Larynx. Arch Otolaryngol Head Neck Surg 132:767–770
22. Gupta AK, Singhal SK, Mann SBS, et al. (1997) Pleomorphic adenoma presenting as a base of tongue mass. J Laryngol Otol 111:1177–1178
23. Harmse JL, Saleh HA, Odutoye T, et al. (1997) Recurrent canalicular adenoma of the minor salivary glands of the upper lip. J Laryngol Otol 111:985–987
24. Howard DJ, Lund VJ (1985) Reflections on the Management of Adenoid Cystic Carcinoma of the Nasal Cavity and Paranasal Sinuses. Otolaryngol Head Neck Surg 93:338–341
25. Huber PE, Debus J, Latz D, et al. (2001) Radiotherapy for Advanced Adenoid Cystic Carcinoma; Neutrons, Photons or Mixed Beam? Radiother Oncol 59:161–167
26. Hyam DM, Veness MJ, Morgan GJ, et al. (2004) Minor salivary gland carcinoma involving the oral cavity or oropharynx. Aust Dental J 49:16–19
27. Isacsson G, Shear M (1983) Intra-oral salivary gland tumors: a retrospective study of 201 cases. J Oral Pathol 12:57–62
28. Jansisyanamont P, Blanchaert RH, Ord RA (2002) Intraoral minor salivary gland neoplasms; a single institution experience of 80 cases. Int J Oral Maxillofac Surg 31:257–261
29. Jenkins DW, Spaulding CA, Constable WC, et al. (1989) Minor Salivary Gland Tumors; The Role of Radiotherapy. Am J Otolaryngol 10:250–256
30. Jones AS, Hamilton JW, Rowley H, et al. (1997) Adenoid Cystic Carcinoma of the Head and Neck. Clin Otolaryngol 22:434–443
31. Jones AS, Beasley NJP, Houghton DJ, et al. (1998) Tumors of the Minor Salivary Glands. Clin Otolaryngol 23:27–33
32. Kessler DJ, Mickel RA, Calcaterra TC (1985) Malignant Salivary Gland Tumors of the Base of the Tongue. Arch Otolaryngol 111:664–666
33. Kokemuller H, Eckardt A, Brachvogel P, et al. (2004) Adenoid Cystic Carcinoma of the Head and Neck–a 20 years Experience. Int J Oral Maxillofac Surg 33:25–31
34. Konno A, Ishikawa K, Numata T, et al. (1998) Analysis of factors affecting Long-term Treatment Results of Adenoid Cystic Carcinoma of the Nose and Paranasal Sinuses. Acta Otolaryngol (Stockh) Suppl 537:67–74
35. Le Q-T, Birdwell S, Terris DJ, et al. (1999) Post-operative irradiation of minor salivary gland malignancies of the head and neck. Radiother Oncol 52:165–171
36. Lee N, Millender LE, Larson DA, et al. (2003) Gamma Knife Radiosurgery for Recurrent Salivary Gland Malignancies Involving the Base of Skull. Head Neck 25:210–216
37. Licitra L, Grandi C, Prott FJ, et al. (2002) Major and Minor Salivary Gland Tumors. Crit Rev Oncol Hematol 45:215–225
38. Lopes MA, Santos GC, Kowalski LP, et al. (1998) Multivariance analysis of 128 cases of oral cavity minor salivary gland carcinomas. Head Neck 20:699–706
39. Lopes MA, Kowalski LP, Santos da C, et al. (1999) A Clinicopathologic Study of 196 intraoral minor salivary gland tumors. J Oral Pathol Med 28:264–267
40. Lopes MA, Perez DE, Alves FA, et al. (2006) Clinicopathologic and Immunohistochemical study on Intraoral Mucoepidermoid Carcinoma. Otolaryngol Head Neck Surg 134:622–626
41. Mahistedt K, Upmuller J, Donath K (2002) Malignant Sialogenic Tumors of the Larynx. J Laryngol Otol 116:119–122
42. Matsuba HM, Simpson JR, Mauney M, et al. (1986) Adenoid Cystic Salivary Gland Carcinoma: A Clinico-Pathologic Correlation. Head Neck Surg 8:200–204
43. Milford CA, Mugliston TA, O'Flynn P, et al. (1989) Carcinoma arising in a Pleomorphic Adenoma of the Epiglottis. J Laryngol Otol 103:324–327
44. Naficy S, Disher MJ, Esclamado RM (1999) Adenoid Cystic Carcinoma of the Paranasal Sinuses. Am J Rhinol 13:311–314
45. Namazie A, Alavi S, Abemayer E, et al. (2001) Adenoid Cystic Carcinoma of the Base of Tongue. Ann Otol Rhinol Laryngol 110:248–253
46. Noghreyan A, Gatot A, Maor E, et al. (1995) Palatal pleomorphic adenoma in a child J Laryngol Otol 109:343–345
47. Parsons JT, Mendenhall WM, Stringer SP, et al. (1996) Management of Minor Salivary Gland Carcinomas. Int J Radiat Oncol Biol Phys 35:443–454

48. Patel SG, Singh B, Polluri A, et al. (2003) Craniofacial Surgery for Malignant Skull Base Tumors. Cancer 98:1179–1187
49. Pinto PX, Coleman N (1997) Regional Metastasis in polymorphous low-grade adenocarcinoma. Int J Oral Maxillofac Surg 26:447–449
50. Pitman KT, Prokopakis EP, Aydogan B, et al. (1999) The Role of Skull Base Surgery for the Treatment of Adenoid Cystic Carcinoma of the Sinonasal Tract. Head Neck 21:402–407
51. Prokopakis EP, Snyderman CH, Hanna E, et al. (1999) Risk Factors for Local Recurrence of Adenoid Cystic Carcinoma: The Role of Post-operative Radiation Therapy. Am J Otolaryngol 20:281–286
52. Prott F-J, Micke O, Haverkamp U, et al. (2000) Results of Fast Neutron Therapy of Adenoid Cystic Carcinoma of the Salivary Glands. Anticancer Res 20:3743–3750
53. Rapidis AD, Givalos N, Gakiopoulou H, et al. (2005) Adenoid Cystic Carcinoma of the Head and Neck: Clinicopathological Analysis of 23 Patients and Review of the Literature. Oral Oncol 41:328–335
54. Rhee C-S, Won T-B, Lee CH, et al. (2006) Adenoid Cystic Carcinoma of the Sinonasal Tract: Treatment Results. Laryngoscope 116:982–986
55. Sawatsubashi M, Tuda K, Tonkunga O, et al. (1997) Pleomorphic Adenoma of the Larynx: A case and a review of the literature in Japan. Otolaryngol Head Neck Surg 117:415–417
56. Schramm VL, Imola MJ (2001) Management of Nasopharyngeal Salivary Gland Malignancy. Laryngoscope 111:1533–1544
57. Schultz-Ertner D, Nikoghosyan A, Didinger B, et al. (2005) Therapy Strategies for Locally Advanced Adenoid Cystic Carcinomas using Modern Radiation Therapy Techniques. Cancer 104:338–344
58. Silverman DA, Carlson TP, Khuntia D, et al. (2004) Role of Postoperative Radiation Therapy in Adenoid Cystic Carcinoma of the Head and Neck. Laryngoscope 114:1194–1199
59. Spiro RH (1998) Management of Malignant Tumors of the Salivary Glands. Oncology 12:671–680
60. Spiro RH, Koss LG, Hadju SI, et al. (1973) Tumors of the Minor Salivary Origin: A Clinicopathologic Study of 492 cases. Cancer 31:117–129
61. Spiro RH, Thaler HT, Hickes WF, et al. (1991) The Importance of Clinical Staging of Minor Salivary Gland Carcinoma. Am J Surg 162:330–336
62. Strick MJ, Kelly C, Soames JV, et al. (2004) Malignant Tumors of the minor Salivary Glands–a 20 year review. Br J Plast Surg 57:624–631
63. Suarez C, Llorente JL, De Leon RF, et al. (2004) Prognostic Factors in Sinonasal Tumors Involving the Anterior Skull Base. Head Neck 26:136–144
64. Szanto PA, Luna MA, Tortoledo ME, et al.. (1984) Histologic grading of adenoid cystic carcinoma of the salivary glands. Cancer 54:1062–1069
65. Tahlan A, Nanda A, Nagarkar N, et al. (2004) Pleomorphic Adenoma of the Nasal Septum. Am J Otolaryngol 25:118–120
66. Tanigaki Y, Mikami Y, Ono M, et al. (2004) Pleomorphic adenoma of the lateral side of the tongue. Acta Otolaryngol 124:694–651
67. van der Wal JE, Snow GB, van der Waal I (1992) Histological reclassification of 101 intraoral salivary gland tumors (new WHO classification). J Clin Pathol 45:834–835
68. vander Poorten VLM, Balm AJM, Hilgers FJM, et al. (2000) Stage as major long-term outcome predictor in minor salivary gland carcinoma. Cancer 89:1195–1204
69. Waldron CA, El-Mofty K, Gnepp DR (1988) Tumors of the intraoral minor salivary glands. A demographic and histologic study of 426 cases. Oral Surg 66:323–333
70. Wang CC, See LC, Hong JH, et al. (1996) Nasopharyngeal adenoid cystic carcinoma: five new cases and a literature review. J Otolaryngol 25:399–403
71. Westra WH (1999) The surgical pathology of salivary gland neoplasms. Otolaryngol Clin North Am 39:919–943
72. Yin ZY, Wu XL, Hu YH, et al. (1986) Cylindroma of the nasopharynx: a chronic disease. Int J Radiat Oncol Biol Phys 12:25–30

Chapter 21

Management of Tumors of the Submandibular and Sublingual Glands

21

Fernando L. Dias, Roberto A. Lima, and Claudio R. Cernea

Contents

Core Features

- Surgical anatomy and practical tips
- Surgical pathology
- Clinical presentation
- Methods of diagnosis and staging
- Surgical treatment of benign tumors
- Surgical treatment of malignant tumors
- Postoperative complications
- Indications for radiation treatment
- Perspectives

Complications to Avoid
- Marginal mandibular nerve injury
- Lingual nerve injury
- Hypoglossal nerve injury

Introduction

Tumors of the submandibular gland are the second most frequent major salivary gland neoplasms after tumors in the parotid gland. Approximately 3–6% of all tumors of the head and neck region occur in the major and minor salivary glands. Sixty-five percent of the tumors arise in the parotid gland, 8% in the submandibular gland, and 27% in the minor salivary glands. In contrast to parotid tumors, approximately half of the tumors of the submandibular gland are malignant. Primary tumors of the sublingual gland are very rare, except for ranulas, which are benign cystic lesions. The submandibular triangle contains several important neurovascular structures, in addition to the submandibular gland: the marginal mandibular branch of the VIIth cranial nerve, the lingual nerve (which is a branch of the third division of the Vth cranial nerve), the XIIth cranial nerve, and the facial artery, as well as lymph nodes that can harbor regional metastases from oral and oropharyngeal primary cancers.

21

Surgical Anatomy and Practical Tips

Submandibular Gland

The submandibular glands, also called submaxillary glands, are 10- to- 15-g walnut-sized glands situated in the submandibular triangle beneath and anterior to the angle of the mandible. They overlie the mylohyoid muscle and extend around its free border in the floor of the mouth along the course of Wharton's duct. These glands lie on the hyoglossus muscle and are in direct contact with the stylomandibular ligament posteriorly. A loosely attached investing fascia encloses the glands. Saliva from the submandibular glands flows into the anterior floor of the mouth through Wharton's duct, the papilla of which opens just lateral to the frenulum of the tongue [1] (Fig. 21.1). The submandibular gland is divided into a superficial and a deep lobe. The superficial lobe lies in the digastric triangle and is bounded anteriorly by the anterior belly of the digastric muscle, posteriorly by the posterior belly of the digastric and stylohyoid muscles, and laterally by the lower border of the mandible and medial pterygoid muscle. Posteriorly, the stylomandibular ligament separates it from the parotid gland. The floor of the submandibular triangle is formed by the mylohyoid muscle anteriorly and the hyoglossus muscle posteriorly. The superficial portion of the submandibular gland is covered by the platysma muscle and is traversed by the anterior facial vein and marginal mandibular nerve. The so-called deep portion of the submandibular gland lies deep to the posterior edge of the mylohyoid muscle. The lingual nerve lies above it and the hypoglossal nerve below it (Fig. 21.2).

The submandibular triangle borders are: anteriorly, the anterior belly of the digastric muscle; inferiorly, hyoid

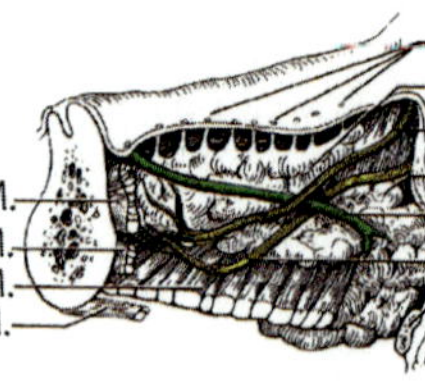

Fig. 21.1: Diagram of normal anatomy of left submandibular and sublingual glands viewed obliquely from the left side. (Reproduced with permission: Som PM. In: Som PM, Bergeron RT (eds) Head and Neck Imaging, ed 2. St. Louis, Mosby, 1991; 281)

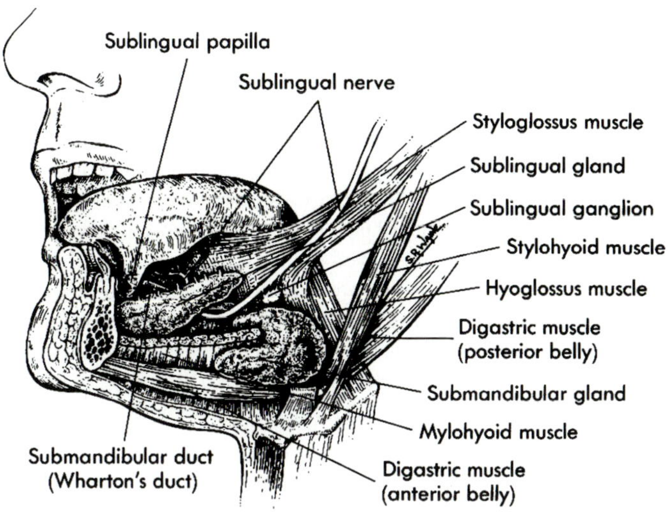

Fig. 21.2: Anatomic relationships of the floor of the mouth with emphasis on the sublingual and submandibular spaces. (Million RR, Cassisi NJ, Clark JR. Cancer of the head and neck. In: DeVita AT Jr, Hellman S, Rosenberg SA (eds) Cancer: Principles and Practice of Oncology, ed 3. Philadelphia, JB Lippincott, 1989; 506)

bone and common digastric tendon; posteriorly, the posterior belly of the same muscle; superiorly, lower mandibular rim; medially, mylohyoid and hypoglossal muscles; and laterally, platysma muscle. Contained within these limits are: lymph nodes of level Ib [2], the submandibular gland, the lingual and facial arteries and veins, the submandibular ganglion, and the marginal mandibular, lingual, and hypoglossal nerves.

There are some practical anatomic tips that can help in the surgical management of submandibular gland tumors.

Marginal Mandibular Branch of the Facial Nerve

This is a very tiny nerve, usually located immediately deep to the platysma muscle. It promotes contraction of mimetic muscles related to the ipsilateral oral commissure (risorius, depressor of lower lip, depressor of angle of the mouth, and mental muscles). Therefore, inadvertent surgical injury during the initial approach to the submandibular triangle should be avoided. One of the most constant landmarks to locate the marginal mandibular branch is the mandibular angle, usually situated 2–5 mm cranially. The nerve runs parallel to the mandibular rim 1–2.5 cm caudally for about 3 cm, turning cranially toward the oral commissure. Generally, there is a close anatomic relationship between the nerve and the facial vessels (which course perpendicularly around the middle third of the body of the mandible). In fact, there is a surgical maneuver, attributed to Hayes Martin: to keep the cranial stumps of these vessels retracted upward during the dissection of the surgical contents of the submandibular triangle, in order to protect the mandibular branch.

Lingual Nerve

The inferior division of V3 is the sensory nerve of the anterior two thirds of the oral tongue; also, it gives parasympathetic supply to the submandibular gland, through a small secretory branch, generally sectioned during excision of the gland. It is situated on the floor of the submandibular triangle, sometimes covered by mylohyoid muscle fibers. It is important to preserve the integrity of this nerve during operations on the submandibular gland; however, when dealing with malignant tumors, especially adenoid cystic carcinomas, it is advisable to get frozen sections from the cranial stump of the severed secretory branch, in order to detect possible perineural invasion.

Hypoglossal Nerve

The XIIth cranial nerve is the main motor supply to the tongue and muscles of the floor of the mouth. It crosses the floor of the submandibular triangle in a very deep position, except near the transition between the posterior belly and the tendon of the digastric muscle. When dissecting the inferior border of the submandibular gland, caution must be exerted at this point to avoid a nerve injury, which causes ipsilateral tongue paralysis.

Facial Artery

The facial artery is the fourth branch of the external carotid artery [1]. It enters the submandibular triangle near the medial aspect of the posterior belly of the digastric muscle (where it can be easily identified and tied), crossing the submandibular gland vertically and, together with the anterior facial vein, running underneath the marginal mandibular branch (see above). This artery is usually ligated twice during excision of the submandibular gland: near the digastric muscle and near the body of the mandible. However, some authors defend the preservation of this artery in selected cases in order to maintain the blood supply to skin flaps that may be used for reconstruction [3].

Wharton's Duct

The duct, also called the submandibular duct, arises from the deep surface of the gland and passes anteriorly for approximately 5 cm to an opening near the midline of the floor of the mouth. It runs between the mylohyoid, hyoglossus, and genioglossus muscles before entering the floor of the mouth. On the hyoglossus muscle, the duct lies between the lingual and hypoglossal nerves but it crosses lateral to the lingual nerve along the anterior border of the muscle [4]. It is important to dissect the duct as close as possible to the floor of the mouth before its ligation/sectioning, carefully protecting the hypoglossal nerve.

Lymphatic System

Numerous lymphatic channels permeate this region, and lymph nodes frequently overlie the submandibular gland itself. Most are situated immediately under the deep cervical fascia, including the prevascular and postvascular nodes adjacent to the facial vessels, and some are located between the gland and the mylohyoid muscle. They represent level I, according to the current staging system of cervical lymph nodes [2]. Recently, they were divided into: submental group (level Ia), located between the anterior belly of the digastric muscles and cephalad to the hyoid bone; and submandibular group (level Ib), located in the triangular area bounded by the anterior and posterior bellies of the digastric muscle and the inferior border of the body of the mandible [5]. The lymph nodes adjacent to the submandibular gland and along the facial artery are included in this group. They are of paramount importance in surgical oncology, because they represent the first echelon for lymph vessels from the nose, lips, and anterior and lateral portions of the tongue and floor of the mouth. When involved secondarily in cancer within the drainage territory, lymph nodes are closely attached to, and sometimes adherent to the substance of the submandibular gland; their removal requires clearing the compartment of its glandular content. These lymph nodes drain to the subdigastric and high midjugular (level II) lymph nodes [2, 6].

Sublingual Gland

The paired sublingual glands, which are the smallest of the major salivary glands, weighing approximately 2 g each, lie immediately below the mucous membrane of the floor of the mouth. According to Batsakis, these poorly encapsulated glands represent not unit organs but, rather, a mosaic composed of a large segment (the major sublingual gland) and a group of 8–30 smaller glands (the minor sublingual glands) [7]. Variations exist in size and location of sublingual ducts (ducts of Rivinus) that pass from the multiple "minor" sublingual glands and drain by way of several openings directly into the oral cavity or into the submandibular duct. Batsakis also noticed that the larger gland (the major sublingual gland) is drained by the sublingual duct (the duct of Bartholin) [7]. The sublingual glands are separated by the paired midline genioglossus and geniohyoid muscles. A crest of mucous membrane, termed the plica sublingualis, along the frenulum represents the projection of the glands and openings of the sublingual ducts. The blood supply to the sublingual gland comes from the sublingual and submental arteries. The nerve supply is from the chorda tympani and lingual nerves [1]. Lymphatic drainage goes into the submental and submandibular lymph nodes (Figs. 21.1, 21.2).

Pathology

There are equal proportions of malignant and benign lesions in the submandibular gland. True sublingual gland tumors are rather unusual, and most are malignant.

Benign Tumors

The most commonly encountered benign tumor of the submandibular gland is the pleomorphic adenoma (benign mixed tumor) which comprises 53–64% of submandibular tumors [8–10]. The histologic features and biologic behavior of pleomorphic adenoma of the submandibular gland are similar to those of the parotid gland. Comparing the frequency of this tumor with the parotid equivalent, the proportion is 1:10, respectively. Typical presentation is that of a slowly growing painless mass (sometimes present for several years). Larger tumors have a multinodular appearance. This benign tumor is usually a pseudoencapsulated and well-demarcated neoplasm containing both epithelial and mesenchymal elements with an inner epithelial layer and an outer myoepithelial layer. The stroma in the tumor varies from mucoid, fibroid, vascular, and chondroid to myxochondroid, the latter two being associated with an increase in recurrence of the tumor. The high recurrence rate associated is believed to be due to pseudopod formations at the periphery of the tumor, as well as to inadequate excision (enucleation). Recurrence may occur months to years following inadequate excision of the tumor. These tumors can also undergo malignant transformation (approximately 2–6%) particularly in long-standing tumors or in those that have recurred. Multicentric tumors are estimated to be 0.5% [10].

Other types of adenomas, such as the basal cell adenoma, are much less common, and other benign tumors, such as Whartin's tumor, oncocytomas, and myoepitheliomas, are very rarely found in submandibular and sublingual glands.

Hemangiomas can involve the major salivary glands. However, 90% are related to the parotid gland. Occasionally, the submandibular gland can be affected, but only as a part of massive facial lesions (Fig. 21.3a, b).

Benign tumors of the sublingual gland are extremely rare entities. Yet, this gland may present a non-neoplastic disease which resembles a submucosal tumor in the floor of the mouth: the ranula. Its name derives from the Latin word *rana* (frog), due to the typical bluish appearance, similar to a frog's belly [11]. There are two different concepts for the pathogenesis of ranula. One is a true cyst due to ductal obstruction with an epithelial lining, and the other is a pseudocyst due to injury of the duct and extravasation of mucus without an epithelial lining [12–14]. Recently, typical ranulas have been considered as an extravasation phenomenon of the sublingual gland [14, 15]. According to the variations of its extension, ranula has

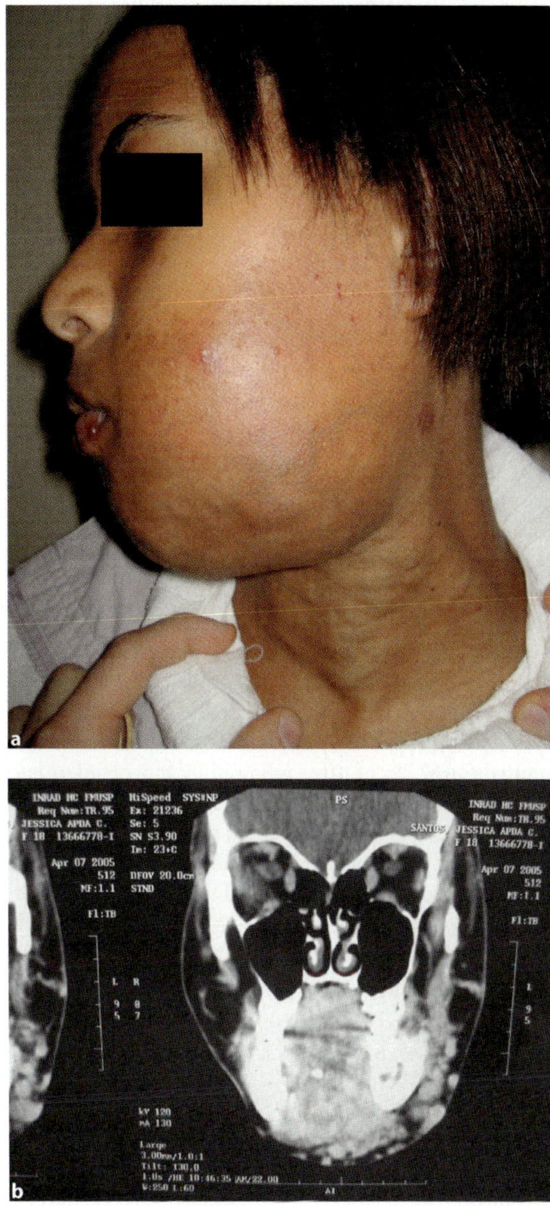

Fig. 21.3: Vascular malformation of the submandibular region. **a** An extensive cavernous hemangioma causing distortion of the left submandibular region and cheek. **b** CT scan, coronal view revealing calcification of the central compartment, phleboliths, and involvement of the suprahyoid muscles

been classified into three clinical types: sublingual type, sublingual-submandibular type, and submandibular type [16]. The sublingual type is a simple ranula while the sublingual-submandibular type and submandibular type are plunging ranulae. The clinical presentation is of a slowly growing submucosal mass in the floor of the mouth, with a cystic appearance (Fig. 21.4a, b). Pathologically, there is a simple or multiloculated cavity filled with amorphous or mucoid material [11].

The most frequent benign tumors are listed in Table 21.1 [8, 17].

Malignant Tumors

Both submandibular and, rarely, sublingual glands may give rise to a wide variety of malignant neoplasms, which can be divided into: primary, secondary, and local manifestations of systemic neoplastic diseases. Among malignant tumors, the most frequent is adenoid cystic carcinoma accounting for 36–63% of cases [9, 10, 18–20]. Bhattacharyya [20] analyzed the data from the Surveillance, Epidemiology and End Results (SEER) database for the period from 1988 to 1998, and found a total of 370 cases of submandibular gland cancers. Adenoid cystic carcinoma accounted for 42.2% of cases followed by mucoepidermoid carcinoma (22.2%), squamous cell carcinoma (17.3%), and adenocarcinoma (15.4%). Adenoid cystic carcinoma usually develops over a short time with rapid growth and is frequently associated with pain and fixation to the mandible. A third of these patients develop regional lymph node metastases. This tumor has a propensity to invade nerves, and due to the anatomic location of the submandibular gland, this poses a risk of perineural spread through the lingual and hypoglossal nerves toward the skull base. Perineural spread may also involve the mandibular or cervical branches of the facial nerve. The risk of distant metastases and the development of late recurrences are similar to those observed in the parotid gland [10].

Table 21.1. Benign neoplasms

Benign epithelial tumors	Soft tissue tumors
Pleomorphic adenoma	Hemangioma
Myoepithelioma	
Basal cell adenoma	
Warthin tumor	
Oncocytoma	
Canalicular adenoma	
Sebaceous adenoma	
Lymphadenoma	
Sebaceous	
Non-sebaceous	
Ductal papillomas	
Inverted ductal papilloma	
Intraductal papilloma	
Sialadenoma papilliferum	
Cystadenoma	

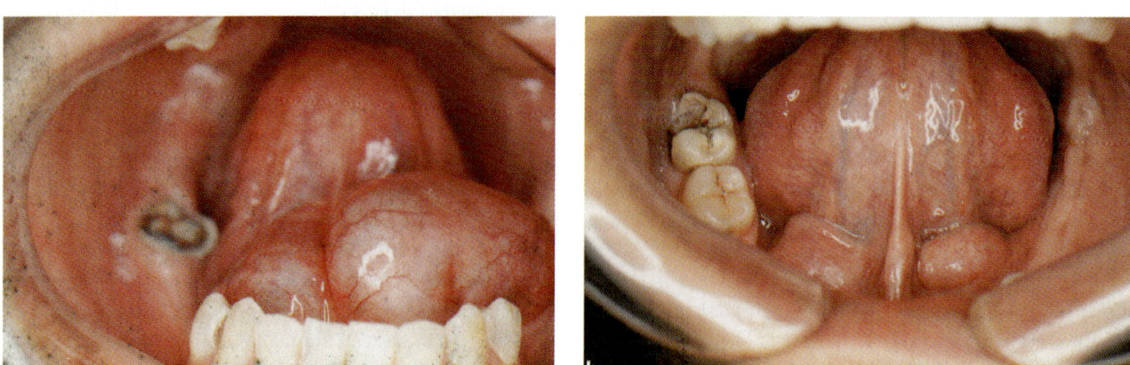

Fig. 21.4: Types of ranula. **a** Plunging ranula, sublingual-submandibular type (unilateral presentation). **b** Simple ranula, sublingual type (bilateral presentation)

The next most common cancer of the submandibular gland is mucoepidermoid carcinoma. These tumors may be low, intermediate, or high grade in their histologic appearance, with eventual outcome dependent upon this grading. Low-grade tumors are usually well circumscribed and are comprised of epidermoid and mucus-secreting cells. Grossly they resemble benign mixed tumors, and have been found to recur after excision in approximately 15% of patients. High-grade tumors are aggressive and invade locally, causing fixation and extension to the nerve. On presentation, up to 50% of patients with high-grade tumors are reported to have lymph node metastases [9, 10]. The propensity for local failure can be as high as 40% [10].

Squamous cell carcinoma usually presents as a hard mass, often fixed, with a short history of 1 year or less. The tumor is often asymptomatic but 20% of patients have a painful mass. Neck metastases occur in nearly 50% of patients. Morphologically the ductal cell is most likely the cell of origin. Due to the frequency of squamous cell carcinoma in other head and neck sites, it is important to ensure that this tumor is a primary tumor of the gland and not a metastatic lesion to the submandibular lymph nodes. Differential diagnosis with mucoepidermoid carcinoma must also be confirmed. Locoregional recurrence can occur in nearly 50% of cases [10]. Adenocarcinoma arises infrequently in the submandibular gland. These very aggressive tumors invariably present with lymph node metastases and massive local extension to soft tissue and invasion of the mandible, resulting in poor local control which adversely affects prognosis [10].

The most frequent cancers are listed in Table 21.2 [8, 17].

Clinical Presentation

Submandibular and Sublingual Glands

Most swellings occurring in the submandibular gland are due to inflammatory processes and calculi [21]. Benign and malignant tumors of the submandibular gland are frequently identified as a painless mass in the submandibular region. The association of pain with submandibular neoplasms is rare, but when it occurs, it suggests malignancy. Usually, a painful submandibular gland enlargement is consistent with a clinical diagnosis of sialadenitis, until proven the contrary. Painless swelling was the presenting symptom in 87% of patients with benign and 69% of those with malignant parotid or submandibular gland tumors in the huge series of 2,200 patients with major salivary gland tumors (including 235 submandibular tumors) published by Spiro [9]. Pain was reported by 10% of those with malignant major salivary gland tumors, but was uncommon with benign tumors in these glands (4%) [9]. Vander Poorten et al. [19] analyzed the clinical data of 43 patients with malignant submandibular gland tumors who were treated at the Netherlands Cancer Institute between 1973 and 1994. All patients presented with submandibular swelling, existing for a median of 13 months (range 1–330 months). The swelling was painless in 72% of patients, whereas 28% experienced local pain. Although skin invasion was difficult to evaluate in patients who underwent previous incisional biopsy or had an inadequate resection (excisional biopsy), visible skin invasion was present in only three (6.9%) patients. The discharge of purulent saliva from the salivary duct is usually diagnostic of an inflammatory glandular process. Nevertheless, it must be kept in mind that a salivary gland tumor can coexist with obstructive sialopathy leading to sialadenitis (Fig. 21.5a–d).

The differential diagnosis of swelling in the submandibular area must include enlargement of lymph nodes not associated with salivary gland diseases. In adults presenting submandibular swelling, metastases from a squamous carcinoma primary of the skin or of the oral cavity must be considered. In addition, other possibilities are atypical mycobacteria infection, cervicofacial actinomycosis, sarcoidosis, Sjögren's syndrome, acquired or congenital cysts, benign follicular hyperplasia of lymph nodes, and cat-scratch disease [22].

Submandibular gland tumors usually present as a firm, lobulated solitary mass. Physical examination, including bimanual palpation, is important in order to evaluate the extension and fixation to adjacent structures. Sensory (lingual nerve) and motor (hypoglossal and marginal mandibular nerves) nerve deficits must be interpreted as evidence of malignancy. Although skin invasion was difficult to evaluate in patients who underwent previous incisional biopsy or had an inadequate resection (excisional biopsy), visible skin invasion was present in only three (6.9%) patients in Vander Poorten's series [19]. In contrast, skin invasion or deep fixation to the mandible or to floor of the mouth muscles were found in a higher percentage (28%) of patients with submandibular cancer in Spiro's series of 217 patients with submandibular gland tumors [23]. Occasionally, these tumors may fungate by direct extension through the

Table 21.2. Malignant neoplasms

Primary tumors	Secondary tumors	Systemic neoplasms
Acinic cell carcinoma	Lymph node metastases:	Hodgkin's lymphoma
Mucoepidermoid carcinoma	Oral cavity cancers	Diffuse large B-cell lymphoma
Adenoid cystic carcinoma	Squamous cell carcinoma	Extranodal marginal zone B-cell lymphoma
Polymorphous low-grade adenocarcinoma	Minor salivary gland tumors	
Epithelial-myoepithelial carcinoma	Skin cancers	
Clear cell carcinoma, not otherwise specified	Malignant melanoma	
Basal cell adenocarcinoma	Squamous cell carcinoma	
Sebaceous carcinoma	Direct extension from adjacent cancers:	
Sebaceous lymphadenocarcinoma	Oral cavity cancers	
Cystadenocarcinoma	Mandibular tumors	
Low-grade cribriform cystadenocarcinoma	Skin cancers	
Mucinous adenocarcinoma		
Oncocytic carcinoma		
Salivary duct carcinoma		
Adenocarcinoma, not otherwise specified		
Myoepithelial carcinoma		
Carcinoma ex-pleomorphic adenoma		
Carcinosarcoma		
Metastasizing pleomorphic adenoma		
Primary squamous cell carcinoma		
Small cell carcinoma		
Large cell carcinoma		
Lymphoepithelial carcinoma		
Sialoblastoma		

skin or in association with dermal lymphatic permeation (Fig. 21.6a, b).

Benign lesions frequently have a long medical history; however, the presence of long-standing symptoms does not exclude a diagnosis of cancer. In a large series published by Spiro [9], most patients with malignant tumors had symptoms within a year of treatment, but in 19% of patients with submandibular gland tumors, the duration of symptoms was longer than 10 years. Although the sexes were almost equally represented with respect to malignant tumors, benign tumors occurred more often in women (64%). The median age of patients with benign tumors was 46 years, whereas the median age for malignant tumors was 54 years in those with malignant neoplasms [9]. Painless swelling was the most frequent presenting symptom (69%) of patients with either benign or malignant tumors of the submandibular gland [9]. Low-grade mucoepidermoid and malignant mixed tumor were the typical histopathology found among these slow-growing malignant tumors. Cervical lymph node metastases, another clear indication that the primary tumor was malignant, was found in 24.9–28% of patients with sub-

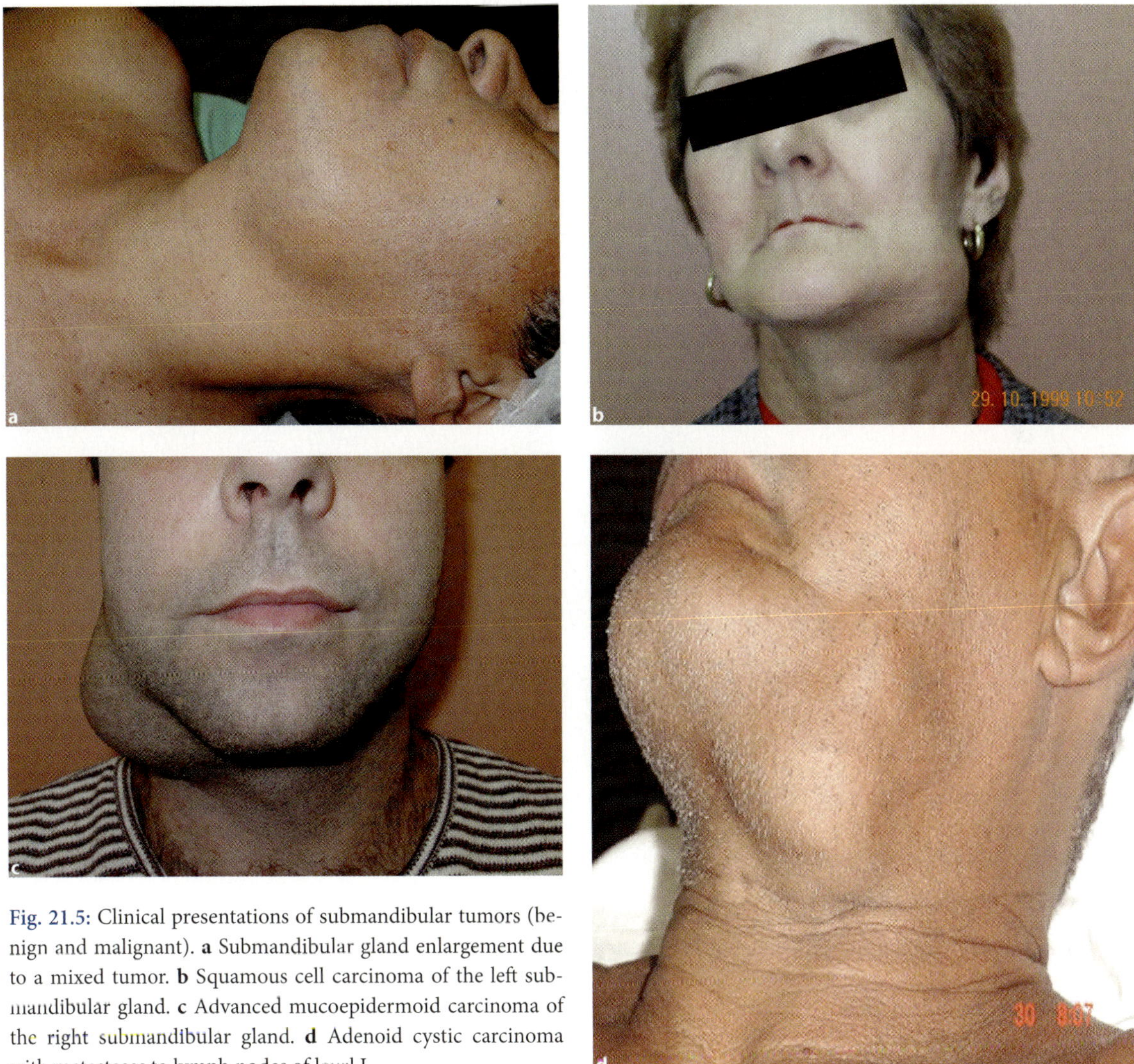

Fig. 21.5: Clinical presentations of submandibular tumors (benign and malignant). **a** Submandibular gland enlargement due to a mixed tumor. **b** Squamous cell carcinoma of the left submandibular gland. **c** Advanced mucoepidermoid carcinoma of the right submandibular gland. **d** Adenoid cystic carcinoma with metastases to lymph nodes of level I

mandibular cancer, according to two major series found in the literature [9, 20]. There is a consensus regarding the similar distribution rates of benign versus malignant neoplasms in the submandibular gland, pleomorphic adenoma being the most common benign neoplasm. Spiro's series of 217 submandibular neoplasms showed that adenoid cystic carcinoma was the most common malignancy, followed by mucoepidermoid carcinoma and malignant mixed tumors [23].

Distribution of 68 patients with malignant submandibular epithelial tumors, according to TNM classification, at first consultation in Spiro's series reveled 41% of stage I, 25% of stage II, and 34% of stage III–IV [9]. Only 36 of the originally 43 patients with submandibular gland cancer in Vander Poorten's series were amenable for staging. They found 6 patients (16.6%) with stage I disease, 11 (30.5%) with stage II, 8 with stage III (22.2%), and 11 with stage IV (30.5%) [19].

Tumors of the sublingual gland, which are very rare, usually present as a mass under the tongue, which may be painless or associated with minimal discomfort. Other symptoms include pain, difficulty with retention of a den-

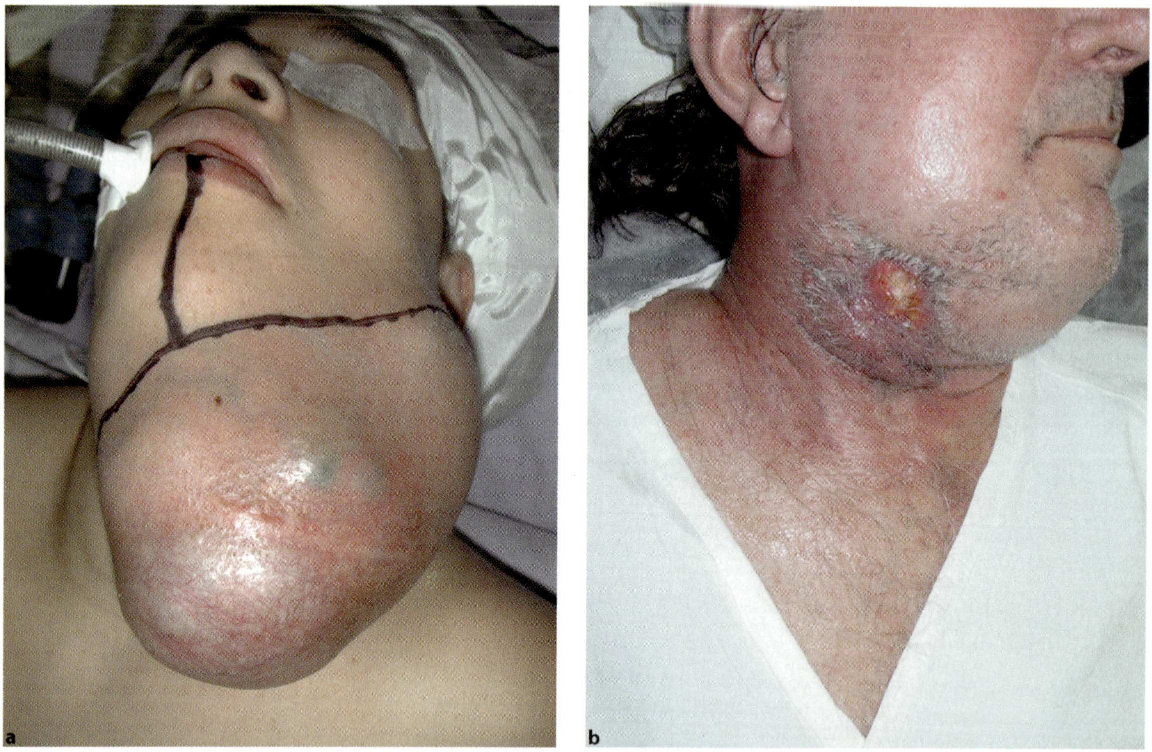

Fig. 21.6: **a** Recurrence of adenoid cystic carcinoma with deep fixation to the mandible, soft tissues of the neck, and with direct extension through the skin of the neck. **b** Recurrent mucoepidermoid carcinoma with deep fixation to the mandible, fungating by direct extension through the skin

tal prosthesis, and numbness of the tongue. A heightened degree of suspicion must be employed for lesions in this region of the floor of the mouth as a neoplasm may be mistaken for ranula or some other benign entity which presents as a submucosal mass in association with the salivary duct system. When they occur, 75% of them are malignant; mucoepidermoid carcinoma and adenoid cystic carcinoma comprise 80% of all carcinomas arising in this region [10] (Fig. 21.7a, b).

Pediatric Neoplasms

Salivary neoplasms are even less common in children. Only 1.7–3.2% of salivary gland epithelial neoplasms occur in patients 16 years old or younger [24]. As in adults, salivary tumors in the pediatric age group usually involve the parotid gland. A review of 587 patients with nonvascular tumors of the salivary glands treated over a 37-year period identified 19 tumors (3.2%) in patients 16 years old or younger [25]. Most of these tumors (63%) were pleomorphic adenomas and the remainder were malignant. Nonepithelial tumors, namely primary hemangioma and lymphangioma, were identified as the most common salivary gland tumor in the pediatric age group, with a total of 17 cases. Evaluating all cases of malignant neoplasms involving major salivary glands in 18-year-old patients or younger extracted from the Surveillance, Epidemiology, and End Results database (1988–2001), Shapiro and Bhattacharyya [26] found 113 primary salivary gland malignancies (103 parotid, 10 submandibular). In agreement with other studies, they found that salivary gland malignancies in the pediatric age group are most commonly found in the parotid gland with a 10:1 ratio between parotid and submandibular gland. Among 10 cancers of the submandibular gland, 3 (30%) were acinic cell carci-

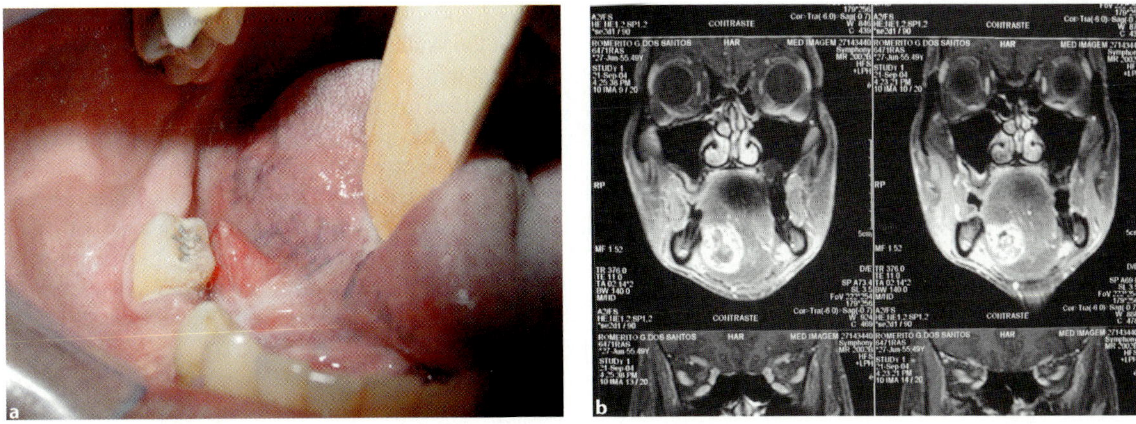

Fig. 21.7: **a** Clinical picture of adenoid cystic carcinoma of the right sublingual gland. **b** A coronal view (T1-weighted) of the same tumor on MRI revealing its relationship with the lingual aspect of the mandible and muscles of the oral tongue and floor of the mouth

noma, 2 (20%) were mucoepidermoid carcinoma, and 2 (20%) were adenocarcinomas. Extraglandular extension was identified in 2 (20%) patients. Interestingly, none of the submandibular gland tumors presented with metastases to the lymph nodes in the neck, whereas 9 (8.7%) parotid gland malignancies had locoregional lymphadenopathy. Only one patient with high-grade mucoepidermoid carcinoma in the entire cohort died at 86 months of follow-up.

Treatment for salivary gland cancer in the pediatric age group of epithelial cell origin is primarily surgical. Addition of adjuvant radiotherapy remains controversial, with some series showing no benefit in long-term outcomes. Because of the rarity of this disease in children, it is difficult to establish sound evidence-based adjuvant treatment, based on tumor histology and site [26].

Methods of Diagnosis and Staging

Physical Examination

Bimanual examination is the method of choice to evaluate size, mobility, and local extension of the tumors of submandibular and sublingual glands. The tumor mass usually is tethered or even fixed to the mandible, unless it is benign or it is small. It is important to mention that loss of mobility may occur with both benign and malignant lesions. Sometimes it is difficult to differentiate between an enlarged submandibular gland with cancer and an enlarged, fixed lymph node harboring metastases. In advanced cases, careful examination of the overlying skin and of the cranial nerves VII and XII is mandatory.

Differential Diagnosis

The differential diagnosis of a submandibular mass includes inflammatory disease, metastatic squamous cell carcinoma to a lymph node, and a primary neoplasm of the submandibular gland. Episodic pain and mass are the hallmark of inflammatory disease, although one third of the lesions may be asymptomatic. Obstructive sialadenitis, due to stricture or calculus in the duct, is a common cause of enlargement of the submandibular gland. In these instances, pain and swelling are associated with eating, receding after several hours. Erythema may occur over the mass, and a stone may be palpated in the duct which can, occasionally, drain purulent saliva when the gland is compressed [21, 22].

A solitary squamous carcinoma metastatic to a submandibular lymph node in the absence of an obvious primary lesion in the oral cavity is rather uncommon. Although a benign or malignant primary tumor of the submandibular gland is a relatively rare event, the recognition of such a condition is important for the initial step in management.

Primary tumors of the sublingual gland, which are very rare, usually present as a painless mass under the lateral aspect of the ventral tongue. These salivary gland tumors can be differentiated from mucosal lesions of the floor of the mouth by their submucosal location. Nevertheless, it is almost impossible to differentiate primary tumors of minor salivary origin in the floor of the mouth from tumors of the sublingual glands [9, 21].

Diagnostic Imaging

The main objectives of imaging of major salivary gland lesions are: (1) to establish whether the mass is intrinsic or extrinsic to the gland; (2) to determine its relationship to the nerves; and (3) to evaluate the full extent of the lesion, with possible signs of invasion of surrounding structures. If there is any radiologic evidence of malignancy, the study is extended to include the neck.

Plane radiographs, sialography, and nuclear scans add very little to the diagnostic information and are seldom indicated for evaluation of submandibular and sublingual gland masses. Although the primary application of ultrasound to salivary gland disease has been the differentiation of solid and cystic masses, some helpful information can be achieved by using this imaging technique. Differentiation between intraglandular and extraglandular nodules can be achieved by ultrasound, as well as important information regarding the contents of the mass, its size, and limits. Nevertheless, there are no definitive ultrasound criteria to differentiate between benign and malignant tumors. Sonographically, pleomorphic adenoma is well circumscribed and usually has homogeneous hypoechogenicity. Sharp, lobulated margins, as well as calcifications, are considered typical. Color Doppler sonography often demonstrates a moderate vascularization with a predominantly peripheral flow pattern. Malignant tumors such as mucoepidermoid carcinomas, particularly those smaller than 2 cm, usually have a homogeneous structure and present with smooth borders, and may be erroneously considered as benign. Highly malignant tumors and large lesions, in contrast, have irregular borders and typical heterogeneous echo pattern. Frequently, irregular necrosis is found. In malignant tumors, color Doppler usually shows enhanced vascularization when compared with the normal parenchyma or with benign tumors. It is noticeable, however, that patterns of extraglandular spread, such as perineural invasion and infiltration of the parapharyngeal space, the base of the skull, and the mandible, are not easily visible at sonography [27].

Computed tomography (CT) and magnetic resonance imaging (MRI) permit better visualization of masses within the salivary glands. CT and MRI are equally satisfactory in differentiating cystic from solid lesions and allow evaluation of the relationship with adjacent structures, including soft tissues and bones. CT scans are especially useful in the assessment of bone erosion, while MRI evaluates soft tissue involvement and may detect tumor extension along cranial nerves.

On CT, most benign mixed tumors are smoothly marginated, spherical tumors, with higher attenuation than the surrounding parenchyma, and with no significant enhancement on postcontrast studies. Smaller lesions are usually quite homogeneous in appearance, whereas larger masses have a heterogeneous appearance, with areas of necrosis, hemorrhage, and cystic degeneration. The larger tumors tend to develop a lobulated appearance, which can be confused with multiple masses. Dystrophic calcification can occasionally be seen, and is highly suggestive of pleomorphic adenoma. On MRI, these tumors have a nonhomogeneous appearance, with intermediate signal intensities on T1-weighted and proton density-weighted images (Wis). On T2-weighted images there is usually a mixture of intermediate and high signal intensities. Areas of hemorrhage appear as regions of high signal intensity on T1-weighted images; however, the regions of focal low attenuation seen on CT may not have directly corresponding sites of either high or low signal intensity on T2-weighted images. The nonhomogeneous MRI appearance is not unique for this tumor and can be seen in other lesions, including malignancies. In MRI studies, dystrophic calcifications cannot be visualized or distinguished from focal areas of fibrosis [28, 29] (Fig. 21.8 and 21.9a, b).

On imaging studies, features of low-grade malignant salivary tumors are nonspecific, whereas high-grade cancers may show imaging characteristics of highly cellular and infiltrating tumors with ill-defined margins. Adenoid cystic carcinoma may appear either as a benign or a malignant process while in its initial stages. Extension to the skull base via cranial nerves may be demonstrated by computed sectional scanning, especially when evaluating postoperative recurrences. The CT findings of mucoepidermoid lesions vary with the grade of the tumor. Low-grade lesions are benign in appearance with apparently well-delineated smooth margins. Cystic areas

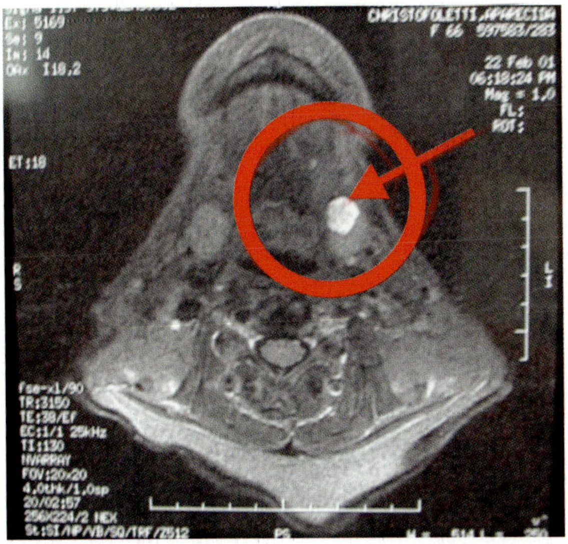

Fig. 21.8: MRI of pleomorphic adenoma of the left submandibular gland revealing an ovoid heterogeneous tumor with irregular borders and areas of dystrophic calcifications, consistent with pleomorphic adenoma

may be present with a low attenuation of 10–18 H. Rarely, focal calcification may be seen. Conversely, high-grade lesions are poorly circumscribed with indistinct infiltrative borders on CT and MRI. If a malignant mixed tumor (carcinoma ex-pleomorphic adenoma) is present, it may look like a large pleomorphic adenoma with no CT evidence of malignancy, or like a benign mixed tumor with an aggressive tumor appearance in a portion of the lesion (necrotic center, thick and irregular walls, and infiltrating margins), or may appear entirely aggressive with no remaining evidence of any benign pleomorphic adenoma (Fig. 21.10a–c). Similar findings may be observed on MRI; however, if a necrotic, thick-walled area is present, it may be poorly represented. Salivary gland primary lymphoma is very rare and this diagnosis can only be made if there is histologic proof of lymphoma in the salivary parenchyma, without any evidence of intra- or extraglandular nodal involvement. In contrast, the presence of lymph node metastases associated with a salivary tumor is highly suspicious for a high-grade cancer (Fig. 21.11a, b). Secondary involvement of the salivary glands is also rare with an estimated incidence of 1–8% of all cases of lymphoma. The CT appearance of secondary lymphoma varies with the pathologic distribution of the disease. Most commonly, the lymphoma is confined to the periglandular nodes, and one or multiple benign masses are identified in the submandibular triangle. Each node is homogeneous and may enhance slightly on postcontrast CT scans. If the parenchyma is involved, a diffuse infiltration will be seen either with poorly defined margins or involving the entire gland. On MRI, the lymphoma has homogeneous intermediate signal intensity on all imaging sequences. In patients with Hodgkin's disease, on CT

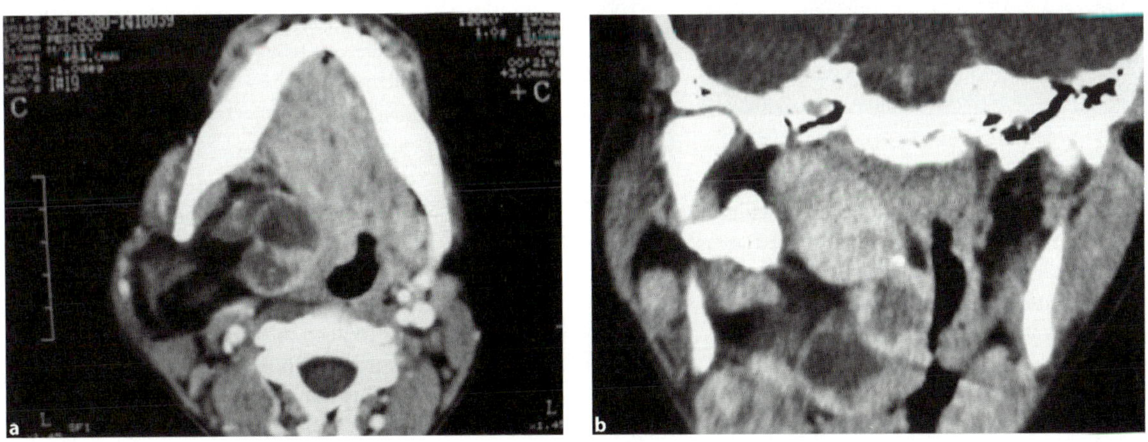

Fig. 21.9: Neurofibromatosis of submandibular region. Axial (**a**) and coronal (**b**) CT scans demonstrate rim-enhancing lesions in close relationship with the mandible, occupying the submandibular, sublingual, and parapharyngeal spaces causing distortion of the oropharynx

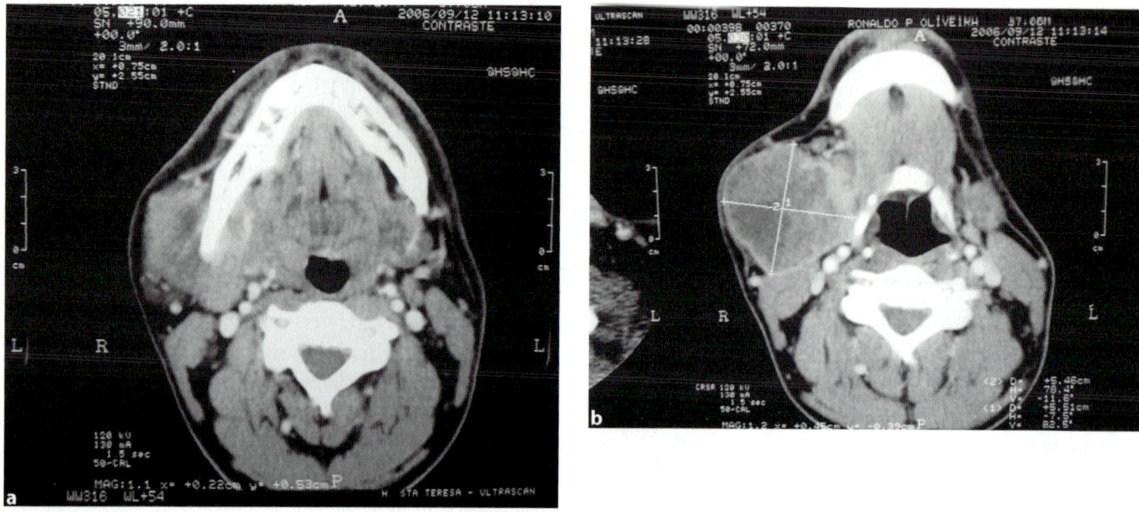

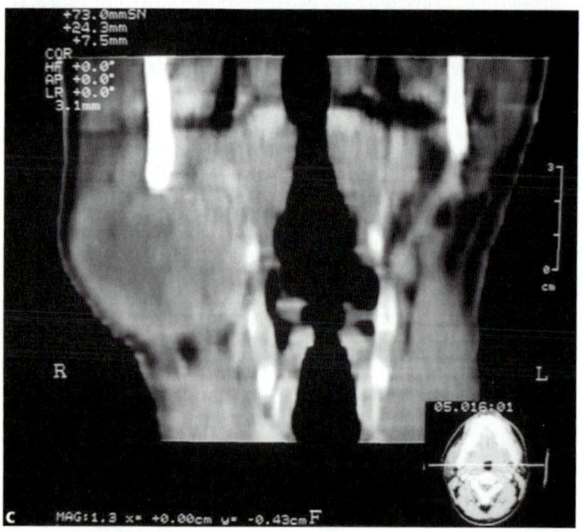

Fig. 21.10: CT scan (axial view) demonstrates a right submandibular mass consistent with a mucoepidermoid carcinoma, involving the subcutaneous tissue and the mandible (**a**), with central necrosis and measuring 7.5 × 5 cm (**b**). CT scan (coronal view) shows the inferior extension of the tumor (**c**)

the nodes may be nonhomogeneous with some sites of enhancement intermixed with scattered areas of low attenuation. This nonhomogeneity can also be seen on MRI of an adenoid cystic carcinoma of the right sublingual gland [28–30] (Fig. 21.12a–d).

Staging

Staging of cancer of the salivary glands is essential for treatment planning and comparison of results. As in other head and neck malignancies, staging of salivary gland tumors considers clinical variables of tumor size, presence or absence of local extension, regional lymph node status, and presence or absence of distant metastases (Tables 21.3, 21.4). This staging system for the major salivary glands includes the parotid, submandibular, and sublingual glands. To keep the classification scheme simple, yet effective, only two clinical variables are used in the assignment of T status: tumor size and local extension of tumor. Absence of local extension is distinguished from the presence of local extension by clinical macroscopic evidence of invasion of skin, soft tissues, bone, or nerve. Staging of regional nodal status (N) and distant metastases (M) is the same for salivary gland cancer as it is for other head and neck mucosal malignancies [10].

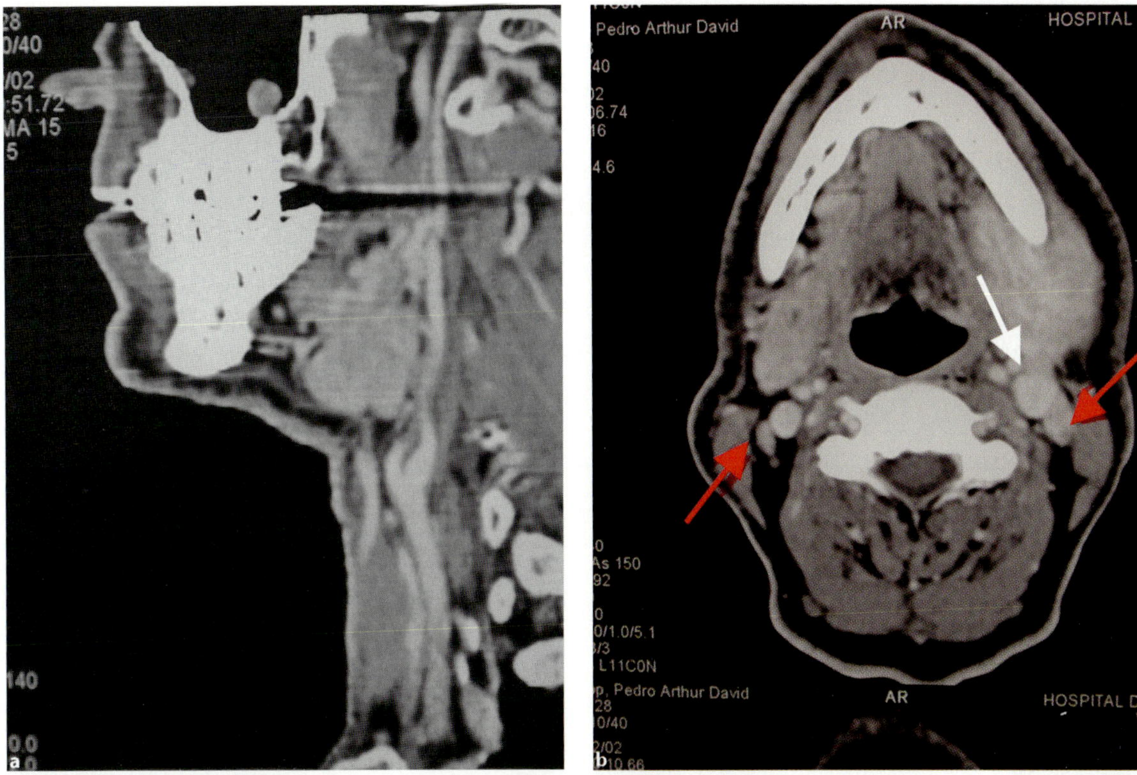

Fig. 21.11: CT scan (sagittal view, **a**) revealing a heterogeneous tumor, with irregular borders, occupying the submandibular area. On axial view (**b**), the tumor reveals its aggressiveness involving the mandible, and invading the sublingual space and the jugular vein (*white arrow*). Bilateral lymph node metastases to levels II (high jugular chain) can also be seen (*red arrows*)

Cytopathologic Diagnosis

Cytologic diagnosis can be established by a fine-needle aspiration biopsy. Aspiration with a no. 21 gauge needle is usually satisfactory in securing tissue for accurate diagnosis. Cytopathologic diagnosis is accurate in over 90–95% of patients in experienced hands [31]. There is a significant potential advantage of using fine-needle aspiration to identify the histology of tumors prior to the initial surgical extirpation of the gland. If the histopathologic type can be determined preoperatively, this information may be used to determine the extent of surgical procedure (with or without neck dissection). In cases of submucosal tumors located on the lateral aspect of the floor of mouth, a transoral fine-needle aspiration biopsy may be employed in order to plan therapy accordingly, especially if malignancy is suspected. High-grade cancers such as adenocarcinomas and squamous cell carcinomas of major salivary glands should be considered for neck dissection based on significant increased rates of occult lymph node metastases. Conversely, sarcomas, adenoid cystic carcinoma, and other histologic types which are unlikely to involve nodal disease may not benefit from elective treatment of the neck [32]. Management of the neck is addressed by Gendron and Ferris in Chapter 25. Diagnosis of pleomorphic adenoma poses no difficulties in cytopathologic specimens. Aspirates from pleomorphic adenoma are highly cellular containing both myxocartilaginous stroma and large sheets or small aggregates of epithelial cells. Individual epithelial cells have uniform, small nuclei and inconspicuous nucleoli. A transition between the epithelial and stromal tissue is quite characteristic of pleomorphic adenoma [33]. The typical aspirate from Warthin's tumor, however, contains oncocytes with abundant granular cytoplasm in an amorphous and granular background. This cytologic "picture" can be accompanied by lymphocytes, histiocytes,

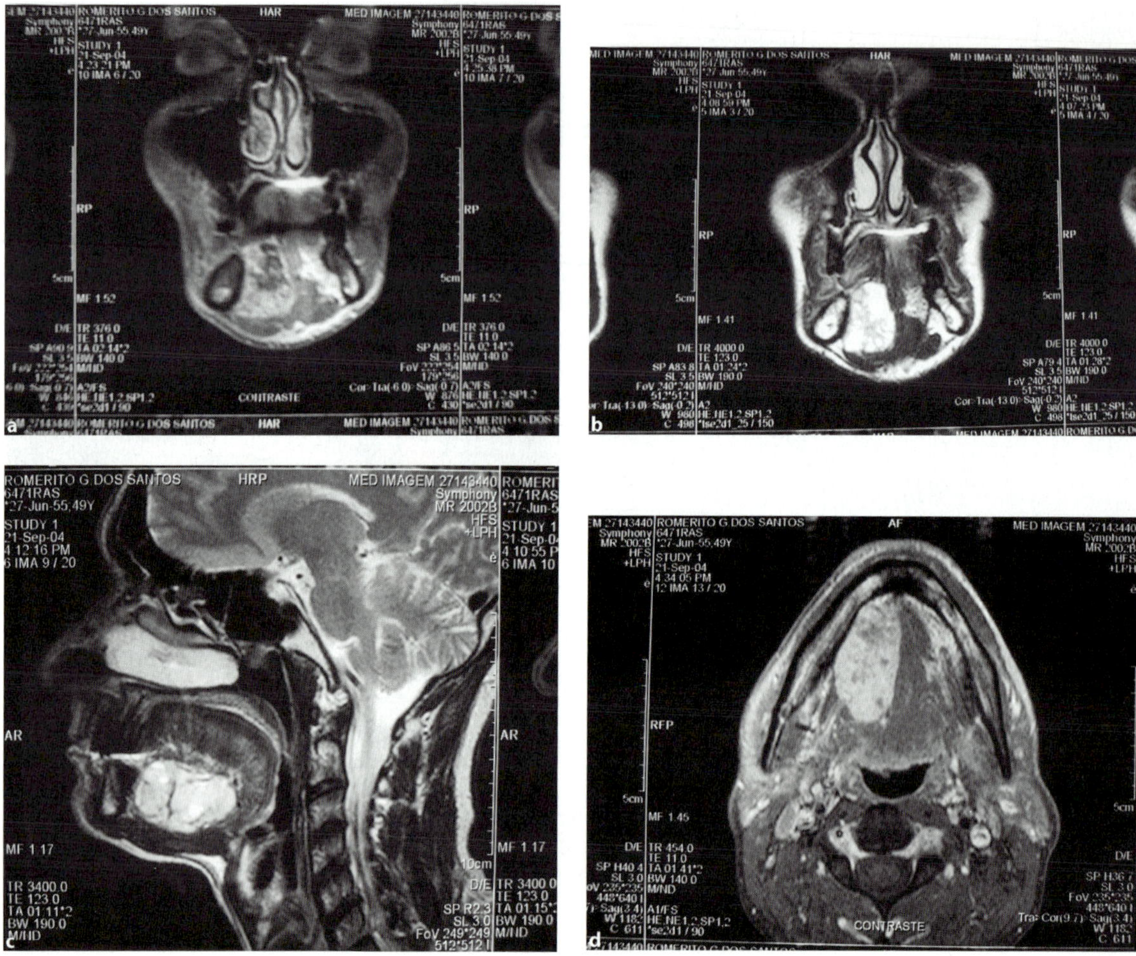

Fig. 21.12: T1-weighted coronal MRI images (with and without contrast) of a heterogeneous sublingual mass in close relationship with the inner part of the mandible (**a**) and involving the suprahyoid muscles (**b**). T2-weighted sagittal MRI images revealing its higher anteroposterior diameter (**c**). T1-weighted axial MRI revealing the relationship of the tumor and the lingual muscles, consistent with an adenoid cystic carcinoma of the right sublingual gland (**d**)

and tingible body macrophages. Because these tumors are frequently cystic, smears may be acellular, giving rise to a false-negative diagnosis [34]. The typical aspirate from adenoid cystic carcinoma contains spherical hyaline globules of basement membrane-like material, sharply demarcated from the surrounding small cuboidal epithelial cells [35]. In high-grade tumors the epithelial cells show nuclear features of malignancy, while in low-grade tumors cells with scant cytoplasm and a round or oval nucleus with a small nucleolus are present. Epidermoid cells, mucin-producing cells, and intermediate cells present in a dirty background of mucus and debris are more likely to be a mucoepidermoid carcinoma. Several aspirates may be necessary to reach the correct diagnosis. Papanicolau's PAS and mucicarmine stains are useful in confirming the keratinizing or mucoid character of the cells [34].

Treatment of Benign Tumors

The need for extension of a resection beyond removal of the gland, including the adjacent structures, depends on the preoperative assessment as well as the findings at the time of surgery. Weber and associates recommend that

Table 21.3. Staging system for major salivary gland malignancy [2, 17]

Primary tumor (T)	
TX	Primary tumor cannot be assessed
T0	No evidence of primary tumor
T1	Tumor 2 cm or less in greatest dimension without extraparenchymal extension[a]
T2	Tumor more than 2 cm but not more than 4 cm in greatest diameter without extraparenchymal extension
T3	Tumor more than 4 cm and/or having extraparenchymal extension
T4a	Tumor invades skin, mandible, ear canal, and/or seventh nerve
T4b	Tumor invades base of skull, pterygoid plates, and/or carotid artery
Regional lymph nodes (N)	
NX	Regional lymph nodes cannot be assessed
N0	No regional lymph node metastases
N1	Metastases in a single ipsilateral lymph node, 3 cm or less greatest dimension
N2	Metastases in a single ipsilateral lymph node, more than 3 cm but not more than 6 cm in greatest dimension, or in multiple ipsilateral lymph nodes, none more than 6 cm in greatest dimension, or in bilateral or in contralateral lymph nodes, none more than 6 cm in greatest dimension
N2a	Metastases in a single ipsilateral lymph node more than 3 cm but not more than 6 cm in greatest dimension
N2b	Metastases in multiple ipsilateral lymph nodes, none more than 6 cm in greatest dimension
N2c	Metastases in bilateral or contralateral lymph nodes, none more than 6 cm in greatest dimension
N3	Metastases in lymph node more than 6 cm in greatest dimension
Distant metastases (M)	
MX	Distant metastases cannot be assessed
M0	No distant metastases
M1	Distant metastases

[a] Extraparenchymalextension is characterized by clinical/macroscopic evidence of soft tissue/nerve invasion, with the exception of those structures listed in T4a and b. Focal microscopic extraparenchymal invasion is not considered for T classification

the routine treatment of submandibular gland tumors include a regional dissection of the submandibular triangle to include the submental (level Ia) and submandibular (level Ib) lymph nodes as well as the gland [36]. This so-called level I neck dissection would provide adequate margins in the treatment of benign tumors and also serve to sample lymph nodes adjacent to the gland in the treatment of malignant tumors [36]. Alternatively, a subfascial dissection may be performed to remove the submandibular gland without a cuff of surrounding normal tissue in cases of benign diseases such as small benign neoplasms (completely included in the parenchyma of the gland) and sialolithiasis or sialadenitis refractory to conservative management. This approach is performed more rapidly and is associated with a lower chance of complication.

Treatment of Recurrent Pleomorphic Adenoma

Local recurrence of a benign mixed tumor of the submandibular gland is a rare event if the initial operation is a complete excision of the submandibular gland. Local recurrence is seen more frequently when the initial

Table 21.4. Stage grouping

Stage	Primary tumor (T)	Regional lymph nodes (N)	Distant metastasis (M)
I	T1	N0	M0
II	T2	N0	M0
III	T3	N0	M0
	T1, T2, T3	N1	M0
IVA	T1, T2, T3	N2	M0
	T4a	N0, N1, N2	M0
IVB	T4b	Any N	M0
	Any T	N3	M0
IVC	Any T	Any N	M1

operation is enucleation or when there is spillage of the tumor during the surgical procedure. These tumors are also called "semi-malignant growths" because of their tendency for recurrence and risk of malignant degeneration [37, 38]. Large series published in the literature have found rates of malignant transformation to be significantly less than 10% [39, 40]. Friedrich et al. analyzing 94 patients with recurrent pleomorphic adenomas found most of the cases in the parotid gland (77.6%) and rarely in other glands [41]. Malignant transformation was noticed in 8.5% of patients.

Local recurrence of a benign mixed tumor may occur in a unifocal or a multifocal fashion (Fig. 21.13). Interestingly, unifocal recurrence is usually seen after incomplete removal of the tumor and multifocal recurrence after the resection of the entire gland. Preparation for reoperation should include a review of the previous operative notes and pathology report, as well as an MRI or CT scan. The operative procedure is relatively easy in unifocal recurrences in comparison with multifocal recurrences. In unifocal type of recurrence, completion of the resection of the gland and tumor associated with dissection of level I is the treatment of choice, but in multifocal recurrence the procedure of level I dissection is technically difficult with significant risk of injury to the mandibular branch of the facial nerve. Usually the skin overlying the multiple foci of recurrence must be excised with the surgical specimen. A slow and meticulous approach to the nerve, helped by electrical monitoring and magnification with loupes or microscope is advisable [42, 43]. Niparko and coworkers reviewed the charts of 48 patients with recurrent pleomorphic adenoma who had been treated at the

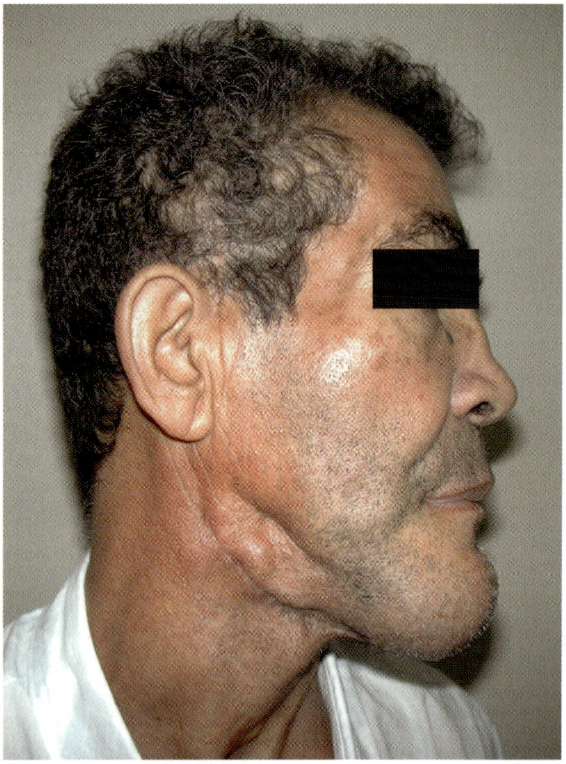

Fig. 21.13: Multiple recurrences of pleomorphic adenoma of the right submandibular gland after an incomplete excision. Observe the multiple foci of recurrence typical of this particular situation

University of Michigan over a 40-year period ending in 1975 [40]. They found recurrences developing at an average of 6.1 years after initial treatment, which is similar to the 7.7- and 9.4-year intervals cited by Fee et al. and Dawson and Orr [39, 44]. Recurrences of pleomorphic adenomas after reoperations can be high. Control rates for retreatment were 14% for 21 patients treated with simple re-excision of the tumor, 38% for 8 patients treated with superficial parotidectomy, 54% for 13 patients treated with total parotidectomy with facial preservation, and 50% for patients who underwent total parotidectomy with facial nerve sacrifice. The high rates of recurrence reported by Niparko and coworkers may reflect expectations of treatment of recurrent pleomorphic adenomas [40]. A more aggressive approach is recommended by some authors, who included postoperative radiotherapy for positive margins, intraoperative tumor spill, and multiple recurrences [45–47]. According to Dawson and Orr [44], re-excision of the recurrence in 28 patients coupled with postoperative radiotherapy resulted in a control rate of 90% for those treated for a first recurrence compared with 50% for those treated for a second recurrence. These controls reflect higher control rates than those reported by others who use surgery alone for treatment of recurrences. Fee and coworkers reported a control rate of 65% for first recurrences and a control rate of 29% for second recurrences with surgery alone [39]. Based on these findings, Dawson and Orr suggested that radiotherapy should be used in patients with second or subsequent recurrences, and in cases in which the tumor has been removed in a piecemeal fashion or residual tumor has been left after surgery [44]. More recently, Douglas et al. published their experience with neutron radiotherapy for recurrent pleomorphic adenomas of major salivary glands. They found an actuarial 15-year locoregional control of 76% for patients with gross residual disease versus 100% for those with microscopic disease with acceptable treatment-related morbidity. Malignant transformation and metastases were uncommon [47].

Surgical Technique: Excision of the Submandibular Gland

The patient is placed on the operating table under general endotracheal anesthesia in a supine position with the neck turned to the opposite side. Marking the skin surface over the angle of the mandible and the submandibular gland is helpful to facilitate the positioning of the line of incision. The skin incision is placed in an upper neck skin crease at least two fingerbreadths below the angle of the mandible to protect the mandibular branch of the facial nerve. As stated earlier in this chapter, the nerve is two fingerbreadths below the angle of the mandible and two fingerbreadths anterior to the angle of the mandible. It runs parallel to the mandibular rim 1–2.5 cm caudally for about 3 cm lying over the surface of the submandibular gland. The skin incision is completed and the platysma muscle is exposed along the length of the incision and then incised and elevated with the overlying skin, up to the level of the lower border of the mandible. The dissection must be carried out close to the inner aspect of the platysma muscle in order to avoid injury of the nerve. At this point, a careful identification, dissection, and preservation of the mandibular branch of the facial nerve which directly overlies the submandibular gland is undertaken. Identification of the posterior facial artery, which is a good landmark to find the nerve, can help to identify the nerve. The vein usually runs almost parallel to the cervical branch of the facial nerve. Both of these structures are divided to facilitate retraction/protection of the mandibular branch cephalad along with the upper skin flap. This is due to the fact that the posterior facial vein lies deep to the mandibular branch of the facial nerve, thus dividing the vein low and retracting its upper stump cephalad will protect the already dissected and mobilized nerve on the upper skin flap. This surgical maneuver is known as "Hayes Martin maneuver."

The gland is now retracted inferiorly, exposing the anterior belly of the digastric muscle in the submental region. During this dissection, small blood vessels overlying the anterior belly of the digastric and the mylohyoid muscles are divided, to gain further exposure of the underlying mylohyoid muscle. The nerve and vessels to the mylohyoid muscle lying over it are individually clamped, divided, and ligated. The facial artery and vein on the posterior aspect of the gland proceeding toward the body of the mandible are dissected next. In most cases the facial artery must be individually clamped, divided, and ligated with the facial vein as well. Division of the facial vessels allows caudal retraction of the submandibular gland, providing full exposure of the underlying mylohyoid muscle.

With the mylohyoid muscle retracted toward the chin of the patient and the submandibular gland gently retracted to the opposite side, the undersurface of the floor of the mouth is brought into view and it is then possible to identify the secretomotor fibers to the submandibular gland as they come off the lingual nerve, as well as Wharton's duct with accessory salivary tissue along the duct. The submandibular ganglion and the secretomotor fibers of the lingual nerve are clamped, divided, and ligated. The remaining attachments of the submandibular gland are Wharton's duct and the vessels running along with it and the proximal part of the facial artery and vein. Wharton's duct is isolated and divided as close as possible to the floor of the mouth. During this dissection , the hypoglossal nerve is seen in a deeper plane to Wharton's duct and should be carefully protected. Further traction of the gland exposes the proximal part of the facial artery deep to the posterior belly of the digastric muscle. It is carefully dissected, clamped, and divided as well as its venae comitantes, when present. After the removal of the surgical specimen, meticulous hemostasis is obtained followed by irrigation with saline solution. A single suction drain is inserted and the wound is closed in layers (Fig. 21.14a–f).

Surgical Technique: Excision of the Sublingual Gland

Different approaches for treating ranulas have been described in the literature according to the different concepts regarding pathogenesis, such as simple incision, cyst extirpation, marsupialization, and excision of sublingual gland [12–15, 48, 49]. Yoshimura et al. [48] compared three methods of ranula treatment in 27 patients, with a recurrence rate of 25% with excision of ranula only, 36% with marsupialization, and 0% with ranula and ipsilateral sublingual excision only. Crysdale et al.'s [49] comparative study in children showed a recurrence rate of 0% with excision of ranula only, 61% with marsupialization, and 0% with ranula and ipsilateral sublingual gland excision. Although extirpation of ranulas themselves was not considered to be essential, since most ranulas are pseudocysts without epithelial lining, excision of the affected sublingual gland has been mostly recommended [12–15, 48, 49].

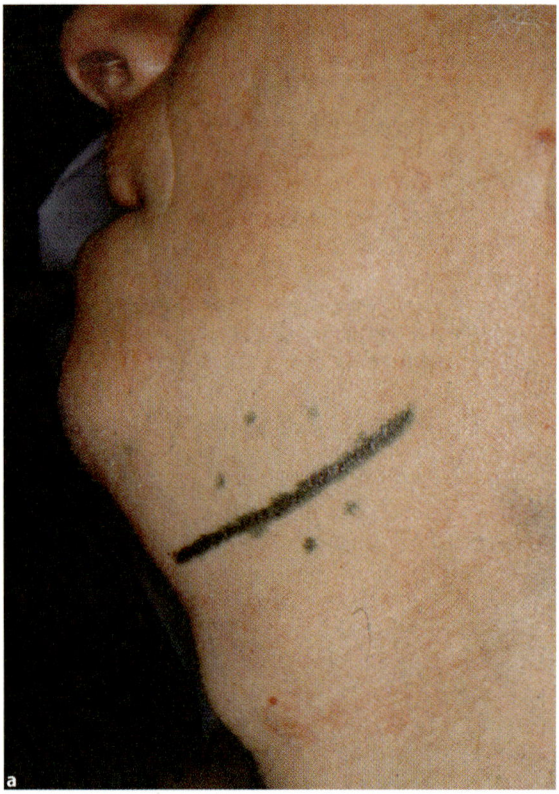

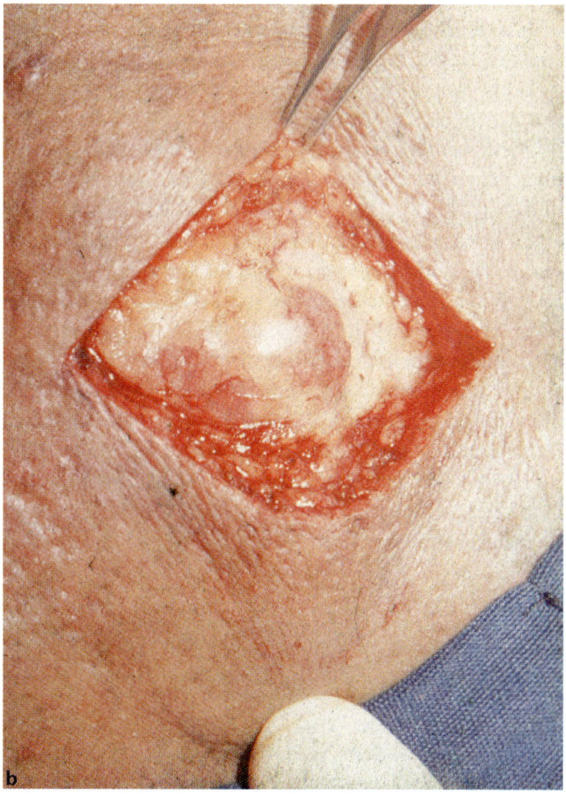

Fig. 21.14a–f: Excision of the right (left) submandibular gland. **a** The skin incision is placed at two fingerbreadths below the angle of the mandible. **b** The skin flaps are elevated and the submandibular gland exposed. **c–f** *(see next page)*

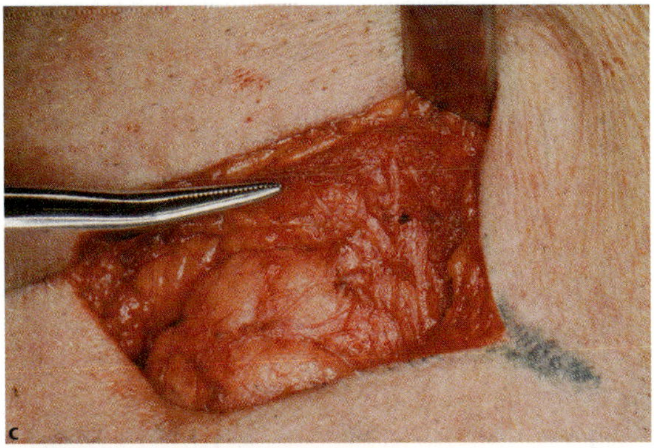

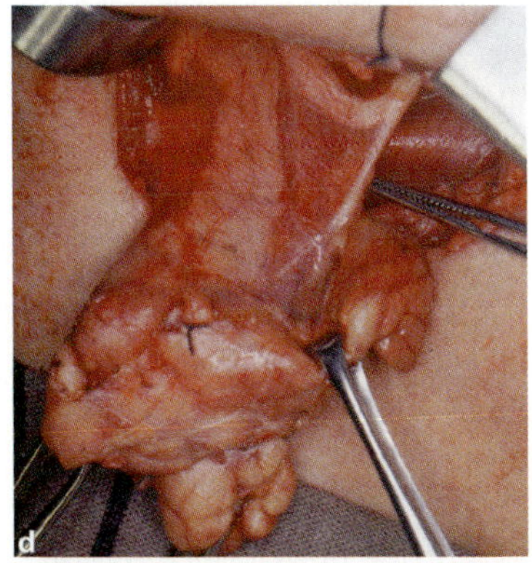

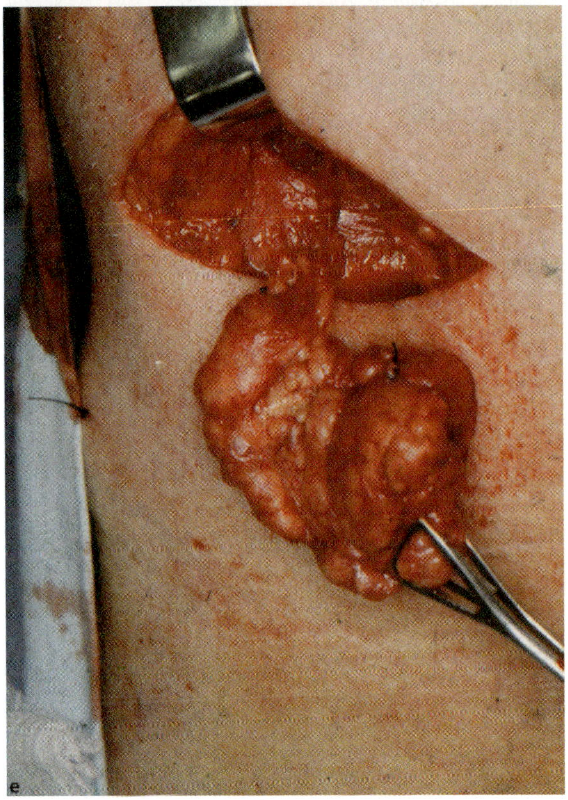

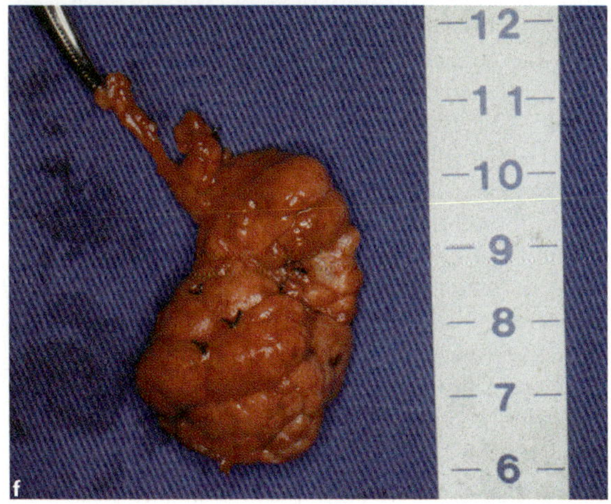

Fig. 21.14a–f: *(continued)* **c** Identification of the mandibular branch of the facial nerve. **d** Identification of the submandibular ganglion and the secretomotor fibers of the lingual nerve. **e** The gland is completely dissected from the submandibular area except by its duct. **f** Surgical specimen including the submandibular gland as well as its salivary duct

The excision of a ranula can be achieved through the oral cavity, with the patient under general anesthesia and nasotracheal intubation. The oral cavity is exposed and opened with a self-retaining mouth retractor. Packing the oropharynx with a humid gauze bolster is also advisable to prevent aspiration during the procedure. An elliptical incision is then made over the curve of the cystic swelling in the floor of the mouth. The mucosal flaps are grasped with mosquito forceps and retracted during exposure of the ranula. The incision is extended anteriorly and posteriorly. The mucosal flap over the cyst is carefully freed from the ranula, both by blunt and sharp dissection with the scissor. The cystic swelling is now grasped with serrated forceps and freed from Wharton's duct by blunt dissection. The cyst is now free from the connective tissue and from its connections with the underlying mylohyoid muscle. All small vessels in the field are sealed with bipolar coagulation forceps. After removing the ranula together with the sublingual gland, the undamaged lingual nerve can be seen lying on the floor of the mouth next to Wharton's duct. After careful hemostasis, the wound is irrigated with saline solution. The mucosa is closed with 3-0 Vicryl sutures. Frequent oral irrigations and rinses with oral antiseptic solutions are advisable to maintain optimal oral hygiene. Feeding by mouth starts with clear liquids and pureed foods (Fig. 21.15a–d).

Treatment of Malignant Tumors

Management of major salivary gland cancers is particularly challenging due to their relative rarity in conjunction with the variety of histologic types and grades. Malignant neoplasms of the submandibular and sublingual glands can be classified into three major categories: (1) tumors of epithelial origin (mucoepidermoid carcinoma, adenoid cystic carcinoma, acinic cell carcinoma, malignant mixed tumor, squamous cell carcinoma, salivary duct carcinoma, etc.); (2) tumors of non-epithelial origin (sarcomas, lymphomas); and (3) secondary tumors. Comprehensive management of these tumors includes definitive treatment of the primary tumor and treatment (therapeutic or elective) of the neck; eventually, only neck observation is advised, as many neoplasms have a low propensity for lymphatic spread. The general guidelines for treatment of submandibular gland cancer are shown in Table 21.5.

Patterns of Spread

Malignant tumors that extend through the capsule of the submandibular gland usually involve the adjacent mandible, invade the mylohyoid muscle and, eventually, the tongue, as well as the lingual and hypoglossal nerves.

Table 21.5. General guidelines for treatment of submandibular gland cancer

	T1 and T2 (N0) Low grade	T1 and T2 (N0 and N1) High grade	T3 and T4 (N0 and N+) Any grade
Tumor type:	Mucoepidermoid (low grade)	Mucoepidermoid (high grade)	Any histologic type
	Acinic cell (low grade)	Acinic cell (high grade)	
	Adenocarcinoma (low grade)	Adenocarcinoma (high grade)	
		Adenoid cystic	
		Ex-pleomorphic adenoma	
		Salivary duct	
		Squamous cell carcinoma	
Treatment:	Level I neck dissection	Supraomohyoid neck dissection (N0)	Supraomohyoid neck dissection (N0)
		Comprehensive neck dissection (N+)	Comprehensive neck dissection (N+)
		Postoperative radiotherapy	Postoperative radiotherapy

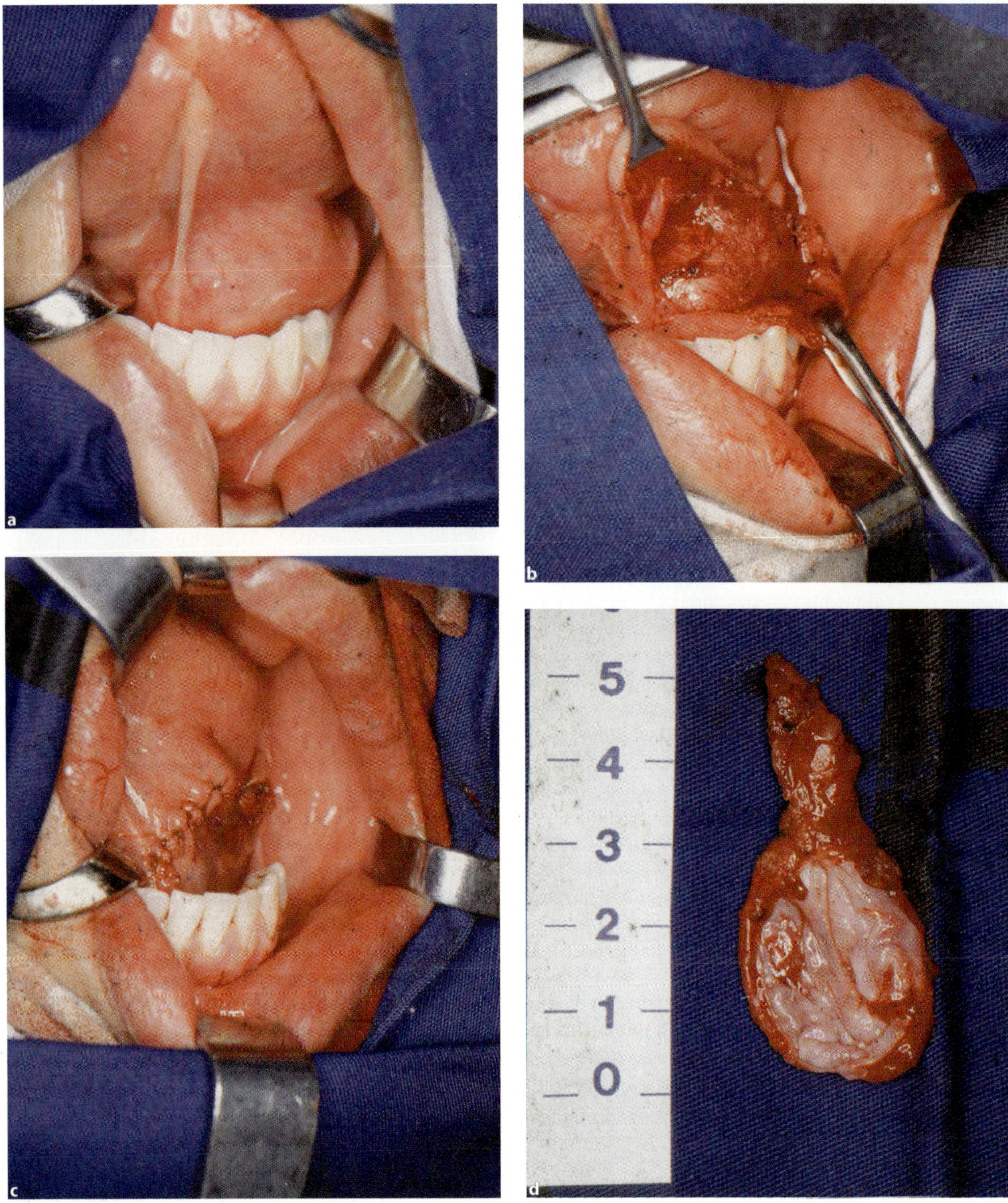

Fig. 21.15: Excision of ranula. **a** Clinical aspect of ranula seen through the mouth. **b** Dissection from the mucosa of the floor of the mouth. **c** Aspect of the floor of the mouth after excision of ranula. **d** Surgical specimen revealing the epithelial lining typical of ranula (true cyst)

Moderate to severe pain is usually associated with advanced tumors, while nerve deficits involving cranial nerves V, VII, and VII can be found in 14% of patients with carcinomas [22, 23]. Extension to the oral cavity is not frequent, but can occur in advanced cases. Skin invasion and, eventually ulceration, occur more frequently in advanced cases with extension through the capsule.

Factors Influencing Selection of Therapy

The size of the primary tumor and histologic grade are the most important tumor factors affecting choice of initial therapy. Clinical (advanced stage and submandibular site) and histologic (higher cancer grade, presence of perineural invasion, presence of lymph node metastases) parameters are considered independent predictors of poorer clinical outcome in most series of major salivary gland malignant tumors published in the literature [9, 19, 20, 23, 36, 50–56]. Vander Poorten et al. [19] found that age at diagnosis ($p = .0006$), T stage ($p = .001$), and clinical skin invasion ($p = .005$) were the most significant predictors of poor survival among his patients. Interestingly, Hocwald et al. [56] found evidence that older patients tend to have a higher incidence of more aggressive tumors in comparison with younger patients (79% versus 56%, respectively). They also observed that men tended to present with higher T stage tumors at diagnosis than did women, 53% compared with 26% ($p = .02$). Using the Surveillance, Epidemiology and End Results (SEER) database for the period of 1988 to 1998, Bhattacharyya [20] identified patients with younger age, decreased tumor grade, and the addition of radiation therapy as factors associated with improved survival ($p < .001$, .005, and .015, respectively) in his series. Factors predicting tumor recurrence in most series include higher TNM stages, perineural growth, and lymph node metastases [9, 10, 19, 20, 23, 36, 50, 56].

Often, most of the clinical variables required to predict survival can be obtained before definitive surgery. Based on findings of clinical evaluation, MRI, and fine-needle aspiration biopsy, patients may be counseled as to surgical approach, need for neck dissection, and need for postoperative radiotherapy.

21

Low-grade, low-stage malignant salivary tumors can be treated by excision of the submandibular gland with dissection of level I. High-grade, high-stage tumors, however, require supraomohyoid neck dissection, in conjunction with the excision of the submandibular gland. When necessary, more radical local resection and neck dissection is indicated for the treatment of advanced (locoregional) submandibular tumors [10, 22, 23, 36, 37]. It is important to mention that the morbidity secondary to sacrifice of hypoglossal, lingual, and marginal branch of the facial nerves is better tolerated than that after loss of the entire facial nerve (Fig. 21.16a–d). Reconstruction with regional, and sometimes microvascular free-flaps, may be necessary (Fig. 21.17a–d). In order to improve local and regional control, adjuvant postoperative radiotherapy may be indicated in selected cases. High-grade malignancies, recurrent tumors, gross or microscopic residual disease, tumor adjacent to the nerves, regional nodal metastases, and invasion of muscle, bone, skin, or nerve are all strong indications for postoperative radiotherapy [50–55]. Advanced unresectable tumors are generally treated by radiotherapy with palliative intent. Treatment with neutron beam therapy is of particular value for adenoid cystic carcinomas.

Surgical Technique for Malignant Submandibular Tumors: Level I Neck Dissection

The patient is placed on the operating table under general endotracheal anesthesia in a supine position with the neck turned to the opposite side. An incision is made approximately 3–4 cm (two fingerbreadths) below the angle of the mandible to protect the mandibular branch of the facial nerve, in a skin crease if possible. The platysma muscle is exposed along the length of the incision and then incised and elevated with the overlying skin up to the level of the lower border of the mandible. The dissection must be carried out close to the inner aspect of the platysma muscle in order to avoid injury to the nerve. At that point a careful identification, dissection, and preservation of the mandibular branch of the facial nerve is performed. As stated in the anatomy section of this chapter, one of the most constant landmarks to locate the nerve is the mandibular angle, usually situated 2–5 mm cranially. The nerve runs parallel to the mandibular rim 1–2.5 cm caudally for about 3 cm, turning cranially toward the oral commissure. Similarly, one may elect to identify the posterior facial vein first, which has a close anatomic relationship with the nerve, located perpendicularly around the middle third of the mandibular body. The vein is divided and its stump used to retract the mandibular branch of the facial nerve (Hayes Martin maneuver).

Dissection now proceeds along the lower border of the body of the mandible. Mobilization of the soft tis-

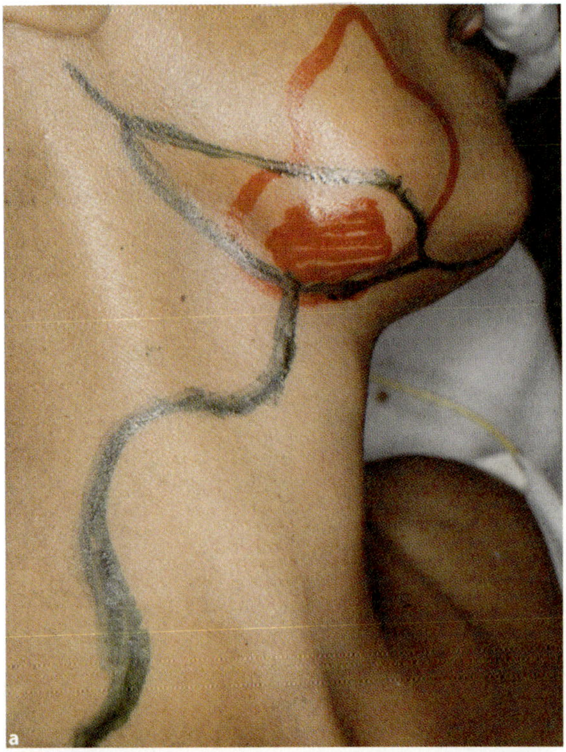

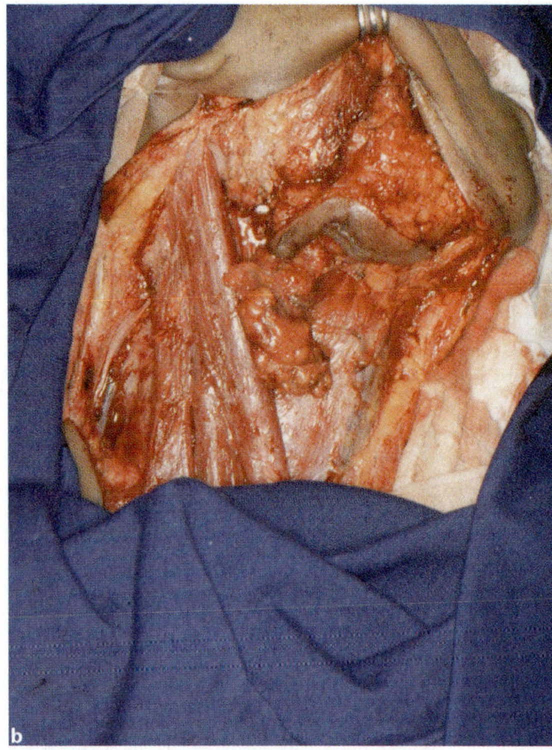

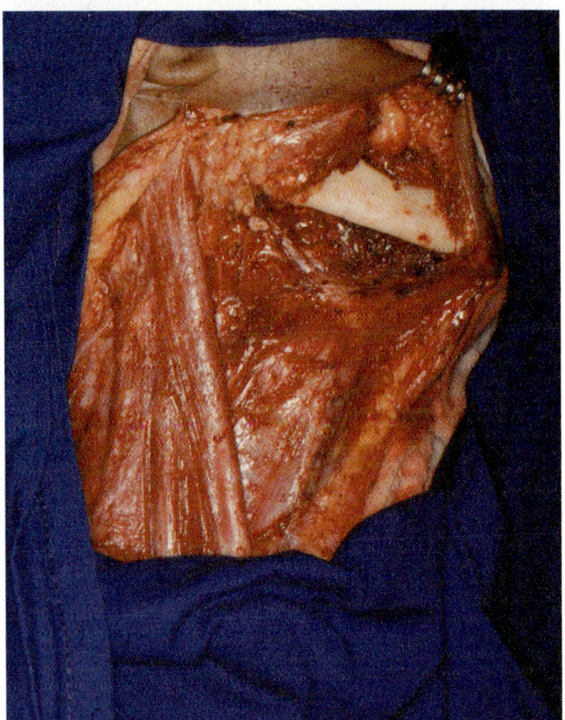

Fig. 21.16a–d: Excision of adenoid cystic carcinoma of the submandibular gland with supraomohyoid neck dissection (SOHND). **a** Aspect of the incision with the inclusion of the skin overlying the tumor and the extension to the neck. **b** Excision "en bloc" of primary tumor and surgical specimen of the neck dissection. **c** Aspect of the surgical field after the resection. The periosteum of the mandible was included in the surgical specimen. **d** *(see next page)*

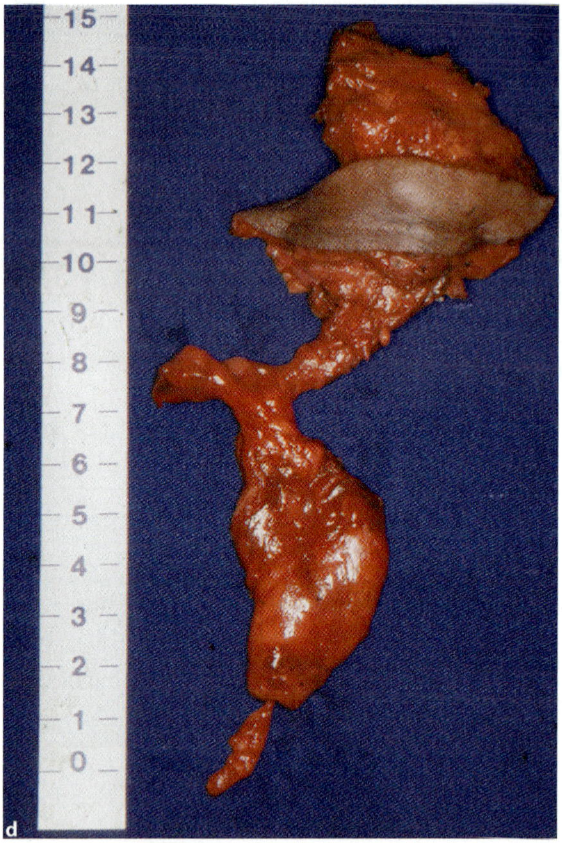

Fig. 21.16a–d: *(continued)* **d** Surgical specimen including the skin overlying the submandibular gland

sues along the lower border of the body of the mandible exposes the prevascular facial lymph nodes, which are carefully dissected and maintained in continuity with the rest of the specimen. The facial artery and its accompanying veins adjacent to those nodes are divided between clamps and ligated. The fascial attachments between the sternomastoid muscle and the angle of the mandible are divided at this time. Dissection continues anteriorly along the lower border of the body of the mandible up to the attachment of the anterior belly of the digastric muscle. At this point, brisk hemorrhage is expected from several vessels that provide blood supply to the anterior belly of the digastric muscle and the mylohyoid muscle. The nerve and vessels to the mylohyoid muscle, which enter parallel to each other in a fascial envelope, must be sacrificed at this moment. After the ligation and division of the nerve and vessels, the muscle comes into full view.

With the mylohyoid muscle retracted medially toward the chin of the patient, and the submandibular gland gently retracted to the opposite side, the undersurface of the floor of the mouth is brought into a view and it is possible to identify the secretomotor fibers to the submandibular gland as they come off the lingual nerve, as well as Wharton's duct with accessory salivary tissue along the duct. At this point, alternate blunt and sharp dissection is necessary to clearly identify Wharton's duct and the lingual and hypoglossal nerves on the floor of the mouth as they enter the tongue. Once the lingual nerve is clearly identified, the secretomotor fibers to the mandibular gland are divided. There is usually a small blood vessel accompanying this nerve so it is divided between clamps and ligated. Similarly, Wharton's duct is divided between clamps and its distal stump ligated.

The entire submandibular gland is now retracted posteroinferiorly, and loose areolar tissue between the gland

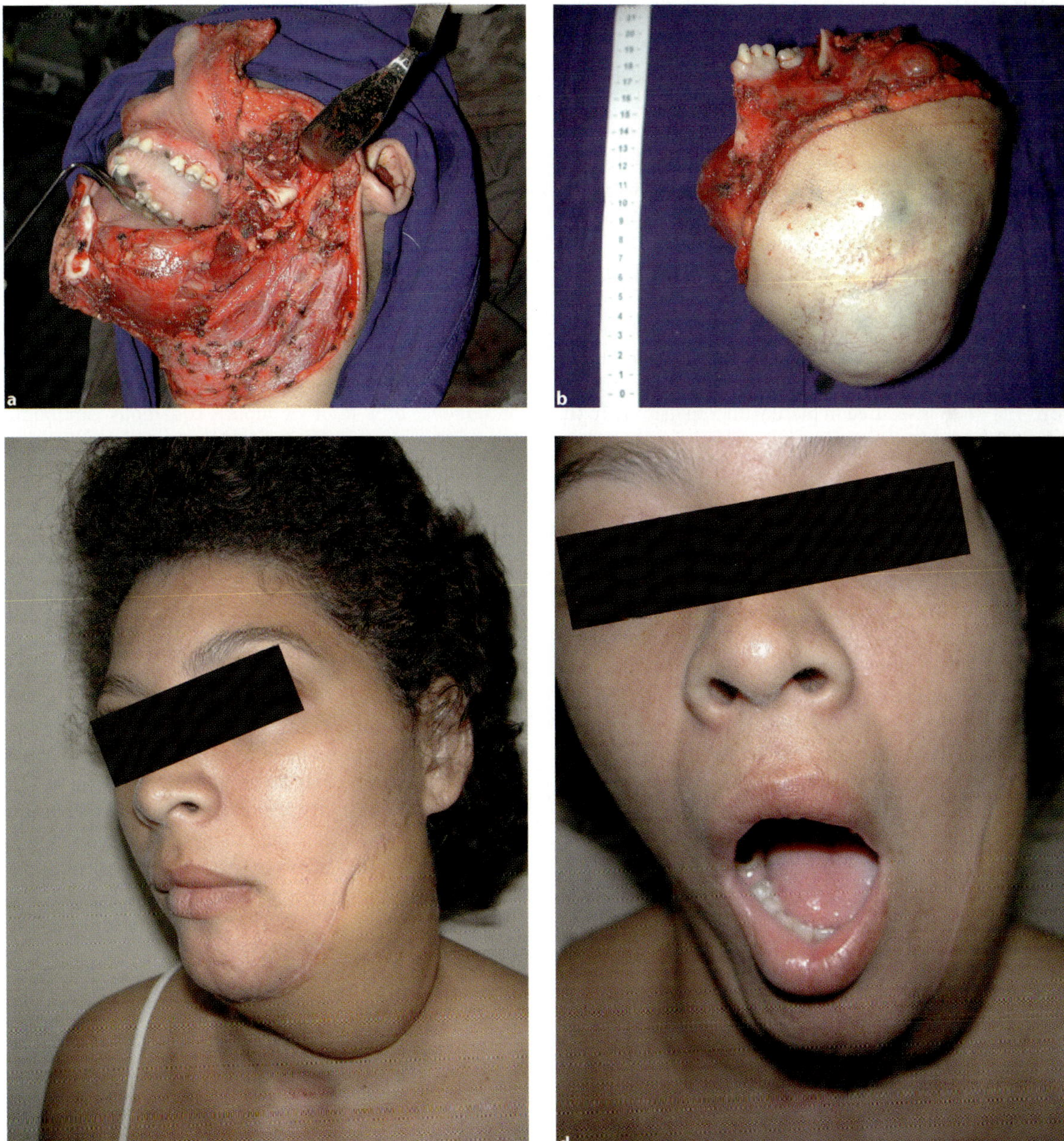

Fig. 21.17: Excision of an extensive recurrent adenoid cystic carcinoma of the left submandibular gland. **a** A composite resection including the mandible, soft tissues of the submandibular area, and skin associated with the dissections of levels I–III. **b** Surgical specimen. **c** Final aspect of the patient with emphasis on free flap reconstruction (with rectus abdominis flap). **d** Patient with good rehabilitation after reconstruction

and the digastric muscle is divided. As one approaches the posterior belly of the digastric muscle, the proximal part of the facial artery as it enters the submandibular gland is exposed, divided between clamps, and ligated. The entire contents of the submandibular triangle are now dissected off the operating field. The surgical field following removal of the specimen must show complete clearance of the submandibular triangle, with preservation of the muscles and nerves as stated above (Fig. 21.18). After careful hemostasis, the wound is irrigated with saline solution and a single suction drain is inserted through the posterior edge of the incision. The incision is closed in two layers using 3-0 Vicryl interrupted sutures for platysma and 2-0 nylon intradermal running suture for the skin. The drain is secured in place with a silk suture to the skin at the site of entry.

Excision of a Sublingual Gland Malignant Neoplasm

The treatment of a malignant tumor of the sublingual gland usually includes the removal of the gland with a surrounding cuff of normal tissue (floor of mouth and lateral aspect of the oral tongue). This is due to the fact that the sublingual gland lies directly beneath the mucosal surface of the anterior floor of the mouth, and close to the inner aspect of the mandible. The development of a soft tissue cuff around a malignant tumor confined to the sublingual gland without extraglandular extension can be accomplished through excision of the mucosa (floor of mouth and small segment of tongue), the mylohyoid muscle, and the periosteum of the mandible. A careful bimanual palpation of the floor of the mouth and submental region with the patient under general anesthesia will often reveal its depth as well as its relationship to the surrounding structures. Although a ductoplasty may permit removal of small benign tumors through the oral cavity, most salivary gland cancers arising in the floor of the mouth are done in concert with at least level I neck dissection, thus removing the submandibular gland. More advanced or recurrent cancer of the sublingual gland is likely to require resection of the floor of the mouth along with a partial glossectomy, mandibulectomy, supraomohyoid structures, and the lingual and hypoglossal nerves. The surgical techniques for resection of cancers of the sublingual glands do not differ significantly from those for removal of a floor of mouth squamous carcinoma (Fig. 21.19a–c).

Surgical Technique: Excision of Sublingual Gland Cancer in Association with the Floor of the Mouth and Marginal Mandibulectomy in Continuity with Neck Dissection (Pull-through Operation)

Excision of moderately advanced sublingual malignant tumors usually implies in a wide exposure for access to the primary tumor and its satisfactory resection. A lower cheek flap approach may be indicated depending on the extension of the primary tumor, particularly if a mandibulectomy (marginal or segmental) is needed. The lower cheek flap approach involves splitting the lower lip and the chin in the midline through its full thickness up to the symphysis of the mandible. The incision continues in the

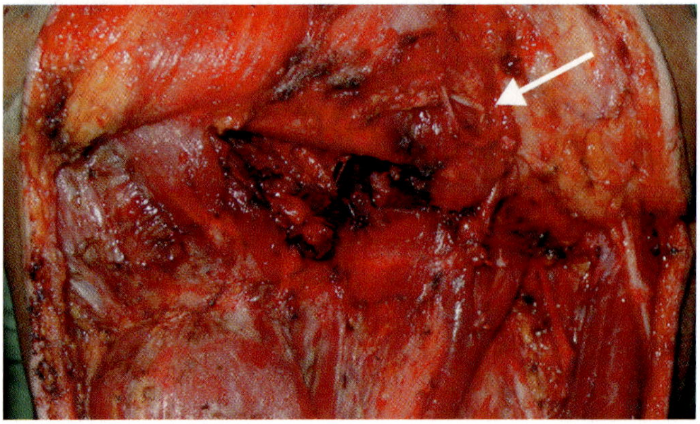

Fig. 21.18: Excision of the submandibular gland and the contents of the submandibular triangle (levels Ia and Ib). *White arrow* points the mandibular branch of the facial nerve dissected and preserved

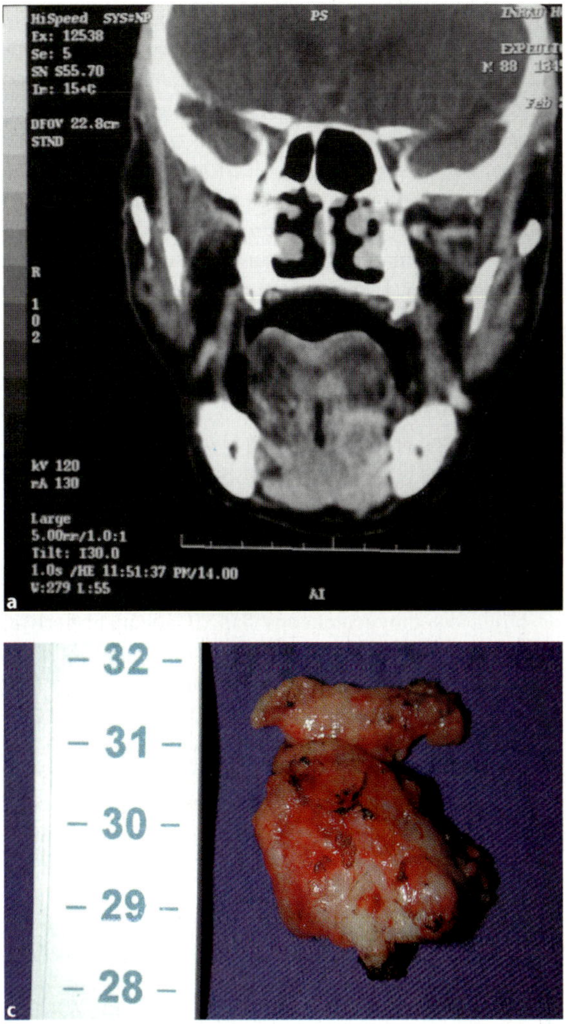

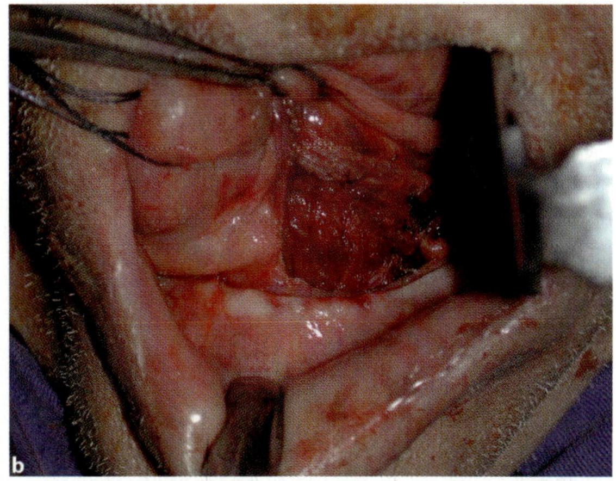

Fig. 21.19: Excision of a sublingual tumor with margins through the mouth. **a** CT scan (coronal view) showing a heterogeneous tumor of the left sublingual gland and its relationship with the muscles of the tongue and floor of the mouth. **b** Aspect of the primary site after resection of sublingual tumor. **c** Surgical specimen

midline up to the thyrohyoid membrane, where it turns toward the ipsilateral neck along an upper skin crease. This transverse component of the incision should be, at least, two fingerbreadths below the body of the mandible to prevent inadvertent injury to the mandibular branch of the facial nerve during elevation of the cheek flap (Fig. 21.20).

The operative procedure planned for a moderately advanced sublingual gland cancer consists of ipsilateral neck dissection (extent of the procedure depends on the presence or absence of lymph node metastases) with resection of the sublingual gland and surrounding tissues (floor of mouth and lateral aspect of the tongue), usually in association with a marginal resection of the mandible. The neck dissection is completed in the usual fashion except for level I, through which the specimen is attached to the primary tumor. All the attachments of the specimen inferior and deep to the digastric tendon are divided at this point. The upper neck flap is already elevated, with careful identification and preservation of the mandibular branch of the facial nerve.

The periosteum of the body of the mandible is exposed, and a close-up view of the primary tumor and its limits with the lingual surface of the mandible and with

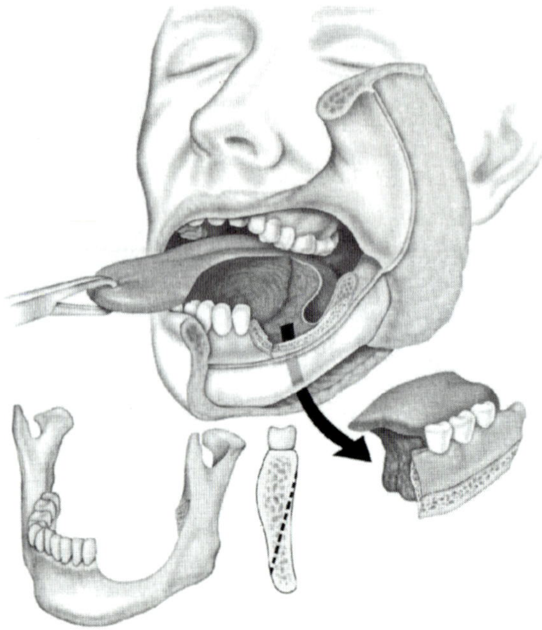

Fig. 21.20: Schematic diagram of excision of a sublingual cancer with partial resection of the anterior and lateral floor of mouth, partial glossectomy, and marginal mandibulectomy through a lower cheek flap. (Dias FL, Lima RA Cancer of the floor of the mouth. In: Myers EN (ed) Surgical Management of Cancer of the Oral Cavity and Oropharynx: Part II. Operative Techniques in Otolaryngology Head and Neck Surgery. 2005; 16 (1): 10-17)

the other intraoral structures facilitates the planning of the three-dimensional resection. In order to outline the extent of intraoral mucosa to be resected, an incision is made in the mucosa of the undersurface of the tongue, extending from the alveolar process of the body of the mandible from one side to another, keeping a generous cuff of normal mucosa around the primary tumor. The musculature is completely divided, and a power saw is used for marginal mandibulectomy. This specimen should include the alveolar process and as much of the lingual plate of the mandible as possible, which is made through an oblique cut. Such an oblique cut permits the resection of the musculature attached to the mandible in a monobloc fashion. Using a skin hook, the portion of the mandible to be resected is elevated from the body of the mandible revealing the deep muscular attachments to the genial tubercle and other parts of the mandible. At this point, a more precise evaluation of the tumor borders (and its relation with the mandible) is possible, confirming or not the indication for a marginal resection instead of a segmental resection. The remaining soft tissue attachments between the surgical specimen and the patient are detached at this point using electrocautery. The excised specimen, in a monobloc fashion, should include a marginal mandibulectomy and through-and-through resection of the sublingual gland tumor with the floor of the mouth and lateral aspect of the oral tongue, in continuity with the submandibular gland and cervical lymph nodes excised by neck dissection. Frozen sections are obtained from appropriate areas of the surgical field. The goals of reconstruction for intraoral defects include the covering of the exposed area of muscle and bone, and releasing the tongue and restoring its mobility for speech, mastication, and swallowing. Primary closure can be used if it does not cause tethering of the tongue. Alternative methods of reconstruction include: (1) nasolabial flaps; (2) a platysma flap; (3) a radial forearm flap; and (4) an iliac crest or fibula osteomyocutaneous flap. If adequate vertical height of the marginally resected mandible is available, the patient should be considered for secondary placement of osseointegrated dental implants and a permanent fixed denture. A tracheostomy is usually necessary and performed at the conclusion of the operation for provision of a satisfactory airway and to facilitate clearance of pulmonary secretions.

Management of the Neck

Treatment of the neck in cancer of the major salivary glands has been somewhat controversial. Although the role of neck dissection in clinically proven metastases in salivary gland cancer is straightforward, routine elective treatment of the negative neck remains controversial. Some investigators recommend neck dissection only for patients with clinically evident regional disease, whereas other authors also recommend elective neck dissection for tumors based on various prognostic factors [9, 10, 20, 36, 37].

Although uncommon, cervical metastases from cancer of the salivary gland is an ominous finding. The incidence of lymph node metastases in submandibular carcinomas at the time of initial presentation varies from 8% to 33% [23, 36, 50, 55].

Data from the Memorial Sloan Kettering Cancer Center in New York demonstrated a decrease in 5-year survival rates from 40% to 9% for submandibular cancer with pathologically positive cervical nodes, which is in line with the results found in the literature [23, 24, 50, 57–61].

The treatment of clinically positive node metastases is surgical. The extent of neck dissection is determined by the grossly involved lymph nodes, and an attempt should be made to spare vital structures. The most common levels of neck involvement in submandibular and sublingual malignant tumors are levels I–III [57, 59]. Because contralateral neck involvement is rare, only the ipsilateral neck is treated. Treatment of the clinically negative neck has been more controversial. The treatment of the N0 neck in major salivary gland cancer has included observation, elective neck dissection, and primary radiation. Currently, treatment of the N0 neck is appropriate when the risk for occult metastases is high. Several authors have attempted to determine predictive factors for cervical metastases in salivary gland malignancy. Armstrong et al. [50] have reported that high-grade tumors demonstrate increased occult node metastases in comparison to low-grade tumors: 49% versus 2% ($p < .00001$). In fact, during recent decades several studies have shown that risk of occult nodal metastases is higher in anaplastic, high-grade mucoepidermoid, squamous cell, adenocarcinoma, and salivary duct carcinoma than in low-grade mucoepidermoid, adenoid cystic, acinic cell carcinoma, and sarcoma [9, 10, 18, 32, 36, 50–52, 57–59]. An increased risk of occult metastases is also associated with advanced-stage primary cancer. Armstrong et al. [50] found that among patients with N0 necks, T4 tumors had a 24% risk of micrometastases in comparison with 16% for T3 tumors and 7% for T1–2 tumors ($p < .00001$). This is in line with many reports in the literature [9, 10, 18, 36, 50, 54, 55, 57–63]. Several authors also found tumors larger than 3 cm as an independent risk for lymphatic micrometastases [50, 56, 57, 59–62]. Extraglandular tumor extent and neural invasion are considered very strong predictors of positive nodal disease, and patients with these clinical factors should be considered for elective treatment of the neck [9, 10, 18, 36, 50–52, 55–63]. Medina [62] adequately summarized the indications found in the literature for elective neck treatment in salivary gland cancers: high-grade tumors, T3–4 tumors, tumors >3 cm, facial nerve (neural) invasion, age >54 years, extraglandular extension, and perilymphatic invasion [9, 10, 15, 18, 36, 50, 55–62]. Analyzing the incidence of occult metastases among patients with submandibular malignant tumors, Armstrong et al. [50] found a 21% rate which was significantly higher in comparison with the 9% rate found among parotid cancer patients ($p = .002$). The anatomic distribution of occult node involvement in submandibular gland cancer was as follows: level I 58.8%; level II 52.9%; level III 47%; level IV 17.6%; and level V 5.8%. In addition to that, 25% of metastases skipped to levels III and IV. Recently, European authors have recommended elective neck dissection in all patients with major salivary gland malignancies based on the concept that frequently the correct histologic tumor type is not ascertained until after the surgery and that most salivary gland tumors have poor radiosensitivity [60, 63]. One group found better rates of disease-free survival among those patients who underwent elective neck dissection for malignant parotid tumors in comparison with those who did not [63] (Fig. 21.21).

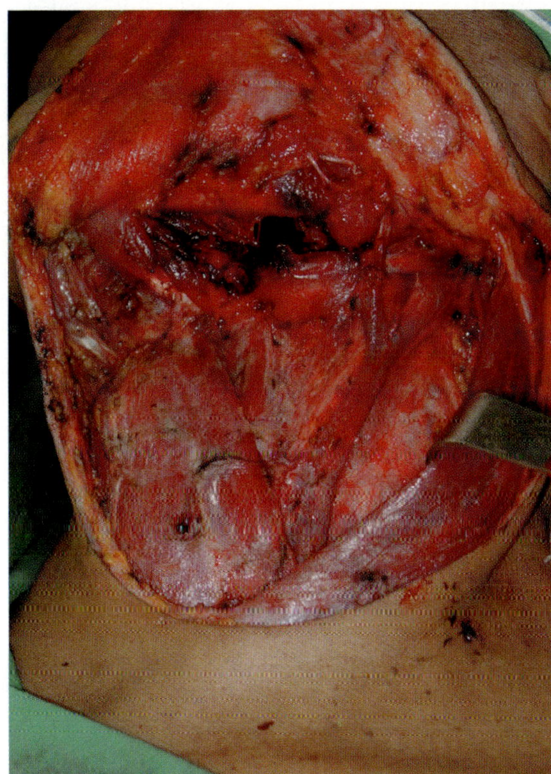

Fig. 21.21: Excision of the submandibular gland in association with a supraomohyoid neck dissection (SOHND)

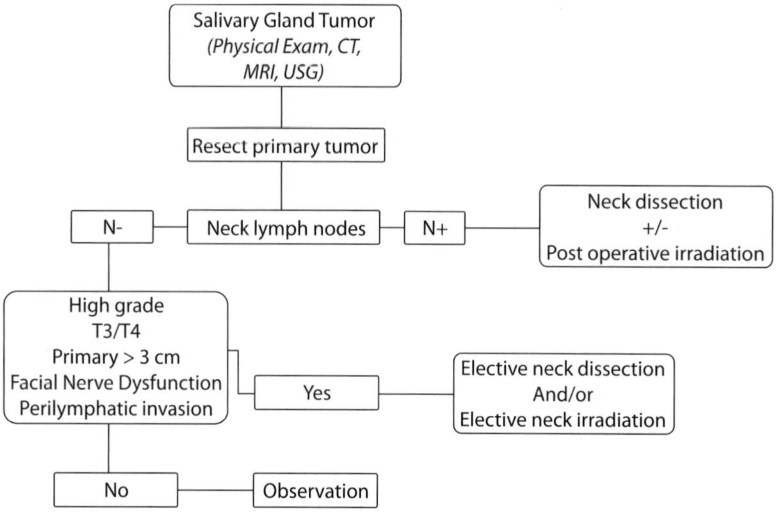

Fig. 21.22: Algorithm for treatment of the neck in major salivary gland malignancy

The current most widely accepted treatment of the neck in major salivary gland malignancy is summarized in Fig. 21.22.

Complications of Surgical Procedures

The most common complication after submandibular gland excision is injury to the marginal mandibular branch of the facial nerve [64]. The incidence of temporary injury (temporary paresis) to the marginal mandibular nerve ranges from 1% to 10%, according to the literature [65–67].

Injury to the lingual nerve is uncommon unless tumor or chronic inflammation presents difficulty in its separation from the gland. Rarer still is injury to the hypoglossal nerve in the course of resection of the contents of the submandibular triangle [66].

The scar that results from cervical incision may be aesthetically unsatisfactory in many patients, particularly those with a slender neck. It is recommended that the incision should be placed at 3 cm below the angle of the mandible to consistently avoid injury to the branches of the facial nerve. Care in order to avoid tension of the surgical wound and the use of intradermal sutures can be helpful to prevent an unsightly scar. Great auricular causalgia and/or the development of amputation neuroma are uncommon complications associated with the resection of submandibular gland [68].

Removal of the sublingual gland is not without potential morbidity, most notably injury to the lingual nerve with subsequent numbness, injury to Wharton's duct with the possibility of obstructive sialadenitis, and ductal laceration causing salivary leakage [15]. Usually incomplete dissection of the lingual nerve before sublingual gland removal is responsible for its inadvertent injury; the lingual nerve needs to be entirely delineated for safe removal of the sublingual gland.

Results and Perspectives

A 41-year experience with submandibular gland tumors encompassing 110 consecutive cases between 1944 and 1985 was reported by Weber and coworkers [36]. Removal of the 24 benign tumors through an approach equivalent to level I selective neck dissection resulted in excision with negative margins in all cases. No recurrences were identified among this group. Recurrences developed in 39 (45%) of 86 patients with malignant submandibular tumors; 21 (53.8%) recurred locoregionally and 18 (46.2%) recurred at distant sites. Among the 86 patients with malignancies, 2- and 5-year survival was 82% and 69%, respectively. Enucleation or excision with a narrow rim of normal tissue in benign mixed tumors of submandibular gland eventually will result in a local recurrence rate of about 20% after 10–15 years of follow-up. Nevertheless, Rafla-Demetrious [69] reported only 2.7% recurrence rate when enucleation or excision was followed by postoperative radiotherapy.

In Vander Porten's series of 43 patients with malignant submandibular gland tumors, the overall 5- and 10-year survival rates were 50%, and the 5- and 10-year disease-specific survival rates were 61% and 51%, which was very similar with the results of treatment for parotid gland malignancies [19]. Seven patients (16.2%), including 4 with an M1 classification at first consultation, remained with residual tumor after treatment. Twelve patients who initially were free of tumor at the end of treatment had a recurrence after a median tumor-free interval of 17 months. Local recurrence occurred in 3 patients, and regional recurrence without local recurrence occurred in 1 patient. The 5- and 10-year recurrence-free survival was 57% and 52%, respectively. Distant metastases occurred eventually in 16 patients (37.2%), of whom 4 had distant metastases at presentation. The organs involved at first diagnosis of distant metastases were the lungs in 7 patients (44%), the skeleton in 4 patients (25%), the liver in 1 patient, and a combination of these in 4 patients. Eight of 18 patients with adenoid cystic carcinomas (44%) developed distant metastases, 1 of 3 acinic cell carcinomas, 1 of 2 mucoepidermoid carcinomas, 4 of 8 adenocarcinomas, and 1 of 4 carcinoma ex pleomorphic adenomas [19].

Wahlberg et al. [70] analyzed the data from the National Swedish Cancer Registry 1960–1995, including 2,465 patients with carcinoma of the parotid or submandibular glands. Four hundred and three patients with a submandibular gland tumor were included in the study. Although without statistical significance, the authors observed an increase in 10-year relative survival rate from 54% for patients treated during the 1960s and 1970s to 65% for the latter two decades ($p = .45$). The more aggressive approach for the treatment of these tumors, with local excision in conjunction with regional lymph node dissection used in more recent years, could explain the improvement obtained in the last two decades [70].

Sykes and coworkers [71] reviewed the charts of 30 patients with histologically confirmed carcinoma of the submandibular gland referred to the Christie Hospital, Manchester, UK, for radiotherapy following primary surgery over a 14-year period. The dose most frequently prescribed was from 50 to 55 Gy in 16 fractions over 3 weeks. Disease-specific survival rates were 79% and 57% at 5 and 10 years, respectively. According to the authors, the continued decrease in cancer-specific survival reflected a number of cases of late relapse seen in patients with adenoid cystic carcinoma. Five patients developed local recurrence of their disease, with only 1 (20%) patient been successfully salvaged with radical surgery. Of the 5 patients who developed a local recurrence, 3 had either incomplete excision of tumor or biopsy only before referral for radiotherapy. Nevertheless, altogether 9 of 12 patients with residual cancer achieved local control with radiotherapy. Six patients (20%) relapsed with lung metastases, in 2 associated with uncontrolled local recurrence. All 6 patients who developed distant metastases had adenoid cystic carcinoma.

Of the original 412 patients with cancer of the submandibular gland studied by Battacharyya [20], 12 (2.9%) cases presented with distant metastases at diagnosis and were excluded from subsequent analysis. From the 370 patients included in the study, 24.9% had lymph node metastases. The results of the Kaplan-Meier 5-year survival analysis for each tumor histopathology was 75.6% for adenoid cystic carcinoma, 55.4% for mucoepidermoid carcinoma, 48.6% for adenocarcinoma, and 34.2% for squamous cell carcinoma.

A study from Denmark spanning a 25-year period ending in 1985 identified 95 patients with malignancies of the submandibular glands, minor salivary glands, and sublingual glands. In this series, only 6 (6.3%) arose in the sublingual glands: 3 patients with adenoid cystic carcinoma, 2 patients with carcinoma ex-pleomorphic adenoma, and 1 patient with adenocarcinoma. These investigators found no difference in survival on the basis of site of the primary lesion, with an overall 5- and 10-year crude survival rates of 62% and 43%, respectively [72].

The role of chemotherapy in the treatment of salivary gland tumors has been limited to the treatment of metastatic disease and to circumstances of palliation of locoregional disease not amenable to either salvage surgery or radiation therapy. Due to the limited number of patients with metastatic or nonsurgical disease, there are no randomized phase III studies examining the best chemotherapeutic regimen.

The most studied single agent in the treatment of salivary gland cancer is cisplatin. Licitra et al. [73] analyzed the results obtained from 25 patients treated for advanced salivary gland carcinoma in a phase II trial

(100 mg/m² of cisplatin every 3 weeks). They observed an 18% response rate in locoregional recurrence but only 7% response rate in metastatic lesions. The median response duration was 7 months and the median survival time was 14 months.

For combination chemotherapy with cisplatin, the most common agents used include 5-fluorouracil, cyclophosphamide, and doxorubicin. A regimen using all four drugs was tested in 17 patients and a 50% objective response rate was observed. The median duration of response was 8 months and medial survival was 18 months [74]. Two studies utilized a regimen of cisplatin with cyclophosphamide and doxorubicin. Dreyfuss et al. [75] treated 13 patients with combination of cyclophosphamide 500 mg/m², doxorubicin 50 mg/m², and cisplatin 50 mg/m² every 28 days. An overall response rate of 46% with a median duration of response of 5 months was observed.

Based on previous promising data extracted from a phase I study with the vinca alkaloid vinorelbine in salivary gland malignancies, Arioldi et al. [76] conducted a randomized phase II trial with 36 patients comparing vinorelbine alone versus the combination of vinorelbine and cisplatin. Vinorelbine appears to have moderate activity in salivary gland cancer with more significant response rates found in the doublet arm with 44% response rate compared to a 20% response rate in the single arm. Complete response rates of 19% and 0% were observed in the doublet and single arms, respectively.

The most recent phase II study in recurrent or metastatic salivary gland malignancies evaluated the combination of cisplatin and mitoxantrone. Fourteen patients entered into the trial and were treated with cisplatin 30 mg/m² on three consecutive days and mitoxantrone 12 mg/m² on the first day of treatment. Treatment was repeated every 28 days for a maximum of six courses. Disease stability was noted in 64% of patients and the overall response rate was 14%. The median duration of stabilization was 15 months and, after 22 months of follow-up, 43% of patients were still alive [77].

Several molecular targets have been identified in salivary gland cancer. C-kit proto-oncogene, EGFR, HER2 proto-oncogene, androgen receptors, p53 protein, and VEGF are examples of recent targets that have been evaluated with varying degrees of expression in salivary gland carcinomas. These and other molecular targets may ultimately provide useful information into diagnosis, biologic behavior, and management of cancer of the salivary glands [78–85].

Take Home Messages

- There are equal proportions of malignant and benign lesions in the submandibular gland. True sublingual gland tumors are rather unusual, and most are malignant.
- Nerves at risk during operations involving the submandibular gland are: mandibular branch of facial nerve, lingual nerve, and hypoglossal nerve.
- The smallest operation for benign tumors of submandibular gland is excision of the whole gland.
- Low-grade, low-stage malignant salivary tumors can be treated by excision of the submandibular gland with dissection of level I. High-grade, high-stage tumors, however, require supraomohyoid neck dissection, in conjunction with the excision of the submandibular gland.

References

1. Janfaza P, Fabian RL. Anatomy of the neck. In: Janfaza P, Nadol JB Jr., Galla RJ, Fabian RL, Montgomery WW (2001) Surgical Anatomy of the Head and Neck. Lippincott Williams & Wilkins
2. American Joint Committee on Cancer Staging Manual – 6th edition (2003). Springer. New York
3. Talmi YP, Wolf M, Bedrin L, et al. (2003) Preservation of the facial artery in excision of the submandibular salivary gland. Br J Plast Surg 2003; 56:156–157
4. Fried LA: Salivary system, in Fried LA (ed): Anatomy of the Head, Neck, Face, and Jaws. Philadelphia. Lea and Febiger, 1980, pp 187–200
5. Robbins KT, Medina JE, Wolf GT et al. Standardizing neck dissection terminology. Arch Otolaryngol Head Neck Surg 1991; 117:601–605
6. McVay CB: Anterior regions of the neck, In: Anson BH and McVay CB (eds): Surgical Anatomy. Philadelphia. Igaku-Shoin/Saunders International Edition, 1985, pp 253–255
7. Batsakis JG. Sublingual gland. Ann Otol Rhinol Laryngol 1991; 100:521–522

8. Peel RL. Diseases of the salivary glands, in Barnes L (ed): Surgical Pathology of The Head and Neck. Marcel Dekker, New York, 2001, pp 634–757
9. Spiro RH. Salivary neoplasms: overview of a 35-year experience with 2.807 patients. Head Neck Surg 1986; 8:177–184
10. Shah JP, Ihde JK. Salivary gland tumors. Curr Probl Surg 1990; Dec: 803–811
11. Verbin RS, Barnes L. Cysts and Cyst-like Lesions of the Oral Cavity, Jaws, and Neck, in Barnes L (ed): Surgical Pathology of The Head and Neck. Marcel Dekker, New York, 2001, pp 1437–1555
12. de Visscher JGM, van der Wall KGH, de Vogel PL. The plunging ranula pathogenesis, diagnosis and management. J Craniomaxillofac Surg 1989; 17:182–185
13. Batsakis GJ. Cyst, pseudocysts, fistulae and sialectsis of the salivary glands. In: Tumors of the Head and Neck. 2nd ed. Baltimore, MD: Waverly Press, 1984, pp. 116–117
14. Davidson MJ, Morton RP, McIvor NP. Plunging ranula: clinical observations. Head Neck 1998; 20:63–68
15. Baurmash HD. Marsupialization for treatment of oral ranula: a second look at the procedure. J Oral Maxillofac Surg 1992; 50:1274–1279
16. Iwata S. Ranula. In: Japan Society of stomato-pharyngology editors. The clinical features of stomato-pharyngology. 1st ed. Tokyo: Igakusyoin; 1998, pp100–101
17. Barnes L, Eveson JW, Reichart P, Sidransky D. Tumors of the Salivary Glands: WHO and TNM classification. In: Barnes L, Eveson JW, Reichart P, Sidransky D. Eds. Pathology and Genetics – Head and Neck Tumors. Lyon. IARC Press, 2005 pp 210–211
18. Sykes AJ, Slevin NJ, Birzgalis AR, Gupta NK. Submandibular gland carcinoma; an audit of local control and survival following adjuvant radiotherapy. Oral Oncol 1999; 35:187–190
19. Vander Poorten VLM, Balm AJM, Hilgers FJM, et al. Prognostic factors for long term results of the treatment of patients with malignant submandibular gland tumors. Cancer 1999; 85:2255–2264
20. Bhattacharyya N. Survival and prognosis for cancer of the submandibular gland. J Oral Maxillofac Surg 2004; 62:427–430
21. Gallia TD, Johnson JT. The incidence of neoplastic versus Inflammatory disease in major salivary gland masses diagnosed by surgery. Laryngoscope 1981; 91:512–515
22. Rice DH. Salivary gland disorders: neoplastic and nonneoplastic. Med Clin North Am 1999; 83:197–218
23. Spiro RH, Hadju SI, Strong EW. Tumors of the submandibular gland. Am J Surg 1976; 132:463–468
24. Castro EB, Huvos AG, Strong EW, et al. Tumors of the major salivary glands in children. Cancer 1972; 29:312–317
25. Schuller DE, McCabe BF. Salivary gland neoplasms in children. Otolaryngol Clin North Am 1977; 10:399–412
26. Shapiro NL, Bhattacharyya N. Clinical characteristics and survival for major salivary gland malignancies in children. Otolaryngol Head Neck Surg 2006; 134:631–634
27. Gritzmann N, Rettenbacher T, Hollerweger A, et al. Sonography of the salivary glands. Eur Radiol 2003; 13:964–975
28. Som PM et al. Benign and malignant parotid pleomorphic adenomas: CT and MR studies. J Comput Assist Tomogr 1988; 12:65–68
29. Mirisch DR, McArdle CB, Kulkarni MV. Benign pleomorphic adenomas of the salivary glands: surface coil MR imaging versus CT. J Comput Assist Tomogr 1987; 11:620–625
30. Johns ME. The salivary glands: anatomy and embryology. Otolaryngol Clin North Am 1977; 110:161–267
31. Stewart CJ, MacKenzie K, McGarry GW, Mowat A. Fine-needle aspiration cytology of salivary gland: a review of 341 cases. Diagn Cytopathol 2000; 22:139–146
32. Luna MA, Tortoledo ME, Ordonez NG, et al. Primary sarcomas of the major salivary glands. Arch Otolaryngol Head Neck Surg 1991; 117:302–306
33. Geisinger KR, Weidner A. Aspiration cytology of salivary glands. Semin Diagn Pathol 1986; 3:219–226
34. Meyers DS, Templer J, Davis WE, et al. Fine needle aspiration biopsy in salivary gland tumors. Clin Otolaryngol 1986; 11:75–77
35. Eneroth CM, Zajieck J. Aspiration biopsy of salivary gland tumors. IV. Morphologic studies on smears and histologic sections from 45 cases of adenoid Cystic Carcinoma. Acta Cytol 1969; 13:59–63
36. Weber RS, Byers RM, Petit B et al. Submandibular gland tumors: adverse histologic factors and therapeutic implications. Arch Otolaryngol Head Neck Surg 1990; 116:1055–1060
37. Batsakis J. Tumors of major salivary glands. In Tumors of the Head and Neck,, 3rd ed. Baltimore, Williams and Wilkins, 1982, pp 1–75
38. Eneroth CM, Zettemberg A. Malignancy in pleomorphic adenoma: a clinical and microspectrophotometric study. Acta Otolaryngol 1974; 77:426–432
39. Fee WE, Goffinet D, Calcaterra T. Recurrent mixed tumors of the parotid gland: results of surgical therapy. Laryngoscope 1978; 88:265–273
40. Niparko JK, Beauchamp ML, Krause CJ, et al. Surgical treatment of recurrent pleomorphic adenoma of the parotid gland. Arch Otolaryngol Head Neck Surg 1986; 112:1180–1184

41. Friedrich RE, Knop J, Giese M, Schmelzle R. Pleomorphic adenoma of the salivary glands: analysis of 94 patients. Anticancer Res 2005; 25:1703–1705
42. Conley JJ. Problems with reoperation of the parotid gland and facial nerve. Otolaryngol Head Neck Surg 1988; 99:480–488
43. Makeieff M, Venail F, Cartier C, et al. Continuous facial nerve monitoring during pleomorphic adenoma recurrence surgery. Laryngoscope 2005; 115:1310–1314
44. Dawson A, Orr J. Long-term results of local excision and radiotherapy in pleomorphic adenoma of the parotid. Int J Radiat Oncol Biol Phys 1985; 11:451–455
45. Debets JMG, Munting JDK. Parotidectomy for parotid tumors: 19-year experience from the Netherlands. Br J Surg 1992; 79:1159–1161
46. Jackson SR, Roland NJ, Clarke RW, et al. Recurrent pleomorphic adenoma. J Laryngol Otol 1993; 107:546–549
47. Douglas JG, Einck J, Austin-Seymour, et al. Neutron radiotherapy for recurrent pleomorphic adenoma of major salivary glands. Head Neck 2001; 23:1037–1042
48. Yoshimura Y, Obara S, Kondoh T, et al. A comparison of three methods used for treatment of ranula. J Oral Maxillofac Surg 1995; 53:280–282
49. Crysdale WS, Mendelson JD, Conley S: Ranulas-mucoceles of the oral cavity: experience in children. Laryngoscope 1988; 98:296–298
50. Armstrong JG, Harrison LB, Thaler HT et al. The indications for elective treatment of the neck in cancer of the major salivary glands. Cancer 1992; 69:615–619
51. Spiro RH. Changing trends in the management of salivary tumors. Semin Surg Oncol 1995; 11:240–245
52. Armstrong JG, Harrison LB, Spiro RH et al. Malignant tumors of major salivary gland origin: a matched pair analysis of the role of combined surgery and postoperative radiotherapy. Arch Otolaryngol Head Neck Surg 1990; 116:290–293
53. Terhaard CHJ, Lubsen H, Rasch CRN, et al. The role of radiotherapy in the treatment of malignant salivary gland tumors. Int J Radiat Oncol Biol Phys 2005; 61:103–111
54. Mendenhall WM, Morris CG, Amdur RJ et al. Radiotherapy alone or combined with surgery for salivary gland carcinoma. Cancer 2005; 103:2544–2550
55. Shah JP. Management of regional metastasis in salivary and thyroid cancer. In: Larson DL, Ballantyne AJ, Guillamondegui M, eds. Cancer of the Neck: evaluation and treatment. New York: MacMillan, 1986:253–256
56. Hocwald E, Korkmaz H, Yoo GH, et al. Prognostic factors in major salivary gland cancer. Laryngoscope 2001; 111:1434–1439
57. Gold DR, Annino DJ. Management of the neck in salivary gland carcinoma. Otolaryngol Clin North Am 2005; 38:99–105
58. Bhattacharyya N, Fied MP. Nodal metastasis in major salivary gland cancer: predictive factors and effects on survival. Arch Otolaryngol Head Neck Surg 2002; 128:904–908
59. Shah JP. Cervical lymph nodes. In: Shah JP, Patel SG eds. Head and Neck Surgery & Oncology 3rd ed. Edinburgh: Mosby 2003:353–394
60. Stennert E, Kisner D, Jungehuelsing M, et al. High incidence of lymph node metastasis in major salivary gland cancer. Arch Otolaryngol 2003; 129:720–723
61. Lima RA, Tavares MR, Dias FL, et al. Clinical factors in malignant parotid gland tumors. Otolaryngol Head Neck Surg 2005; 133:702–708
62. Medina JE. Neck dissection in the treatment of cancer of major salivary glands. Otolaryngol Clin North Am 1998; 31:815–822
63. Zbaren P, Schupbach J, Nuyens M, et al. Carcinoma of the parotid gland. Am J Surg 2003; 186:57–62
64. Eisele DW, Johns ME. Complications of surgery of the salivary glands. In Eisele DW (ed): Complications in Head and Neck Surgery. St Louis: Mosby, 1993, pp 183–200
65. Milton CM, Thomas BM, Bickerton RC. Morbidity study of submandibular gland excision. Ann R Coll Surg Engl 1986; 68:148–150
66. Kennedy PJ, Poole AG. Excision of the submandibular gland: Minimizing the risk of nerve damage. Aust N Z J Surg 1989; 59:411–414
67. Goh YH, Sethi DS. Submandibular gland excision: A 5 year review. J Laryngol Otol 1998; 112:269–274
68. Nusair YMH, Dickenson AJ. Great auricular causalgia: an unusual complication of excision of the submandibular gland. Br J Oral Maxillofac Surg 2003; 41:334–335
69. Rafla-Demetrious S. Submaxillary gland tumors. Cancer 1970; 26:821–826
70. Wahlberg P, Anderson H, Biorklund A, et al. Carcinoma of the parotid and submandibular glands – a study of survival in 2465 patients. Oral Oncol 2002; 38:706–713
71. Sykes AJ, Slevin NJ, Birzgalis AR, Gupta NK. Submandibular gland carcinoma; An audit of local control and survival following adjuvant radiotherapy. Oral Oncol 1999; 35:187–190
72. Andersen LJ, Therkildsen MH, Ockelmann HH, et al. Malignant epithelial tumors in the minor salivary glands, the submandibular gland, and the sublingual gland: Prognostic factors and treatment results. Cancer 1991; 68:2431–2437

73. Licitra L, Marchini S, Spinazze S, et al. Cisplatin in advanced salivary gland carcinoma. A phase II study of 25 patients. Cancer 1991; 1:1874–1877
74. Dimery IW, Legha SS, Shirinian M, Hong WK. Fluorouracil; doxorubicin. Cyclophosphamide, and cisplatin combination chemotherapy in advanced or recurrent salivary gland carcinoma. J Clin Oncol 1990; 8:1056–1062
75. Dreyfuss AI, Clark JR, Fallon BG, et al. Cyclophosphamide, doxorubicin, and cisplatin combination chemotherapy for advancer carcinomas of salivary gland origin Cancer 1987; 60:2869–2872
76. Airoldi M, Pedani F, Succo G, et al. Phase II randomized trial comparing vinorelbine versus vinorelbine plus cisplatin in patients with recurrent salivary gland malignancies. Cancer 2001; 91:541–547
77. Gedlicka C, Schull B, Formanek M, et al. Mitoxandrone and cisplatin in recurrent and/or metastatic salivary gland malignancies. Anticancer Drugs 2002; 13:491–495
78. Dodd RL, Slevin NJ. Salivary gland adenoid cystic carcinoma: A review of chemotherapy and molecular therapies. Oral Oncol 2006; 42:759–769
79. Harari PM, Huang SM. Modulation of molecular targets to enhance radiation Clin Cancer Res 2000; 6:323–325
80. Vered M, Braunstein E, Buchner A. Immunohistochemical study of epidermal growth factor receptor in adenoid cystic carcinoma of salivary gland origin. Head Neck 2002; 24:632–636
81. Sugano S, Mukai K, Tsuda H, et al. Immunohistochemical study of c-erbB-2 oncoprotein overexpression in human major salivary gland carcinoma: an indicator of aggressiveness. Laryngoscope 1992; 102:923–927
82. Nagler RM, Kerner H, Ben-Eliezer S, et al. Prognostic role of apoptotic, Bcl-2, erbB-2, and p53 tumor markers in salivary gland malignancies. Oncology 2003; 64:389–398
83. Nasser SM, Faquin WC, Dayal Y. Expression of androgen, estrogen, and progesterone receptors in salivary gland tumors. Frequent expression of androgen receptor of malignant salivary gland tumors. Am J Clin Pathol 2003; 119:801–806
84. Nemunaitis J, Khouri F, Ganly I, et al. Phase II trial of intratumoral administration of ONYX-015, a replication-selective adenovirus, in patients with refractory head and neck cancer. J Clin Oncol 2001; 19:289–298
85. Kaban K, Herbst RS. Angiogenesis as a target for cancer therapy. Hematol Oncol Clin North Am 2002; 16:1125–1171

Chapter 22

Management of Cancer Metastatic to the Parotid Gland

22

Jonathan Clark, Lorna Sneddon, Christopher O'Brien

Contents

Core Features

- Pathology of metastatic cancer to the parotid
- Investigation and staging of cancer metastatic to the parotid
- Surgery for cancer metastatic to the parotid
- Adjuvant therapy for cancer metastatic to the parotid

Complications to Avoid

- Wound related:
  - Skin flap necrosis due to inappropriate incision design or flap elevation, particularly after radiotherapy
  - Skin flap "button-hole"
  - Avoid unreliable local or regional skin flaps in patients who require timely adjuvant radiotherapy
- Tumor related:
  - Inappropriate surgery due to inadequate preoperative investigation (e.g., excision biopsy by neglecting to perform an FNA or omitting neck dissection in patients with concomitant neck disease who did not undergo imaging)
  - Tumor rupture due to dissection of tumor on facial nerve or excessive retraction
  - Local tumor recurrence due to not performing a lateral temporal bone resection where indicated
- Gland related:
  - Salivary fistula and sialocele due to preserving parotid tissue when the parotid duct is ligated

Complications to Avoid *(continued)*

- Nerve related:
- Facial nerve injury
- Frey's syndrome (gustatory sweating)
- Great auricular nerve neuroma

Pathology of Cancer Metastatic to the Parotid Gland

Carcinoma metastatic to the parotid gland is a region-specific disorder where the relative incidence of the various histopathological types (Table 22.1) is dependent on geographical location. In Australia, metastatic cutaneous squamous cell carcinoma (SCC) is the most common malignancy seen in the parotid, including primary cancer of the parotid gland [12]. This contrasts with many other areas of the world, including North America and Europe where primary cancer of the parotid gland is more frequent [61]. In Australia, the crude rate of basal cell carcinoma (BCC) is 1,752 per 100,000 persons (2,093 per 100,000 men and 1,456 per 100,000 women) and the crude rate for SCC is 819 per 100,000 persons (1,053 for men and 615 for women) [53]. In Northern Australia this incidence may rise up to 1,300 per 100,000. This compares with the USA where the age-adjusted incidence of SCC is approximately 150 per 100,000 [1]. Melanoma affects approximately 31 to 41 per 100,000 population per year (women and men, respectively) [14], with the incidence of melanoma increasing with proximity to the equator. Although metastatic cancer to the parotid is relatively infrequent worldwide, in 40% of patients with this disease it will be the first manifestation of skin cancer [32].

Squamous Cell Carcinoma

The precise rate of cervical and/or parotid nodal metastases is not known for SCC. However it is estimated that 5% of cutaneous SCCs metastasize to regional lymph node basins, including the parotid [37]. Current evidence suggests that between 25% and 50% of patients with nodal metastases to the parotid from SCC will also have cervical nodal disease, either clinical or pathological [37]. Clinicopathological features that increase the risk of nodal metastases are listed in Table 22.2. In high-risk SCC the associated risk of nodal metastases is up to 20% [4].

22

Overall mortality for cutaneous SCC is low at 3.4% but increases substantially in patients with regional metastatic disease [27]. In a multicenter study of 325 patients with metastatic SCC to the parotid there was a 27% rate of synchronous neck disease and overall survival was 72% at 5 years [3]. Locoregional control in metastatic SCC of the parotid is high with the exception of patients with highly invasive disease (bone or other deep structures) or extensive perineural invasion. Cutaneous SCC has a high predilection for perineural invasion, which may affect both motor (facial) and sensory (auriculotemporal/V3) nerves within the parotid and surrounding tissue.

Melanoma

Ten to 20% of cutaneous melanoma arises in the head and neck [35] and approximately 20% of patients develop regional metastases [31]. Current evidence suggests that patients with clinically palpable metastatic melanoma in the parotid have a high rate of occult neck disease, ranging from 28% to 58% [7, 13, 37]. The overall mortality for cutaneous melanoma of the head and neck is high, with 10-year survival rates ranging from 45% to 72%. This falls to 34% for patients with proven nodal metastases and further decreases with increasing number of positive nodes [39, 40]. Clinicopathological features that predict for nodal disease and mortality are listed in Table 22.3.

Other

Other malignancies metastasizing to the parotid are uncommon and often form the subject of case reports. Merkel cell carcinoma is a rare and aggressive neuroendocrine cutaneous malignancy with a high potential for regional and distant metastases. The largest reported series of head and neck Merkel cell carcinoma demonstrated pathological nodal metastases in 48 of 110 patients. Locoregional control is most effective when surgery is combined with radiotherapy [16, 59], particularly for primary tumors greater than 1 cm in size. Evidence to date does not support the routine use of adjuvant chemotherapy, although a number of agents have been trialed including carboplatin, cisplatin, etoposide, and alkaloids [45].

Mucosal cancer, including SCC, infrequently metastasizes to the parotid gland. Nasopharyngeal cancer has been reported as a primary site when there is advanced neck disease [29] and extensive sinonasal cancers involving the subcutaneous tissue of the cheek and orbit may disseminate to the parotid gland. In addition advanced oropharyngeal cancers may invade directly through the parapharyngeal space to involve the parotid gland. Renal

Table 22.1. Pathology of metastatic cancer to the parotid gland

Cutaneous and mucosal primary	Solid organ	Lymphoproliferative
Squamous cell carcinoma	Renal cell carcinoma	Lymphoma
Melanoma	Lung	
Merkel cell carcinoma	Other rare	
Sinonasal carcinoma		
Nasopharyngeal carcinoma		
Other rare (MFH, dermatofibrosarcoma, metastatic BCC)		

Table 22.2. Clinicopathological features that increase risk of nodal metastases

High-risk squamous cell carcinoma
Size > 2 cm
Invasion into subcutaneous fat
Depth > 5 mm
Poorly differentiated tumors
Perineural invasion
Lymphovascular invasion
Site: ear or lip
Incomplete excision
Local recurrence
Immunosuppression

Table 22.3. Clinicopathological features that predict for nodal disease and metastases

High-risk cutaneous melanoma
Tumor thickness (> 1 mm)
Tumor ulceration
Site (scalp)
Level of invasion (Clark level IV)
Gender (male)
Age (increasing age)

cell carcinoma is the most common solid organ cancer to metastasize to this site and appears to have a peculiar predilection for the parotid [18]. Frequently renal cell carcinoma is misdiagnosed as acinic cell cancer on fine-needle aspiration (FNA) and is particularly vascular at parotidectomy.

Investigation and Staging of Cancer Metastatic to the Parotid Gland

Clinical Assessment

In all head and neck malignancy a thorough examination of the head and neck is essential for accurate diagnosis and staging. For patients with cancer metastatic to the parotid, all potential cutaneous and mucosal sites need examination. This includes fiberoptic examination of the nasopharynx and oropharynx. Particular care is necessary when inspecting potential cutaneous sites since cutaneous malignancies may be small relative to the bulk of regional disease (Fig. 22.1). Inconspicuous lesions hiding in the hair, behind the ear, nasal vestibule, and in the external auditory canal are easily overlooked. Non-pigmented nodular lesions are difficult to diagnose and may represent amelanotic melanoma or Merkel cell cancer.

Examination should include assessment of fixation, parapharyngeal extension, synchronous cervical disease, and facial nerve grading as standard. The great auricular nerve may be involved directly causing ear lobule/angle of mandible dysesthesia and the trigeminal nerve (V3) may be involved via branches of the auriculotemporal nerve. Hence sensation in the distribution of both these nerves should also be assessed.

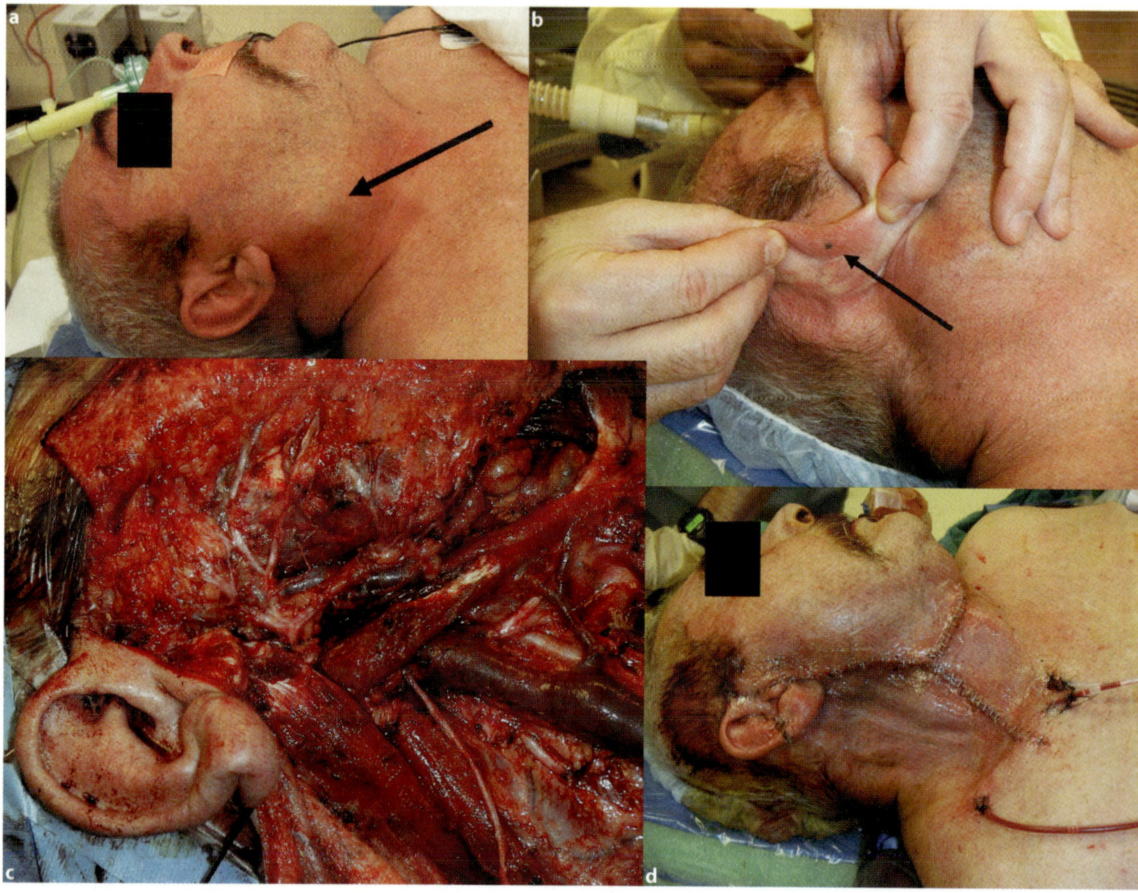

Fig. 22.1: **a** Metastatic melanoma right parotid. **b** Inconspicuous primary helix of right ear. **c** Parotidectomy and neck dissection. **d** Contour defect from extensive dissection of parotid and neck

A thorough history of previous cutaneous surgery is essential. Patients frequently do not consider minor excisions to be of importance and fail to disclose or recall this information. Potential lesions may have been treated with topical 5-fluorouracil, cryotherapy, or removed without pathological diagnosis and in these cases no histological confirmation may be obtainable. Alternatively patients may have multiple cutaneous SCCs removed over many years and confirming that the primary has been treated may be impossible using standard pathological techniques. Pathology reports should be obtained and the original pathology slides may need to be reviewed by an experienced pathologist to confirm unusual primary lesions such as poorly differentiated SCC, Merkel cell carcinoma, spindle cell tumors, and even melanoma.

Investigations

Fine-needle aspiration biopsy is recommended for all parotid tumors and is useful for planning the extent of surgery and stratifying urgency for intervention [46]. Certainly all clinically malignant parotid tumors need cytological confirmation and FNA is reliable in the detection of metastatic SCC [2]. Cytology for primary and uncommon secondary parotid cancers requires a level of expertise and pathological review should be sought where there is doubt.

Standard imaging depends on institutional expertise. Our preference in patients with and without fixed disease is high resolution multislice computerized tomography (CT) scanning with intravenous contrast. This allows assessment of the parotid and surrounding structures, including the parapharyngeal space. Bone windows are used to determine cranial or mandibular invasion. CT examines both potential mucosal sites and the neck to detect subclinical synchronous nodal disease. A dedicated temporal bone CT is obtained where there is fixation or facial nerve deficit.

Magnetic resonance imaging (MRI) can be substituted for CT and is particularly useful in patients with parapharyngeal extension and neurotrophic cancers. However, in general it is more expensive, less readily obtained, poorly tolerated by patients due to confinement and length of procedure, and provides poor cortical bone definition. Cervical node assessment with MRI is equivalent to multislice CT and we reserve MRI for selected patients with nerve deficit or extensive disease. Ultrasound has been reported to be highly specific and sensitive for cervical node disease in selected series [49] and can be combined with ultrasound-guided FNA. However, ultrasound requires technical expertise to achieve these high rates of accuracy and is resource intensive to acquire the necessary detail. Ultrasound is inferior to CT or MRI in patients with extensive parotid disease, in particular patients with facial paresis.

There are few Data examining the role of positron emission tomography (PET) in metastatic cancer to the parotid gland is limited despite this. PET and PET-CT is being used more frequently as a standard investigation and has a role in the assessment of regional and distant metastatic disease. It is unlikely to detect small cutaneous primaries that were unseen on thorough examination. Distant metastases are uncommon in cutaneous SCC, including patients with nodal metastases. PET is more established and more likely to be positive in patients with melanoma where distant disease is common. 18F-FDG PET is superior to other modalities in the detection of distant metastases and in patients with recurrent disease where the sensitivity and specificity ranges from 70% to 100% [9]. However, PET is relatively insensitive (0–40%) in the detection of regional metastases in patients with early-stage disease when compared to sentinel node biopsy. Detection of distant metastases has both prognostic and therapeutic value, since isolated distant disease is amenable to surgical resection [22]. Regardless of distant disease status, locoregional control is of value for symptomatic relief since the rate of disease progression is unpredictable. Evidence for the utility of PET in rare secondary parotid malignancies is unlikely to ever exceed that of small retrospective case series.

Staging for Cutaneous Metastatic Squamous Cell Carcinoma

The current staging system stages all patients with cutaneous SCC and nodal metastases to the parotid as N1 regardless of the extent or volume of disease [57]. O'Brien [36] has proposed a revised staging system which has demonstrated prognostic value as shown in Table 22.4.

Staging for Melanoma

Staging for melanoma is listed in Table 22.5. Parotid metastases are included as regional nodal disease. There is no separate staging for parotid disease.

Table 22.4. Revised staging of metastatic SCC of the head and neck

Parotid		Neck	
P0	No clinical parotid disease	N0	No clinical neck disease
P1	Metastatic node < 3 cm	N1	Single ipsilateral neck node < 3 cm
P2	Metastatic node > 3 cm but < 6 cm	N2	Single node > 3 cm
	Multiple parotid nodes		Multiple or contralateral neck nodes
P3	Metastatic node > 6 cm		
	Multiple or contralateral neck nodes		

Table 22.5. American Joint Committee on Cancer staging for cutaneous melanoma

Tumor		Node		Metastasis	
T1	< 1 mm thick	N1	Single nodal or parotid metastases	M1a	Distant skin, subcutaneous or distant nodal metastases
T2	1–2 mm thick	N2	2–3 nodal metastases	M1b	Lung metastases
T3	2–4 mm thick	N3	> 3 nodal metastases	M1c	Other visceral metastases or any distant metastases with elevated LDH
T4	> 4 mm thick				
a	No ulceration	a	Micronodal metastases		
b	Ulceration	b	Macronodal metastases		

LDH Lactate dehydrogenase

Surgery for Cancer Metastatic to the Parotid Gland

Ablative Surgery

The extent of surgery in both the parotid and the neck is an ongoing area of controversy (Table 22.6). Current evidence does not indicate that more extensive surgery is associated with either improved disease control or survival [21]. This may reflect the frequent use of adjuvant radiotherapy [38] which is effective for control of microscopic nodal disease in both the parotid and neck. This is applicable for both SCC and melanoma, although melanoma traditionally is considered to be radioresistant [6].

The extent of parotidectomy and neck dissection is decided on an individual basis. The standard parotid dissection is a superficial parotidectomy carried out superficial to the plane of the facial nerve. There is no evidence to suggest that a limited or more aggressive approach is preferable. Parotid lymphatics and lymph nodes are present throughout the parotid substance, both superficial and deep to the plane of the facial nerve. However, superficial lymph nodes are more numerous and more likely to harbor metastatic disease. McKean et al. [33] examined this issue and found between two and 22 nodes in the superficial lobe compared with less than five in the deep segment. Graham [24] suggests that the retromandibular vein should be the appropriate depth of dissection, rather than the facial nerve and this is supported by Batsakis [8].

Total parotidectomy with facial nerve sacrifice (radical parotidectomy) is highly morbid and current trends are toward more conservative surgery where possible [60]. Aesthetic and functional consequences of radical parotidectomy are described in Table 22.7. More extensive parotid dissection is indicated in invasive parotid metastases or recurrent disease and may necessitate facial nerve sacrifice with or without temporal bone resection and resection of adjacent structures involved by the cancer such as the skin, mandible, and skull base.

Resection of skin is relatively simple and can be restored using a number of standard techniques such as a cervicofacial rotation flap [34] or free flap where indicated. In more advanced disease the likelihood of local control needs to be balanced against the morbidity of surgery. As more radical procedures are undertaken the rate of positive surgical margins also increases [28] hence more radical surgery does not necessarily confer disease control. An argument can be made for more radical parotid surgery where radiotherapy is contraindicated, such as recurrent disease, or where radiotherapy may be avoided by adequate surgery, such as single small nodal metastasis with no extracapsular extension or neck disease. Techniques of parotidectomy and temporal bone resection are the topic of other chapters in this text and will not be reviewed here. At our institution we perform all temporal bone resections as a combined procedure with the (neuro)otologist, unless minimal, and recommend early preoperative consultation.

Neck dissection may be combined with parotidectomy as an elective or therapeutic procedure. Therapeutic neck dissection is appropriate to maximize disease control [28] and should incorporate all at risk nodal basins. This depends on the location of the primary and the extent of

Table 22.6. Ablative surgery for metastatic cancer to the parotid gland

Parotidectomy	Neck dissection (elective and therapeutic)
Limited parotidectomy	Selective
Superficial parotidectomy	Comprehensive
Total parotidectomy with nerve preservation	Extended
Radical parotidectomy	
Extended parotidectomy	
Skin resection	
Mandibulectomy	
Lateral temporal bone resection	

Table 22.7. Functional and aesthetic consequences of radical parotidectomy

Functional	Aesthetic
Visual disturbance (brow ptosis - frontalis)	Contour defect
Corneal exposure and ulceration (orbicularis oculi)	Brow ptosis
Oral incompetence (orbicularis oris, depressor anguli oris, depressor labii inferioris)	Eyelid paralysis
Speech impairment (buccinator, orbicularis oris)	Ectropion
	Nasal collapse
	Upper lip asymmetry
	Lower lip asymmetry

nodal metastasis. In general terms a comprehensive neck dissection incorporating level I to V is standard, however in low volume neck disease a selective dissection of levels II to V is appropriate for posterior primaries or levels I to IV for anterior lesions [36]. Resection of non-lymphatic structures, such as the sternomastoid muscle and internal jugular vein is indicated where disease is suspected to involve them directly.

Consideration needs to be given to nodal groups that are not traditionally encompassed in neck dissection for mucosal SCC. This includes external jugular lymph nodes which are at high risk for any malignancy involving the parotid and should be included routinely [36]. Level II b should be routinely dissected. Occipital and retroauricular lymph nodes are at high risk in posterior scalp malignancy and lesions involving the pinna. Perifacial lymph nodes are at high risk in cheek, lip, and nasal primaries.

Elective neck dissection has not been shown to confer improved disease control or survival despite the substantial rate of occult neck disease. Presumably this is due to the frequent use of adjuvant radiotherapy [37, 42]. Selective neck dissection of levels II and III may be appropriate as a staging procedure in selected patients, however this depends on the location of the primary. Morbidity associated with these highly selective dissections is minimal and can be performed readily through a modified Blair incision with minimal or no extension. The relative merit of this approach is unproven but is useful where adjuvant therapy, such as radiation may not be necessary. Certainly in patients where adjuvant radiotherapy is not possible a more comprehensive neck dissection should be combined with parotidectomy.

Elective parotidectomy in patients with cervical disease is not generally employed. However parotid nodes are frequently involved in patients with cervical disease from primary cutaneous malignancy, in particular primary melanoma and SCC of the ear, face, and anterior scalp. Shah et al. [47] found that 33 of 57 elective parotidectomies for neck disease had melanoma involving the parotid and adjacent nodes. This is supported by the high rate of sentinel nodes biopsies occurring in the periparotid region [15], however other series have not replicated this high rate of positive metastases to the parotid [58] (Table 22.8). There may be a role for lymphoscintigraphy to determine whether the parotid contains any sentinel nodes for the primary.

Table 22.8. Complications of parotid surgery for metastatic malignancy

Facial nerve paralysis or paresis—increased in malignancy
Lip depressor weakness—increased when combined with neck dissection
Great auricular neuroma or dysesthesia
Frey's syndrome
Sialocele
Salivary fistula
Wound infection or necrosis

Reconstructive Surgery

Reconstruction following radical parotid surgery is frequently required and preoperative consultation with the head and neck reconstructive surgeon should be performed to optimize functional and aesthetic outcomes. The most common structure sacrificed is skin followed by the facial nerve. The method of cutaneous reconstruction depends on the extent of the cutaneous defect, type of neck dissection, additional structures sacrificed, and whether radiotherapy has been given previously. In patients with moderate-sized defects where neck dissection is combined, a cervicofacial rotation flap [51] is an excellent method of cutaneous reconstruction, particularly for elderly patients not concerned about the contour deformity that arises from extensive parotid surgery. The deep plane cervicofacial flap [51] is favored in patients where the facial artery is preserved due to its reliability and lesser dissection. The submental island flap is also a very useful reconstructive technique due to the excellent color match with the cheek [44], however it requires planning with regards to incisions and the pedicle needs to be carefully dissected. We do not consider it suitable in patients where perifacial nodes are at risk and where a level I neck dissection is indicated since the pedicle runs through this tissue (Figs. 22.2, 22.3).

Many patients are best managed with free tissue reconstruction for a number of reasons, in particular, patients with prior irradiation or extensive cutaneous defects where a cervicofacial flap is insufficient or likely to fail. This is important in patients with exposed bone and where postoperative radiotherapy or chemoradiation is planned and marginal flap necrosis will delay the onset of radiotherapy, which should be commenced within 6 weeks after surgery. Free flap failure is uncommon, particularly with reliable flaps such as the radial forearm where failure rates are less than 1% in many series [5, 19]. The additional time associated with harvest is minimal using a two team approach. With regards to optimal donor site, the radial forearm has been used extensively with great success, however the donor site morbidity is substantial where large flaps are harvested and the color match with the head and neck is poor. Color match is important in the face and is best obtained by using flaps located in proximity of the head and neck. We have used the parascapular flap for this reason, however depending on ethnicity other flaps are preferred. Patients of Asian descent are more easily managed with low morbidity flaps such as the anterolateral thigh which can be easily harvested using a two team approach (Figs. 22.4–22.6).

Following radical parotidectomy there are several components to optimal reconstruction which can be performed primarily (ideally) or secondarily. These include the cutaneous defect (if present), contour defect, bone defect, facial nerve, brow ptosis, eyelid paralysis, ectropion, and lip paralysis. There are many options in reconstructing these complex problems depending on individual or institutional expertise (Table 22.9). We have not used dynamic reconstructions (other than facial nerve graft) because of inconsistent outcomes; however remarkable outcomes can be achieved in expert hands using facial reanimation techniques such as the gracilis free flap [23]. We have favored static reconstructions and prefer to perform most components primarily as described below.

Facial Nerve

Where the proximal facial nerve can be accessed in the temporal bone without disease a cable nerve graft can be performed using sural, saphenous, or antebrachial cutaneous nerve. Facial nerve function following neu-

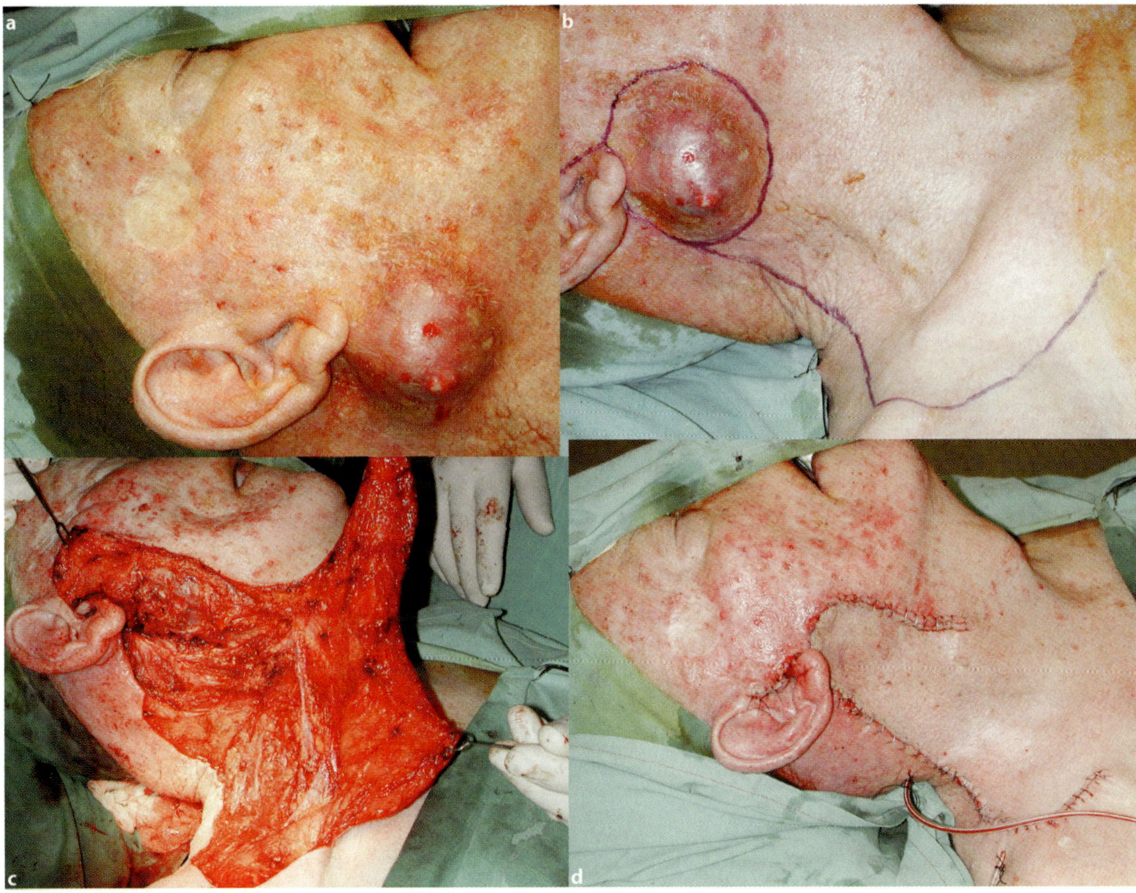

Fig. 22.2: **a** Metastatic SCC right parotid involving overlying skin. **b** Design of excision and cervicofacial rotation flap. **c** Limited parotidectomy with cervicofacial rotation flap raised. **d** Inset cervicofacial flap

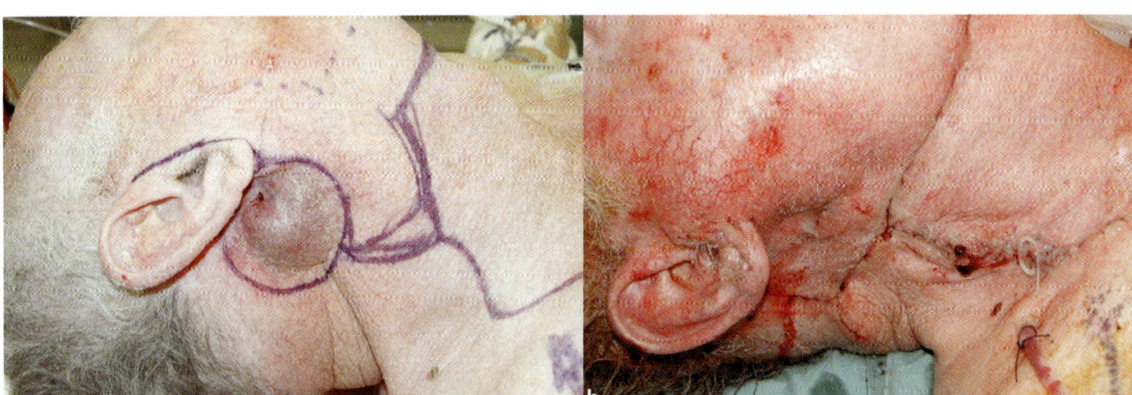

Fig. 22.3: **a** Retroauricular metastatic SCC involving tail of parotid. Design of deep plane cervicofacial flap based on perforators from facial artery. **b** Inset deep plane cervicofacial flap following parotidectomy and neck dissection

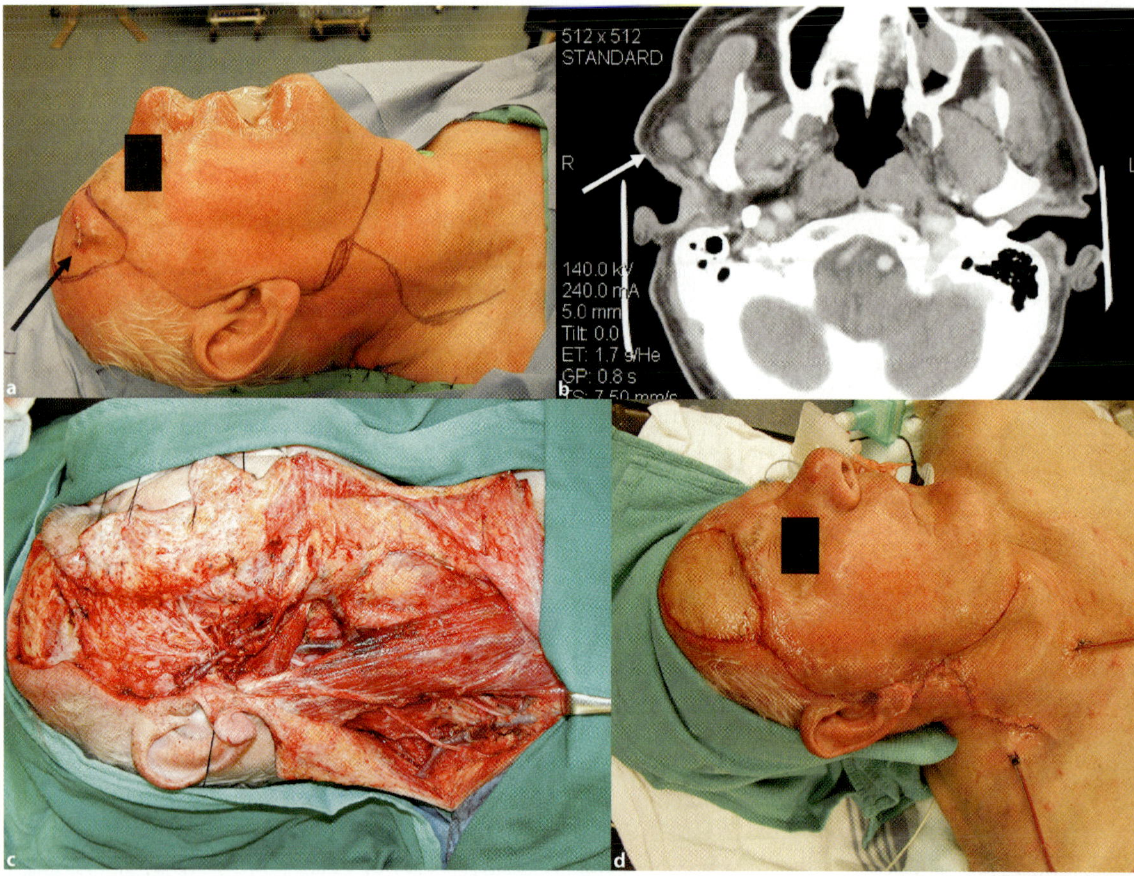

Fig. 22.4: **a** Recurrent melanoma and intransit metastases right forehead. **b** Nodal metastases right parotid (CT scan). **c** Wide local excision, subtotal parotidectomy with resection of subcutaneous lymphatics and functional neck dissection (cervical plexus sparing). **d** Reconstruction using anterolateral thigh free flap

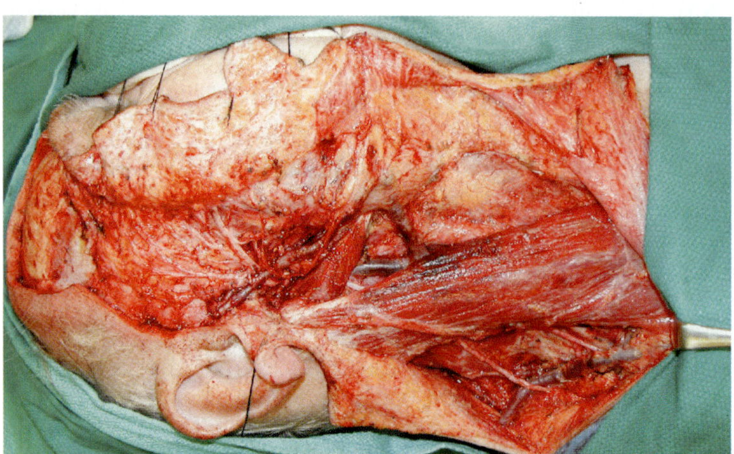

Fig. 22.5: Close up of Fig. 22.4c

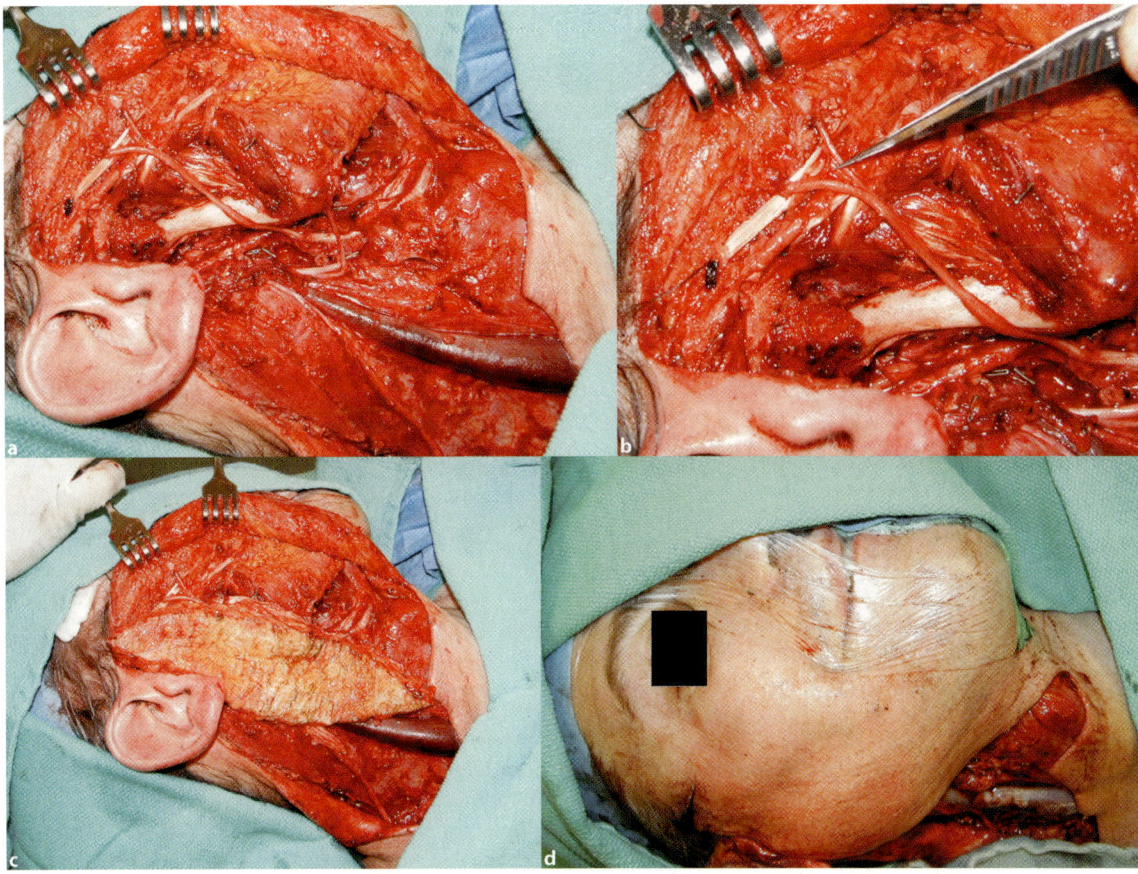

Fig. 22.6: **a** Radical parotidectomy with plantaris static sling. **b** XII–VII facial nerve graft using sural nerve. **c** Contour reconstruction of parotid and neck using de-epithelialized anterolateral thigh free flap. **d** Contour reconstruction and lateralization of oral commissure

rorrhaphy is unlikely to be better than a House Brackmann grade III and some synkinesis is unavoidable [56]. Furthermore facial nerve recovery is likely to take 6–12 months and hence static reconstruction is important in the interim.

Contour

The contour defect is well corrected using a de-epithelialized fasciocutaneous free flap such as parascapular or anterolateral thigh. A temporoparietal flap can be used as a pedicled flap for small defects. Muscle flaps should be avoided since the ultimate volume is unpredictable.

Static Reconstruction

The upper eyelid is managed using a gold weight and the lower eyelid using a tendon sling to prevent ectropion with or without canthoplasty. Using this combination a lateral tarsorrhaphy, which is aesthetically inferior, is usually unnecessary. The oral commissure is lateralized using a woven tendon sling (plantaris or palmaris). This is favored over fascia lata which tends to stretch over time. The commissure and lip is suspended from the zygomatic arch using multiple passes to recreate the appropriate vectors. The lip is overcorrected initially (lateralized) to create a more natural lip position in the long term. The lower lip can be everted and depressed using the anterior

Table 22.9. Reconstructive surgery for metastatic cancer to the parotid gland

Cutaneous reconstruction	Bone reconstruction	Contour restoration	Facial reanimation		
			Facial nerve neurorrhaphy	Static reanimation	Dynamic reanimation
Skin graft	Reconstruction plate	Regional flap	Direct coaptation	Eyelid	Regional muscle transfer
Local flap	Bone graft	Free tissue transfer	Cable graft	Tarsorrhaphy	Temporalis
Regional flap	Osseous free flap		Crossover graft	Gold weight	Masseter
Free tissue transfer	Osteocutaneous free flap		XII–VII graft	Canthoplasty	Digastric
				Eyelid sling	Free muscle transfer
				Lip	Gracilis
				Tendon or fascial sling	Pectoralis minor
				Forehead	Latissimus
				Brow lift	

belly of digastric as a semidynamic reconstruction [56]. All of these components are undertaken primarily. Other minor corrections can be performed secondarily such as a brow lift, revision canthoplasty, or tarsorrhaphy and flap revision to remove excess bulk.

Adjuvant Therapy for Cancer Metastatic to the Parotid Gland

Squamous Cell Carcinoma

Adjuvant therapy for metastatic SCC to the parotid includes:

- Radiotherapy,
- Concurrent chemotherapy.

Traditionally the parotid was regarded as radioresistant and there is limited data regarding primary radiotherapy treatment for metastases to the parotid. One such study [30] reported a 2-year local control rate of 50% in 14 patients. After 5 years the figure dropped to 20%. The sole use of radiotherapy should be restricted to those in whom surgery is not possible. In patients with bulky disease radiotherapy is likely to be palliative only.

Presently, in patients with metastatic SCC to the parotid, the vast majority will undergo adjuvant radiotherapy. However, it was not until 1970 that Fletcher reported the first compelling argument in favor of combining radiotherapy with surgery. Most contemporary series have demonstrated that local failure rates with combined therapy are approximately one third of those with surgery alone. Guillamondegui et al. [25] showed a reduction in local recurrence from 30% to 9% and Taylor et al. [52] found a similar reduction from 27% to 11% with combined surgery and radiotherapy.

Recent data from the TransTasman Oncology Group Post-Operative Skin Trial (POST study) [54] has high-

Table 22.10. High-risk nodal disease with any T-stage

- Presence of extracapsular extension
- Intraparotid nodal metastasis regardless of size or number
- ≥ 2 cervical nodes or > 3 cm cervical node(s)

Table 22.11. Standard radiation therapy for metastatic SCC to the parotid gland

Clinical target volume (CTV)	The volume including the site of resected gross disease, surgical bed/scar, and next echelon of draining lymph nodes with a minimum of a 0.5-cm margin in all dimensions
Planning target volume	Defined as CTV 1 with a minimum of a 1.0-cm margin in all dimensions
Radiation dose	50–60 Gy in 25–30 fractions, 2 Gy per fraction, 5 fractions per week

lighted metastasis to the parotid in the high-risk group for adjuvant therapy comparing surgery and radiotherapy with surgery and chemoradiation (Table 22.10). Various radiation schedules have been used for metastatic cancer to the parotid, however standard fractionation has been advocated as described (see Table 22.11) [54].

Data from MD Anderson demonstrated that for high-risk SCC of the head and neck, increasing the postoperative dose beyond a biologically effective dose of 60 Gy increased the risk of late complications, with no increased benefit in locoregional control [43]. Where parotid metastases have occurred 12 months or more following definitive treatment to the index lesion, consideration should be given to including the primary site and intervening dermal lymphatics in the treatment volume.

Concurrent Chemoradiotherapy

It is well documented that concurrent radiotherapy and chemotherapy is superior over radiotherapy alone for advanced mucosal SCC. Recent data have also demonstrated improved locoregional control and survival with concurrent chemoradiation in the postoperative setting [26] for high-risk mucosal cancer. This is at the cost of a substantial increase in both early and late adverse effects. At present there is no compelling data to suggest that the same benefit is present in cutaneous SCC and this is the subject of several trials [17]. Although there is significant morbidity associated with this, if the survival benefit could be demonstrated in metastatic parotid disease, the risks may be justified.

Current therapeutic agents have included cisplatin and fluorouracil in conjunction with radiotherapy. Brizel et al. [11] reported on hyperfractionated irradiation with or without concurrent chemotherapy. For mucosal cancer Cisplatin was given for 5 days at a dose of 12 mg/m^2 of body surface area per day and 600 mg/m^2 of fluorouracil per day during weeks 1 and 6 of irradiation. Two cycles of cisplatin and fluorouracil were given after the completion of radiotherapy. Locoregional control at 3 years was 70% in the combined group and 44% in radiotherapy alone. There was no statistically significant difference in overall complications of the two groups, although the rates of nasogastric feeding or gastrostomy feeding tubes were higher in the combined treatment group.

More recently, trials using carboplatin rather than cisplatin have been used in an attempt to minimize the toxicity, particularly for elderly patients who are most commonly affected by advanced cutaneous disease. For the POST trial, carboplatin is given once per week for 6 weeks, 30 min prior to radiotherapy. The dose is calculated according to Calvert formula and based on glomerular filtration rate (GFR).

Melanoma

Adjuvant therapy for metastatic melanoma includes:

Radiotherapy,
Chemoimmunotherapy.

Radiotherapy has an established role, in the management of metastatic melanoma to the parotid gland following surgical excision. With those patients in whom radiotherapy is employed, this is associated with improved locoregional control but not with overall survival benefits [41]. Despite the high incidence of distant metastases, locoregional control is a vital component in the management plan. Parotid metastases fall into the high-risk group for regional relapse (Table 22.12).

Table 22.12. Significant risk of regional disease

> 1 parotid node
> 2 neck or axillary nodes
> 3 groin nodes

Differing schedules of radiotherapy have been proposed. Hypofractionated schedules are thought to improve the therapeutic ratio for melanoma [10]. In one such study [48] a postoperative hypofractionated radiotherapy regimen was utilized. Indications for irradiation included microscopically involved or close surgically resected margins, neurotrophic desmoplastic histopathology, perineural spread, or tumor satellites. With a starting date for the majority of patients less than 6 weeks postsurgery, they received 30–36 Gy in six fractions over 18 days. Parotid and neck lymph node fields were treated with direct electron fields or photon wedge pair fields. Infield recurrence was the only significant predictor of survival. 5-year survival with infield recurrence was 0%, and without at 46%.

Currently, our attention is focused on determining the benefits of adjuvant radiotherapy using randomized clinical trials. One such trial [55] is looking at the group of patients with nodal metastatic melanoma at risk of relapse following surgical resection. They are proposing a schedule of 48 Gy delivered in 20 fractions over 30 days. Outcome measures include regional metastasis, as well as morbidity, patterns of relapse, and overall survival.

Chemoimmunotherapy

The role of chemotherapeutic agents and immunotherapy has yet to be established in the treatment of locally advanced or metastatic melanoma. There are various trials underway to test hypotheses regarding drug therapy. It is proposed that interferon-alfa may interfere with the growth of tumor cells [20] and this is an active trial ECOG-1697 recruiting patients with stage II and III disease. Also being investigated is whether there may be a synergistic role with interferon-alfa and interleukin-2 (IL-2) in combination. IL-2 is thought to stimulate white blood cells to mount a response to melanoma cells [50]. It is hoped that colony-stimulating factors such as sargramostim may result in increased immune cells in bone marrow and peripheral blood, and also the use of vaccines has been postulated. However, it should be emphasized that these therapeutic interventions are at present limited to phase III clinical trials, and their efficacy has not been proven.

Take Home Messages

- History – previous cutaneous SCC or melanoma
- Examination – operative scars, current lesions of the head and neck, associated lymphadenopathy, fiberoptic nasoendoscopy, sensation
- Investigations – FNA (may need expert interpretation), CT, MRI, PET-CT
- Staging – O'Brien et al. and American Joint Committee on Cancer (AJCC)
- Treatment options
- Surgery – ablative/reconstructive
- Radiotherapy – indicated for SCC and melanoma
- Chemotherapy – indicated for SCC
- Chemoimmunotherapy – may have a role in the management of metastatic melanoma

References

1. Alam M, Ratner D. Cutaneous squamous cell carcinoma. N Engl J Med 2001;344(13):975–983
2. Alphs HH, Eisele DW, Westra WH. The role of fine needle aspiration in the evaluation of parotid masses. Curr Opin Otolaryngol Head Neck Surg 2006;14(2):62–66
3. Andruchow J, O'Brien CJ, et al. Implications for clinical staging of metastatic cutaneous squamous carcinoma of the head and neck based on a multicenter study of treatment outcomes. Cancer 2006;106:1078–1083
4. Audet N, Palme C, Gullane P, Gilbert R, Brown D, Irish J, Neligan P. Cutaneous metastatic squamous cell carcinoma to the parotid gland: analysis and outcome. Head Neck 2004;26:727–732
5. Bae YC, Zuker RM, Manktelow RT, Wade S. A comparison of commissure excursion following gracilis muscle transplantation for facial paralysis using a cross face nerve graft versus the motor nerve to the masseter nerve. Plast Reconstr Surg 2006;117(7):2407–2413

6. Ballo MT, Ang KK. Radiation therapy for malignant melanoma. Surg Clin North Am 2003;83:323–342
7. Barr LC, Skene AI, Fish S, et al. Superficial parotidectomy in the treatment of cutaneous melanoma of the head and neck. Br J Surg 1994;81:64–65
8. Batsakis JG. Parotid gland and its lymph nodes as metastatic sites. Ann Otol Rhinol Laryngol 1983;92:209–210
9. Belhocine TZ, Scott AM, Even-Sapir E, et al. Role of nuclear medicine in the management of cutaneous malignant melanoma. J Nucl Med 2006;47:957–967
10. Bentzen SM, Overgaard J, Thames HD, Overgaard M, Vejby, et al. Clinical radiobiology of malignant melanoma. Radiother Oncol 1989;16:169–182
11. Brizel D, Albers M, Fisher S, Scher R, et al. Hyperfractionated irradiation with or without concurrent chemotherapy for locally advanced head and neck cancer. N Engl J Med 1998;338:1798–1804
12. Bron L, Traynor MD, McNeil E, O'Brien CJ. Primary and metastatic cancer of the parotid: comparison of clinical behavior in 232 cases. Laryngoscope 2003;113:1070–1075
13. Caldwell CB, Spiro RH. The role of parotidectomy in the treatment of cutaneous head and neck melanoma. Am J Surg 1988;156:318–322
14. Cancer Institute New South Wales Statistics 2006
15. Chao C, Wong SL, Edwards MJ, et al. Sentinel lymph node biopsy for head and neck melanomas. Ann Surg Oncol 2003;10:21–26
16. Clark JR, Veness MJ, Gilbert R, O'Brien CJ, Gullane PJ. Merkel cell carcinoma of the head and neck: Is adjuvant radiotherapy necessary? Head Neck (in press)
17. Cooper J, Pajak T, Forastiere A, Jacobs J, et al. Postoperative concurrent radiotherapy and chemotherapy for high risk squamous cell carcinoma of the head and neck. N Engl J Med 2004;350(19):1937–1944
18. Coppa GF, Oszczakiewicz M. Parotid gland metastasis from renal carcinoma. Int Surg 1990;75(3):198–202
19. Disa JJ, Pusic AL, Hidlago DH, Cordeiro PG. Simplifying microvascular reconstruction: A rational approach to donor site selection. Ann Plast Surg 2001;47(4):385–389
20. ECOG Trial National Cancer Institute Sponsor. US ECOG-1697 2005
21. Eicher S, Clayman G, Myers J, Gillenwater A. A prospective study of intraoperative lymphatic mapping for head and neck cutaneous melanoma Arch Otolaryngol Head Neck Surg 2002;128:241–246
22. Essner R. Surgical treatment of malignant melanoma. Surg Clin North Am 2003;83(1):109–156
23. Gidley Gantz PW, Rubinstein JT. Facial nerve grafts: from cerebellopontine angle and beyond. Am J Otol 1999;20(6):781–788
24. Graham JW. Metastatic cancer in the parotid lymph nodes. Med J Aust 1965;2:8–12
25. Guillamondegui OM, Byers RM, Luna MA. Aggressive surgery in treatment for parotid cancer; the role of adjuvant postoperative radiotherapy. Am J Roentgentol 1975;123:49–53
26. Jassem J, Bartelink H. Chemotherapy in locally advanced head and neck cancer: a critical reappraisal. Cancer Treat Rev 1996;21:447–462
27. Joseph MG, Zulueta WP, Kennedy PJ. Squamous cell carcinoma of the skin of the trunk and limbs: the incidence of metastases and their outcome. Aust N Z J Surg 1992;62(9):697–701
28. Khurana VG, Mentis DH, O'Brien CJ, et al. Parotid and neck metastases from cutaneous squamous cell carcinoma of the head and neck. Am J Surg 1995;170:446–450
29. King AD, Ahuja AT, Leung SF, et al. Neck node metastases from nasopharyngeal carcinoma: MR imaging patterns of disease. Head Neck 2000;22(3):275–281
30. Krengli M, Pisani P, Pia F. Exclusive radiotherapy of parotid metastases. Results in 14 cases. Radiol Med 1993;86(5)684–686
31. Mack L, McKinnon G. Controversies in the management of metastatic melanoma to regional lymphatic basins. J Surg Oncol 2004;86:189–199
32. Malata C, Camilleri I, McLean N, Piggott T, Soames J. Metastatic tumors of the parotid gland. Br J Oral Maxillofac Surg 1998;36:190–195
33. McKean ME, Lee K, McGregor IA. The distribution of lymph nodes in and around the parotid gland: an anatomical study. Br J Plast Surg 1985;38:1–5
34. Moore BA, Wine T, Netterville JL. Cervicofacial and cervicothoracic rotation flaps in head and neck reconstruction. Head Neck 2005;27(12):1092–1101
35. Myers JN. Value of neck dissection in the treatment of patients with intermediate-thickness cutaneous malignant melanoma of the head and neck. Arch Otolaryngol Head Neck Surg 1999:125:110–115
36. O'Brien CJ. The parotid gland as a metastatic basin for cutaneous cancer. Arch Otolaryngol Head Neck Surg 2006;131:551
37. O'Brien CJ, McNeil ED, McMahon JD. Incidence of cervical node involvement in metastatic cutaneous malignancy involving the parotid gland. Head Neck 2001;23(9):744–748
38. O'Brien CJ, Peterson-Schaefer K, McCarthy W, et al. Adjuvant radiotherapy following neck dissection and parotidectomy for metastatic malignant melanoma. Head Neck 1997;19:589–594

39. O'Brien CJ, Petersen-Schaefer K, Ruark D, et al. Radical, modified and selective neck dissection for cutaneous malignant melanoma. Head Neck 1995;17:232–241
40. O'Brien CJ, Coates AS, Petersen-Schaefer K, et al. Experience with 998 cutaneous melanomas of the head and neck. Cancer 1993;71:751–758
41. Overgaard J. The role of radiotherapy in recurrent and metastatic malignant melanoma: a clinical radiobiological study. Int J Radiat Oncol Biol Phys 1986;12:867–872
42. Pedraza V, Guerrero MR, Luna del Castillo JD. Time-dose-response relationship in postoperatively irradiated patients with head and neck squamous cell carcinomas. Radiother Oncol 2001;60:137–145
43. Peters LJ, Goepfert H, Ang KK, et al. Evaluation of the dose for post-operative radiation therapy of head and neck cancer: First report of a prospective randomized trial. Int J Radiat Oncol Biol Phys 1993;26:3–11
44. Pistre V, Pelissier P, Martin D, et al. 10 years experience with the submental flap. Plast Reconstr Surg 2001;108(6):1576–1581
45. Poulsen M. Merkel-cell carcinoma of the skin. Lancet Oncol 2004;5:593–599
46. Seethala RR, LiVolsi VA, Baloch ZW. Relative accuracy of fine-needle aspiration and frozen section in the diagnosis of the parotid gland. Head Neck 2005;27(3):217–223
47. Shah JP, Kraus DH, Dubner S, et al. Patterns of regional lymph node metastases from cutaneous melanomas of the head and neck. Am J Surg 1991;162:320–323
48. Stevens G, Thompson J, Firth I, O'Brien CJ, McCarthy W, Quinn M. Locally advanced melanoma. Cancer 2000;88:88–94
49. Stuckensen T, Kovacs AF, Adams S, et al. Staging of the neck in patients with oral cavity squamous cell carcinomas: a prospective comparison of PET, ultrasound, CT and MRI. J Craniomaxillofac Surg 2000;28(6):319–324
50. SWOG Trial National Cancer Institute Sponsor. SWOG S0008 2005
51. Tan ST, MacKinnon CA. Deep plane cervicofacial flap: a useful and versatile technique in head and neck surgery. Head Neck 2006;28(1):46–55
52. Taylor BW, Brant TA, Mendenhall NP, Mendenhall WM. Carcinoma of the skin metastatic to parotid area lymph nodes. Head Neck 1991;13:427–433
53. The 2002 national non-melanoma skin cancer survey. A report by the National Cancer Control Initiative Non-melanoma Skin Cancer Working Group for the state and territory cancer councils. November 2003
54. Trans-Tasman Radiation Oncology Group. TROG 05.01. Post-operative concurrent chemo-radiotherapy versus post-operative radiotherapy in high-risk cutaneous squamous cell carcinoma of the head and neck. Version 1: 11 march 2005
55. Trans-Tasman Radiation Oncology Group Inc. Australia and New Zealand melanoma trials group. A randomized clinical trial of surgery versus surgery plus adjuvant radiotherapy for regional control in patients with completed resected macroscopic nodal metastatic melanoma TROG 02.01 ANZMTG Trial 1–02 July 2003
56. Tulley P, Webb A, Chana JS, et al. Paralysis of the marginal mandibular branch of the facial nerve: treatment options. Br J Plast Surg 2000;53(5):378–385
57. UICC TNM Staging 2003
58. Vaglini M, Belli F, Santinami M, et al. The role of parotidectomy in the treatment of nodal metastases from cutaneous melanoma of the head and neck. Eur J Surg Oncol 1990;16:28–32
59. Veness MJ, Morgan GJ, Gebski V. Adjuvant locoregional radiotherapy as best practice in patients with Merkel cell carcinoma of the head and neck. Head Neck. 2005;27(3):208–216
60. Veness M, Morgan G, Palme C, Gebski V. Surgery and Adjuvant radiotherapy in patients with cutaneous head and neck squamous cell carcinoma metastatic to lymph nodes: combined treatment should be considered best practice. Laryngoscope 2005;115:870–875
61. Woods JE, Chong GC, Beahrs OH. Experience with 1360 primary parotid tumors. Am J Surg 1975;130:460–462

Chapter 23

Temporal Bone Resection

23

Moisés A. Arriaga, Christian Hall, Daniel Nuss, and Melda Kunduk

Contents

Core Features

- Anatomic relationship between the parotid gland and the temporal bone
- Clinical signs suggestive of a temporal bone malignancy
- The usefulness of diagnostic testing
- The staging of temporal bone malignancies
- Indications and techniques for temporal bone resection
- The utility of neoadjuvant and adjuvant therapy

Complications to Avoid

- Treatment delays due to missed diagnosis
- Incomplete work-up
- Inadequate staging of disease
- Failure to clear a resectable surgical margin
- Surgical error
- Lack of necessary soft tissue protection against postoperative radiation therapy
- Delayed initiation of postoperative radiation therapy
- Failure to address the sequelae of lower cranial nerve lesions

Introduction

Neoplasms involving the temporal bone present a rare and difficult problem for the patient and treatment team. Tumors involve the temporal bone through primary growth, direct extension, and metastatic spread. The latter two mechanisms are most significant when we consider salivary gland pathology in the temporal bone. The pathologic consequences include morbidity due to anatomic remodeling, intracranial extension, perineural spread, vascular encasement, dural invasion, and ultimately death. Historically, carcinoma of the temporal bone was an ominous diagnosis. Advancements in diagnostic and surgical technique have demonstrated greatly improved outcomes. The successful resection of T1 disease has demonstrated survival outcomes of up to 95%, and the treatment of T2 and T3 disease has demonstrated survivals up to 85% when a clear surgical margin is combined with postoperative radiation therapy [14].

A multidisciplinary approach to the diagnosis and treatment of these lesions offers the best possible outcome. Surgery and radiation represent the principal treatment arms; however, increasing interest is developing in a possible combined role for chemotherapy [25]. The type of resection needed is determined by the extent of disease. A sound oncologic resection can be achieved through a lateral temporal bone resection, subtotal temporal bone resection, and total temporal bone resection with parotidectomy, facial nerve resection, mandibulectomy, and cervical lymphadenectomy as indicated. Once the surgery has been planned, reconstructive options should be explored. Over the past century great strides have been made in the surgical and non-surgical management of temporal bone neoplasms, but they remain a significant treatment challenge.

Temporal Bone Malignancy

While neoplastic lesions of the temporal bone can arise from diverse histologic cell types, they tend to be of epithelial, mesenchymal, or salivary gland origin [11, 22]. Salivary gland tumors can originate from ectopic rests of salivary tissue within the middle ear (pleomorphic adenoma has been described in that location), or from minor salivary glands within the external auditory canal (EAC), but both are rare [11, 28]. Salivary gland tumors are more likely to involve the temporal bone through direct extension from the parotid gland. The anatomic relationship between the temporal bone and parotid gland is responsible for this tendency. The parotid gland is located in close proximity to the mastoid and tympanic portions of the temporal bone. It communicates directly with the cartilaginous EAC through the fissures of Santorini and foramen of Huschke [31]. The stylomastoid foramen, carotid canal, jugular foramen, petrotympanic fissure, and eustachian tube provide avenues for intratemporal extension. Ninety percent of tumors of the parotid gland originate in the superficial lobe with the remaining 10% being deep lobe in origin [24]. Tumors of the parotid gland originating within or extending to the deep lobe make contact with the lateral skull base via the parapharyngeal space. Tumors of the superficial lobe access the parapharyngeal space after traversing the stylomandibular tunnel.

Tumors of the temporal bone carry an incidence of 200 new cases per year with a frequency of 6 cases per million. Eighty-six (86%) percent of these tumors are squamous cell carcinoma (SCCA). Basal cell carcinoma, adenoid cystic carcinoma, adenocarcinoma, and ceruminous carcinoma occur less frequently [23, 25, 33]. Tumors of mesenchymal origin are as rare, with rhabdomyosarcoma occurring most frequently [22]. The reporting of tumors of salivary gland origin of the temporal bone is sporadic, making their study difficult.

Although benign parotid tumors rarely involve the temporal bone, it does occur, and is more likely when patients have previously undergone parotidectomy. Advanced or recurrent cases of pleomorphic adenoma and Warthin's tumor have been reported [17]. In these rare cases of temporal bone involvement by benign tumors of the parotid gland, symptoms of a facial mass, trismus, or compression of the parapharyngeal space by tumor usually precede temporal bone involvement. Additionally, benign masses have a tendency to compress or remodel adjacent tissue, rather than invade it. This allows for extirpation of a benign parotid neoplasm, in some cases, without requiring a formal temporal bone resection. These lesions can be removed through traditional parotidectomy techniques. Disarticulation of the mandibular condyle, resection of the EAC, or mastoidectomy may be necessary to assist with resection. Pleomorphic adenoma of the tail of the parotid gland can present as a subcutaneous mass of the floor of the lateral portion of the EAC. This situation is best managed with combined superficial parotidectomy with mastoidectomy and postauricular canalplasty.

Malignancies of salivary gland origin are more aggressive and involve adjacent tissue more readily. They can develop insidiously and relatively asymptomatically with 75% presenting as a painless mass and only 6–13% presenting with facial nerve palsy [35]. Symptoms may not be present until after temporal bone invasion has occurred. Pain, dysphagia, and dysphonia can present after direct invasion of the skull or involvement of the lower cranial nerves at the jugular foramen. Direct extension into bone, fissures, and foramen are potential routes of spread. Mass lesions of the poststyloid parapharyngeal space can traverse the carotid canal and jugular foramen, and neurotrophic tumors such as adenoid cystic carcinoma follow the facial nerve as an avenue toward the stylomastoid foramen. Additionally, carcinoma of the auricle, anterior scalp, or face that has spread to the intraparotid lymphatics can involve the temporal bone in a similar fashion.

Mucoepidermoid carcinoma, adenoid cystic carcinoma, and adenocarcinoma are the most common salivary malignancies. High-grade adenocarcinoma is known for its aggressiveness and low survival rates. Adenocarcinoma occurs in the parotid gland with a frequency of 28% and 5- and 10-year survival rates of 45% and 39%, respectively [35]. In a review of 27 cases of advanced and recurrent parotid neoplasms requiring temporal bone resection, Leonetti et al. found that adenocarcinoma occurred most commonly followed by adenoid cystic carcinoma and mucoepidermoid carcinoma [17].

Malignancies involving the temporal bone present a formidable problem. Without treatment these lesions result in a high incidence of morbidity and almost certain death. Extension into the otic capsule and petrous bone can result in hearing loss, vestibulopathy, cranial neuropathies, and hemorrhage. Malignant spread into the middle and posterior fossa and extension into the petroclival region or cavernous sinus portend a grim prognosis even with aggressive surgical efforts. In cases of distant metastatic disease a temporal bone resection may still be indicated for palliation.

History and Physical Examination

A thorough history and physical are indispensable for proper diagnosis and treatment planning. Patients with tumors of the parotid gland involving the temporal bone present with diverse symptoms, signs, and medical backgrounds. On initial presentation, the diagnosis may not be readily evident. It has been reported that 30% of patients with advanced parotid cancer are without pain [17]. Additionally, otologic inflammation due to tumor can, and frequently does, masquerade as an infectious process. A missed diagnosis could be responsible for treatment delays that result in the progression of disease. The experienced examiner can avoid this by taking a thorough history and performing a complete head and neck examination with special attention to the cranial nerves. Past treatment failures, asymmetry of the parotid area, trismus, lymphadenopathy, and facial nerve palsy are highly suggestive of malignancy and the need for further work-up (Table 23.1).

Biopsy

Once a mass lesion has been identified, tissue should be obtained for histologic study. Fine-needle aspiration biopsy (FNAB) provides a quick and efficient means for di-

Table 23.1. Clinical presentation of temporal bone cancer

	Leonetti et al. [17][a] Number (%)	Kuhel et al.[b, c] (%)	Pensak et al. [27] (%)
Symptoms:			
Pain	19 (74)	51	60
Hearing loss	18 (69)	29	20
Headache	12 (46)		
Facial numbness	8 (31)		
Hoarseness	3 (12)		
Dysphagia	1 (4)		
Vertigo/tinnitus		15	
Signs:			
Ear canal mass	26 (100)	37	
Bloody otorrhea	18 (69)	61	60
Facial paralysis	13 (5)	16	35
Cranial nerve defects	8 (31)		10
Parotid, neck mass	7 (27)		
Temporal mass	4 (15)	19	

[a] 26 cases
[b] 442 cases
[c] Adapted from Kuhel WI, Hume CR, Selesnick SH (1996) Cancer of the external auditory canal and temporal bone. Otolaryngol Clin North Am 29(5):827-852

agnosing salivary tumors. The accuracy of FNAB in salivary disease "ranges from 54% to 98%. FNAB of salivary malignancy has a sensitivity of approximately 60% to 73% for detection of malignancy [35]." If biopsy of the EAC or middle ear is needed, imaging of the temporal bone should be obtained first. This can prevent disasters related to biopsy of an encephalocele, an aberrant carotid artery, or a dehiscent jugular bulb.

Diagnostic Testing

Imaging studies and audiometric testing are also of critical importance. Magnetic resonance imaging (MRI) and computed tomography (CT) provide accurate information helpful in the staging of disease and determining the extent of resection needed. A preoperative hearing assessment will establish a functional baseline, the need for postoperative middle ear reconstruction when appropriate, and the potential for postoperative deficits. Angiography should be performed in all cases where the carotid artery is at risk. When carotid resection is anticipated cerebral blood flow analysis should be used to determine resectability and the need for revascularization. Consideration should also be given to embolization when intraoperative hemorrhage is a concern. Once the work-up is complete the proper staging can take place.

The close proximity of vital structures within and adjacent to the temporal bone requires an accurate assessment of the involved anatomy. CT and MRI are indispensable in this regard. The ability of CT to detail bony structures and the superb soft tissue contrast offered by MRI play complementary roles during work-up. Together, CT and MRI are helpful in establishing tumor extent, the involvement of critical structures, and the best surgical plan [8, 10].

The use of high resolution CT with fine cuts is recommended. Images with a thickness of 0.625–1.25 mm will produce the best assessment of the skull base. Direct axial and coronal scans should be obtained. When advanced scanning technologies are available reconstructed images provide resolution that is equivalent to the original data set [10]. CT is essential to preoperative staging. Arriaga et al. demonstrated that CT can "achieve 98% accuracy in predicting pathologic involvement in temporal bone resection specimens [2]." CT scans are not without limitation, however. Distinguishing mucosal inflammation from tumor and the extension of tumor without bony erosion remains difficult [1] (Fig. 23.1).

Magnetic resonance imaging should be used to examine tumor relative to dura, brain, cerebrospinal fluid, and skeletal muscle [10]. MRI also offers the advantage of imaging in multiple planes. This is useful when evaluating lesions that traverse the skull base through direct extent or perineural spread [10]. T1, T2 and fat-saturated sequences should be obtained. T1 images help to determine spatial relationships and bone marrow involvement while T2 images help to delineate tumors. Post-gadolinium T1-weighted images with fat saturation should also be obtained to determine the presence and extent of perineural involvement. This can manifest as foraminal widening or enhancement, replacement of fat density, or increased signal intensity [8, 10].

In previously operated areas, positron emission tomography (PET)-CT combined imaging has proven useful for distinguishing scar from neoplasm in identifying tumor recurrence and guiding treatment.

Audiologic testing demonstrates the functional status of the middle and inner ear. This information is useful during surgical planning and preoperative patient counseling. Conductive losses may be attributable to the presence of a malignancy in the external or middle ear. Anacusis, tinnitus, and vertigo suggest inner ear involve-

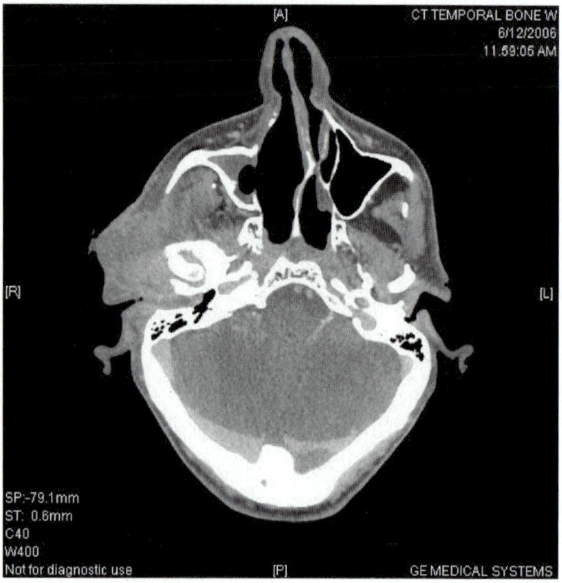

Fig. 23.1: Axial CT scan demonstrating neoplastic invasion of the temporal bone by SCCA of the parotid gland (pt at UMC-Lafayette)

23

ment. If a reduction or elimination of hearing is anticipated the patient should be informed in advance. Ossicular chain reconstruction or a bone-anchored hearing aid may be indicated when conductive hearing is sacrificed, but sensorineural hearing is spared.

A four vessel angiogram with venous runoff should be used in cases of carotid encasement or when disease mandates dissection of the petrous carotid. Arterial stenosis and contour irregularity at the site of the lesion are suggestive of malignant involvement. Close inspection of the carotid canal on CT as well as CT angiography are useful for carotid assessment. Temporary balloon occlusion coupled with a cerebral blood flow quantification study helps to determine when carotid sacrifice will be tolerated. Quantification studies include PET, functional MRI, and xenon-CT. Xenon-CT is the best studied modality [22]. An occlusional cerebral blood flow < 30 ml/100 g per min requires prophylactic or intraoperative saphenous grafting. Cerebral blood flow < 20 ml/100 g per min or the development of neurologic symptoms during the test are indicative of a high risk of perioperative stroke. These findings either preclude the surgical option or require that prophylactic revascularization be done if surgery is performed [23].

Staging

The American Joint Committee on Cancer states "that a staging system should provide a sound basis for therapeutic planning for cancer patients by describing the survival and resultant treatment of different groups in comparable form [1]." A lack of uniformity regarding preoperative staging and treatment plans has made the study of temporal bone cancer difficult. This has changed with the demonstration that CT imaging accurately predicts the degree of neoplastic involvement. The supplementation of these observations with clinical findings enabled the formation of a reliable system for staging carcinoma of the EAC [2]. Attempts to modify this system have been made. Moody et al. propose upstaging patients with preoperative facial nerve paralysis or paresis to T4 status when the primary tumor originates in the EAC. They propose that the extension of tumor through tissue separating the facial nerve and EAC, and tumor involving the horizontal segment of the nerve, are ominous signs [24]. While this and other modifications to the original system by Arriaga et al. have been suggested, the original system has provided a useful framework for staging these lesions and validation of the various systems are still pending [1] (Table 23.2).

This system can be used to plan the surgical management of the temporal bone when involved secondarily by a cancer of the parotid gland. Although the data are not as clear for salivary gland cancers extending to the temporal bone as for primary temporal bone lesions, the same staging criteria should be applied to decisions regarding the extent of the anatomic resection and the need for radiation therapy. Patients can be counseled about prognosis and survival based on results with primary cancer arising in the temporal bone.

Surgical Treatment

The surgical management of temporal bone tumors varies depending upon the extent of disease. When tumors involve the temporal bone secondarily through direct extension, temporal bone resection accompanies the surgical management of the primary tumor. The medial exten-

Table 23.2. University of Pittsburgh staging system for cancer of the external auditory canal (adapted from reference 2)

T1 status	Tumor limited to the external auditory canal without bone erosion or evidence of soft tissue extension
T2 status	Tumor with limited external auditory canal bone erosion (not full thickness) or radiographic finding consistent with limited (< 0.5 cm) soft tissue involvement
T3 status	Tumor eroding the osseous external auditory canal (full thickness) with limited (< 0.5 cm) soft tissue involvement, or tumor involving middle ear or mastoid, or patients presenting with facial paralysis
T4 status	Tumor eroding the cochlea, petrous apex, medial wall of middle ear, carotid canal, jugular foramen or dura, or with extensive (> 0.5 cm) soft tissue involvement
N status	Involvement of lymph nodes is a poor prognostic finding and automatically places the patient in an advanced stage (i.e., stage III (T1, N1) or stage IV (T2, 3, and 4, N1) disease)
M status	Distant metastasis indicates a poor prognosis and immediately places patients in the stage IV category

sion of tumor dictates the indication for partial temporal bone resection, subtotal temporal bone resection, and total temporal bone resection (Fig. 23.2).

Partial temporal bone resection includes removal of the entire external auditory meatus. It is indicated for cancer of the temporal bone which is limited to the external canal. The facial nerve provides the medial limit of resection. The procedure begins by performing a complete mastoidectomy. The mastoid air cells are completely removed. The tegmen and sigmoid sinus are identified. The course of the facial nerve is dissected from the lateral semicircular canal to the stylomastoid foramen. An extended facial recess approach provides wide access to the middle ear space. Drilling of the auditory canal continues inferior to the external canal. The dissection proceeds anteriorly toward the glenoid fossa and medially through the hypotympanum toward the jugular bulb and carotid artery. The zygomatic air cells are also dissected. Drilling proceeds superiorly from the antrum toward the zygomatic root and through the epitympanum. The bone between middle fossa dura and the remaining EAC is removed. Superior to the external canal the dissection proceeds lateral to the incus and malleus. The surgeon takes care to avoid middle fossa dura by remaining close to the superior aspect of the external canal. Once the superior and inferior approaches to the glenoid fossa have been completed, the incudostapedial joint is separated, the tensor tympani is cut, and the ligamentous attachments of the ossicles are divided. At this point the anterior portion of the external canal is its only remaining attachment. This bone is fractured free of the carotid with gentle pressure or tapping with an osteotome. If a chisel is used it is important to angle the instrument lateral to the carotid so that inadvertent injury of the vessel can be avoided. Once the specimen has been removed and the middle ear fully exposed, the eustachian tube is obliterated [33] (Figs. 23.3, 23.4).

During the procedure it is important to remain cognizant of the tumor, being careful that it is avoided during the dissection. While drilling the epitympanum it is important to remain lateral to the geniculate ganglion and medial to the annulus. An intact tympanic membrane should be preserved with the specimen for tumors limited to the external canal [14]. This reduces the likelihood of tumor spillage. When involvement of the facial nerve is present, specimens of the proximal margins should be examined histologically with sufficient tissue resection until the margins are free of tumor. If the nerve is sacrificed an interposition graft connects the proximal and distal tumor-free portions of the nerve. The sural nerve

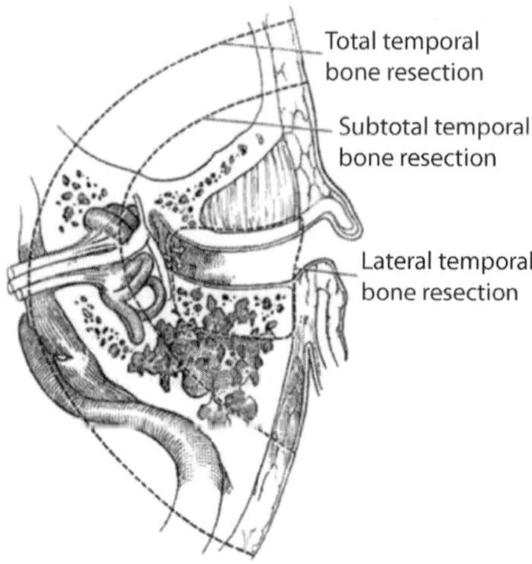

Fig. 23.2: Margins of resection for lateral temporal bone, subtotal temporal bone, and total temporal bone resection

and the greater auricular nerve serve as excellent donor sites. The greater auricular nerve is used more often because of its proximity to the surgical field, but if there is malignant lymphadenopathy in the neck, the sural nerve should be used instead. Care is necessary during graft orientation to position the graft so regenerating fibers are not lost through side branching, orienting the graft with the distal end of the graft in apposition with the proximal segment.

If the temporal bone has been involved secondary to direct extension from the parotid gland, the involved parotid tissues should be removed in continuity. Resection of the mandibular condyle and zygomatic root facilitates dissection of the infratemporal and parapharyngeal spaces and prevents the violation of soft tissue attachments between the parotid, temporomandibular joint, and EAC [21]. Consideration should also be given to management of the cervical lymphatics. In general, primary temporal bone cancers rarely metastasize to the cervical lymphatics; however, primary cancers of salivary gland origin have inherently different lymphatic drainage than the temporal bone making dissection of the cervical lymph nodes prudent.

Involvement of the middle ear space requires a subtotal temporal bone resection. The dissection extends medially into the otic capsule and petrous portions of the temporal bone in order to obtain negative margins. The medial extent of dissection is defined by the internal auditory canal (IAC). Control of the internal carotid artery (ICA) and

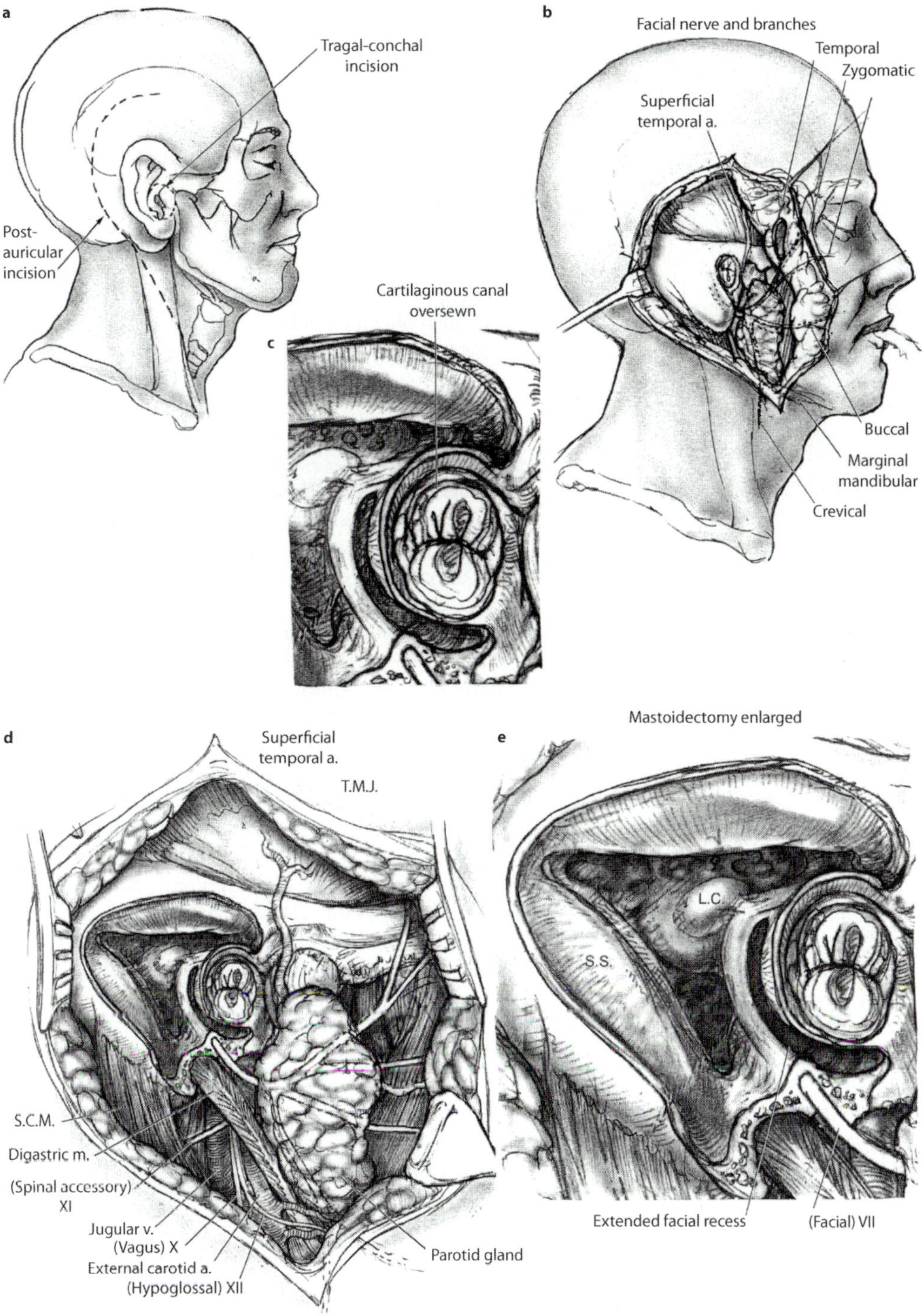

Fig. 23.3: Surgical approach for the lateral temporal bone resection. **a** Incision. **b** Exposure of facial nerve. **c** Oversewing the cartilaginous canal. **d** Exposure including mastoidectomy. **e** Extended facial recess approach

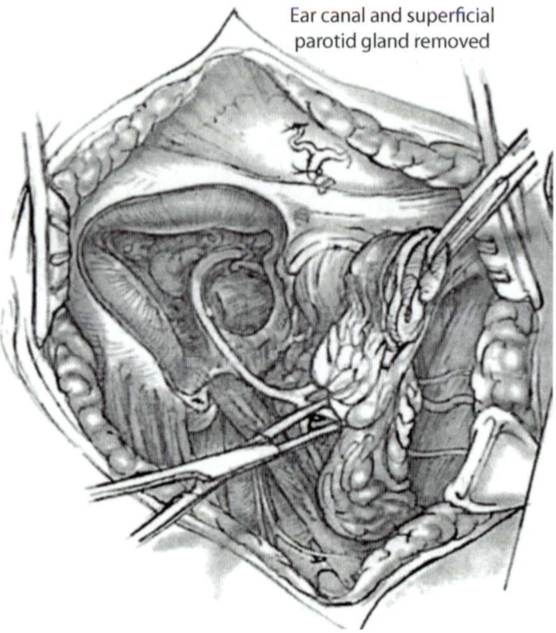

Fig. 23.4: Lateral temporal bone resection. Removal of ear canal and superficial lobe of parotid

jugular vein is obtained inferiorly. The vertical portion of the petrous internal carotid is identified by dissecting through the glenoid fossa and eustachian tube. The sigmoid sinus and jugular bulb are carefully freed from the temporal bone. Brisk bleeding from the inferior petrosal sinus and condylar vein occurs with opening of the jugular bulb, and the surgeon should be prepared. Ligation of the sigmoid sinus and jugular vein permits packing of the bulb in cases of excessive bleeding. An additional strategy to prevent bleeding from the jugular bulb is preoperative coil embolization of the openings of the inferior petrosal sinus and condylar vein [5]. The osteotomy proceeds along the floor of the middle fossa connecting the glenoid fossa, IAC, and posterosuperior mastoid [23].

When the cancer has progressed beyond the limits of a subtotal temporal bone resection, a total temporal bone resection may be indicated. Total temporal bone resection is rarely performed due to the high level of morbidity and a lack of well-documented survival benefit [32]. The surgery involves freeing the temporal bone at the petrous apex. Prior to extirpation the intratemporal portion of the ICA must be dissected to the foramen lacerum, and the internal jugular vein ligated. Sacrifice or reconstruction of the ICA may be performed based on the results of preoperative testing. A subtemporal craniotomy is performed exposing the transverse sinus. The dura covering the cerebellum is incised and the transverse sinus is ligated and divided near the superior petrosal sinus. The tentorium is divided sharply along the petrous bone in a plane superior and parallel to the superior petrosal sinus. The VIIth, and VIIIth cranial nerves are divided at the IAC. With the cerebellum retracted medially an intradural incision is used to divide the IXth, Xth, and XIth cranial nerves and free the specimen at its posterior dural attachment. Once the surrounding structures have been freed, a chisel is placed in the foramen ovale and directed posteriorly in a trajectory lateral to foramen lacerum. This will free the temporal bone at its apex [14, 23, 27] (Fig. 23.5).

Reconstruction

Reconstructive options should be explored preoperatively, but as in all oncologic surgeries, the reconstructive plan must never compromise the completeness of oncologic resection. Consideration should be given to cosmesis and the durability of the repair. Intraoperative findings might dictate a more complex reconstruction than anticipated. Careful planning improves the preparation for a variety of potential defects.

Resections of the temporal bone limited to the external canal and mastoid are successfully reconstructed with a split-thickness skin graft following the removal of cerumen-forming adnexa. The graft should be placed to line the ear canal and mastoid bowl. Its medial extent can be carefully draped over the oval window or stapes remnant. Reconstruction of the ossicular chain can take place at a later time. If the treatment plan includes radiation therapy, the middle ear should not be reconstructed.

A more extensive resection of the temporal bone requires added soft tissue to obliterate dead space, prevent the leakage of cerebrospinal fluid (CSF), and provide protection against complications related to radiation therapy, the most serious of which is osteoradionecrosis [7]. Smaller wounds involving resection of the pinna and external canal may be closed by a posterior scalp or cervicofacial advancement flap. If additional bulk is needed, a muscle or myocutaneous flap can be rotated on a vascularized pedicle, or inset via microvascular anastomosis.

Smaller defects may be amenable to closure using a temporalis muscle rotation flap. A trapezius, latissimus, or pectoralis major muscle rotational flap may become necessary as the size of the defect increases. Extensive defects may require a rectus abdominis muscle or perforated-

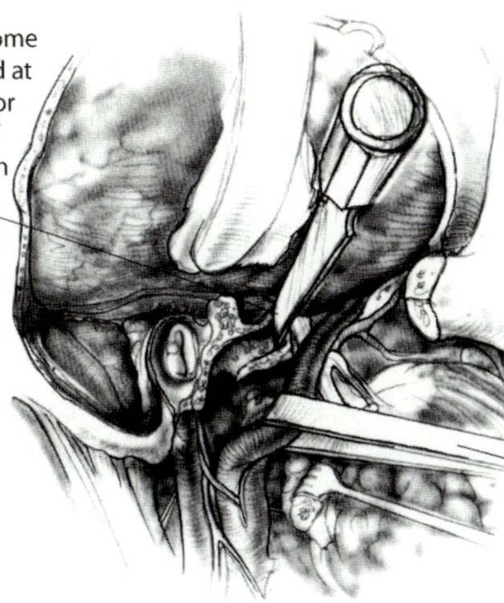

Fig. 23.5: Total temporal bone resection. An osteotome, inserted at the horizontal petrous carotid canal just posterior to the foramen ovale, is directed slightly posteriorly to avoid entry into the foramen lacerum. This releases the total temporal bone specimen

based adipose free flap for closure. The arterial and venous anastomosis should be sutured to the external carotid artery and jugular vein, respectively. In wounds requiring additional skin, a split-thickness skin graft can be placed over the muscular portion of the reconstructive flap. If dura is resected, the dural defect and eustachian tube must be obliterated. This is accomplished with abdominal fat or free tissue transfer, and serves to shield the central nervous system from environmental insult [14, 22, 33].

Complications

Hemorrhage is a common consequence of lateral temporal bone resection. Venous bleeding can be responsible for massive blood loss, and losses up to 2,500 ml can be encountered. As mentioned previously, excessive bleeding most commonly occurs at the inferior petrosal sinus, but this bleeding can be controlled with proper technique. After the jugular vein has been tied in the neck, the proximal sigmoid sinus is occluded with extraluminal oxidized cellulose. The sigmoid sinus is entered distal to this point. Here, bleeding from the inferior petrosal sinus and condylar vein can be encountered. The bleeding can be controlled by advancing oxidized cellulose packing to the jugular bulb. Preoperative coil embolization to occlude the condylar vein and inferior petrosal sinus can be used to reduce bleeding during this portion of the surgery. The excessive use of packing at the jugular foramen can result in injury to cranial nerves IX, X, and XI, so this should be done with caution [4].

Injury to the carotid artery should be managed with direct pressure and placement of temporary clips proximal and distal to the insult. Systemic and intra-arterial heparin should be given. The injury should be repaired with 8-0 monofilament suture. If minor leaks persist following closure, topical hemostatic agents can be applied. If successful repair of the vessel cannot be achieved, the preoperative balloon occlusion test should be used to guide management [14]. Vascular surgery and neurosurgical consultation are imperative. If there is significant carotid involvement, then preoperative stent placement has been demonstrated to avoid vascular complications [34].

Facial nerve sacrifice or excessive manipulation of the nerve can result in facial asymmetry and inadequate eye closure. During the immediate postoperative period the eye should be protected with lubrication, use of a moisture chamber, or mechanical lid closure. If the nerve is sacrificed an interposition graft using the ipsilateral greater auricular nerve or sural nerve should be performed. If the great auricular nerve is unavailable the sural nerve can be used in its place. Successful nerve interposition can restore function to a House-Brackmann scale grade III, but may take 12–18 months to occur. Placement of a gold weight implant or spring, lateral tarsorrhaphy, or tensing of the lower eyelid may be necessary during the reinnervation period. Facial-hypoglossal anastomoses can also help restore facial function. When lower cranial nerve deficits exist, this should be done with caution. A loss in the function of the XIIth nerve can have devastating consequences on an already impaired swallowing apparatus.

Tumor involving the jugular foramen may result in pre- or postoperative paresis or palsy of the IXth and Xth nerves. Such lesions can manifest in airway and nutritional difficulty. Temporary or permanent tracheotomy and the placement of a gastrotomy tube may be necessary to compensate for the associated deficits. The combination of an insensate supraglottis, vocal fold motion impairment, or inadequate swallow reflex can result in aspiration with fatal consequences. Vocal fold medialization may restore safe deglutition. In more severe cases of swallowing or laryngeal dysfunction a laryngotracheal separation may be necessary.

If dura has been excised or violated the resulting defect must be repaired immediately. Primary closure should be instituted whenever possible. If necessary the dural defect should be obliterated with fat, fascia, or free tissue transfer. Postoperative leakage of CSF can be managed conservatively for up to 7–10 days with appropriate measures. Bed rest, elevation of the head of the bed, stool softeners, and placement of a lumbar drain can be useful in reducing intracranial pressure [26]. If the leak persists beyond this period the wound should be explored surgically and closure of the dural defect should be reattempted [14, 18, 33].

Radiation

Plans for the use of postoperative radiation should be made during the preoperative work-up. The use of adjuvant radiation should be anticipated whenever the middle ear is involved with disease. If intraoperative findings confirm the need for radiation it should be given in a timely fashion. Radiation therapy should not be delayed, or withheld in lieu of a recurrence. This can result in decreased therapeutic efficacy [15]. Closure of the surgical defect with viable, durable tissue is necessary to prevent development of osteoradionecrosis, which can be a devastating and sometimes fatal complication. In addition, careful postoperative hygiene and maintenance (cleaning and debridement with otomicroscopy) of the reconstructed area is essential to reduce likelihood of chronic infection that can predispose to osteoradionecrosis. Dosages typically range from 5,000 to 6,000 rads and fields should be designed to include the area of resection and involved nodal groups [15, 19]. The rarity of temporal bone malignancy makes the study of treatment protocols difficult, but encouraging results have been reported. T1 lesions successfully treated with surgery alone have a 95% 5-year survival, with no benefit from the addition of radiation. Some T2 and T3 lesions treated with radiation following complete surgical removal have shown an 85% 5-year survival. The 5-year survival of patients with more advanced lesions drops below 50% [14]. Cancer requiring a total temporal bone resection carries a dismal prognosis, with a 50% 1-year survival and 0% 2-year survival [33] (Fig. 23.6)

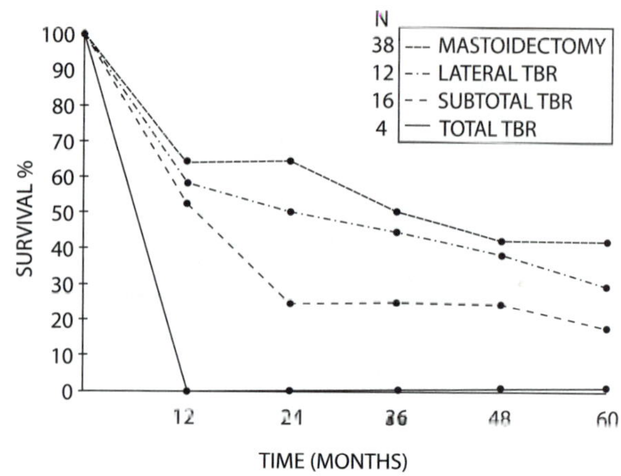

Fig. 23.6: Treatment-specific survival for patients with carcinoma extending to the middle ear. *TBR* Temporal bone resection

Chemotherapy

23

The role of chemotherapy in the treatment of temporal bone malignancy has not been determined, but interest in its use is growing. Because of the relatively low incidence and the histologic diversity of temporal bone malignancies, few meaningful studies have been conducted. Temporal bone malignancies of salivary gland origin, like salivary malignancies in other sites, do not usually respond to currently available chemotherapeutic agents. SCCA of the temporal bone may respond to platinum-based agents, but typically the results are not durable and other modalities must be used. For these reasons, most patients with temporal bone cancer are treated with surgery, radiation, or a combination of the two, and chemotherapy is usually reserved for palliation in patients with distant metastases or recurrences. Nakagawa et al. have published data that suggest a possible role for preoperative chemoradiation therapy (CRT) in the treatment of T3 and T4 SCCA when staged according to the Arriaga system. The radiation enhancing effect of chemotherapy may be useful in reducing the tumor burden and improving control of the surgical margin. Nakagawa et al. have demonstrated improved survival rates for T4 lesions not involving dura, pyramidal apex, carotid canal, or lymph nodes that are as good as those in patients with T3 lesions [25]. The poor outcomes associated with the treatment of advanced temporal bone malignancy mandate further investigation into the possible role of chemotherapy as a treatment modality.

Rehabilitation of Lower Cranial Nerve Deficits

The size and specific location of temporal bone tumors will determine the outcome of speech, voice, and swallowing function of the patient. Surgery and radiation of these tumors, especially when they involve the parapharyngeal space, can cause damage to cranial nerves IX, X, and XII, even if the tumor itself has not directly affected them. These cranial nerves provide sensory and motor innervation to tongue, pharynx, and larynx, and are essential for airway protection during swallowing and intact speech and voice production. Therefore, multiple cranial nerve injury can have debilitating effects resulting in aspiration, dysphonia, and significantly reduced intelligibility of speech. This may necessitate extensive rehabilitation following the intervention. The involvement of a speech and language pathologist (SLP) specialized in voice and swallowing function both preoperatively and postoperatively will contribute to achieving a comprehensive rehabilitative management plan for the patient.

Preoperative evaluation of the patient's voice, speech, and swallowing functions may include both subjective and objective tests to determine the functional level of the patient pre-intervention. The objective tests of swallowing may include modified barium swallow test (MBS) or fiberoptic endoscopic evaluation of swallowing (FEES) [16]. The quality of the patient's voice and its resonance can be examined via perceptual, endoscopic, acoustic, and aerodynamic methods. In addition, the patient's cognitive status and support systems should be examined to determine his/her capability to carry out the rehabilitative intervention for the expected voice, speech, and swallowing dysfunctions which will follow surgical and radiation treatment.

Postoperatively, in order to develop an effective treatment plan, a thorough assessment of speech, swallowing, and voice structures and the degree of their dysfunction needs to be reestablished. Further, the impact of the dysphonia, dysphagia, and speech problems on the patient's quality of life should be determined. Deficits involving one or more of cranial nerves IX, X, and XII will have varying effect on speech, voice, and swallowing mechanism. The degree of the impact can vary from mild and short term to long term and debilitating to life threatening caused by aspiration pneumonia [6, 29, 30].

During the evaluation of voice, close attention should be paid to the presence of hypernasality, weak voice, and the duration of voice. The hypernasality will indicate velopharyngeal dysfunction which can also result in nasal regurgitation of food during swallowing. A weak, breathy voice with reduced duration can indicate insufficient glottic closure and this could be due to vocal fold motion impairment. A flexible nasopharyngoscopic and videostroboscopy evaluation can establish the presence of palatal, pharyngeal, and laryngeal insufficiencies resulting from cranial nerve X involvement. The maximum phonation time (MPT) can also give information regarding the effectiveness of glottic closure during phonation [13]. Management of voice problems might include surgery to medialize the vocal fold, behavioral voice therapy, and use of amplification devices [6]. Velopharyngeal dysfunction can be addressed by collaborative work between the SLP and the prosthodontist for the appropriateness and best fitting of a palatal prosthesis for the patient, and occasionally may involved surgical treatment including palatoplasty or palatopexy.

Cranial nerve IX, X, and XII deficits can have an overwhelming effect on oral and pharyngeal stages of swallowing resulting in aspiration before, during, and after swallowing [19]. The extent and mechanism of these deficits will be determined best by using one or more of the following tests administered postoperatively; the clinical examination (does not detect the silent aspiration), MBS, FEES, and flexible endoscopic evaluation of sensory testing (FEESST) [3]. The SLP will determine the compensatory, behavioral or dietary modification strategies during the administration of the test/s in order to determine the safest method of oral intake for the patient. When this is not possible immediately after the surgery, an alternative means of nutrition and hydration via nasogastric or gastrostomy tube placement is established and a swallowing treatment program with realistic goals is established for the patient. Jennings et al. found that in the acute state, oropharyngeal dysfunction reduced laryngeal elevation and pharyngeal residue resulted in aspiration in 78% of the patients who underwent skull base surgery [12]. Oral intake was possible in 58% of these patients in 2 weeks with the help of compensatory swallow techniques and diet modifications.

Cranial nerve XII deficiency could also result in reduction in rate and accuracy of the tongue movements. This could lead to an altered speech pattern of the patient. Speech intelligibility difficulties occurring following the surgery can be addressed by intensive speech therapy focusing on tongue motion exercises and articulation therapy [9].

Xerostomia is one of the most common acute and long-term side effects of the radiation. It can have a severe effect on the quality of life and swallowing skills of the patients. If patients are capable of oral intake of food, during and after radiation, they often complain about needing to wash the food down with water while eating, food getting stuck in the mouth and throat, and alteration in taste [20]. These problems can still be present many months after irradiation [15]. Recommending dietary changes can alleviate problems. Mild oral antiseptic and antifungal mouth washes have also been found to be helpful with these symptoms [15]. Patients should be aware of the importance of good oral hygiene in order to prevent further complications.

Rehabilitation of voice and swallowing dysfunction demands a team approach for the best outcome. The patient is part of the team and his/her needs and goals should guide the rehabilitation efforts. Preoperative and postoperative evaluation of swallowing, voice, and speech function will facilitate the recognition of deficits and timely initiation of rehabilitation, which will lead to improved quality of life.

Take Home Messages

- Advanced parotid neoplasms can invade the temporal bone.
- Malignancies involving the temporal bone can be mistaken for infection.
- CT and MRI are complementary and indispensable during work-up of temporal bone malignancy.
- The University of Pittsburgh staging system is reliable and effective for staging temporal bone malignancy.
- The goal of surgery should be a tumor-free margin.
- Reconstruction should provide soft tissue protection against radiation therapy.
- Postoperative radiation therapy provides survival benefit for advanced disease.
- The sequelae of lower cranial nerve lesions can be dire.
- Chemoradiation therapy shows promise as a neoadjuvant therapy.

References

1. Arriaga MA, et al. (1991) The role of preoperative CT scans in staging external auditory meatus carcinoma: Radiologic-pathologic correlation study: Otolaryngol Head Neck Surg 105(1):6–11
2. Arriaga MA, et al. (1990) Staging proposal for external auditory meatus carcinoma based on preoperative clinical examination and computed tomography findings. Ann Otol Rhinol Laryngol 99(9):714–721
3. Aviv JE, Kim T, Goodhart K, et al. (2000) The safety of flexible endoscopic evaluation of swallowing with sensory testing (PEESST): An analysis of 500 consecutive evaluations. Dysphagia 15:39–44
4. Brackmann DE, Arriaga MA (1994) Surgery for glomus and jugular foramen tumors. In: Brackmann D (1994) Otologic Surgery, Saunders
5. Carrier D, Arriaga MA, Dahlen R (1997) Preoperative embolization of anastomosis of the jugular bulb: A new adjuvant in jugular foramen surgery. Am J Neuroradiol 18:1252–1256
6. Colton RH, Casper JK (2005) Understanding voice problems: A physiological perspective for diagnosis and treatment (3rd edition) Baltimore; William and Wilkins
7. Day TA, Davis BK (2001) Skull base reconstruction and rehabilitation. Otolaryngol Clin North Am 34(6):1241–1257
8. Durden D, Williams D (2001) Radiology of skull base neoplasms. Otolaryngol Clin North Am 34(6):1043–1064
9. Eibling DE, Boyd EM (1997) Rehabilitation of lower cranial nerve deficits. Otolaryngol Clin North Am 30:865–875
10. Glenn L (2005) Innovations in Neuroimaging of skull base pathology. Otolaryngol Clin North Am 38(4):613–629
11. Goodwin JW, Jesse HR (1980) Malignant neoplasms of the external auditory canal and temporal bone. Arch Otolaryngol 106:675–679
12. Jennings KS, Siroky D, Jackson CL (1992) Swallowing problems after excision of tumors of the skull base: diagnosis and management in 12 patients. Dysphagia 7(1):40–44
13. Kent RD, Kent JF, Rosenbek JC (1987) Maximum performance tests of speech production. J Speech Hear Disord 52:367–387
14. Kinney SE, Malignancies of the temporal bone – Limited temporal bone resection. In: Brackmann DE et al. (eds) (1994) Otologic Surgery. Saunders
15. Koukourakis MI, Danieldis V (2005) Preventing radiation induced xerostomia. Cancer Treat Rev 31:546–554
16. Langmore SE, Schatz K, Olsen N (1988) Fiberoptic endoscopic examination of swallowing safety: A new procedure: Dysphagia 2:216–219

17. Leonetti JP, Smith PG, Anand V, et al. (1993) Subtotal petrosectomy in the management of advanced parotid neoplasms. Otolaryngol Head Neck Surg 108:270–276
18. Lewis JS (1975) Temporal bone resection review of 100 cases. Arch Otolaryngol 101:23–25
19. Logemann JA (1997) Evaluation and treatment of swallowing disorders (2nd edition) Pro-ed, Austin, Texas
20. Logemann JA, Smith CH, Pauloski BR, et al. (2001) Effects of xerostomia on perception and performance of swallow function. Head Neck 23(4):317–321
21. Manolidis S, Pappas D Jr, Doerslen P, et al. (1998) Temporal bone and lateral skull base malignancy: experience and results with 81 patients. Am J Otol 19(16 Suppl):S1–15
22. Marsh MM, Jenkins HA: Temporal bone neoplasms and lateral cranial base surgery: In: Cummings CW, et al. (eds) (2005) Cummings Otolaryngology – Head and Neck Surgery Mosby
23. Moffat D, De la Cruz A, Evans PHR, Management of tumours of the temporal bone. In: Evans PHR (2003). Principles and Practice of Head and Neck Oncology. Martin Dunitz
24. Moody SA, Hirsch BE, Myers EN (2000) Squamous cell carcinoma of the external auditory canal: an evaluation of a staging system. Am J Otol 21(4):582–588
25. Nakagawa T, Kumamoto Y, Natori Y, et al. (2006) Squamous cell carcinoma of the external auditory canal and middle ear: An operation combined with preoperative chemoradiotherapy and a free surgical margin. Otol Neurotol 27(2):242–249
26. Nuss DW, Constantino PD (1993) Cerebrospinal fluid leaks: Comprehensive diagnosis and management. Otolaryngol Head Neck Surg 108(5):539
27. Pensak M, Willging JP: Tumors of the temporal bone. In: Jackler R (ed) (1994) Neurotology. Elsevier Mosby, Philadelphia
28. Peters BR, Maddox HE, Batsakia JG (1988) Pleomorphic Adenoma of the middle ear and mastoid with posterior fossa extension. Arch Otolaryngol Head Neck Surg 114:676–678
29. Peterson KL, Fenn J (2005) Treatment of dysphagia and dysphonia following skull base surgery. Otolaryngol Clin North Am 38(4):809–817
30. Pou A, Carrau RL, Skull base surgery. In (ed) (1999) Comprehensive management of swallowing disorders. Singular publishing group, London UK
31. Prasad M, Kraus D (2004) Acinic cell carcinoma of the parotid gland presenting as an external auditory canal mass. Head Neck 26:85–88
32. Prasad S, Janecka IP (1994) Efficacy of surgical treatments for squamous cell carcinoma of the temporal bone: A literature review. Otolaryngol Head Neck Surg 110(3):270–280
33. Prasad S, Janecka IP, Malignancies of the temporal bone – radical temporal bone resection. In: Brackmann DE, et al. (eds) (1994) Otologic surgery Saunders
34. Sanna M, Khrais T, Menozi R, et al. (2006) Surgical removal of jugular paraganglioma after stenting of the intratemporal internal carotid artery: A preliminary report. Laryngoscope 116(5)742–6
35. Simental A, Carrau R, Malignant neoplasms of the salivary glands. In: Cummings C, et al. (eds) (2005) Cummings Otolaryngology – Head and Neck Surgery. Mosby

Chapter 24

Facial Nerve Reconstruction

24

Eberhard Stennert

Contents

Core Features

- Implications of facial nerve damage on related central and peripheral structures
- Time schedule for facial nerve repair
- Decision criteria for facial nerve reconstruction
- Importance of normal function of the trigeminal nerve in cases of hypoglossal-facial reanimation (basic functional triad between Vth, VIIth, and XIIth cranial nerves)
- Disadvantages of cross-face anastomosis

General Aspects

Before going into detail of the different surgical techniques available, it is necessary to outline some basic facts that should be considered.

Consequences of Facial Nerve Damage Leading to Axon Degeneration

The facial nerve itself is the structure to be operated on and, although it is important, it is a relatively simple "connecting cable" between the central nervous system (CNS) and the facial mimic musculature, thus being only a small part within a much more complex system. Not only the morphology of the nerve but also the vital condition of the central and peripheral structures of this threefold system have to be taken into account, especially in cases of delayed reconstruction.

As a consequence of any severe facial nerve damage leading to axon degeneration, this degeneration results:

a) Centrally, in retrograde changes to the motoneurons and their cellular environment [2, 7–11, 15, 30, 31] and
b) Peripherally, in the degeneration of muscle fibres [6, 12].

The reversibility or irreversibility of these degenerative processes depends on the time that has elapsed between nerve injury and reinnervation of the musculature.

Time Schedule for Facial Nerve Repair

Since the relationship between the elapsed time and the extent of these retrograde and anterograde morphological (and as a consequence, functional) changes differs for each species, it is not possible to draw any conclusions relating to human beings from animal experiments. Our knowledge is therefore limited to clinical experience. Based on our considerable empirical experience, we would make the recommendations compiled in the table about the time schedule for facial nerve repair (Table 24.1).

However, for recovery of facial expression following partial or subtotal resection of the facial nerve and/or the peripheral nerve plexus, an immediate surgical reconstruction should be performed when at all possible for the following reasons:

1. The surgeon should be aware that facial expression, with its unique arbitrary and spontaneous nature, plays an extremely important role in the social life of humans. Thus if it is lost or distorted this can have profound psychological consequences.
2. As already mentioned above, reconstructive nerve surgery should be performed as a one-stage operation together with tumour resection or, if a histomorphological analysis of the specimen is necessary, within 10–14 days at most, otherwise the rapid development of scar tissue may jeopardise the success of this delicate surgery.
3. The general health of the patient is to be considered, since with a reduced tolerance to anesthesia, more complex and therefore longer procedures must be replaced with simpler methods.
4. The biological age of the patient plays a role in the choice of procedure. With advancing age, the regeneration strength diminishes in nerve tissue, and preference is to be given to procedures that make a safe and fast reinnervation of the paralysed musculature possible. These are all procedures with end-to-end anastomoses, thus avoiding the use of interposition grafts.

24

Table 24.1. Time schedule for facial nerve repair

Duration of paralysis (years[a])	Functional recovery of facial musculature
0–1	Absolutely certain
1–2	Expected, therefore recommendable
2–3	Probable, with delay and decrease in function
3–5	Increasingly questionable, patient must be notified
5+	Improbable, therefore not to be recommended

[a] Timeinterval between onset of denervation and probable reinnervation

5. The same decision criteria apply to patients who are particularly psychologically unstable, and may find it more difficult to live with a failed procedure than more stable or indifferent individuals.
6. The length of the interposition graft has a substantial influence on the final functional result after reconstruction. In principle, the rule can be applied that the longer the graft, the worse the final outcome will be, particularly when the graft is longer than 4–5 cm. The main reason for this is that the axons need more time to penetrate the endoneural tubes, while at the same time, degeneration of the Schwann cells and fibrosis occurs. In particular the penetration of the distal anastomosis will be handicapped through meanwhile development of scar tissue.

Fundamental Questions Prior to Nerve Surgery

In cases of delayed nerve reconstruction, the following questions should be addressed before planning the surgery.

Peripheral Nervous System (Facial Nerve and Plexus)

a) To what extent has the nerve plexus been resected? In other words, is there still enough nerve tissue of the main branches in situ to perform successful anastomoses?

b) How realistic are the chances of identifying and isolating the branches within the scar tissue from the injury or the previous operation?
c) Is there enough suitable nerve material available for free nerve transplantation?
d) If the hypoglossal nerve is to be used for anastomosis, are the XIIth and also the Vth cranial nerves intact in their extracranial course? (In this context see explanation below under "Central Nervous System".)
e) In cases of tumour resection, is the remaining facial nerve tissue free from tumour infiltration?

Central Nervous System

a) What is the general condition of the brain? I.e., is the patient intellectually or emotionally limited by cerebrosclerosis or other diseases of the CNS?
b) Is the trigeminal nerve as well as the hypoglossal nerve functioning normally? If the hypoglossal nerve is to be used as a donor graft for facial nerve reconstruction, it is important to take into consideration that there is a functional relationship, based on tight neuroanatomical connections, between the cranial nerves V, VII, and XII. The function of both motor nerves (N VII, N XII) depends on the common afferent input from the trigeminal nerve. The hypoglossal-facial nerve anastomosis only leads to good results if this triad is intact as a whole [13, 23].

Musculature

a) Is it still vital enough to regain its contractibility? (See also Table 24.1)
b) Is it free from tumour infiltration?
c) Is it free from infection?

Methods for Reconstruction of the Extratemporal Facial Nerve Plexus

Due to longstanding clinical experience the following methods for reconstruction of the extratemporal facial nerve plexus are recommended [27]:

1. End-to-end anastomosis
2. Free nerve transplantation (interposition graft)
3. Hypoglossal-facial anastomosis (HFA) as end-to-end anastomosis
4. Hypoglossal-facialis jump anastomosis (HFJA) as an end-to-side anastomosis
5. Combined approach (facio-facial anastomosis combined with HFA)

In comparison to the overall excellent functional outcome of the abovementioned techniques that allow a sufficient reanimation of the mimetic musculature in nearly all cases, the cross-face anastomosis has several disadvantages leading to only suboptimal or bad results:

- The need to harvest the sural nerve is time consuming and leads to decreased sensation at its innervation area.
- The implantation of two to three transplants across the face are again time consuming and bothersome to the patient.
- The anastomosis with facial nerve branches of the opposite side destroys healthy structures.
- The long transplants need much more time for reinnervation.
- Long transplants always result in a worse outcome compared to short grafts and especially to end-to-end anastomoses.

Therefore we have not used this technique for the last three decades.

Take Home Messages

- For careful indicated nerve reconstruction, not only the nerve itself but also the vital conditions of the CNS and the paralysed muscles have to be taken into account, especially in cases of delayed reconstruction.
- Reconstruction beyond a 5-year interval between onset of denervation and expected reinnervation seems not recommended.
- Reconstructive nerve surgery must be performed as soon as possible, either as a one-stage operation together with tumour resection or, if a histomorphological analysis of the specimen is necessary, within 10–14 days at most because of the rapid development of scar tissue.

Take Home Messages

- Good results of hypoglossal-facial reanimation depend on normal function of the trigeminal nerve.
- Cross-face anastomosis has several disadvantages.

End-to-end Anastomosis

Core Features

- Recommendation for how to get a tension-free anastomosis
- Recommendation for correct "trimming" of nerve endings
- Critical remarks on fascicular sutures

In the majority of cases, a "clean-up" of the nerve is unavoidable, which requires a shortening of the nerve endings. Lack of tension in the anastomosis is an important prerequisite for a good, functioning result, and a tension-free suture can only be achieved after mobilisation of the central and peripheral nerve stumps.

According to our experience, the possibilities for such a mobilisation are limited, and the following procedure is therefore recommended to relieve tension from the anastomosis. Before performing the nerve suture, insert a suture of strength 7-0 or 8-0 through the epineurium of one or both of the nerve stumps a few millimetres from the anastomosis to the right and left, and pull these sutures with moderated pressure towards the anastomosis, securing it in the underlying base of the incision. (Such a procedure is naturally only possible when the nerve branches are of sufficient size.)

Regarding the suture technique for end-to-end anastomoses, there are two false statements that are frequently found in the literature, supported by unrealistic diagrams [4]. First, according to these opinions, the epineurium should be trimmed back at the ends of the fascicles. Although the epineurial sheath is moveable to a certain extent, suture of the epineurium of both nerve endings leads to an additional shortening of this surrounding structure. This can easily lead to an intrafascicular rejection of the fascicle endings, which in turn leads to a correct adaptation of the fascicles being prevented. The resultant "bulging" of the fascicles within the anastomosis can often be felt against the bordering nerve section through soft palpation with microinstruments alone. Conversely, suture of epineuria that overlap the ends of the fascicles leads to an intraneural separation, creating an "empty space". As a consequence it is recommended that the nerve endings be "cleaned up" by one sharp section through the entire nerve.

Second, claims that a fascicular suture can be performed for facial nerve surgery are particularly unrealistic. This is impossible for three reasons:

1. In contrast to peripheral nerves, which consist of individual fascicles well separated from each other by the perineurium (polyfascicular form), cranial nerves do not show any clear individual fascicles (monofascicular form).
2. The consistency of the alleged fascicles is so soft that they would tear while trying the knot on even the most gentle of sutures.
3. The suture material used for such a technique would shift inward, where it would be perceived as a foreign body and interfere with the healing process by inducing granulation tissue.

Take Home Messages

- Tension-free anastomosis is essential for good functional outcome.
- Nerve endings should simply be trimmed by one sharp section through the whole nerve or nerve branch.
- Fascicular sutures are impossible to perform in cranial nerves.

Free Nerve Transplantation (Interposition Graft)

Core Features

- The tree-like branching out of the facial plexus leads at the same time to numerical and size discrepancies between its central and peripheral parts
- Advantage of greater auricular nerve and disadvantage of sural nerve as donor grafts
- Description of a reliable technique for overcoming the numerical and size discrepancies

In the context of surgery of the parotid gland (and here principally as a consequence of resection of malignant tumours), nerve defects arise in the region of the facial nerve plexus (pes anserinus). This has a tree-like branching out which is unique in the entire human organism. The most significant problem to deal with when attempting to overcome material loss of the pes anserinus comes from this tree-like branching out. This causes two problems when trying to overcome severe material defects in the central region of the nerve plexus (Fig. 24.1):

1. Due to the tree-like branching out, there are only a few (or one) central nerve stump(s) compared with numerous peripheral endings, causing a numerical discrepancy.
2. At the same time, the central nerve stumps have a larger diameter than the very thin peripheral nerve endings, causing a size discrepancy.

The extraction of a single graft that imitates this division satisfactorily is only possible in exceptional cases, and one must therefore almost always opt for several individual grafts. Usually nerve transplants cannot imitate the tree-like branching out of the facial fan.

The common donor graft is the greater auricular nerve, which has two advantages:

1. It is easy to extract because it is already within the area being operated upon for the parotid gland surgery.
2. Like the facial nerve and its plexus branches, it is monofascicular.

We recommend that the greater auricular nerve be followed as far as possible into the parotid gland at the start of the parotidectomy, because there is occasionally a suitable branching in the posterior pole of the parotid.

As a further possible donor, the sural nerve is usually considered, which has two considerable disadvantages:

1. Its extraction is very costly.
2. The bifurcations of its nerve branches are very far apart.

Overcoming the Discrepancy in Number and Size by Using Interposition Graft(s)

We have had excellent functional results in many cases using the following techniques [25, 27].

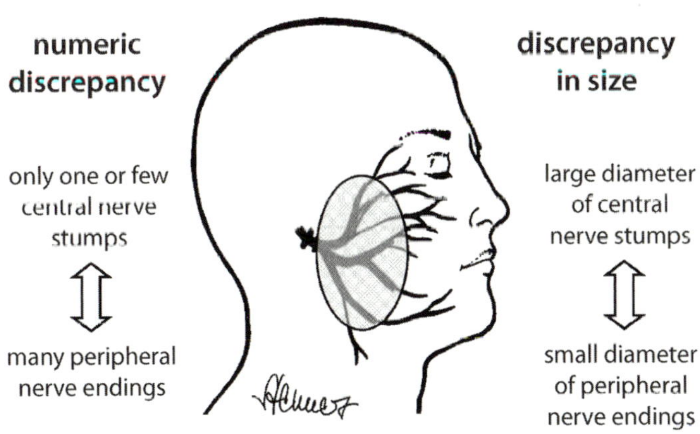

Fig. 24.1: Two main problems for reconstruction of central parts of the facial nerve plexus with interposition graft(s): numerical discrepancy and discrepancy in size between central and peripheral nerve endings

Interventions at the Peripheral Nerve Branches

The ends of the nerve in the region of the peripheral resection are mobilised sufficiently that each of the two neighbouring nerve branches can be positioned with their proximal ends about 5 mm alongside each other. If possible, the epineuria at the contact edges are dissected and, finally, the edges are bound together with a 10-0 suture. In this way, a new nerve branch is created from two peripheral nerve branches, now consisting of two fascicles. This allows the number of peripheral branches to be halved, while at the same time doubling their size, resulting in the defect being more easily repairable with a graft (Fig. 24.2).

This technique can be taken further when required, using, for example, three or four neighbouring nerve branches to make a new large nerve branch.

Interventions with the Graft

When a suitable graft is chosen, its peripheral ends can also be split into individual fascicles, which has a branching effect in addition to the interventions taken at the peripheral nerve endings (so-called diversification).

The combination of both methods results in the most suitable synergistic double-effect: the reduction of number and increase in size of the peripheral nerve structures and the increase in number and reduction of size of the central nerve structures.

Take Home Messages

- Effective overcoming of the numerical and size discrepancies between central and peripheral parts of the tree-like branching out of the facial nerve plexus can be reached twice:

  1. In the periphery by unifying neighbouring nerve branches to one new branch, thus decreasing their number and increasing their size; and
  2. Centrally by splitting suitable grafts into individual fascicles, thus increasing their number and decreasing their size.

Hypoglossal-Facial Nerve Anastomosis (HFA)

Core Features

- Critical comments on postulated disadvantages
- Outline of possible functional results
- Importance of an adequate mimic training in order to take advantage of brain plasticity

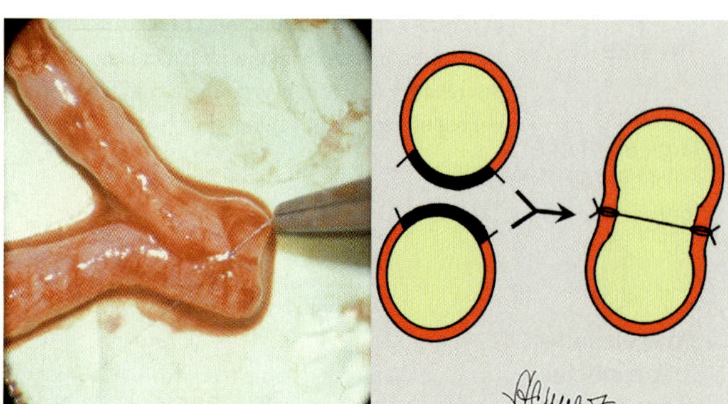

Fig. 24.2: Technique for reduction in number and increase in size. After mobilisation and adaptation of amputated nerve endings, the epineurium at the site of contact is resected, the edges are bound together with a 10-0 suture and thereby the numbers of peripheral branches are halved, while at the same time doubled in their size

Dr. W. Körte, who was at that time head of the ENT department at the Charité in Berlin, performed this anastomosis in 1901 for the very first time in humans. Two years later, Körte reported unexpectedly good results from this operation. After Bernhard, a neurologist, had critically observed and documented the patient's postoperative course, Körte noted: "It is a most remarkable physiological fact that ganglion cells of the hypoglossal or the accessory nerve nucleus can acquire under voluntary influence the ability to induce contractions of muscles originally innervated from other nerve centres. We cannot yet decide whether there are connections between the two areas of nerve ganglia, or whether by willpower the nerve center can adapt or become accustomed to stimulating a newly acquired muscle system" [14].

In the past, our study group, consisting of otorhinolaryngologists and neuroanatomists, has done extensive clinical and experimental research on the central nervous connections between these two cranial nerves. It could be demonstrated that there are multiple preformed correlations which gave answers to Körte's question and can explain the excellent results of this anastomosis [19–22, 26].

Hypoglossal-facial nerve anastomosis was often criticised and rejected, because of the following postulated disadvantages:

1. Hemiparesis of the tongue leads to problems when talking and eating.
2. Facial movements are only possible through deliberate movements of the tongue.
3. These deliberate movements of the tongue lead to uncontrolled grimacing.
4. Spontaneous emotional expression will never be regained.

These criticisms are by no means justified. To begin with, it must be stated that the HFA is technically easy to perform; success is assured; and it leads to a rapid reinnervation of the paralytic musculature because of its peripheral localisation. With respect to the possible functional results, experience has shown that:

1. The partial atrophy of the tongue, which varies in degree but is always restricted to the lateral aspect of the involved side, does not lead to substantial problems with talking and eating.
2. Intended movements of facial musculature become independent from deliberate movements of the tongue.
3. Separate activation of different facial muscle groups can be gained, e.g. selective innervation can be achieved.
4. Limited emotional facial expression is possible (e.g. spontaneous smile).

The quality of these possible functional results depends on:

1. The intensity and duration of facial expression rehabilitation by an adequate mimetic training program in order to take advantage of brain plasticity [1, 3, 5]
2. The vitality of brain function
3. The duration of denervation (atrophy of facial musculature and retrograde changes in the CNS)
4. The surgical quality of the anastomosis

Take Home Messages

- Criticisms are by no means justified.
- Excellent results are based on preformed anatomical connection between both cranial nerves on all levels of the CNS.
- The quality of the final functional outcome depends very much on the duration and quality of a postoperative mimic training in order to take advantage of brain plasticity.

Hypoglossal-Facial Nerve Anastomosis as End-to-end Anastomosis

Core Feature

- Indications

The classic HFA as end-to-end anastomosis between the two cranial nerves is restricted to the following few situations in parotid surgery:

Early tumour infiltration into the nerve stem followed by growth (spreading) proximally into the mastoid is observed, especially in adenoid cystic carcinomas, which develop deep in the parotid gland. A free transplant is required for the reconstruction of the dissected nerve section. Since the wallerian degeneration caused by either the tumour or the surgery extends to the motor end plates, reanimation of the facial musculature can take many months.

In such cases, a direct HFA as an end-to-end anastomosis can be indicated, particularly for older patients with a tendency for rapid drooping of the facial musculature. This is because the direct anastomosis is relatively more peripheral, leading to a much quicker reinnervation and thus to a more rapid recovery of muscle tone.

A direct HFA is indicated in the same way in cases where an attempt at rehabilitation using a free graft has failed.

Take Home Messages

- HFA as an end-to-end anastomosis has advantages:
  1. It is technically easy to perform and therefore is not time consuming;
  2. It is an end-to-end anastomosis and therefore a safe procedure; and
  3. The anastomosis lies relatively far peripherally, thus leading to an early reinnervation (3–4 months).
- HFA as an end-to-end anastomosis is therefore particularly indicated:
  a. For older patients with a tendency for rapid drooping of the facial musculature;
  b. In cases where an attempt at rehabilitation using a free graft has failed; and
  c. In cases in which an early postoperative radiation is mandatory.

Hypoglossal-Facial Nerve Anastomosis with "Jump" Anastomosis (HFJA)

Core Features

- Description and illustration of the surgical technique
- Special indications

This is a very valuable alternative to the classic HFA. Figure 24.3 illustrates the procedure. This technique was popularised by M. May [18]. However, it is worthwhile to note that the first HFA performed by W. Körte in 1901 was also an end-to-side anastomosis [14].

The hypoglossal nerve is exposed in the retromandibular fossa and a diagonal incision made into its ventral circumference, half way through the axons and through the epineurium, leaving an open V-shaped wound. A graft (usually from the greater auricular nerve) is then sutured into this V-shaped incision so that its ends anastomose with the proximal stumps of the dissected axons of the hypoglossal nerve. Finally, the peripheral end of the graft can be sutured with the facial nerve stem as well as with each branch of its plexus. In the plexus region, for overcoming discrepancy in number and size, the same techniques can be used as those described above.

In comparison to direct anastomosis between the two nerve trunks, this technique is more time consuming and delicate to perform because of the additional need of harvesting and interposing a free nerve graft. However, in the hands of a well-trained microsurgeon this technique is also a safe method leading to excellent functional results [16, 17]. Since the functional deficits of the tongue are negligible, the method is especially indicated for all patients with speech occupation and for rehabilitation of irreversible facial palsy after the removal of an acoustic neurinoma, which might be the first manifestation of a Morbus Recklinghausen (type II) disease and then may later also develop on the contralateral side!!!

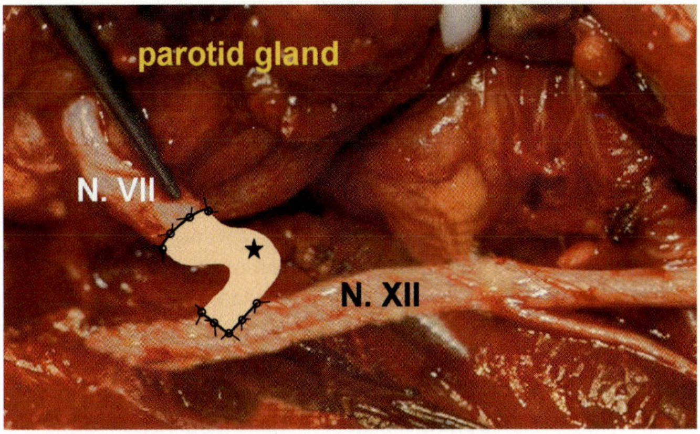

Fig. 24.3: Technique of a "hypoglossal-facial jump anastomosis". The hypoglossal nerve is exposed in the retromandibular fossa and a diagonal incision is made into half of its ventral circumference. The distal end of the interposed nerve transplant has to be directed towards the proximal stumps of the dissected axons of the hypoglossal nerve

Take Home Messages

- The indirect HFA with interposition graft is a safe method leading to excellent functional results.
- The method is especially indicated:
  a. For all patients with speech occupation; and
  b. For rehabilitation of irreversible facial palsy after the removal of an acoustic neurinoma, which might be the first manifestation of a Morbus Recklinghausen (type II) disease, which later may also develop on the contralateral side!!!

Extended Hypoglossal-Facial Nerve Anastomosis

Core Features

- Discussion of indications
- Description and illustration of the surgical technique

This is the method of choice for all tumours that require extensive resection of the facial plexus, which are in general malignant. It has recently been recognised that malignant tumours of the parotid gland show a high tendency towards lymphogenous metastasis, and as with all other malignant tumours of the head and neck region, simultaneous neck dissection is indicated [28].

For reconstruction of a facial plexus that has been extensively dissected peripherally, HFA offers an ideal solution to many of the problems described above, while at the same time having considerable advantages:

1) The hypoglossal nerve is already exposed within the region being operated upon for surgery of malignant tumours, especially when combined with a neck dissection, meaning that the preparation of a nerve transplant from another region of the body is not necessary.
2) The following recommendations are made for preparation of the hypoglossal nerve:
   a) Initially it is exposed to its entrance into the musculature of the floor of the mouth, until its arborisation into peripheral branches can be identified. Beyond this arborisation the nerve is dissected.
   b) With sufficient magnification under the microscope, the stumps of the peripheral branches can now be isolated retrograde from the connective tissue, and if necessary followed as single fascicles further into the main stem.
   c) This is followed by step-by-step retrograde mobilisation of the hypoglossal nerve (main trunk) towards the skull base. In the meantime, it is possible to check at which point the resected ends of the

transpositioned hypoglossal nerve reach the facial plexus nerve stumps without tension.

d) Separation of the ansa hypoglossi is also necessary when mobilising the hypoglossal nerve to overcome expansive defects. The ansa should also be separated as far peripherally as possible to be used as a further anastomosis.

3) After such an extensive mobilisation, it is possible to twist the hypoglossal nerve ventrocranially to such an extent that even nerve endings of extremely peripherally located facial branches can be reached.
4) This allows a multiple tension-free end-to-end anastomosis to be made, and guarantees instant axonal growth through the anastomosis (Fig. 24.4).
5) Because the anastomoses are far peripheral, there is rapid reinnervation of the musculature. This is particularly important for malignant tumours with the necessity of additional radiotherapy.
6) This method is much less time-consuming than the removal and transplantation of many individual grafts, and is therefore less of a strain on both patient and surgeon.
7) If necessary, this method can also be combined with the procedure described above to overcome the discrepancy between central and peripheral nerve stumps regarding their number and size by combining the stumps of the facialis branches that remain in situ (Fig. 24.4).
8) Because longer free nerve grafts are avoided and the end-to-end anastomosis is far peripheral, postoperative radiotherapy has no negative effect on the functional result.

All abovementioned points are of particular advantage especially for older patients. Experience has shown that, as a rule, after 4 months the facial muscle tone is already more balanced in a relaxed state, and within the following 2 months the motor function for intended movements becomes rapidly stronger. This should then be followed by about 2 years of a mimetic training.

Take Home Messages

- It is the method of choice for all malignant tumours that require extensive resection of the facial plexus, especially when combined with a neck dissection.
- It allows multiple tension-free end-to-end anastomosis to be made, and guarantees instant axonal growth through the anastomoses.
- Because the anastomoses are far peripheral, there is rapid reinnervation of the musculature. This is particularly important for malignant tumours with the necessity of additional radiotherapy.
- Preparation of nerve transplants from other bodily regions are not necessary, which makes the method much less time consuming than the removal and transplantation of several individual grafts, and is therefore less of a strain on both patient and surgeon.
- If necessary, this method can also be combined with the procedure described above to overcome the discrepancy between central and peripheral nerve stumps regarding their number and size.

Combined Approach (= Diversification Technique = Facio-Facial Anastomosis Combined with Hypoglossal-Facial Nerve Anastomosis)

Core Features

- Hint to the functional anatomy of the facial musculature
- Description and illustration of method

This reconstruction method is also to be considered for patients with total loss of facial expression, but only when the resection defect is restricted to the central portion of the pes anserinus (facial plexus), i.e. nerve trunk, bifurcation, temporofacial and cervicofacial main branch and immediately adjacent sections of branches extending

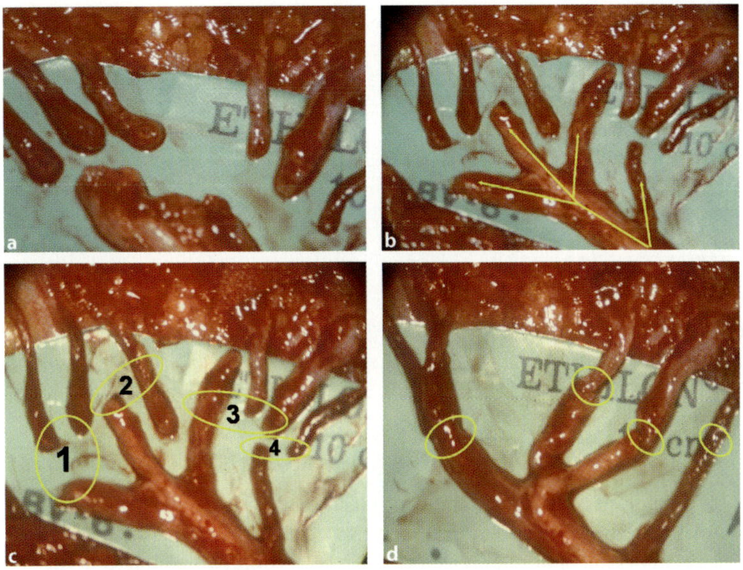

Fig. 24.4: Extended HFA for reconstruction of the facial plexus. **a** The situs shows in the upper part the endings of the preserved facial nerve branches, and in the lower part the distal stump of the hypoglossal nerve resected deep in the floor of the mouth at the beginning of its branching. **b** Same situs after diversification (separation) of N XII branches. **c** End-to-end anastomoses 1 and 3 are made by combining the facial branches, and anastomosis 3 by additional shortening of the hypoglossal branch. Anastomoses 2 and 4 are made by direct end-to-end anastomoses after shortening of the facial branch in anastomosis 2. **d** End result of the HFA which allowed a large defect of the facial plexus to be bridged over after tumour resection, allowing invariable end-to-end anastomosis

from this region. The method pays particular attention to the functional anatomy of the facial musculature, which consists of an ocular and oral sphincter system [24, 29]. Experience with the HFA has shown that good functional rehabilitation of the musculature of the oral sphincter system can be achieved using the hypoglossal nerve. For this reason, nerve branches that innervate the perioral musculature are supplied either directly or with a jump anastomosis by the hypoglossal nerve.

To innervate the musculature of the ocular sphincter system, a facio-facial anastomosis between the nerve trunk and the cranial nerve branches is made using a free nerve transplant. In this way, the motor neurons (reflex fibres) that are responsible for the blink reflex will have a chance for a more targeted reinnervation of the orbicularis oculi muscle. Here also, the method described above for overcoming discrepancy in number and size can be applied for the peripheral anastomoses. Using both cranial nerves at the same time leads to a physiologically "diversified" innervation of both independently operating sphincter systems. This leads to a significant reduction in synkineses and especially in the so-called mass movements [29] (Fig. 24.5).

Take Home Messages

- This combined approach leads to excellent results in cases where the resection defect is restricted to the central portion of the pes anserinus (facial plexus).
- The method pays particular attention to the functional anatomy of the facial musculature, which consists of an ocular and an oral sphincter system.
- Good functional rehabilitation of the musculature of the oral sphincter system is achieved using the hypoglossal nerve.
- To innervate the musculature of the ocular sphincter system, a facio-facial anastomosis between the nerve trunk and the cranial nerve branches is made using a free nerve transplant. In this way, the motor neurons (reflex fibres) that are responsible for the blink reflex will have a chance for a more targeted reinnervation of the orbicularis oculi muscle.

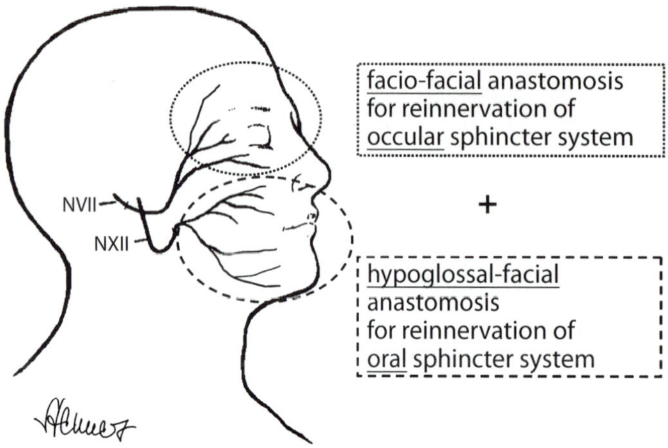

Fig. 24.5: Principle of the combined approach: the method pays attention to the functional anatomy of the mimic musculature, which consists of an ocular and oral sphincter system. Reanimation of the ocular system via a facio-facial anastomosis with an interposition nerve transplant and at the same time reanimation of the oral system via a hypoglossal-facial anastomosis leads to a physiologically "diversified" innervation of both independently operating sphincter systems, thus leading to a significant reduction in synkineses ("mass movements")

References

1. Beurskens CHG (2005) Mime therapy: contents and evidence. In: Beurskens CHG, van Gelder RS, Heymans PG, Manni JJ, Nicolai J-PA (eds) The Facial Palsies. Lemma, Utrecht, pp 285–293
2. Blinzinger K, Kreutzberg G (1968) Displacement of synaptic terminals from regenerating motoneurons by microglial cells. Z Zellforsch Mikrosk Anat 85:145–157
3. Bongers-Janssen HMH, Buck MJI, Kleine-Snijders ATH, Neetesen-Lobé HJ, Seelen HAM (2005) Multidisciplinary treatment of patients with a peripheral facial nerve lesion. In: Beurskens CHG, van Gelder RS, Heymans PG, Manni JJ, Nicolai J-PA (eds) The Facial Palsies. Lemma, Utrecht, pp 309–320
4. Burgess LPA, Goode RL (1994) Reanimation of the Paralyzed Face. Thieme, Stuttgart, p 16
5. Coulson SE (2005) Physiotherapy rehabilitation following facial nerve paresis. In: Beurskens CHG, van Gelder RS, Heymans PG, Manni JJ, Nicolai J-PA (eds) The Facial Palsies. Lemma, Utrecht, pp 263–274
6. Goebel HH, Schneider I, Tews DS, Gunkel A, Stennert E, Neiss WF (1994) Morphologic studies on human and rodent facial muscles. Eur Arch Otorhinolaryngol Dec:S24–S27
7. Graeber MB, Kreutzberg GW (1986) Astrocytes increase in glial fibrillary acidic protein during retrograde changes of facial motor neurons. J Neurocytol 15:363–373
8. Graeber MB (1994) The role of astrocytes in facial nerve regeneration. Eur Arch Otorhinolaryngol Dec:S75–S77
9. Guntinas-Lichius O, Gunkel A, Stennert E, Neiss WF (1994) Astroglial response in facial and hypoglossal-facial anastomoses in the rat. Eur Arch Otorhinolaryngol (Suppl) S557
10. Guntinas-Lichius O, Gunkel A, Stennert E, Neiss WF (1994) Synaptic stripping in facial and hypoglossal nucleus after hypoglossal-facial anastomoses in the rat. Eur Arch Otorhinolaryngol (Suppl) S558
11. Guntinas-Lichius O, Irintchev A, Streppel M, Lenzen M, Grosheva M, Wewetzer K, Neiss WF, Angelov DN (2005) Factors limiting motor recovery after facial nerve transection in the rat: combined structural and functional analyses. Eur J Neurosci 21:391–402
12. Irintchev A, Wernig A (1994) Denervation and reinnervation of muscle: physiological effects. Eur Arch Otorhinolaryngol Dec:28–30
13. Kivelitz R, Loew F, Hübner H (1974) Perspectives on the indications and contraindications of various nerve transplant techniques in cases of facial nerve paralysis after pontine angle tumor operations. Chir Plast (Berl) 2:161–167
14. Körte W (1903) Ein Fall von Nervenpfropfung: Des Nervus facialis auf den Nervus hypoglossus. Deutsch Wschr 17
15. Kreutzberg GW (1982) Acute neural reaction to injury. In: Nicholls JG (ed) Repair and Regeneration of the Nervous System. Springer, Berlin Heidelberg New York, pp 57–69

16. Manni JJ, Beurskens CHG, Velde van de C, Stokroos RJ (2001) Reanimation of the paralyzed face by indirect hypoglossal-facial nerve anastomosis. Am J Surg 182:268–273
17. Manni JJ (2005) Reanimation of the hemiparalysed face with the hypoglossal-facial nerve interpositional graft anastomosis. In: Beurskens CHG, van Gelder RS, Heymans PG, Manni JJ, Nicolai J-PA (eds) The Facial Palsies. Lemma, Utrecht, pp 177–185
18. May M, Sobol SM, Mester SJ (1991) Hypoglossal-facial nerve interpositional-jump graft for facial reanimation without tongue atrophy. Otolaryngol Head Neck Surg 104:818–825
19. Neiss WF, Schulte E, Guntinas-Lichius O, Gunkel A, Stennert E (1994) Response of Nissl substance in the facial and hypoglossal nucleus after hypoglossal-facial anastomoses in the rat. Eur Arch Otorhinolaryngol (Suppl) S559
20. Streppel M, Popratiloff A, Angelov DN, Guntinas-Lichius O, Hilgers RD, Stennert E, Neiss WF (1998) Significance of trigeminal sensory input on regrowth of hypoglossal and facial motoneurons after hypoglossal facial anastomosis in rats. Acta Otolaryngol 118:790–796
21. Streppel M, Popratiloff A, Gruart A, Angelov DN, Guntinas-Lichius O, Delgado-Garcia JM, Neiss WF, Stennert E (2000) [Morphological connections between the hypoglossal and facial nerve in the brain stem of the rat.] Morphologische Verbindungen zwischen N. hypoglossus und N. facialis im Hirnstamm der Ratte. HNO 48:911–916
22. Stennert E (1979) Hypoglossal facial anastomosis: its significance for modern facial surgery. II. Combined approach in extratemporal facial nerve reconstruction. Clin Plast Surg 6:471–486
23. Stennert E, Limberg CH (1982) Central connections between fifth, seventh and twelfth cranial nerves and their clinical significance. In: Graham MD, House WF (eds) Disorders of the Facial Nerve. Raven, New York, pp 57–65
24. Stennert E (1982) Das Autoparalytische Syndrom – ein Leitsymptom der postparetischen Fazialisfunktion. Arch Otorhinolarygol 236:97–114
25. Stennert E (1992) Prinzipien der Nervenrekonstruktion. In: Naumann HH, Helms J, Herberhold C, Kastenbauer E (eds) Oto-Rhino-Laryngologie in Klinik und Praxis. Thieme, Stuttgart pp 744–747
26. Stennert E (1997) Neurophysiologische und neuroanatomische Untersuchung zur Hypoglossus-Facialis-Anastomose und ihre klinische Bedeutung. Jahrbuch 1996 der Deutschen Akademie der Naturforscher Leopoldina, Halle/Saale. Leopoldina (R. 3) 42:363–385
27. Stennert E, Jungehülsing M (2001) Chirurgie der Glandula parotis einschließlich rekonstuktiver Fazialis-Chirurgie: Standard und Qualitätssicherung. Laryngorhinootologie 80(suppl 1):156–197
28. Stennert E, Kisner D, Jungehülsing M, Guntinas-Lichius O, Klussmann JP (2003) High incidence of lymph node metastasis in major salivary gland cancer. Arch Otolaryngol Head Neck Surg 129:720–723
29. Stennert E (2005) Synkineses and the Autoparalytic Syndrome. In: Beurskens CHG, van Gelder RS, Heymans PG, Manni JJ, Nicolai J-PA (eds) The Facial Palsies. Lemma, Utrecht, pp 117–133
30. Streit WJ (1994) The role of microglia in regeneration. Eur Arch Otorhinolaryngol Dec:S69–S70
31. Tetzlaff W, Graeber MB, Kreutzberg GW (1986) Reactions of motoneurons and their microenvironment to axotomy. Exp Brain Res (Suppl) 13:3–8

Chapter 25

Management of the Neck in Cancer of the Salivary Glands

25

Kristin B. Gendron and Robert L. Ferris

Contents

Core Features

- Discussion of risk factors for metastasis from cancer of the salivary glands
- Algorithm for management of the clinically negative (N0) neck in cancer of the salivary glands based upon clinical assessment, fine-needle aspiration biopsy, and frozen section pathology
- Management of the clinically positive (N+) neck, including neck dissection and postoperative radiation therapy
- Future directions in understanding salivary gland tumorigenesis and cervical metastasis, such as using molecular markers for prognosis and developing targeted therapy

Complications to Avoid

- Lack of awareness of specific risk factors associated with a high risk of metastasis will result in inadequate treatment of the regional lymphatics in salivary gland malignancy.
- Although the overall complication rate of elective neck dissection is low, there is associated risk to the lingual, hypoglossal, spinal accessory, and marginal mandibular nerves as well as vascular structures. In the absence of extensive clinical metastasis, sacrifice of named structures during neck dissection is not necessary during surgical excision of regional nodal disease.

Complications to Avoid *(continued)*

- Fine-needle aspiration biopsy usually does not provide adequate pathologic information to support treatment of the neck. Frozen section is often sufficient to guide treatment, but at times the decision must be deferred until the final pathology results are available.
- In the setting of a salivary gland mass and associated lymphadenopathy, lymphoma and metastatic skin cancer must be included in the differential diagnosis to prevent over- or undertreatment.

Introduction

Management of the neck in cancer of the salivary glands is a crucial component of oncologic care. Cancers of the salivary glands have a low incidence, representing only 1–3% of all malignancies in the head and neck [6]. Only a fraction of these cancers have clinically apparent nodal metastases at presentation. These cancers include a diverse group of histologic types found in several anatomic sites. For these reasons, there have been no randomized, controlled studies to evaluate the indications and efficacy of treatment of the neck with either surgery or radiation for occult or apparent metastases. The reported incidence of metastasis varies widely according to tumor type, grade, and primary salivary site. It is important to develop an understanding of the behavior of these cancers and adopt a standardized approach to the treatment of the neck because nodal metastasis correlates with a poor prognosis. As in other cancers of the head and neck, the presence of nodal metastasis decreases mean survival by greater than 50% [6, 47]. In addition, patients who develop recurrent disease in the neck have a low rate of surgical salvage (12–30%) [24]. Thus, thorough evaluation of the neck in the setting of cancers of the salivary glands is an important component of accurate staging and helps to optimize treatment.

We believe that the neck should be addressed if there is clinically apparent metastasis or if the primary tumor has a significant risk for occult metastases. However, the most appropriate management of the clinically negative neck in cancer of the salivary glands is controversial. The true frequency of nodal metastasis is difficult to assess due to the common practice of local sampling of lymph nodes as opposed to formal neck dissection. Lymph nodes removed in the process of attaining surgical exposure to the primary tumor may be pathologically negative in cases in which comprehensive neck dissection would reveal metastatic cancer. Several changes over the years in the evaluation of cancer of the salivary glands complicate the interpretation of retrospective studies. Evolution in the interpretation of pathology of the salivary glands (Chapter 3, Pathology of Salivary Gland Disease) has altered the classification of some cancers, making it difficult to interpret certain aspects of studies that span decades of experience. Other considerations include disparities between different centers in the histologic nomenclature, the overlap of multiple risk factors in relatively small studies (i.e., high grade and large tumor size), and grouping of salivary tumor sites, making interpretation of individual risk factors problematic.

Despite inherent limitations, previous studies have provided valuable information about indications for treatment of the neck in salivary gland cancer, highlighting a number of risk factors associated with increased incidence of neck metastases. Careful consideration of tumor type, grade, size, T stage, and other factors can help select high-risk patients who require accurate staging, which is best accomplished by doing a neck dissection. Accurate staging of the neck is important for evaluating prognosis and guiding adjuvant therapy. It is accepted that patients with positive nodal disease should be treated with a combination of neck dissection and postoperative radiation, which is described in detail in Chapter 27, Role of Radiotherapy in the Treatment of Tumors of the Salivary Glands. Currently, chemotherapeutic options are under clinical investigation, as described in Chapter 28, Chemotherapy in the Management of Malignant Tumors of Salivary Gland Origin. Current research investigating molecular markers and cellular receptors involved in salivary tumorigenesis may facilitate the application of targeted therapies.

Evaluation

History and Physical Examination

Although cancer of the salivary glands cannot be distinguished from benign salivary tumors on physical examination, a thorough evaluation may reveal signs and symptoms suggestive of malignancy. A history of rapid growth, pain, and facial weakness, or an ipsilateral scalp melanoma or squamous cell carcinoma increases the suspicion of cancer. Physical findings of facial weakness or ipsilateral cervical lymphadenopathy are concerning for a high-grade cancer. A careful survey of the skin of the scalp and face is important because a metastasis to the parotid gland may be the initial presentation of a skin cancer (see Chapter 1, Anatomy, Function, and Evaluation of the Salivary Glands).

Pathologic Evaluation

Fine-needle Aspiration Biopsy (FNAB)

Needle biopsy is a low-risk diagnostic procedure that is commonly used in the evaluation of salivary gland lesions. In a review of 341 cases of benign and malignant salivary gland aspirates, Stewart et al. found that FNAB has a sensitivity, specificity, and accuracy of 92%, 100%, and 98%, respectively [55]. However, diagnosis of salivary malignancy by FNAB can be challenging, reflected by diminished sensitivity, specificity, and accuracy (reported to be 55% to 95%, 86% to 100%, and 84% to 97%, respectively). In addition, the accuracy of determining the specific tumor type is even lower, with a reported range from 29% to 84% [63]. Despite the limitations of cytopathologic analysis, diagnosis of a cancer of the salivary gland by FNAB can help guide the treatment algorithm for the neck (Fig. 25.1).

Cystic masses and tumors with overlapping histologic characteristics can be particularly difficult to diagnose using FNAB. Reactive atypical squamous metaplasia associated with benign cystic lesions can lead to a false-positive diagnosis, and cystic low-grade mucoepider-

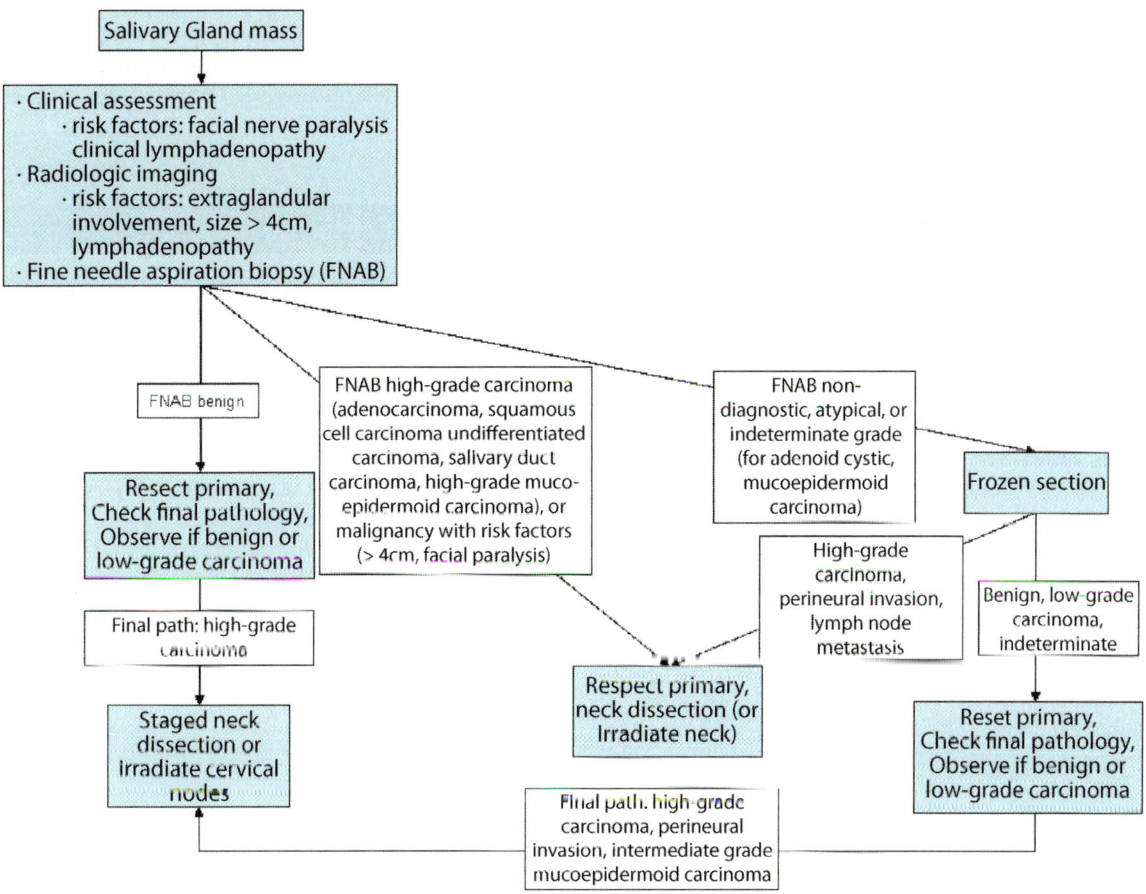

Fig. 25.1: Algorithm for management of the neck in salivary malignancies. Decision making is based on clinical history and risk factors, radiographic findings, and pathologic features in the primary tumor

moid carcinoma can look similar to ductal obstruction, resulting in a false-negative diagnosis [30, 53]. Other tumor types that can be challenging to diagnose by FNAB include acinic cell carcinoma, polymorphous low-grade adenocarcinoma, adenoid cystic carcinoma, metastatic lesions, and salivary basal cell or small cell tumors [12, 53, 55]. These challenging neoplasms represent a minority of salivary gland lesions, but they are a potential source of cytologic misdiagnoses (see Chapter 3).

Tumor grade is difficult to determine from FNAB specimens. In a review of 63 cases of cancer of the salivary glands, Zbaren et al. found that only about half of the malignancies could be correctly graded using FNAB [63]. Of the remainder, nine (14%) were incorrectly graded, and seven of these were downgraded based upon final histologic evaluation of the resected tumor. Although this is a small study, others have shown similar limitations of FNAB. It is important to recognize that, in the absence of clinical features that are associated with a high risk of nodal metastases or concerning frozen section pathology, an equivocal FNAB result can lead to overtreatment.

Intraoperative Frozen Section and Analysis

Intraoperative frozen section analysis is a useful adjunct to fine-needle aspiration cytology. In general, frozen section is less sensitive but more specific than FNAB [45]. Frozen section is particularly useful in evaluating tumor grade. According to a study by Zbaren et al., tumor grading based upon frozen section was correct, false, or not mentioned in 81%, 5%, and 14% of true-positive specimens, respectively [63]. Thus, frozen section is superior to FNAB for indicating high-grade cancer. If the FNAB shows atypia, malignancy of indeterminate tumor type, or a malignancy for which grade is important in determining the treatment of the neck (e.g., mucoepidermoid carcinoma), frozen section is useful in directing the treatment algorithm (Fig. 25.1). Findings of a high-grade carcinoma, involvement of the facial nerve, or cancer within intraparotid or other regional lymph nodes on frozen section are indications for neck dissection.

Radiographic Imaging

Radiographic imaging is useful in the preoperative evaluation of salivary gland cancers and the ipsilateral neck. Either contrast-enhanced computed tomography (CT) or magnetic resonance imaging (MRI) with gadolinium can help to define the extent of the primary cancer and evaluate for cervical lymphadenopathy. Several studies have also indicated that positron emission tomography (PET) can be useful in the evaluation of cancer of the salivary glands [9, 39, 61]. PET has a high level of sensitivity for salivary cancer, but the false-positive rate is too high to use PET to discriminate between malignancies and benign lesions [25]. In the setting of biopsy-proven cancer however, preliminary studies have shown that PET is useful in evaluating for regional and distant metastases [9, 39]. Larger studies need to be performed before routinely incorporating PET scanning into the evaluation of cancers of the salivary glands. But in the future, FDG-avid lesions consistent with distant metastases may lead to further work-up before planning an elective neck dissection. As in other cancers of the head and neck, a potential pitfall of PET scanning is that false-positives may increase complications and delay definitive locoregional therapy for the documented disease (see Chapter 2, Imaging of the Salivary Glands).

Management of the N0 Neck

Risk Factors for Occult Nodal Metastasis

Many tumor characteristics have been associated with increased risk of occult metastasis to the ipsilateral neck. Due to the limitations of retrospective studies, there remains some debate over which tumor features correlate with a risk for metastasis that is sufficient to warrant treatment of the neck. In spite of variations in reported incidences of nodal metastases, there are several factors that have consistently proven to help predict regional spread of disease. Careful evaluation of tumor type, grade, size/stage, and various other factors can help determine which patients are at high risk for nodal metastases, and therefore are candidates for staging neck dissection.

Tumor Type

There is a consensus that certain histologic tumor types confer a high risk of nodal metastasis, including undifferentiated (or anaplastic) carcinoma, high-grade mucoepidermoid carcinoma, squamous cell carcinoma, adenocarcinoma, and salivary duct carcinoma [6, 17, 19, 44, 48, 54]. Of note, the use of the term "adenocarcinoma" has diminished as pathologic techniques such as immunohistochemical staining have advanced, allowing many of these to be otherwise categorized [17]. Most studies indicate that patients with adenoid cystic carcinoma, low-grade mucoepidermoid carcinoma, acinic cell carcinoma, myoepithelial carcinoma, and sarcomas are at low risk for developing nodal metastasis [3, 6, 19, 44].

The metastatic potential of a number of tumor types continues to be controversial. Malignant mixed tumors may fall into the high-risk category, with multiple reports of regional metastatic rates of up to 35% [40, 44]. However, some studies indicate that the rate of occult metastasis is much lower than this [3, 19, 22, 36]. These inconsistencies may be due in part to discrepancies in nomenclature used at different institutions. Some use the terms "malignant mixed tumor" and "carcinoma ex-pleomorphic adenoma" interchangeably, whereas others treat them as separate entities. Adenoid cystic carcinoma has a number of unique clinical and pathologic characteristics. In a review of the 242 cases of adenoid cystic carcinoma treated at Memorial Sloan Kettering Cancer Center between 1939 and 1963, Spiro found that this tumor type is more commonly associated with distant disease than cervical metastasis. Only 15% of cases had cervical metastasis, and of these, half were clinically apparent at the time of initial presentation. Cancers arising from the oral cavity, oropharynx, or major salivary glands have a higher rate of regional metastases than those in the larynx and nasopharynx [51, 58]. Contrary to the behavior of most other tumor types, the rate of cervical metastasis does not appear to vary with size of tumor. Due to the low rate of occult metastasis, Spiro did not advocate elective treatment of the neck for adenoid cystic carcinoma [51].

Stennart et al. have challenged the high- and low-risk categories put forth by others. This group performed a neck dissection on all patients with cancer of the salivary glands and found that even "low risk" cancers, including adenoid cystic, acinic cell, basal cell, carcinoma ex-pleomorphic adenoma, and myoepithelial carcinomas, had positive lymph nodes in more than 20% of cases [54]. This study raises the question as to why the nodal failure rate is not higher in other studies if untreated necks have a significant rate of positive nodes on pathologic examination.

Finally, it is important to note that there may be a significant risk of nodal metastases from low-risk tumor types, particularly if other risk factors are present. For example, acinic cell carcinoma is considered to be a low-risk tumor type, but a small number of these tumors are poorly differentiated and do have a high risk of regional nodal metastases [29] (Fig. 25.2). Likewise, certain histologic features of adenoid cystic carcinoma (solid histologic type) may confer a greater likelihood of regional metastasis, and merit consideration of elective therapy of the neck. Due to the potential for aggressive behavior by some "low-risk" tumor types, we advocate treatment of the neck if any of the risk factors discussed below are present (high grade, large size, extraglandular extension, and facial nerve paralysis).

Tumor Grade

High-grade cancer is a strong indicator of risk for nodal metastasis. In a multivariate analysis of SEER (Surveillance, Epidemiology and End Results) data gathered by the National Cancer Institute from 1988 to 1998, Bhattacharyya and Fried found high-grade cancer to have an odds ratio of 1.99 for presence of nodal disease [6]. Other authors have had similar findings in smaller studies [3, 16, 19]. Severe desmoplasia was also identified as a predictor of lymph node metastases [44].

Grading correlates most closely with clinical behavior for mucoepidermoid carcinoma, adenocarcinoma, acinic cell carcinoma, and squamous cell carcinoma [31]. The relationship of clinical behavior, and specifically the incidence of regional metastasis, to grading of adenoid cystic carcinoma (solid being high grade) is controversial. Spiro felt that clinical behavior could not be reliably predicted by grade of adenoid cystic carcinoma, but others have correlated the solid type of the tumor with increased risk of nodal metastasis [51].

The level of risk incurred by intermediate-grade mucoepidermoid carcinoma is difficult to evaluate because relatively few studies address the different grades of this tumor, and most do not include an intermediate-grade category. Of those authors who discuss the intermediate grade, Kelley and Spiro advocate treatment of the neck, citing up to a 30% risk of cervical nodal metastases [24, 50]. On the contrary, Frankenthaler et al. and Regis de Brito Santos et al. categorize it as low risk, with only an 11% incidence of occult metastasis [19, 44]. These differences highlight the problem of inter-institutional variability in diagnostic classification.

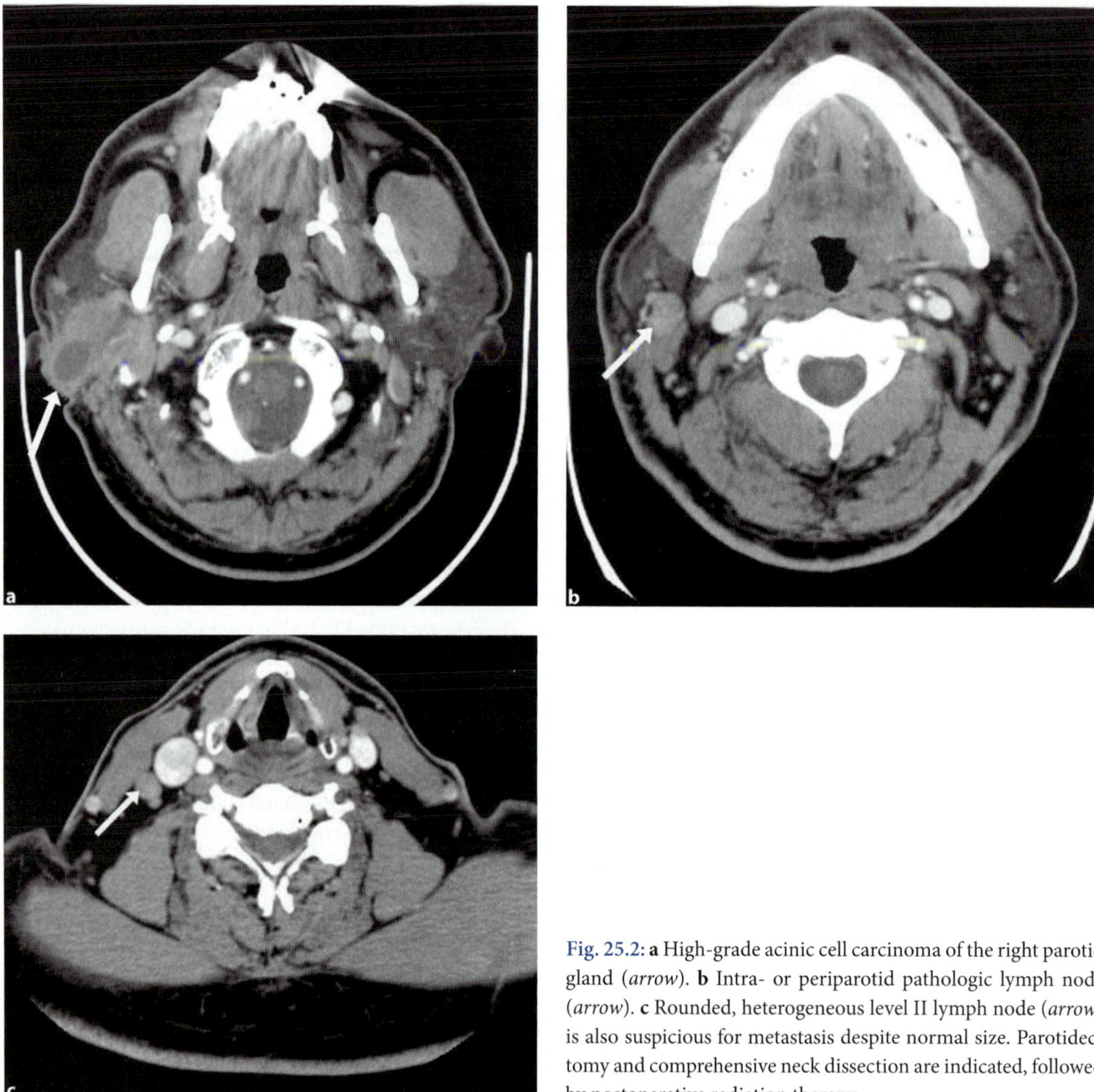

Fig. 25.2: **a** High-grade acinic cell carcinoma of the right parotid gland (*arrow*). **b** Intra- or periparotid pathologic lymph node (*arrow*). **c** Rounded, heterogeneous level II lymph node (*arrow*) is also suspicious for metastasis despite normal size. Parotidectomy and comprehensive neck dissection are indicated, followed by postoperative radiation therapy

Tumor Stage

T stage (T3 or T4), size > 4 cm, and extraparenchymal extension have collectively and individually been associated with a high risk of nodal metastasis. T stage takes both size and extraparenchymal involvement into account, and some debate remains over which of these factors is more important. According to Bhattacharyya, multivariate analysis supports primary tumor size as a predictor of lymph node metastasis, but it only becomes a strong predictor once the size exceeds 5 cm. However, extraglandular involvement had an odds ratio for nodal metastasis of 1.71 [6]. Other authors have found a size of 4 cm or larger, extraglandular involvement, and T3 to T4 tumor stage to carry a 20% risk of occult metastasis [3, 10, 17, 19, 24, 52, 54, 59]. In addition, Poulsen et al. found T3 and T4 cancer of the parotid gland to be at increased risk of nodal recurrence [43] (Fig. 25.3).

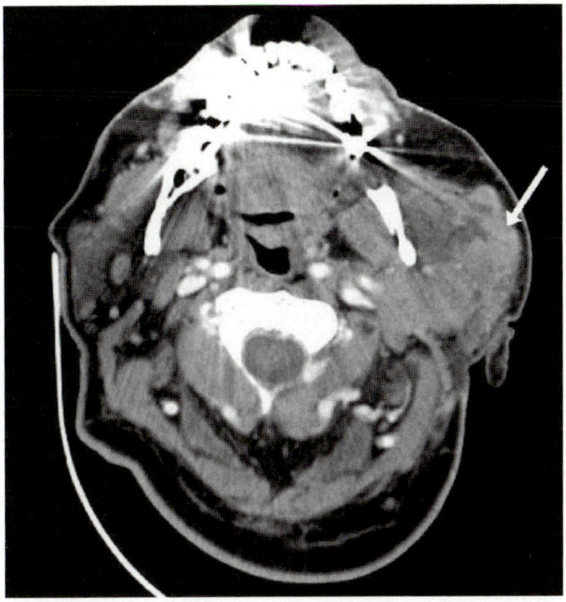

Fig. 25.3: Six-centimeter left parotid mass without evidence of cervical metastasis (*arrow*)

Other Risk Factors

Some authors propose that weakness of the facial nerve, age > 54 years, perineural spread, and lymphatic invasion are predictors of lymph node metastasis [6, 10, 17, 19, 24, 44]. Of these, facial nerve paralysis appears to be the most significant [6, 19].

Intraparotid metastasis from skin cancer is associated with a high incidence of occult cervical lymph node metastasis. Metastatic deposits of squamous cell carcinoma and melanoma within intraparotid lymph nodes are associated with occult regional metastatic rates of 35% and 27%, respectively [40] (Fig. 25.4).

Finally, site may be an important factor for nodal metastasis, perhaps due to proximity of lymphatic drainage. The literature suggests that cancers of the submandibular gland are higher-grade, more aggressive, and have lethal metastases more often than cancer of the parotid gland [5]. The incidence of metastasis is 21–46%, though the incidence of clinically apparent metastasis to the neck is only 8% [3, 59, 62]. It is possible that the interpretation of direct extension of primary tumors into adjacent lymph nodes, as can be seen with adenoid cystic carcinoma, has

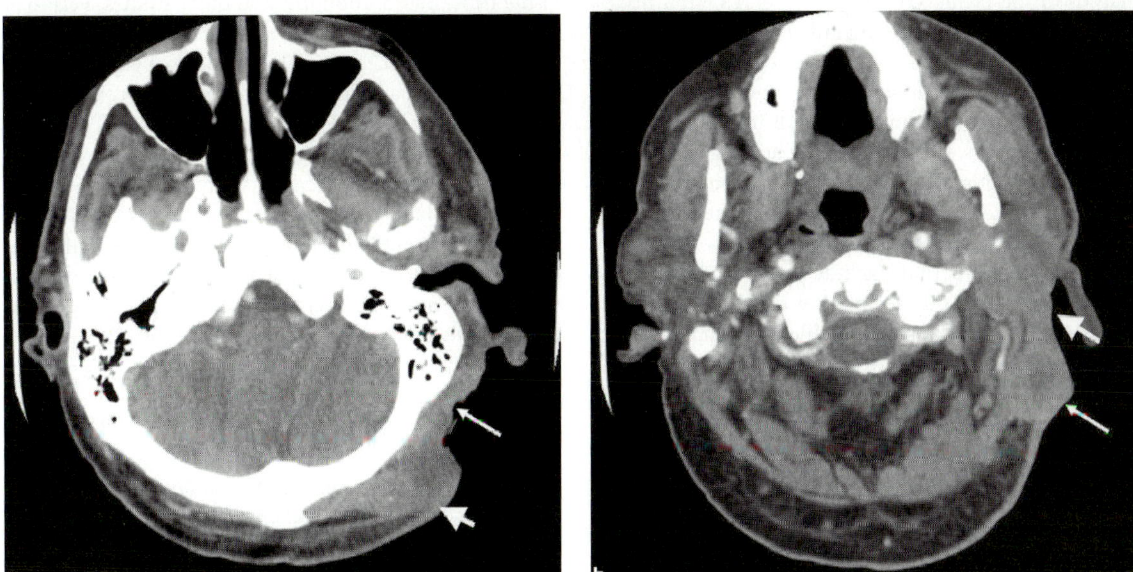

Fig. 25.4: **a** Squamous cell carcinoma of the left scalp. Note the surgical defect from initial resection (*fine arrow*) and the adjacent soft tissue abnormality with replacement of fat representing recurrent cancer (*heavy arrow*). **b** Dermal metastasis from squamous cell carcinoma of the scalp (*fine arrow*) with direct extension into the left parotid gland (*heavy arrow*). Although no cervical lymph nodes meet pathologic criteria by imaging, a neck dissection is indicated

elevated the rate of metastasis attributed to these cancers. However, several studies show the rate of metastasis from cancer of the submandibular gland to be two to three times higher than from cancer of the parotid gland of the same histologic type [3, 5, 8]. Squamous cell carcinoma and high-grade glandular carcinomas (adenocarcinoma, mucoepidermoid, and undifferentiated) as well as those exhibiting perineural invasion have the highest rates of metastasis. Therefore, we believe that elective treatment of the neck is indicated in all but the earliest and least aggressive submandibular lesions [59].

Surgical Treatment of the N0 Neck

Data on the long-term outcome of different approaches to the N0 neck are limited, and as a result a wide range of approaches has been advocated. These approaches range from neck dissection for every patient with a cancer of the salivary glands [54] to selective neck dissection or irradiation of the neck for cancers with risk factors for nodal metastasis [6, 10, 17, 19, 24, 36, 44]. The decision as to which approach to take has been based upon the characteristics of the primary cancer, frozen section analysis of the primary cancer or level II lymph nodes, and whether a neck dissection enhances the exposure of the primary tumor [4, 27, 28]. Due to the retrospective nature of these relatively small, non-randomized studies, no approach has been shown to result in a survival benefit over the others. Because accurate staging of cancer of the salivary glands is essential, we are strong proponents of performing selective neck dissection at the time of definitive surgical resection of any cancer with risk factors for metastasis. Exceptions include patients who are poor surgical candidates due to medical conditions or those who have a cancer in an unfavorable location. For example, cancer arising in minor salivary gland tissue in the base of the tongue is difficult to access, has the potential to metastasize to bilateral necks, and its exposure is not enhanced by lymphadenectomy. In such a case, surgery has fewer advantages over radiation therapy than in the setting of cancers of the major salivary glands.

There are several advantages to performing a neck dissection along with resection of the primary cancer: exposure of the primary cancer may be improved, it ensures accurate staging, and it often spares patients with pathologically N0 necks the morbidity of radiation therapy. In addition, for cancer of the parotid and submandibular glands, the incision and dissection required to remove the nodes most likely to harbor metastases is minimally greater than that required for resection of the primary tumor. Furthermore, accurate staging will become increasingly important in the future as patients with cancer of the salivary glands are enrolled in prospective clinical trials of novel therapeutic strategies. One caveat is that some cancers lack high-risk clinical and cytopathologic characteristics, but are diagnosed as high-risk cancer on final pathology. In this case, either staged neck dissection or irradiation of the neck is a reasonable approach.

Parotid Gland

Selective neck dissection, rather than modified radical neck dissection, is the preferred procedure for the N0 neck in cancer of the parotid gland. According to Armstrong et al., the incidence of occult metastasis from cancer of the parotid gland by level is: 53% in intra- or periparotid nodes, 10% in level I, 27% in level II, 23% in level III, 20% in level IV, and 3% in level V [3]. Although skip metastases to levels III and IV can be observed, evaluation of levels II and III is adequate to identify occult disease 90% of the time. Based upon this and other studies, Ferlito et al. recommend including levels IB, II, III, and upper V in selective neck dissections for parotid malignancies [17]. Of necks with pathologic lymph nodes, approximately a quarter involve levels IV or V [59]. When a selective neck dissection reveals pathologically positive nodes, adjuvant radiation therapy is indicated. With the possible exception of an isolated small metastasis with no extracapsular spread, the potential for failure in levels IV or V after selective neck dissection as well as the benefits of adjuvant therapy for advanced stage cancers support the use of postoperative radiation therapy (see Chapter 27).

Submandibular Gland

Prior to 1965, most surgeons took an aggressive approach to submandibular malignancies, resecting the submandibular gland en bloc with a radical neck dissection and resection of the floor of the mouth with a marginal mandibulectomy. Since then, the trend has evolved toward resection of the primary tumor with an ipsilateral selective neck dissection [49]. Cancer of the submandibular gland drains primarily to levels I through III, with 59% of node-positive malignancies having metastasis in level I, 53% in level II, 47% in level III, 18% in level IV, and 6% in level V [3, 5]. Because skip metastases to level IV or V are rare, selective neck dissection of levels I through III will detect the vast majority of occult metastases [3]. The presence of occult metastasis is an indication for postoperative irradiation of the neck as was noted for cancer of the parotid gland. In contrast to cancer of the parotid gland, where a single intraparotid or cervical nodal metastasis without extracapsular spread may not require radiation therapy of the neck, all cancers of the submandibular gland with nodal metastasis should be treated postoperatively with radiation to the primary site and the ipsilateral neck (see Chapter 27).

In most cases, adenoid cystic carcinoma of the submandibular gland warrants treatment of the neck. Although the risk of nodal metastases from adenoid cystic carcinoma is relatively low, this tumor has a propensity for infiltration of adjacent lymph nodes and soft tissue. In some cases it is difficult to distinguish between direct invasion of adjacent lymph nodes and true metastasis [8]. This locally aggressive behavior is reflected in a recurrence rate of 35–85%, approximately four times greater than with cancer of the parotid gland of the same stage [5, 8]. Due to its tendency toward infiltration of local tissue, treatment of adenoid cystic carcinoma of the submandibular gland calls for a wide local resection of lymph nodes and soft tissue in addition to the submandibular gland followed by radiation therapy [8].

Sublingual Gland and Minor Salivary Glands

Neoplasms of the sublingual glands constitute only 1% of major salivary gland tumors [5]. It has long been observed that risk of malignancy increases inversely with the size of the salivary gland. Approximately 80% of sublingual gland tumors are malignant, most commonly mucoepidermoid carcinoma, followed by adenoid cystic carcinoma. Because these malignancies are rare and at times difficult to distinguish from minor salivary cancers of the floor of the mouth, the available data are not adequate to indicate risk factors for occult metastasis. Carcinoma of the minor salivary glands is found in many locations, the hard and soft palate being the most common, followed by other oral cavity and oropharynx subsites, and other locations within the upper aerodigestive tract. Mucoepidermoid carcinoma and adenoid cystic carcinoma are the most common histologic types, although many others can be found in the minor salivary glands. Studies often group sublingual and minor salivary gland or major and minor salivary gland malignancies together, making it difficult to draw conclusions regarding clinical behavior of sublingual or oral cavity minor salivary gland cancers.

The incidence of nodal metastases from cancers of the minor salivary glands is approximately 9–16% overall [11, 33, 34]. According to Chou et al., this number reaches 65% for patients with stage III or IV disease. The histologic tumor types associated with lymphatic metastasis were, in order of frequency; acinic cell, adenoid cystic, undifferentiated, and mucoepidermoid carcinomas, adenocarcinoma, carcinoma ex-pleomorphic adenoma, and papillary cystadenocarcinoma. In this study, the highest survival rate was observed in patients treated with primary excision and neck dissection. We advocate neck dissection for patients with stage III or IV cancer of the minor salivary glands or those with high-risk histology. Due to the diversity of sites and relative rarity of these tumors, data on patterns of regional lymphatic metastases are lacking. Therefore, the nodal basins removed in a selective neck dissection for clinically negative necks, as well as whether the contralateral neck needs to be addressed, may be considered analogous to squamous cell carcinoma of the same site.

Management of the N+ Neck

A comprehensive neck dissection of levels I through V followed by radiation therapy is the most widely accepted treatment for clinically positive disease (Fig. 25.4). The benefits of a comprehensive approach to cervical lymph node metastasis include reduction of gross disease to optimize the effect of radiation therapy, obtaining additional prognostic information, and reducing the need for reoperation in the surgical and/or radiation fields if recurrence develops. Some surgeons believe that a selective neck dissection is appropriate for removal of early macroscopic disease when used in conjunction with radiation therapy to treat residual microscopic disease, but this approach is controversial [16].

In the absence of adjuvant therapy, carcinoma of the submandibular gland with adverse features (i.e., extraglandular extension, positive margins, locally recurrent, perineural invasion, advanced nodal disease) have a locoregional control rate of less than 50% [56]. For tumors that do recur in the neck, surgical salvage is rarely successful. As the rate of locoregional control falls, so does overall and disease-free survival. Therefore, cancer of the submandibular gland with high-risk features should be treated aggressively with surgery and postoperative radiation therapy encompassing the cervical nodal basins at risk (see Chapter 27).

Postoperative Radiation Therapy

Although cancer of the salivary glands was once felt to be relatively radioresistant, current data indicate that radiation therapy can help improve outcome over surgery alone [60]. Most head and neck oncologists agree that pathologically positive necks should receive adjuvant radiation therapy postoperatively. Indications for radiation therapy of salivary cancers include close or positive margins, extraglandular disease extension (T3 or T4), perineural invasion, and intraglandular or cervical nodal disease. Studies have shown that locoregional control is significantly improved when radiation therapy is added to surgical management for these indications [20, 22, 59]. Combined therapy may also improve survival for advanced disease, but this conclusion is controversial and difficult to prove without prospective, randomized trials [3, 41]. Of note, in Terhaard's study, even N1 disease had better locoregional control with postoperative radiation therapy [59]. Failure rates are worse among patients with five or more involved lymph nodes, male gender, major (named) nerve involvement, or extraglandular extension. Of patients with nodal disease, more than 50% have three or more positive nodes. Levels IV or V are involved in half of patients with three or more positive nodes, so it is important to treat levels I through V. The need to treat all levels is further supported by the increased incidence of nodal recurrence after radiation therapy of only the upper cervical lymph nodes [43]. There is some question of whether postoperative radiation therapy to the neck is necessary if only one positive node without extracapsular spread is identified, but studies have not adequately determined the risk of failure in levels IV and V in this situation.

Even for patients with clinically negative necks, there is a trend toward improved regional control with combined therapy over surgery alone [3, 59]. This approach should directly reduce distant failure of tumor control. In Armstrong et al. series of 474 patients, of the patients who underwent elective neck dissection, a recurrence rate of nearly 30% was observed among those who did not receive postoperative radiation therapy, and a 0% recurrence rate was found among those who were irradiated [3]. However, the numbers in this cohort are too low to reach statistical significance. In the MD Anderson Cancer Center experience with postoperative radiation therapy for minor salivary gland malignancies, Garden et al. report a low rate of regional failure. Three of the 13 patients who presented with node-positive disease had regional failures, but only 5% of those with N0 necks failed regionally regardless of the elective neck treatment [21].

For more information regarding postoperative irradiation, please refer to Chapter 27.

Future Directions

Molecular Markers and Systemic Therapies

Recent studies have identified molecular markers that may help us better differentiate similar tumor types, understand salivary gland tumorigenesis, and predict prognosis. A p53 homolog, p63, is found in basal duct cells and myoepithelial cells, and is expressed in tumors derived from these cell types [7, 23, 46]. Immunohistochemical staining for p63 in adenoid cystic carcinoma and basaloid squamous cell carcinoma, which can be difficult to distinguish by morphology alone, produces unique staining patterns [13]. Differential expression of p63 isotypes also may help distinguish different tumor types and explain their neoplastic transformation. For example, the DeltaNp73L isoform of p63 is present in salivary gland neoplasms, with greater expression in malignant than benign lesions, but not normal salivary gland tissue. On the contrary, TAp63 is highly expressed in benign salivary lesions but not in carcinomas [18, 35]. Thus, refinement of immunohistochemical staining for p63 isoforms may enhance our ability to distinguish high- from low-risk cancers and achieve a greater understanding of tumorigenesis.

A multitude of genetic alterations and patterns of protein expression associated with cancer of the salivary glands are now being described. Alterations in expression of proteins that regulate the cell cycle, such as p21 (WAF1/CIP1) and p27 (KIP1), have been found in a number of cancers [1]. Promoter hypermethylation of RB1, loss of heterozygosity at various loci, and acetylation of histones have all been found in salivary gland carcinomas, and may prove to be important in tumorigenesis [26]. Salivary duct carcinoma, which has been compared to prostate cancer on histologic grounds, frequently expresses androgen receptor, epidermal growth factor receptor (EGFR), and transforming growth factor alpha (TGF-alpha) [15]. Carcinoma ex-pleomorphic adenoma and basal cell adenocarcinoma also express the androgen receptor, raising the possibility that anti-androgen or other targeted therapies may improve the success of systemic therapies for selected salivary malignancies [38].

Several molecular markers have been linked with prognosis. Overexpression of p53, vascular endothelial growth factor (VEGF), and c-erbB-2 (HER2/neu) as well as positive TUNEL assays correlate with clinically aggressive tumors and poor clinical outcomes [14, 32, 37, 42, 57].

Systemic therapy for salivary gland carcinomas has had minimal success. The response rates are low, and the duration of response less than 1 year [2] (see Chapter 28). As the molecular profiles of metastatic cancer of the salivary glands are further elucidated, prediction of metastasis and application of targeted therapy may be pursued.

Conclusion

Cervical metastasis of salivary gland carcinoma, as in other tumors, is associated with a significant decrease in quality of life, tumor control, and survival. In addition, neck recurrence is difficult to salvage, with a success rate of less that 30% [3, 43]. In order to accurately stage and manage these malignancies, we advocate neck dissection if the primary tumor has risk factors for occult cervical metastasis. For positive nodal disease, a comprehensive neck dissection is indicated, followed by radiation therapy. After treatment, patients should be routinely evaluated for recurrence using standard clinical and radiographic techniques. Many of these cancers can lead to recurrence of disease, particularly distant metastasis, years to decades after initial diagnosis, and thus warrant long-term follow-up. Future molecular studies and prospective clinical trials hold promise for application of more efficacious techniques for prediction of metastasis and use of targeted systemic therapeutic agents.

Take Home Messages

- Neck dissection can provide valuable information for staging and prognosis, and reduce tumor burden of high-risk salivary gland carcinomas malignancies.
- An algorithm incorporating clinical presentation, risk factors, fine-needle aspiration biopsy, and intraoperative frozen section pathology can help direct appropriate treatment of the clinically negative (N0) neck in cancer of the salivary glands.
- If one or more risk factors are identified in the primary tumor, elective dissection of the ipsilateral neck is warranted, including levels IB through III ± upper level V for parotid tumors and levels I through III for submandibular tumors. If elective neck irridation is employed in lieu of neck dissection, levels I through V should be addressed.
- Clinically apparent cervical metastases should be treated with a comprehensive neck dissection and postoperative radiation therapy (with the possible exception of a small solitary positive node without extracapsular spread).

References

1. Affolter A, Helmbrecht S, Finger S, Hormann K, Gotte K (2005) Altered expression of cell cycle regulators p21, p27, and p53 in tumors of salivary glands and paranasal sinuses. Oncol Rep 13(6):1089–194
2. Agulnik M and Siu LL (2004) An update on the systemic therapy of malignant salivary gland cancers: role of chemotherapy and molecular targeted agents. Curr Med Chem Anticancer Agents 4(6):543–551
3. Armstrong JG, Harrison LB, Thaler HT, Friedlander-Klar H, Fass DE, Zelefsky MJ, Shah JP, Strong EW, and Spiro RH (1992) The indications for elective treatment of the neck in cancer of the major salivary glands. Cancer 69(3):615 619
4. Bardwil J (1967) Tumors of the parotid gland. Am J Surg 114:498–502

5. Batsakis JG (1986) Carcinomas of the submandibular and sublingual glands. Ann Otol Rhinol Laryngol 95(2 Pt 1):211–212
6. Bhattacharyya N and Fried MP (2002) Nodal metastasis in major salivary gland cancer: predictive factors and effects on survival. Arch Otolaryngol Head Neck Surg 128(8):904–908
7. Bilal H, Handra-Luca A, Bertrand JC, and Fouret PJ (2003) P63 is expressed in basal and myoepithelial cells of human normal and tumor salivary gland tissues. J Histochem Cytochem 51(2):133–139
8. Bosch A, Brandenburg JH, and Gilchrist KW (1980) Lymph node metastases in adenoid cystic carcinoma of the submaxillary gland. Cancer 45(11):2872–2877
9. Bui CD, Ching AS, Carlos RC, Shreve PD, and Mukherji SK (2003) Diagnostic accuracy of 2-[fluorine-18]fluro-2-deoxy-D-glucose positron emission tomography imaging in nonsquamous tumors of the head and neck. Invest Radiol 38(9):593–601
10. Califano L, Zupi A, Massari PS, and Giardino C (1993) Indication for neck dissection in carcinoma of the parotid gland. Our experience on 39 cases. Int Surg 78(4):347–349
11. Chou C, Zhu G, Luo M, and Xue G (1996) Carcinoma of the minor salivary glands: results of surgery and combined therapy. J Oral Maxillofac Surg 54(4):448–453
12. Darling MR, Schneider JW, and Phillips VM (2002) Polymorphous low-grade adenocarcinoma and adenoid cystic carcinoma: a review and comparison of immunohistochemical markers. Oral Oncol 38(7):641–645
13. Emanuel P, Wang B, Wu M, and Burstein DE (2005) p63 Immunohistochemistry in the distinction of adenoid cystic carcinoma from basaloid squamous cell carcinoma. Mod Pathol 18(5):645–650
14. Etges A, Pinto DS, Jr., Kowalski LP, Soares FA, Araujo VC (2003) Salivary duct carcinoma: immunohistochemical profile of an aggressive salivary gland tumour. J Clin Pathol 56(12):914–918
15. Fan CY, Melhem MF, Hosal AS, Grandis JR, and Barnes EL (2001) Expression of androgen receptor, epidermal growth factor receptor, and transforming growth factor alpha in salivary duct carcinoma. Arch Otolaryngol Head Neck Surg 127(9):1075–1079
16. Ferlito A, Pellitteri PK, Robbins KT, Shaha AR, Kowalski LP, Silver CE, Anniko M, Rinaldo A, Medina JE, Bradley PJ, and Byers RM (2002) Management of the neck in cancer of the major salivary glands, thyroid and parathyroid glands. Acta Otolaryngol 122(6):673–678
17. Ferlito A, Shaha AR, Rinaldo A, and Mondin V (2001) Management of clinically negative cervical lymph nodes in patients with malignant neoplasms of the parotid gland. ORL J Otorhinolaryngol Relat Spec 63(3):123–126
18. Foschini MP, Gaiba A, Cocchi R, Pennesi MG, and Pession A (2005) p63 expression in salivary gland tumors: role of DeltaNp73L in neoplastic transformation. Int J Surg Pathol 13(4):329–335
19. Frankenthaler RA, Byers RM, Luna MA, Callender DL, Wolf P, and Goepfert H (1993) Predicting occult lymph node metastasis in parotid cancer. Arch Otolaryngol Head Neck Surg 119(5):517–520
20. Garden AS, el-Naggar AK, Morrison WH, Callender DL, Ang KK, and Peters LJ (1997) Postoperative radiotherapy for malignant tumors of the parotid gland. Int J Radiat Oncol Biol Phys 37(1):79–85
21. Garden AS, Weber RS, Ang KK, Morrison WH, Matre J, and Peters LJ (1994) Postoperative radiation therapy for malignant tumors of minor salivary glands. Outcome and patterns of failure. Cancer 73(10):2563–2569
22. Johns ME (1980) Parotid cancer: a rational basis for treatment. Head Neck Surg 3(2):132–141
23. Kawahara A, Harada H, Yokoyama T, and Kage M (2005) p63 Expression of clear myoepithelial cells in epithelial-myoepithelial carcinoma of the salivary gland: a useful marker for naked myoepithelial cells in cytology. Cancer 105(4):240–245
24. Kelley DJ and Spiro RH (1996) Management of the neck in parotid carcinoma. Am J Surg 172(6):695–697
25. Keyes JW Jr., Harkness BA, Greven KM, Williams DW, 3rd, Watson NE Jr., and McGuirt WF (1994) Salivary gland tumors: pretherapy evaluation with PET. Radiology 192(1):99–102
26. Kishi M, Nakamura M, Nishimine M, Ikuta M, Kirita T, and Konishi N (2005) Genetic and epigenetic alteration profiles for multiple genes in salivary gland carcinomas. Oral Oncol 41(2):161–169
27. Korkmaz H, Yoo GH, Du W, Hocwald E, Otero-Garcia JE, Volkan Adsay N, Shibuya T, and Jacobs JR (2002) Predictors of nodal metastasis in salivary gland cancer. J Surg Oncol 80(4):186–189
28. Krause CJ (1981) The management of parotid neoplasms. Head Neck Surg 3(4):340–343
29. Laskawi R, Rodel R, Zirk A, and Arglebe C (1998) Retrospective analysis of 35 patients with acinic cell carcinoma of the parotid gland. J Oral Maxillofac Surg 56(4):440–443
30. Layfield LJ and Gopez EV (2002) Cystic lesions of the salivary glands: cytologic features in fine-needle aspiration biopsies. Diagn Cytopathol 27(4):197–204

31. Licitra L, Grandi C, Prott FJ, Schornagel JH, Bruzzi P, and Molinari R (2003) Major and minor salivary glands tumours. Crit Rev Oncol Hematol 45(2):215–225
32. Lim JJ, Kang S, Lee MR, Pai HK, Yoon HJ, Lee JI, Hong SP, and Lim CY (2003) Expression of vascular endothelial growth factor in salivary gland carcinomas and its relation to p53, Ki-67 and prognosis. J Oral Pathol Med 32(9):552–651
33. Lopes MA, Santos GC, and Kowalski LP (1998) Multivariate survival analysis of 128 cases of oral cavity minor salivary gland carcinomas. Head Neck 20(8):699–706
34. Ma DQ and Yu GY (1987) Tumours of the minor salivary glands. A clinicopathologic study of 243 cases. Acta Otolaryngol 112:106–109
35. Maruya S, Kies MS, Williams M, Myers JN, Weber RS, Batsakis JG, and El-Naggar AK (2005) Differential expression of p63 isotypes (DeltaN and TA) in salivary gland neoplasms: biological and diagnostic implications. Hum Pathol 36(7):821–827
36. McGuirt WF (1989) Management of occult metastatic disease from salivary gland neoplasms. Arch Otolaryngol Head Neck Surg 115(3):322–325
37. Nagler RM, Kerner H, Ben-Eliezer S, Minkov I, and Ben-Itzhak O (2003) Prognostic role of apoptotic, Bcl-2, c-erbB-2 and p53 tumor markers in salivary gland malignancies. Oncology 64(4):389–398
38. Nasser SM, Faquin WC, and Dayal Y (2003) Expression of androgen, estrogen, and progesterone receptors in salivary gland tumors. Frequent expression of androgen receptor in a subset of malignant salivary gland tumors. Am J Clin Pathol 119(6):801–806
39. Otsuka H, Graham MM, Kogame M, and Nishitani H (2005) The impact of FDG-PET in the management of patients with salivary gland malignancy. Ann Nucl Med 19(8):691–694
40. Pedersen D, Overgaard J, Sogaard H, Elbrond O, and Overgaard M (1992) Malignant parotid tumors in 110 consecutive patients: treatment results and prognosis. Laryngoscope 102(9):1064–1069
41. Pohar S, Gay H, Rosenbaum P, Klish D, Bogart J, Sagerman R, Hsu J, and Kellman R (2005) Malignant parotid tumors: presentation, clinical/pathologic prognostic factors, and treatment outcomes. Int J Radiat Oncol Biol Phys 61(1):112–118
42. Potencz E, Cornianu M, Muntean C, and Sotiriadis S (1998) The expression of p53 protein in salivary gland carcinomas. Rom J Morphol Embryol 44(1–4):109–115
43. Poulsen MG, Tripcony LB, and Kynaston B (1991) Nodal recurrence in primary malignant epithelial tumours of the parotid gland. Australas Radiol 35(2):169–173
44. Regis De Brito Santos I, Kowalski LP, Cavalcante De Araujo V, Flavia Logullo A, and Magrin J (2001) Multivariate analysis of risk factors for neck metastases in surgically treated parotid carcinomas. Arch Otolaryngol Head Neck Surg 127(1):56–60
45. Seethala RR, LiVolsi VA, and Baloch ZW (2005) Relative accuracy of fine-needle aspiration and frozen section in the diagnosis of lesions of the parotid gland. Head Neck 27(3):217–223
46. Seethala RR, LiVolsi VA, Zhang PJ, Pasha TL, Baloch ZW (2005) Comparison of p63 and p73 expression in benign and malignant salivary gland lesions. Head Neck 27(8):696–702
47. Shah JP (1990) Cervical lymph node metastases-diagnostic, therapeutic, and prognostic implications. Oncology (Williston Park) 4(10):61–9; discussion 72, 76
48. Spiro RH (1986) Salivary neoplasms: overview of a 35-year experience with 2,807 patients. Head Neck Surg 8(3):177–184
49. Spiro RH (1995) Changing trends in the management of salivary tumors. Semin Surg Oncol 11(3):240–245
50. Spiro RH, Huvos AG, Berk R, and Strong EW (1978) Mucoepidermoid carcinoma of salivary gland origin. A clinicopathologic study of 367 cases. Am J Surg 136(4):461–8
51. Spiro RH, Huvos AG, and Strong EW (1974) Adenoid cystic carcinoma of salivary origin. A clinicopathologic study of 242 cases. Am J Surg 128(4):512–520
52. Spiro RH, Huvos AG, and Strong EW (1975) Cancer of the parotid gland. A clinicopathologic study of 288 primary cases. Am J Surg 130(4):452–459
53. Stanley MW (2002) Selected problems in fine needle aspiration of head and neck masses. Mod Pathol 15(3):342–350
54. Stennert E, Kisner D, Jungehuelsing M, Guntinas-Lichius O, Schroder U, Eckel HE, and Klussmann JP (2003) High incidence of lymph node metastasis in major salivary gland cancer. Arch Otolaryngol Head Neck Surg 129(7):720–723
55. Stewart CJ, MacKenzie K, McGarry GW, and Mowat A (2000) Fine-needle aspiration cytology of salivary gland: a review of 341 cases. Diagn Cytopathol 22(3):139–146
56. Storey MR, Garden AS, Morrison WH, Eicher SA, Schechter NR, and Ang KK (2001) Postoperative radiotherapy for malignant tumors of the submandibular gland. Int J Radiat Oncol Biol Phys 51(4):952–958
57. Sugano S, Mukai K, Tsuda H, Hirohashi S, Furuya S, Shimosato Y, Ebihara S, and Takeyama I (1992) Immunohistochemical study of c-erbB-2 oncoprotein overexpression in human major salivary gland carcinoma: an indicator of aggressiveness. Laryngoscope 102(8):923–927

58. Sung MW, Kim KH, Kim JW, Min YG, Seong WJ, Roh JL, Lee SJ, Kwon TK, and Park SW (2003) Clinicopathologic predictors and impact of distant metastasis from adenoid cystic carcinoma of the head and neck. Arch Otolaryngol Head Neck Surg 129(11):1193–1197
59. Terhaard CH, Lubsen H, Rasch CR, Levendag PC, Kaanders HH, Tjho-Heslinga RE, van Den Ende PL, and Burlage F (2005) The role of radiotherapy in the treatment of malignant salivary gland tumors. Int J Radiat Oncol Biol Phys 61(1):103–111
60. Theriault C and Fitzpatrick PJ (1986) Malignant parotid tumors. Prognostic factors and optimum treatment. Am J Clin Oncol 9(6):510–516
61. Uchida Y, Minoshima S, Kawata T, Motoori K, Nakano K, Kazama T, Uno T, Okamoto Y, and Ito H (2005) Diagnostic value of FDG PET and salivary gland scintigraphy for parotid tumors. Clin Nucl Med 30(3):170–176
62. Vander Poorten VL, Balm AJ, Hilgers FJ, Tan IB, Loftus-Coll BM, Keus RB, and Hart AA (1999) Prognostic factors for long term results of the treatment of patients with malignant submandibular gland tumors. Cancer 85(10):2255–2264
63. Zbaren P, Nuyens M, Loosli H, and Stauffer E (2004) Diagnostic accuracy of fine-needle aspiration cytology and frozen section in primary parotid carcinoma. Cancer 100(9):1876–1883

Chapter 26

Reconstruction After Excision of Cancer of the Salivary Glands

26

Ahmed Afifi and Frederic W.-B. Deleyiannis

Contents

Core Features

- When tumors extend beyond the confines of the salivary gland (i.e., involving the skin, soft tissues, mandible, and/or facial nerve), reconstruction will likely be needed to restore the structure and function of the composite defect.
- A critical analysis of the defect (i.e., what structures are missing) and of the functional consequences will guide the most appropriate reconstruction.
- Two of the relatively minor sequelae of a parotidectomy that may be alleviated with reconstruction are Frey's syndrome and the concavity at the site of the parotidectomy.
- An ideal option for reconstructing cutaneous defects after radical resection of a tumor of the parotid or submandibular gland is the use of cervicofacial or cervicodeltopectoral flaps.
- Free flaps are the ideal reconstructive technique in the reconstruction of parotidectomy and submandibular defects with extensive skin loss and involvement of the mandible.
- Procedures for facial reanimation at the time of parotidectomy are presented.

Complications to Avoid

- Performing a neck dissection with a parotidectomy through a transverse cervical incision may prevent the design of a cervicodeltopectoral flap that could be used for cutaneous reconstruction.
- Harvesting a pectoralis myocutaneous flap with a vertical incision from the cutaneous paddle to the clavicle may also prevent the design of a cerviodeltopectoral flap.
- Flap harvest should only be initiated when the extent and anatomy involved in the defect are defined.
- Vessel selection for microvascular anastomosis should be discussed with the extirpative team to avoid unnecessary ligation during neck dissection.
- The optimal time for nerve grafting is at the time of facial nerve resection.

Introduction

Dramatic advancements in the management of salivary gland malignancies have taken place in the last decade, including the acceptance of standardized classification systems, a better understanding of the behavior and genetic basis, and newer adjuvant treatments [5, 26, 55]. However, these are rare tumors with a diverse histology and a wide spectrum of biological behavior, and until we have more insight into their pathogenesis and alternate treatments, complete surgical excision is likely to remain the mainstay of treatment [48, 54]. The presence or absence of malignant cells at the margins of surgical resection is considered by many to be the single most important factor influencing prognosis [5, 49, 55, 58]. Therefore, when the tumor extends beyond the confines of the salivary gland, the resection must include removal of adjacent tissues, including the skin, soft tissues, mandible, maxilla, and/or facial nerve, leaving a composite defect with functional, structural, and aesthetic deficiencies. The confidence of the extirpative surgeon in the ability to achieve reliable reconstruction in these cases should allow him/her the freedom to achieve a wide local resection with negative margins. Reports from the MD Anderson Cancer Center state that local control is possible by radiotherapy to involved surgical margins, but even in these cases reliable reconstruction should be achieved to withstand the effect of radiation [23]. Regardless of whether the resection is palliative or curative, successful reconstruction has a major effect on the health-related quality of life of the patient.

Incidence of Reconstructive Needs

According to the National Cancer Data Base, cancers of the salivary glands account for 0.3–0.9% of all cancers in the USA [29]. Many salivary gland malignancies require extended radical resection, defined as excision of tissues beyond the salivary gland. De Vincentiis et al. reported the excision of the facial nerve or an adjacent structure in 19 patients out of 363 with a parotid tumor [14]. Tullio et al., who included only patients with malignant parotid tumors, reported resections beyond the parotid gland in 16% of their patients [55]. Bell et al. required a reconstructive modality in 27 out of 44 patients with malignant parotid tumors, while Nouraei et al. needed a reconstructive modality in 25% of 28 patients with carcinoma ex-pleomorphic adenoma of the parotid [5, 45]. These studies all focused on the parotid, the gland with the highest incidence of tumors and the lowest percentage of malignancies. When other salivary gland tumors are considered, the probability of malignancy and its extension to surrounding structures, and therefore the need for reconstruction, rise considerably.

Preoperative Assessment

Ideally, the patient is seen by both the extirpative and reconstructive surgeon together. Although it is mainly the characteristics of the defect that will determine the reconstructive modality, a preoperative assessment of patient and tumor variables can assist the reconstructive surgeon in predicting the defect and planning the reconstruction.

Patient Variables

There are several aspects to consider in evaluating the patient, including age, social and cognitive functions, occupation, and lifestyle. Severe comorbid conditions can independently impact perioperative morbidity, expected survival, and the type of reconstruction [16]. Perhaps one of the most important aspects of the preoperative visit is for the physician to understand the patient's needs and expectations, and to make sure these expectations are realistic. Showing the patient pictures of previous cases with similar conditions, and possibly their contact information if they are willing to share their experiences, can boost the patient's morale and confirm that he/she understands what to expect after surgery.

Tumor Variables

The assessment of the tumor before surgery serves two purposes: the first is an estimation of the size and boundaries of the anticipated defect for its obvious impact on the reconstructive decision. The second reason is to estimate the prognosis of the patient, as reconstruction for a palliative resection in a morbid patient mainly aims to alleviate symptoms, such as pain, and potentially to avoid any perioperative morbidity in a patient with an anticipated shortened life-span. There are several determinants of prognosis, in particular TNM stage, histological grade, and the ability to achieve clear margins [26, 48, 49, 54, 58]. Assessment of the tumor includes clinical, radiological, and pathological examination.

Clinical

Inspection and palpation of the tumor will define its limits and detect invasion of surrounding skin, mucosa, and bone with a high degree of accuracy. Similarly, examination for facial nerve paralysis or weakness is important in anticipating facial nerve resection.

Radiological

A high-quality spiral computed tomography (CT) scan or magnetic resonance imaging (MRI) should yield all the necessary information, including size and extent of the tumor and invasion of surrounding structures. CT scans are more widely available, less costly, and are more accurate in detecting bone invasion. MRI is more accurate in detecting perineural spread, which can have a major impact on the extent of the resection, such as sacrifice of the facial nerve, and the approach to the reconstruction.

Pathological

Certain tumors have peculiar patterns of growth, spread, and/or aggressiveness, which can influence the size of resection margins and the decision about sacrificing or preserving the facial nerve. For example, adenoid cystic carcinoma has a tendency for perineural spread, which is reported to occur in 20–80% of cases.

The Neck

Another important factor to consider is the status of the neck and whether a neck dissection is needed or has been previously done. Neck dissection can influence the reconstructive decision in many ways, including the need to cover the vessels of the neck (i.e., if neck skin has been resected) and the choice and side of inflow and outflow vessels for a free flap. In addition, the reconstructive surgeon can design the neck dissection incision to incorporate a cervical rotation-advancement flap for cutaneous defects, as will be discussed below.

Analyzing the Defect and Reconstructive Priorities

To choose the most suitable method of reconstruction, one first has to critically and methodically analyze the defect. The following is a simple and logical approach to analyze the defect and to plan the reconstruction that can be applied to most defects following salivary gland resection.

The first step is essentially determining the anatomy of the defect (i.e., what structures are missing). For example, in a parotid malignancy, it is essential to determine if it is only a subcutaneous tissue defect causing a concavity of the masseteric area, or if there is a defect of skin, mucosa, bone, and/or the facial nerve. For each, the extent or size of the defect should be identified and documented (e.g., the size of skin defect in centimeters or the extent of the bone defect in relation to the different anatomical parts of the mandible). In a maxillary defect, an exact knowledge of the missing anatomy, including which walls of the maxillary antrum have been excised, is essential for planning and executing the reconstruction.

The second step is defining the sequelae of the missing structures, both functionally and aesthetically. Functional aspects to consider are speech, mastication, deglutition, facial movements, and separation of cavities. Aesthetic aspects are also important for the patient's sense of well-being and for a return to his/her social life and occupation. For example, without bone reconstruction of a lateral mandibular defect malocclusion and mandibular deviation toward the side of resection will develop, while resection of the facial nerve will lead to aesthetically disfiguring facial asymmetry and functional consequences regarding speech and incomplete eye closure.

The third step is setting and prioritizing the reconstructive goals based on the previous findings. First, life-threatening conditions should be reliably resolved, such as coverage of the carotid vessels after neck dissection and skin resection. The second priority is restoration of integrity of the upper aerodigestive tract and wound closure. Subsequent priorities include restoration of articulation, mastication, and facial movements. Once the goals of reconstruction are known and arranged in order of importance, and in the context of the preoperative assessment described above, the surgeon should decide which reconstructive techniques will achieve these goals in each particular patient.

Tumors of the Parotid Gland

Malignancies of the parotid gland are the most common of all salivary gland tumors. In spite of their relatively accessible position, it is not uncommon that these present in late stages requiring extended radical parotidectomy [5, 14, 45, 55]. The scope of the defects from such surgery includes defects of skin, bone, and/or mucosa. When all three are missing, a through and through cheek defect is created that makes the necessary reconstruction more complex. In addition, reconstructive surgery may be needed for filling of the concavity that results from removal of the parotid gland or for reconstruction after facial nerve resection.

Reconstruction of the Concavity and Frey's Syndrome

Two of the relatively minor complications of parotidectomy that may be alleviated by a reconstructive procedure are Frey's syndrome and hollowing at the site of parotidectomy. Frey's syndrome consists of sweating, flushing, and a sense of warmth over the preauricular and temporal areas associated with mastication. It is believed to be due to aberrant reinnervation from the postganglionic secretomotor fibers to the parotid gland (arising from the otic ganglion) that communicate with the postganglionic sympathetic fibers supplying the sweat glands of the skin (that have been denervated during the parotidectomy). Its incidence varies markedly depending upon subjective testing and objective response by the patients. In addition, many patients who do develop Frey's syndrome are not bothered by it [9, 38]. Depression around the masseteric region is another complication that may be especially bothersome to patients. There have been many attempts to prevent these two symptoms by several modalities. The principle of these modalities is to transfer tissues (autogenous or alloplastic) into the site of the parotidectomy effectively replacing the soft tissue volume and separating the skin from the parotid bed to prevent the aberrant innervation responsible for Frey's syndrome [19].

Sternocleidomastoid Flap

The method most commonly used to prevent the concavity and Frey's syndrome after parotidectomy is the sternocleidomastoid muscle flap [19]. The sternocleidomastoid muscle arises from two distinct bellies from the sternum and the medial end of the clavicle. These two heads unite one third up the length of the muscle, although some surgeons advocate that they remain separated along the whole length of the muscle but enclosed in a fibrous sheath. In either case, the muscle is usually split in the upper part of the neck along its long axis preferably along a line of cleavage between the two heads, whether that line is found or artificially created. The anterior part of the muscle is then pedicled superiorly (Fig. 26.1) or inferiorly and transposed into the site of the parotidectomy [20]. Occasionally, it is left bipedicled and pushed anteriorly, or the muscle is opened like a book to reach the defect [47].

No particular technique seems to be superior to another. The value of the sternocleidomastoid flap in correcting the aesthetic defect and preventing Frey's syndrome is disputed. Many retrospective studies and more recent prospective studies have failed to show a definite advantage for using this muscle after parotidectomy, and currently its use should be left to the discretion of the reconstructive surgeon [32, 34].

Superficial Temporal Fascia Flaps, Dermal Fat Grafts, and Alloderm

Several other techniques have been used to augment the site of parotidectomy. The use of a superficial temporal fascia flap (temporoparietal fascia) increases operative time considerably and may have its own cosmetic complications (i.e., injury to hair follicles superficial to the harvest site), and therefore has never gained popularity [10, 32]. Dermal fat grafts were reported to have several merits, including low rates of infection and extrusion, low cost, and technical simplicity. However, their survival or resorption is unpredictable, and due to their need for revascularization from the surrounding recipient site, can only be of a limited size [27]. Recently, alloderm (cadaveric skin substitute, Fig. 26.2) emerged as a suitable alternative, as it is a simple option that does not increase operative time, has no donor site morbidity, is well tolerated by the body, and is incorporated into the recipient tissues. However, to fill the resultant concavity after surgery, a costly amount of alloderm is needed, and the use of alloderm is associated with a significantly increased risk of seroma [24, 52].

Superficial Musculoaponeurotic System (SMAS) Flaps

The growing experience of surgeons with face lifts and a better understanding of the anatomy of the SMAS have stimulated surgeons to modify the incision for parotidectomy and to use the SMAS to fill parotid defects [32, 43]. The preauricular incision curves around the lobule of the ear, up along the auriculomastoid groove then turns down along the occipital hairline. With this design, the visible incision in the neck along the anterior border of

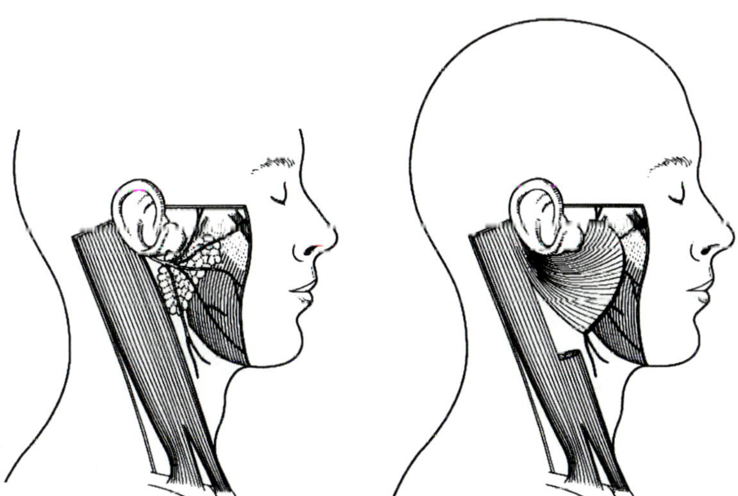

Fig. 26.1: Sternocleidomastoid (SCM) flap used to fill the depression created by a superficial parotidectomy. A superiorly based SCM flap can be rotated onto the deep lobe of the parotid gland. (Reprinted with permission from: Sood S, Quraishi MS, Jennings CR, Bradley PJ (1999) Frey's syndrome following parotidectomy: prevention using a rotation sternocleidomastoid muscle flap. Clin Otolaryngol 24:366, Blackwell)

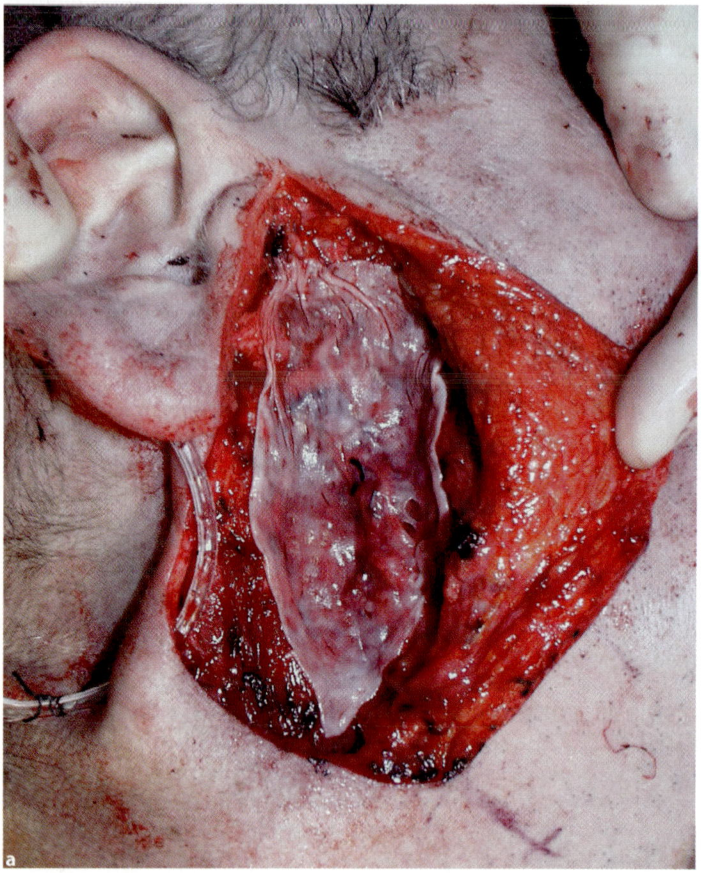

Fig. 26.2a,b: Alloderm to prevent Frey's syndrome. **a** Alloderm has been placed as an onlay graft on the parotidectomy defect. **b** *(see next page)*

the sternomastoid is eliminated. A skin flap is raised in the subfollicular plane (superficial to the SMAS). The SMAS/platysma is then incised along the preauricular groove, extending for a few centimeters below the mandibular border. The SMAS is elevated as a distinct layer in continuity with the platysma in the neck by dissecting it from the parotidomasseteric fascia and the parotid capsule. Once the desired amount of SMAS and platysma is mobilized, the parotidectomy can proceed as usual. Just as there have been many theories and techniques for SMAS lifting in rhytidectomy, there are several methods by which the SMAS can be used to recontour the parotidectomy site. If part of the SMAS has been removed with the tumor, then the remaining SMAS/platysma flap can be simply pulled backward and upward and sutured to the mastoid, zygomatic arch, and the sternomastoid muscle (Fig. 26.3). Otherwise, the SMAS can be used in many different ways to provide soft tissue volume, including transposition and plication. The platysma can be transposed into the cheek to gain extra volume. Some authors believe that the SMAS is too thin to fill the contour deformity, and that it should be sutured under considerable tension so as to act as a membrane for guided tissue regeneration, with a hematoma/seroma forming underneath it and later organizing to fill the defect [6, 30]. The value of using the SMAS to fill parotidectomy defects is disputed, as the limited benefit it provides may not justify the increased operative time and technical complexity.

Reconstruction of Defects of the Skin and Parotid

Excision of skin clinically invaded by a parotid cancer will usually lead to cutaneous defects of considerable size that cannot be adequately covered by skin grafts or local

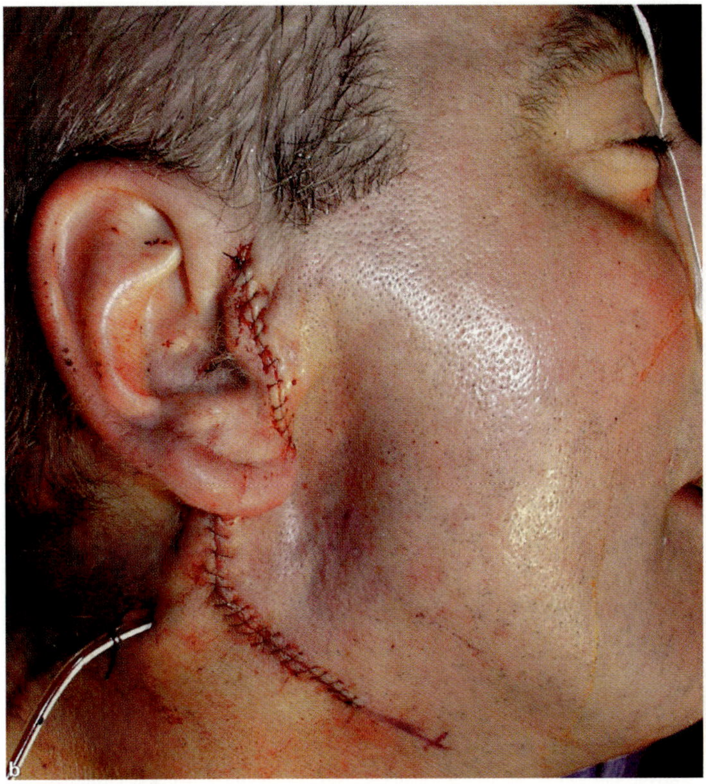

Fig. 26.2a,b: *(continued)* **b** A visible contour defect remains after placement of the alloderm

flaps from the cheek. Skin grafts are usually not applicable due to the high aesthetic demands of the face, while local flaps can only provide a limited amount of skin that will seldom suffice. The most important factors in cheek reconstruction are restoring skin color and texture and cheek volume. Other factors to consider include avoidance of distortion of adjacent structures (e.g., avoid causing ectropion of the lower lid), provision of flexible and thin skin to allow appreciation of facial movement, and replacement of hair-bearing skin in men [42].

Cervicofacial and Cervicodeltopectoral Flaps

The best option for resurfacing of the skin of the cheek is the use of adjacent normal skin because of the ideal color and texture match. One of the simplest and most aesthetically pleasing options is the use of cervicofacial and cervicodeltopectoral flaps (Fig. 26.4). These flaps make use of the laxity of skin in the neck to cover the defect. For the preauricular and lateral cheek defect, the incision usually begins from the posterolateral edge of the defect, goes down along the preauricular groove, under the lobule of the ear, and up to the mastoid process (similar to a parotidectomy incision). For more anterior defects, the incision starts at the superior edge of the defect and first arches upward at or above the zygomatic arch before descending along the preauricular crease. From the mastoid process the incision descends along the hair line and then along the anterior edge of trapezius, ensuring that the flap extends posteriorly enough to allow rotation into the face. The inferior incision can be placed in the lower neck, along the clavicle, or placed further inferiorly on the chest. The chest incision should include the internal mammary perforators of the second

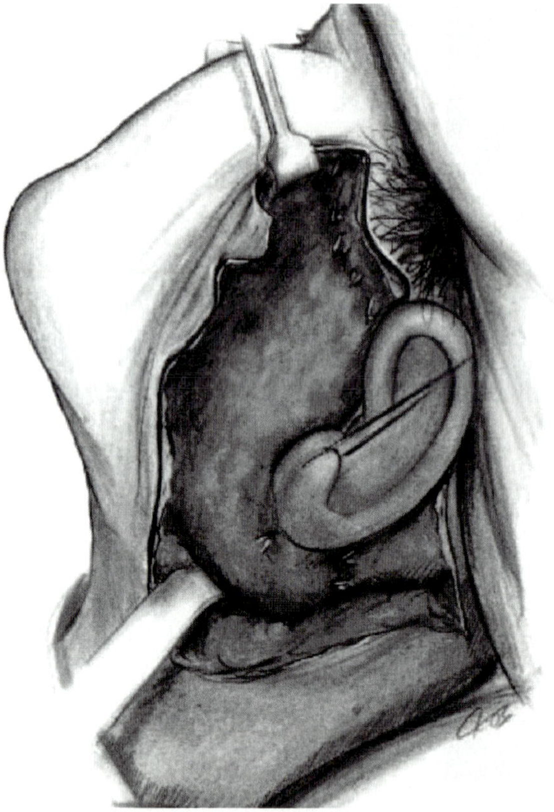

Fig. 26.3: Superficial musculoaponeurotic system (SMAS) flap to fill the parotidectomy contour defect. The SMAS flap has been advanced superiorly and posteriorly to the zygomatic arch, mastoid, and SCM muscle. (Reprinted with permission from: Honig JF (2004) Facelift approach with a hybrid SMAS rotation advancement flap in parotidectomy for prevention of scars and contour deficiency affecting the neck and sweat secretion of the cheek. J Craniofac Surg 15:800, Lippincott Williams and Wilkins)

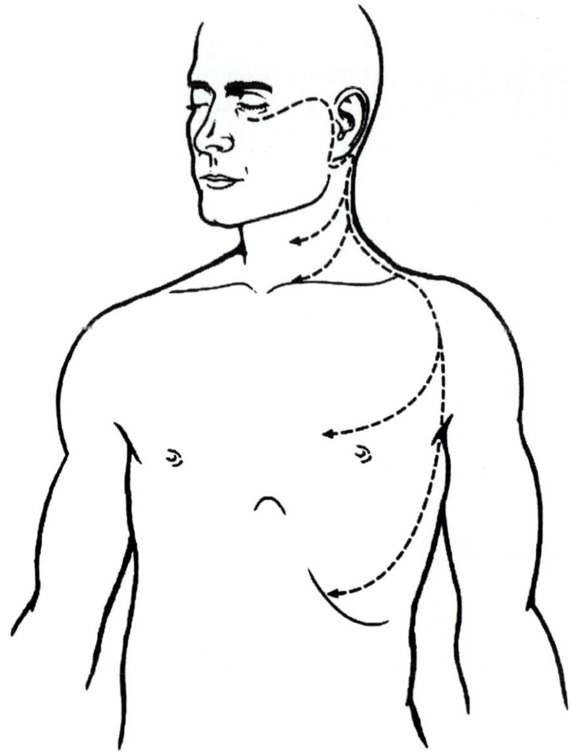

Fig. 26.4: Possible designs of cervicofacial and cervicodeltopectoral flaps for cheek and neck reconstruction. (Reprinted with permission from: Moore BA, Wine T, Netterville JL (2005) Cervicofacial and cervicothoracic rotation flaps in head and neck reconstruction. Head Neck 27:1093, Wiley)

and third intercostals spaces (similar to a deltopectoral flap, flap dissection should stop 2 cm lateral to the sternal edge). The flap is raised to include the platysma in the neck and the deltopectoral fascia in the chest. Undermining usually allows primary closure of the donor site. A skin graft to the chest wall may be needed in large flaps [33, 44].

The cervicofacial and cervicodeltopectoral flaps also allow access to the neck for neck dissection (the reconstructive surgeon should therefore plan the incision with the extirpative surgeon before the surgery) and allow simultaneous or later use of other flaps (e.g., pectoralis major) or anastomosis of free flaps in the exposed neck.

Pectoralis Major (PMF) and Other Pedicled Flaps

In many situations the demands of the defect cannot be met by cervicofacial flaps. This is most commonly seen in deeper or composite defects where a second lining (mucosa) or soft tissue volume is needed. The pectoralis major flap (PMF) has been a popular choice in these situations [1, 13]. Compared to free flaps, a PMF offers several advantages. It is faster and simpler to raise than a free flap and does not require a microvascular anastomosis. It also provides one or two skin paddles for skin/intraoral resurfacing and ample soft tissue volume to fill defects. Even in centers where free flaps are preferred over a PMF, the PMF still has an important role especially in two circumstances. The first is as a salvage flap for failed, unsuccessful, or unfeasible free flaps. The second is in conjunction with a free flap for composite or large defects. The PMF can also be combined with a cervicofacial flap to provide extra skin or soft tissue volume (Fig. 26.5).

Several other pedicled flaps have been used for these defects, most notably the latissimus dorsi flap [3]. The latissimus dorsi shares many of the advantages of a PMF, including a large arc of rotation, reliable vascularity, and the possibility of including a large skin island. However, it necessitates turning the patient to harvest the flap, and is generally a second choice to the PMF flap in cheek reconstruction.

Free Flaps

Free flaps are often the ideal technique in the reconstruction of parotidectomy defects with extensive skin loss. The concept of the reconstructive ladder, in which free flaps are used when pedicled flaps are not available, has been challenged in the last decade, with preference being given to a better functional and cosmetic result rather than simplicity of the procedure. The most commonly used free flaps for skin reconstruction after salivary tumor excision are the anterolateral thigh flap, scapular

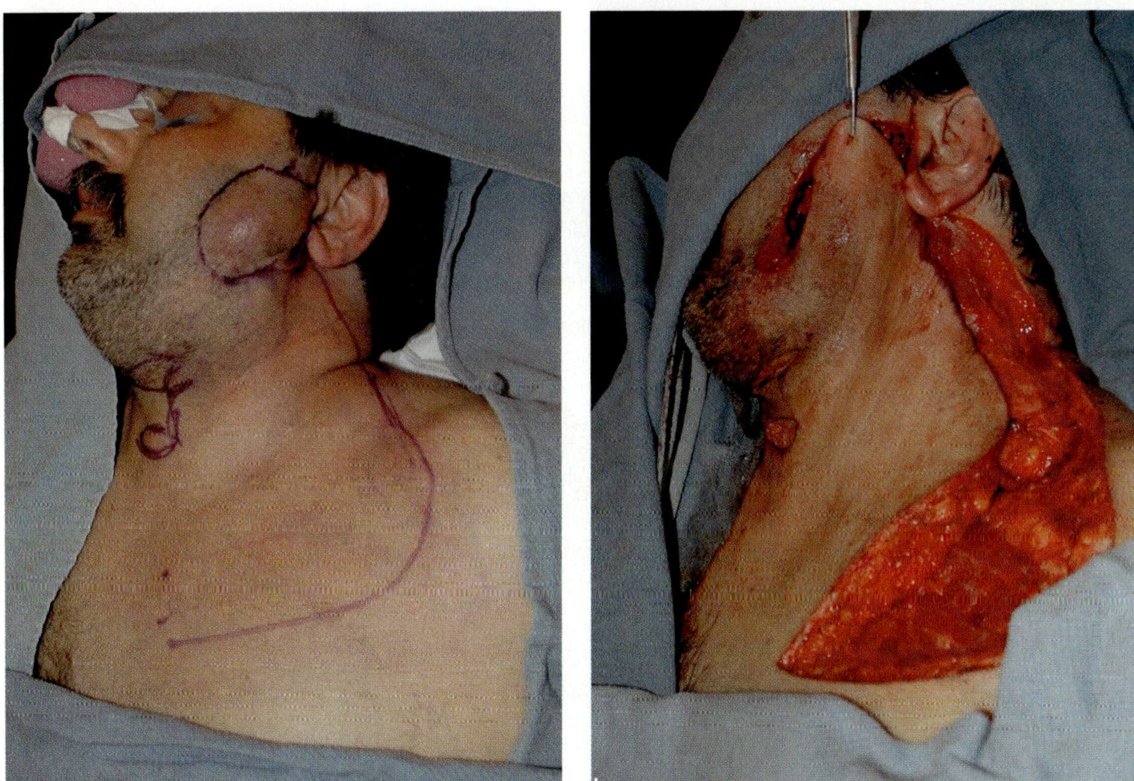

Fig. 26.5a–f: Combined use of a cervicodeltopectoral (CDP) flap and pectoralis myocutaneous (PMC) flap. **a** The expected cheek skin excision and design of a CDP flap. **b** Rotation-advancement of the CDP flap for cheek reconstruction. **c–f** *(see next page)*

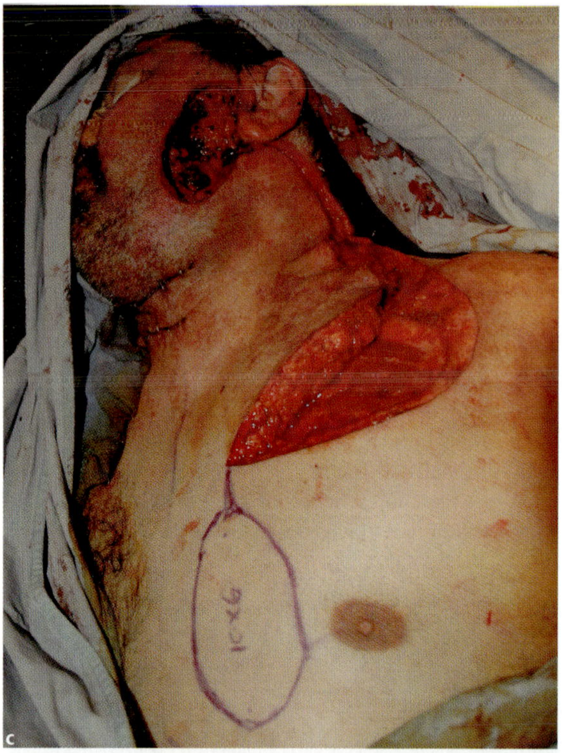

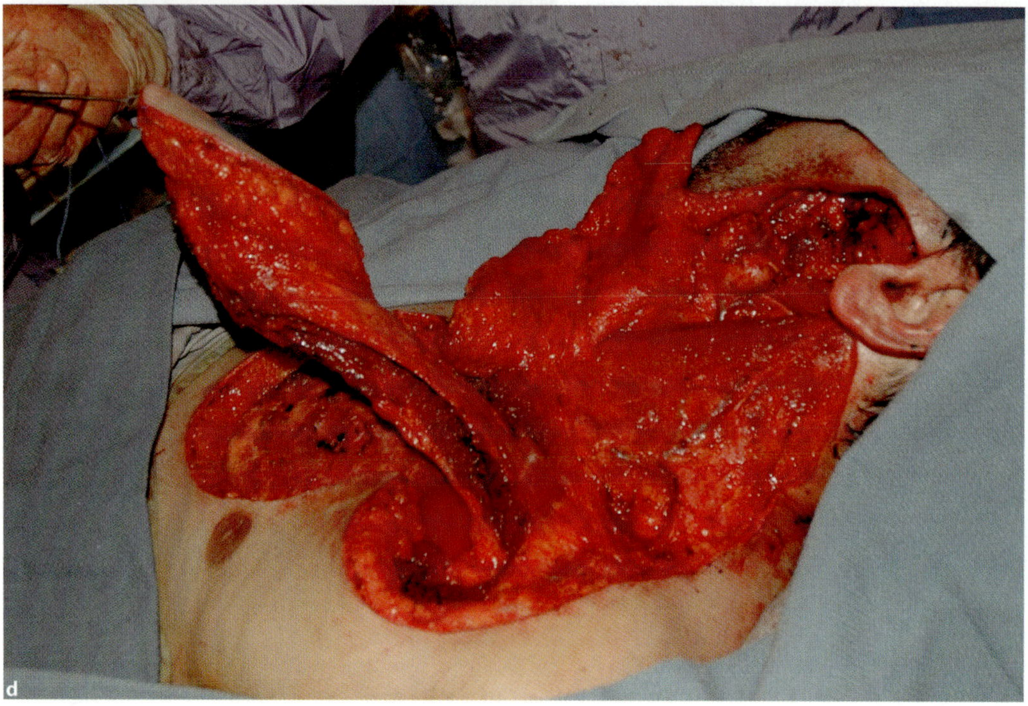

Fig. 26.5a–f: *(continued)* **c** Design of a PMC flap for soft tissue bulk to fill the lateral mandible and parotid defect. **d** PMC flap raised. **e–f** *(see next page)*

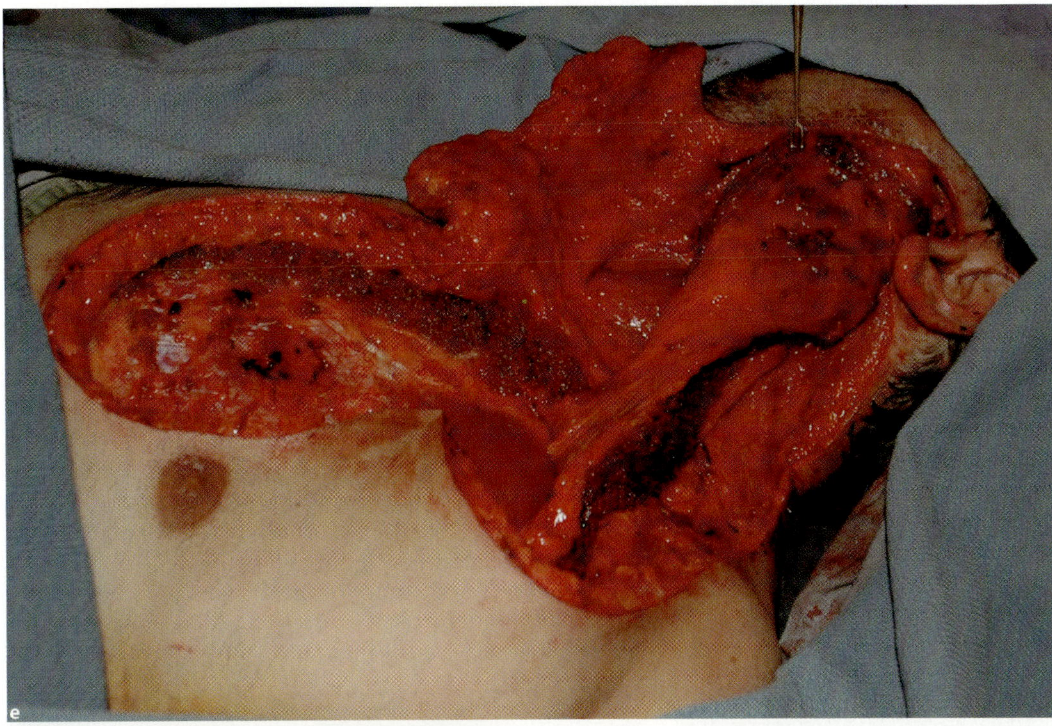

e

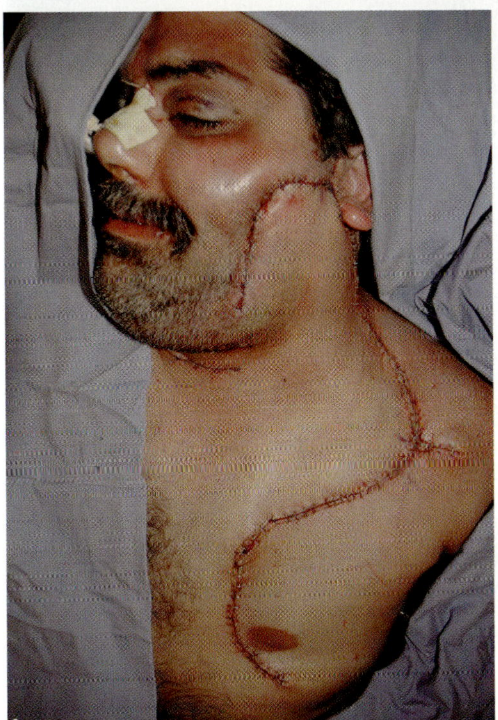

f

Fig. 26.5a–f: *(continued)* **e** Skin paddle of the PMC de-epithelialized; pectoralis flap with subcutaneous fat inset into the parotid and lateral mandible defect. **f** Inset of flap

flap, the rectus abdominis flap, and the radial forearm free flap.

Anterolateral Thigh (ALT) Flap

The anterolateral thigh flap [61] has recently gained popularity in soft tissue reconstruction of the head and neck. It is a perforator flap, derived from the descending branch of the lateral circumflex femoral artery. Its advantages include a long pedicle with a suitable vessel diameter and the possibility of harvesting the flap with thigh musculature (the vastus lateralis muscle, rectus femoris muscle, and/or the tensor fasciae lata) or as a sensate flap (by incorporating the anterior branch of the lateral cutaneous nerve of the thigh). Because of its distance to the head and neck, the harvest can be performed simultaneous with tumor extirpation.

Flap elevation begins by mapping the cutaneous perforators with a pencil Doppler probe. These perforators are located by first marking the midpoint between the anterior superior iliac spine and superolateral corner of the patella (Fig. 26.6). A circle centered at this midpoint is then drawn with a radius of 3 cm. The majority of the cutaneous perforators are located in the inferolateral quadrant of this circle. The flap is then harvested with its center over these perforators and its long axis parallel to that of the thigh. The flap can be elevated with or without the fascia lata (suprafascial dissection). The flap's skin and subcutaneous tissue are raised until the perforator(s) to the skin is defined. Once the skin vessel(s) is seen, it is dissected until the main pedicle is reached. If the skin vessel(s) is a musculocutaneous perforator(s) (the majority of patients), then the harvest includes an intramuscular dissection through the vastus lateralis muscle. If the skin vessel is a septocutaneous perforator, then the dissection is simpler and proceeds between the vastus lateralis and rectus femoris muscles [36]. The length of the pedicle is 8–16 cm, with a vessel diameter of larger than 2 mm.

A skin defect of less than 9 cm in width can be closed primarily without any reported evidence of compartment syndrome. Larger defects require skin grafting. A distinct disadvantage is the thickness of the flap in overweight in-

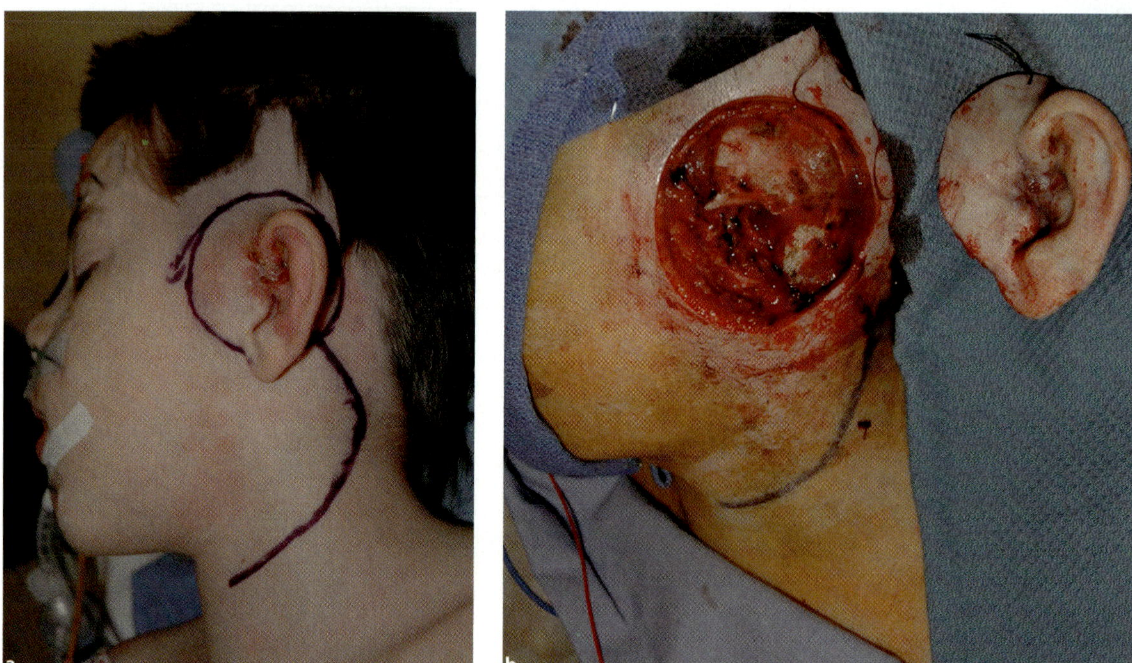

Fig. 26.6a–g: Anterolateral thigh (ALT) flap for cutaneous reconstruction. **a** Expected cheek skin, parotid, and auricular resection. **b** Surgical defect. **c–g** *(see next page)*

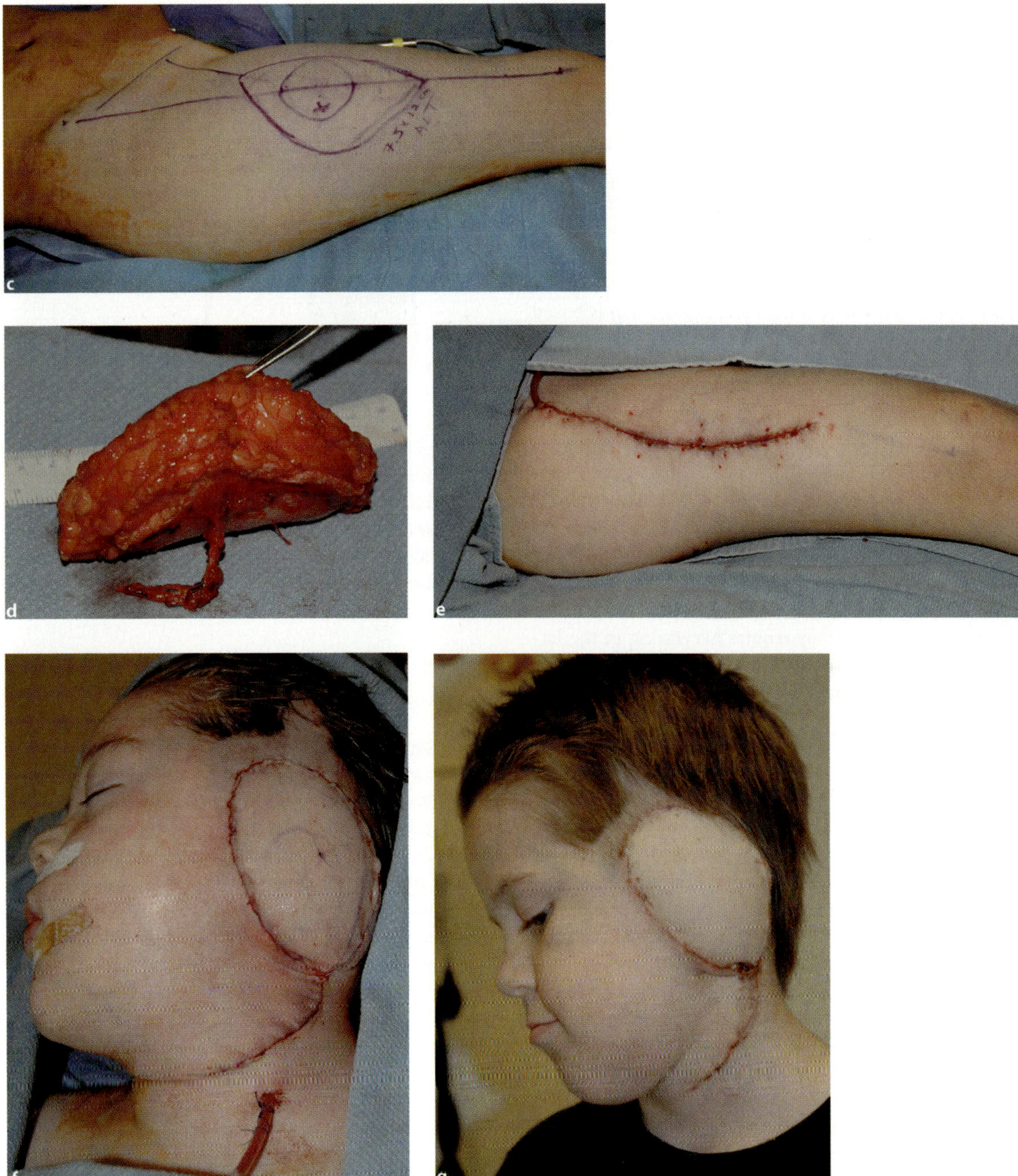

Fig. 26.6a–g: *(continued)* **c** Design of an ALT flap with skin perforators marked. **d** ALT flap harvested. **e** Primary closure of the donor site. **f** ALT inset. **g** Postoperative appearance

dividuals. However, the flap can be trimmed to the subdermal fat level for use as a thinner flap (4 mm).

Scapular and Parascapular Flaps

The branching pattern of the circumflex scapular artery and vein permits the harvest of either a scapular or parascapular fasciocutaneous flap for cheek cutaneous reconstruction [56]. The scapular flap is based on the horizontal cutaneous branch of the circumflex scapular artery (Fig. 26.7), whereas the parascapular flap is based on the descending cutaneous branch of the circumflex scapular artery. The circumflex scapular artery is a branch of the subscapular artery that approaches the lateral border of the scapula, supplies the periosteum of the bone and adjacent muscles, and then traverses the triangular space bounded by the teres major, the teres minor, and long head of the triceps to supply the overlying skin. If the thoracodorsal artery is included in the common vascular pedicle of the subscapular artery and vein, the latissimus dorsi and serratus anterior muscles can also be harvested with the scapular flap. The two disadvantages of these flaps are that they require harvesting in the lateral position and that the skin on the back can also be the thickest in the body. In obese patients these flaps may be too thick.

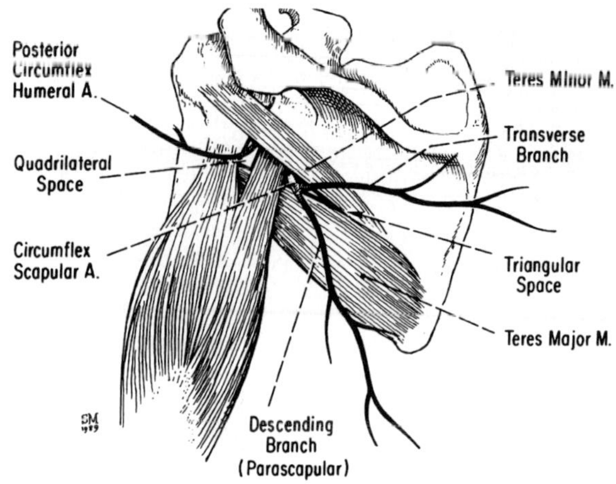

Fig. 26.7: Scapular flaps. Within the triangular space, the circumflex scapular artery emerges close to the long head of the triceps and bifurcates into the transverse (scapular) and descending (parascapular) branches. (Reprinted with permission from: Upton J, Albin RE, Mulliken JB, Murray JE (1992) The use of scapular and parascapular flaps for cheek reconstruction. Plast Reconstr Surg 90:960, Lippincott Williams and Wilkins)

Rectus Abdominis Musculocutaneous Flap

The rectus abdominis free musculocutaneous flap is based on periumbilical perforators from the deep inferior epigastric arteries. Incorporation of the periumbilical perforators permits an orientation of the skin paddle virtually in any direction from the midline. After the perforators are identified, the anterior rectus sheath is incised medial to the linea semilunaris and lateral to the linea alba. To preserve the strength of the abdominal wall, the anterior rectus sheath should not be harvested below the arcuate line. Inferiorly the anterior rectus sheath is incised vertically to completely expose the rectus muscle. The deep inferior epigastric pedicle is identified after the rectus muscle is bluntly dissected free from the posterior rectus sheath. The vascular pedicle, up to 15 cm in length, is exposed all the way to the origin of the vessels from the external iliac artery and vein. The intercostal nerves that supply the rectus muscle and overlying skin are mixed sensory and motor nerves, but microanastomosis to a sensory nerve in the head and neck has not yet resulted in a report of restoration of sensation. Closure of the abdominal wall can be accomplished with direct approximation of the residual anterior fascial margins. Most surgeons would agree that unless patients are engaged in vigorous physical activities, harvest of a unilateral rectus muscle has little impact on function.

Probably the biggest disadvantage of using the rectus abdominis flap is its bulk. However, for parotidectomy defects which involve a large loss of midface volume (i.e., after resection of cheek skin, parotid gland, lateral mandible, and muscles of mastication), the rectus abdominis [17, 37] can be a useful option (Figs. 26.8, 26.9).

Radial Forearm Free Flap (RFFF)

The RFFF is a fasciocutaneous free flap deriving it blood supply from branches of the radial artery that run in the intermuscular septum between the brachioradialis and flexor carpi radialis muscle. The major advantage of the RFFF is the large amount of thin forearm skin that can be

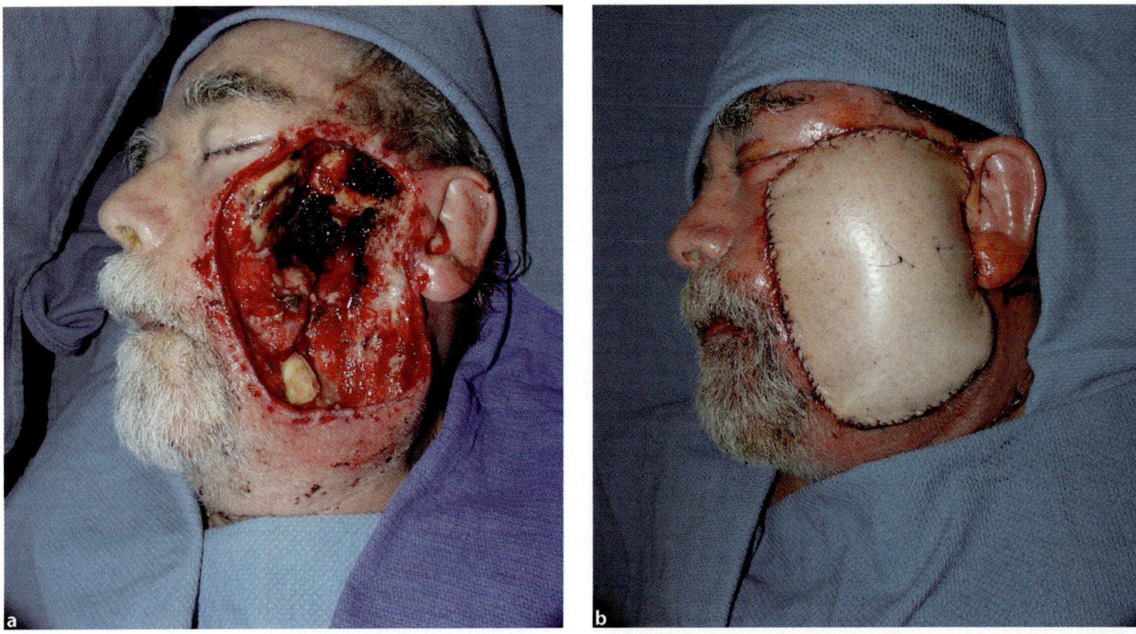

Fig. 26.8: Rectus abdominis free flap for reconstruction of a large volume resection of the midface, parotid, and cheek skin (type III lateral mandibular defect). **a** Lateral segmental mandibulectomy with resection of the parotid gland, infratemporal fossa, zygomatic arch, and cheek skin. **b** Inset of rectus abdominis flap; buccal mucosa closed primarily

harvested for reconstruction. For through and through cheek defects the RFFF can be folded to create separate skin paddles for cutaneous and oral mucosa reconstruction [51]. Compared to an anterolateral thigh flap or scapular flap, an RFFF is thinner, and thus, reconstruction of a parotid and cutaneous defect with an RFFF may still leave the patient with a contour depression at the site of the parotidectomy.

Reconstruction of Defects of the Skin, Parotid, Mandible, and Oral Mucosa

Parotid malignancies requiring resection of the mandible are almost always accompanied by resection of the overlying skin and buccal mucosa creating a through and though defect. The reconstructive challenge becomes threefold: reconstruction of the oral cavity to prevent salivary fistula, restoration of mandibular continuity, and cutaneous coverage [39]. A key element in their reconstruction is deciding the best course for dealing with the mandibular defect.

Mandible Reconstruction

Reconstruction of the mandible has undergone dramatic improvement in the last two decades, with the older modalities, such as nonvascularized grafts and pedicled bone grafts, being replaced by dependable, free vascularized bone flaps [28, 41]. There have been many classification schemes for mandibular defects, and each center or surgeon will usually favor a certain classification. A simple and logical classification is to divide them into defects of the symphysis, body, ramus, and/or condyle. Boyd et al. [7] classified mandibular defects into three types:

1. H defects: lateral defects including the condyle but not crossing the midline,
2. L defects: similar to H defects but with an intact condyle, and
3. C defects: defects of the entire symphysis.

Mandibular defects due to parotid surgery will usually be lateral defects with or without resection of the condyle (i.e., H or L defects). Deleyiannis et al. [17] stressed the importance of the volume and location of the soft tis-

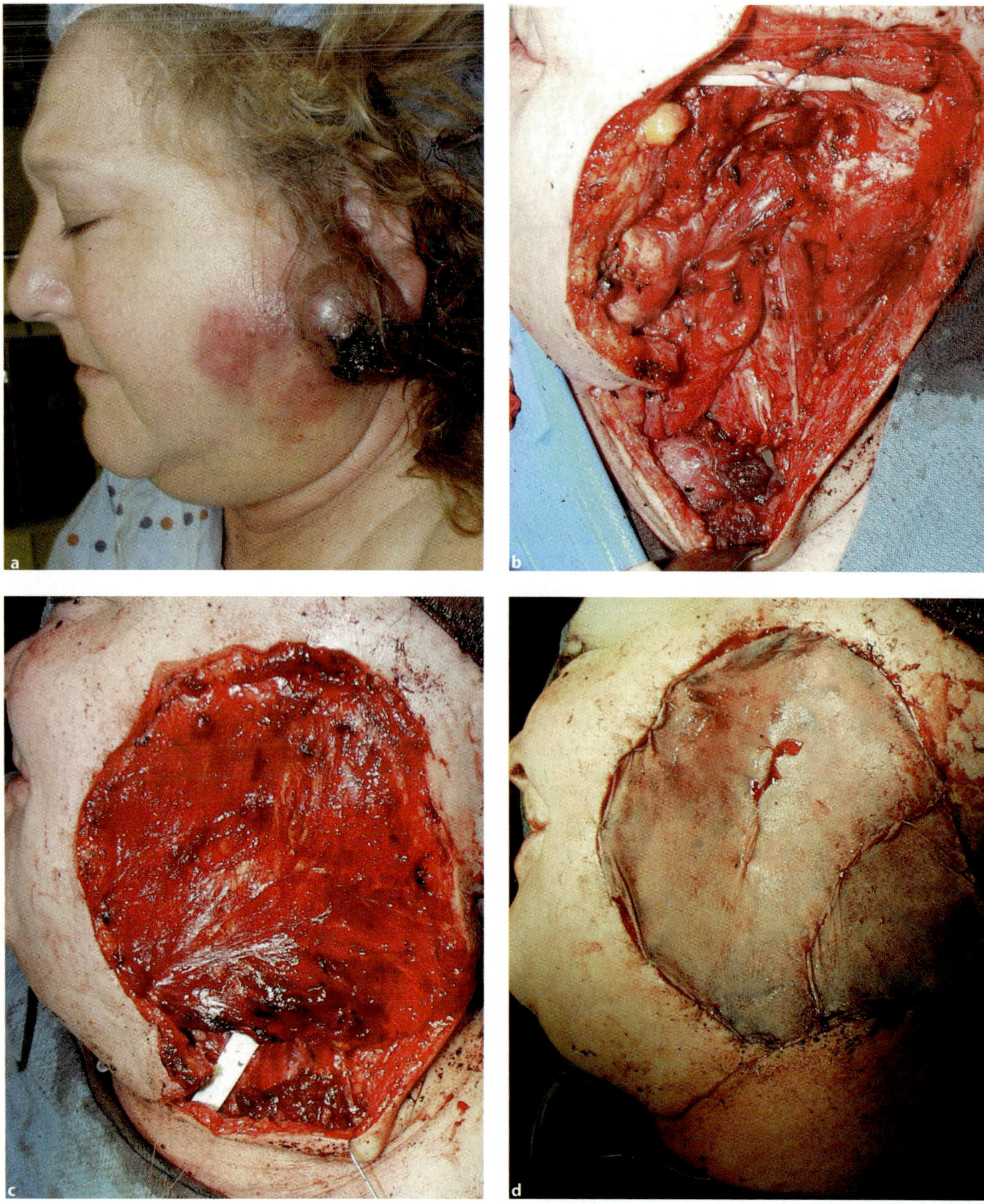

Fig. 26.9: Rectus abdominis free flap for reconstruction of a large volume resection of the midface, parotid gland, and cheek skin (type III lateral mandibular defect). **a** Melanoma with invasion into the parotid gland. **b** Defect; Alloderm placed as a static sling from the modiolus to the malar body. **c** Inset of rectus myofascial free flap. **d** Skin graft to rectus flap for cutaneous coverage

sue defect and the presence of comorbid conditions (i.e., prognosis) in deciding the method for reconstruction of lateral mandibular defects (H or L defects), and classified these lateral defects into:

Type I defects: mandibular defects with a soft tissue resection limited to the oral cavity and oropharynx

Type II defects (Fig. 26.10): through and through defects of the lower face (skin overlying the mandible) or neck

Type III defects (Fig. 26.11): those defects associated with a large volume resection of the midface, parotid, and cheek skin

Extended radical parotidectomy will usually result in a type III defect, whereas a malignant tumor of the submandibular gland that has invaded the lateral mandible and submandibular skin would result in a type II defect. The options for reconstruction in these cases include soft tissue reconstruction without bony mandibular reconstruction or a free osseous flap (with or without a second flap for soft tissue reconstruction).

Soft Tissue Reconstruction Only

Acceptable function, including mastication and speech, can be achieved with soft tissue reconstruction only in lateral mandibular defects. Because these patients do not have restoration of their mandibular continuity with a reconstruction plate or an osseous free flap, they do have malocclusion of their remaining dentition and mandibular deviation to the reconstructed side with mouth opening. However, on frontal view facial symmetry is well preserved.

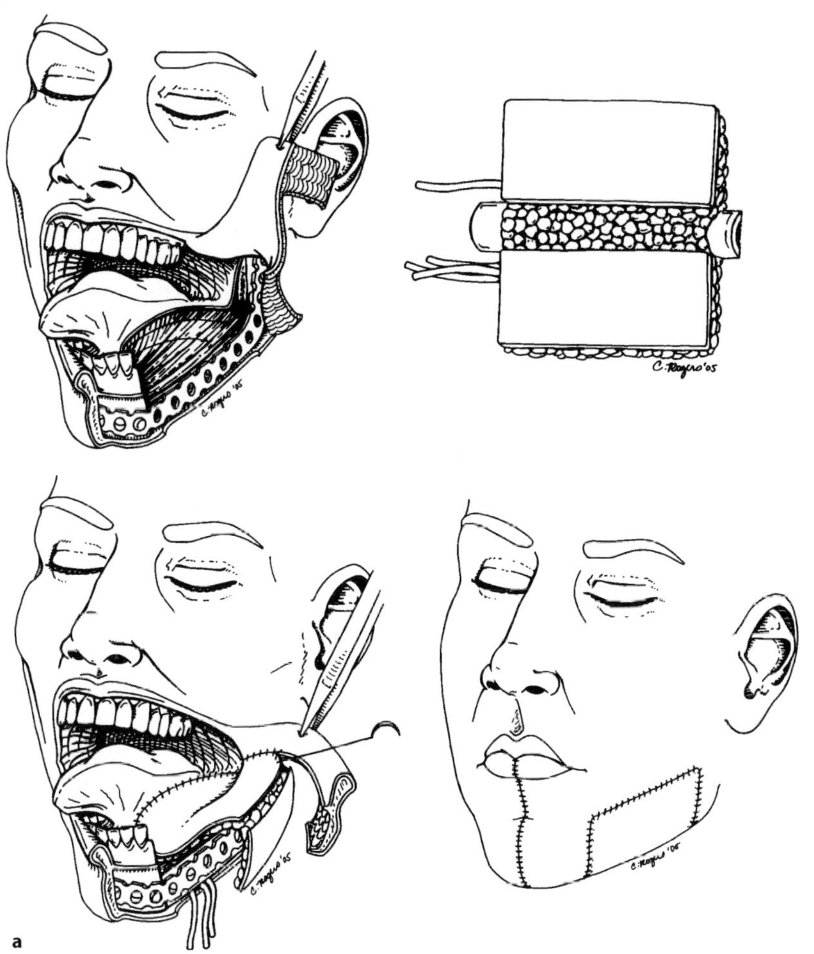

a

Fig. 26.10a,b: Type II lateral mandibulectomy defect: a through and through defect of the lower face (skin overlying the mandible) and/or neck. **a** *Upper left* Through and through defect (skin resected overlying the mandible and neck). *Upper right* Osteocutaneous radial forearm (RFFF) de-epithelialized to create two skin paddles. An osteocutaneous fibular free flap with two skin paddles could also be used. *Lower left* Oral cavity inset done; paddle draped over the radius (or fibula) and reconstruction plate. *Lower right* - Cutaneous inset. **b** *(see next page)*

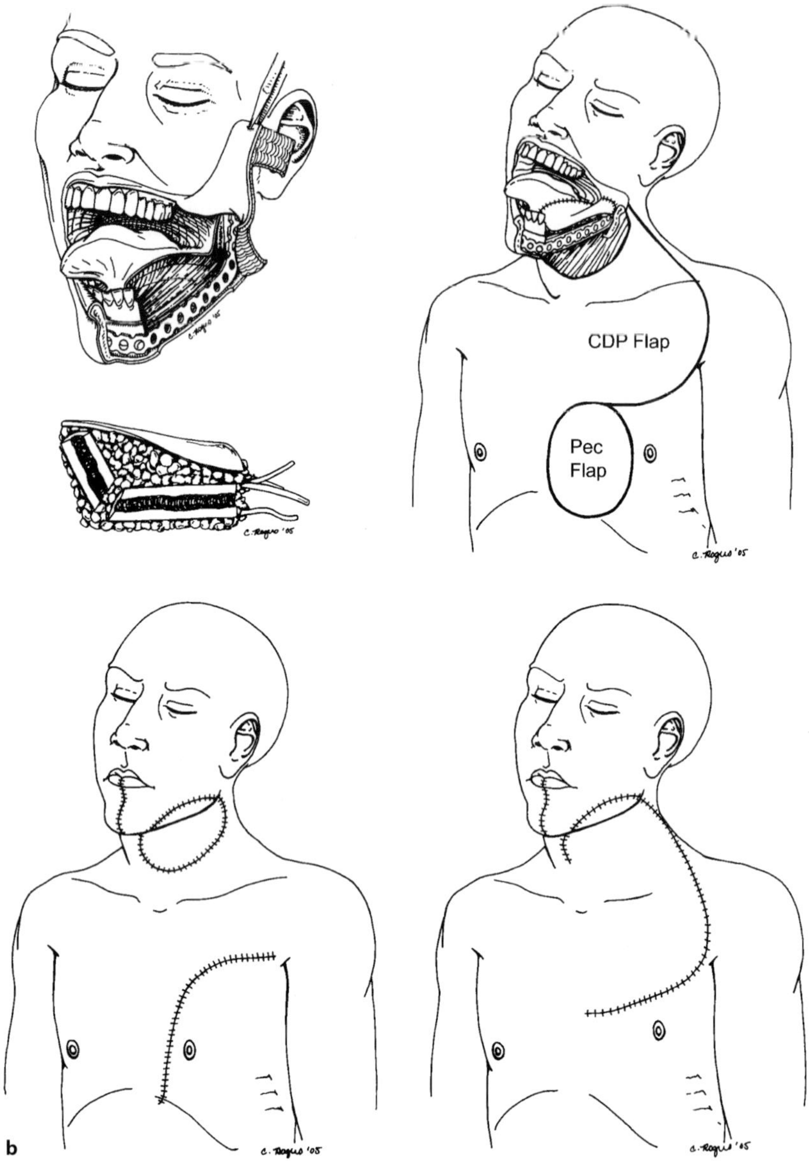

Fig. 26.10a,b: *(continued)* **b** *Upper left* Through and through defect (skin resected overlying the mandible and neck). *Middle left* Osteocutaneous RFFF. *Upper right* Osteocutaneous RFFF used for mandible and oral cavity reconstruction; design of a cervicodeltopectoral (CDP) and pectoralis major (Pec) flap. *Lower right* CDP used for cutaneous reconstruction. *Lower left* Pectoralis flap used for cutaneous reconstruction

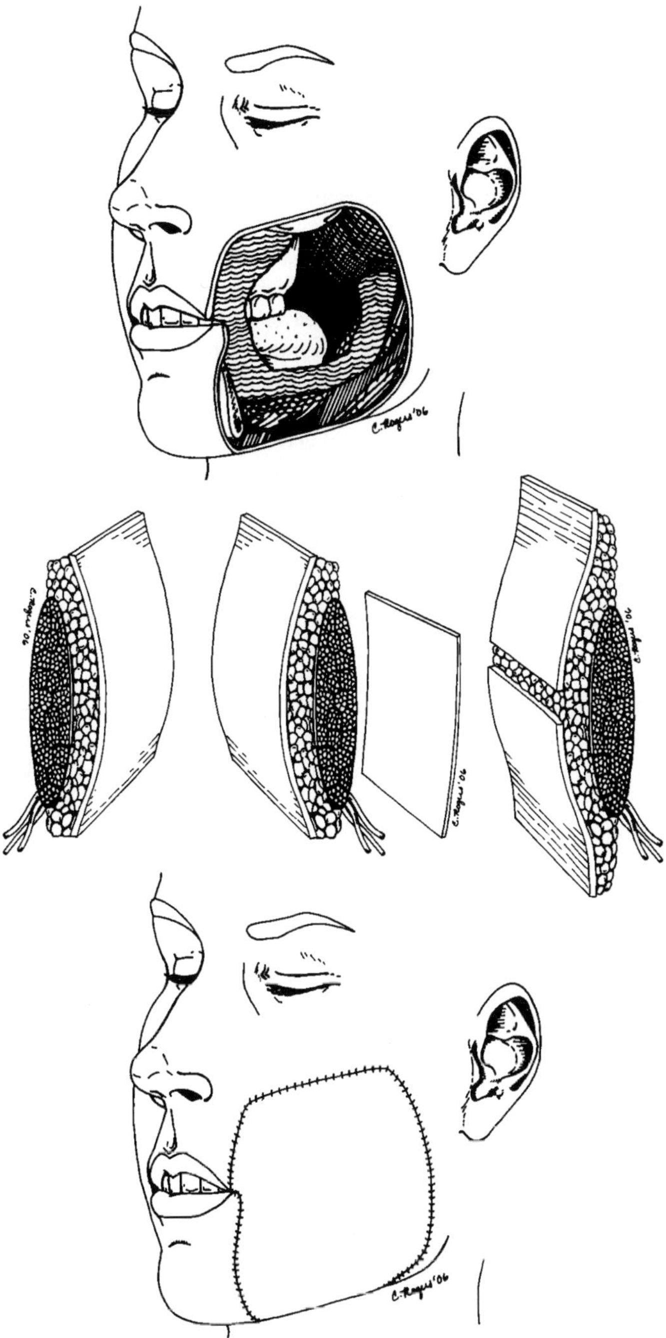

Fig. 26.11: Type III defect: lateral defect with an associated large volume resection of the midface, parotid gland, and/or cheek skin. *Upper* Through and through defect of the cheek and midface. *Middle* Rectus abdominis free flap with a single skin paddle, skin graft, or two skin paddles. *Lower* Flap inset; buccal mucosa closed primarily or with the skin paddle of the rectus flap; cutaneous reconstruction done with a skin paddle of the rectus flap or with a skin graft on the rectus abdominis muscle

A rectus abdominis free flap is our preferred method of reconstructing large volume defects that include buccal mucosa, mandible, muscles of mastication, parotid tissue, and cheek skin. A rectus free flap provides ample bulk to fill the soft tissue defect and a reliable skin island for cheek or buccal mucosal reconstruction. The rectus free flap can be folded on itself to place one skin paddle inside the mouth and another externally, or a skin graft can be placed directly on the rectus muscle to provide external skin coverage (Figs. 26.8–26.10). Because of the low risk of flap failure, low incidence of donor site morbidity, the frequent absence of a functioning temporomandibular joint, and the desire to minimize the complexity of the surgical procedure, the rectus free flap is often our first choice of reconstruction [17].

Free Osteocutaneous Flaps, Alone or with a Second Flap (Pedicled or Free)

A free osteocutaneous flap, in particular a fibular free flap (FFF) or an osteocutaneous radial forearm free flap (ORFFF), can also be used to reconstruct through and through defects caused by parotid malignancies. To reconstruct the associated skin and oral mucosa defects, the flap can be raised as an osteocutaneous flap with two skin paddles or combined with a second flap [1, 17].

The fibular osteocutaneous free flap offers the advantages that it can provide a vascularized bone graft greater than 20 cm in length, that the cross-sectional area of the fibula approximates the cross-sectional area of the mid-body of the mandible, and that it is ideally suited for placement of osseointegrated implants for dental rehabilitation. As the bone is supplied by both the nutrient artery and periosteal branches, multiple corticotomies can be made in the fibula to conform to the shape of the resected mandible. A large skin paddle, based on the posterior septocutaneous perforators, can be harvested with a fibular free flap. Jones et al. have reported the routine harvest of fibular skin paddles from the mid-posterior leg to the lateral border of the tibia for reconstruction of through and through defects [31]. Harvesting the soleus muscle in conjunction with fibula can be utilized to fill soft tissue defects. In addition, as the flap is remote from the head and neck, it can be raised with the patient in the supine position during the extirpative surgery.

The radial forearm osteocutaneous flap can provide up to 12 cm of vascularized bone. It is especially suitable for reconstruction of mandibular defects that are more posteriorly situated with a limited bone defect and a large soft tissue loss [59]. The bone of the ORFFF is not suitable for implants. However, posterior mandibular defects will usually do well without implants due to their posterior position and small size. The cutaneous component of the radial forearm flap can be used to reconstruct the cheek and/or oral mucosa. A double skin paddle flap can be designed to cover both sides of a through and through defect (Fig. 26.10).

Other flap options exist for extensive through and through defects (type II and III). Wei et al. published their preference for double free flaps, in particular a fibular osteocutaneous flap with either a fasciocutaneous RFFF, ALT flap, or myocutaneous rectus abdominis flap [60, 62]. According to the authors, the use of a second free flap allows easier insetting and better reproduction of the three-dimensional anatomical boundaries, such as the buccal sulcus and the trigonal area. The disadvantages of using two free flaps include the extra time needed to harvest two flaps and perform the additional microanastomoses, the possible lack of a second pair of recipient vessels in those patients with a history of previous radiotherapy or neck surgery, and a second donor site morbidity.

The scapular osteocutaneous flap and internal oblique-iliac crest osteomyocutaneous flap have been advocated as a single flap option [18, 57]. The scapular osteocutaneous flap may be combined with a parascapular flap or latissimus dorsi myocutaneous flap on the same subscapular vascular pedicle for independent reconstruction of internal lining, mandibular bone, and external skin. The disadvantages of these flaps are that they require harvesting in the lateral position, the lateral border of the scapula is quite thin, and the segmental periosteal blood supply may be compromised if multiple osteotomies are required. The internal oblique muscle of the internal oblique-iliac crest osteomyocutaneous flap can be used to separately reconstruct the oral cavity mucosal defect. However, femoral nerve injury, hernia, gait disturbance, pain, and abdominal wall denervation are potential donor site morbidities [21].

Facial Reanimation: Procedures Done at the Time of Parotidectomy

Radical parotidectomy with resection of the facial nerve remains one of the common causes of facial nerve palsy. In spite of the many innovations and refinements in facial nerve reconstruction, it remains a difficult problem, with many functional and aesthetic consequences. When part of the nerve has been removed due to tumor infiltration, immediate nerve grafting while the patient is anesthetized and the nerve ends are clearly identified is the ideal option [2]. Other procedures may be added, such as static slings and/or placement of an upper eyelid gold weight.

Nerve Grafting

For facial nerve grafting, a cable graft is performed from the proximal facial nerve stump to the distal branches. The three common donor sites for nerve grafts are the sural nerve, cervical cutaneous nerves (mainly the greater auricular nerve), and the medial or lateral antebrachial nerve. The sural nerve is the most common donor site for nerve grafts due to its length, acceptable donor site morbidity, and ease of harvest (Fig. 26.12). The greater auricular nerve and other cutaneous branches of the cervical plexus if not involved with tumor have the advantage of being in the surgical field and having an extensive arborization pattern, allowing a single nerve sutured to the proximal stump to be anastomosed to several distal branches [2]. The cutaneous nerves of the forearm can also be used, but because of donor site morbidity (numbness in the forearm and the forearm scar), they are usually the last option.

The surgeon should aim to reinnervate as many distal branches as possible. A number of factors can potentially worsen the prognosis, such as the age of the patient, inadequate vascularity of the bed, use of radiotherapy, preoperative facial palsy, and an associated skin defect. It is widely believed that nerve regeneration is worse in old age, but the effect of radiotherapy is debatable. Radiotherapy was classically believed to retard nerve regeneration, but several authors have shown similar results in patients who had and did not have radiotherapy [40, 50]. The use of a vascularized nerve graft might be applicable in those

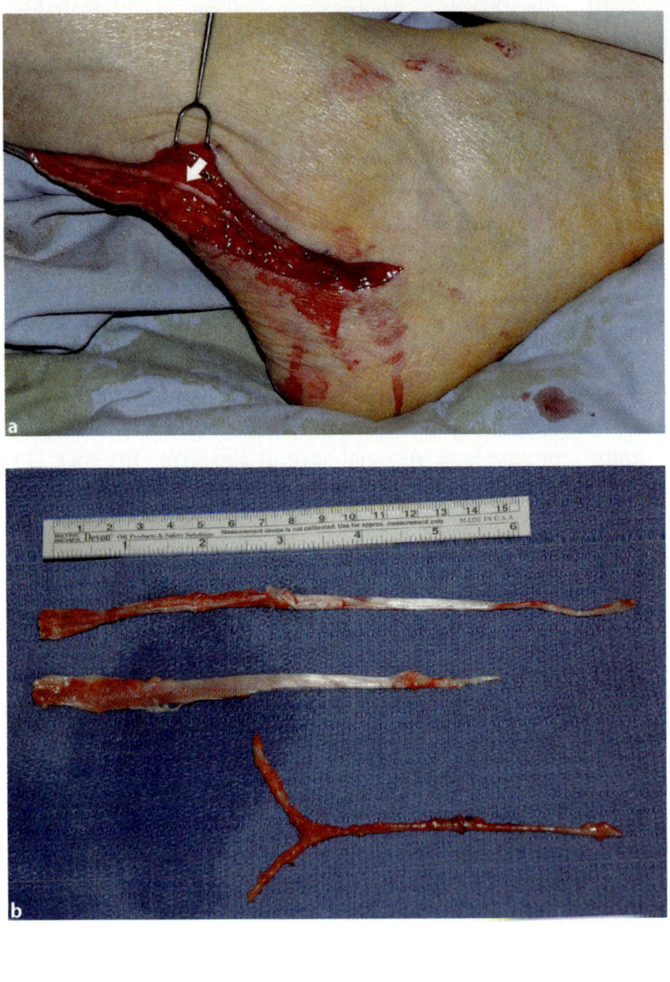

Fig. 26.12a–d: Facial nerve reconstruction at the time of parotidectomy and facial nerve resection. **a** The sural nerve is initially located between the lateral malleolus and Achilles tendon. **b** The sural nerve distally arborizes into at least two branches that can be used for anastomosis. Fascia lata (superior two strips in the image) from the lateral thigh can be harvested at the same time for static sling reconstruction. **c–d** *(see next page)*

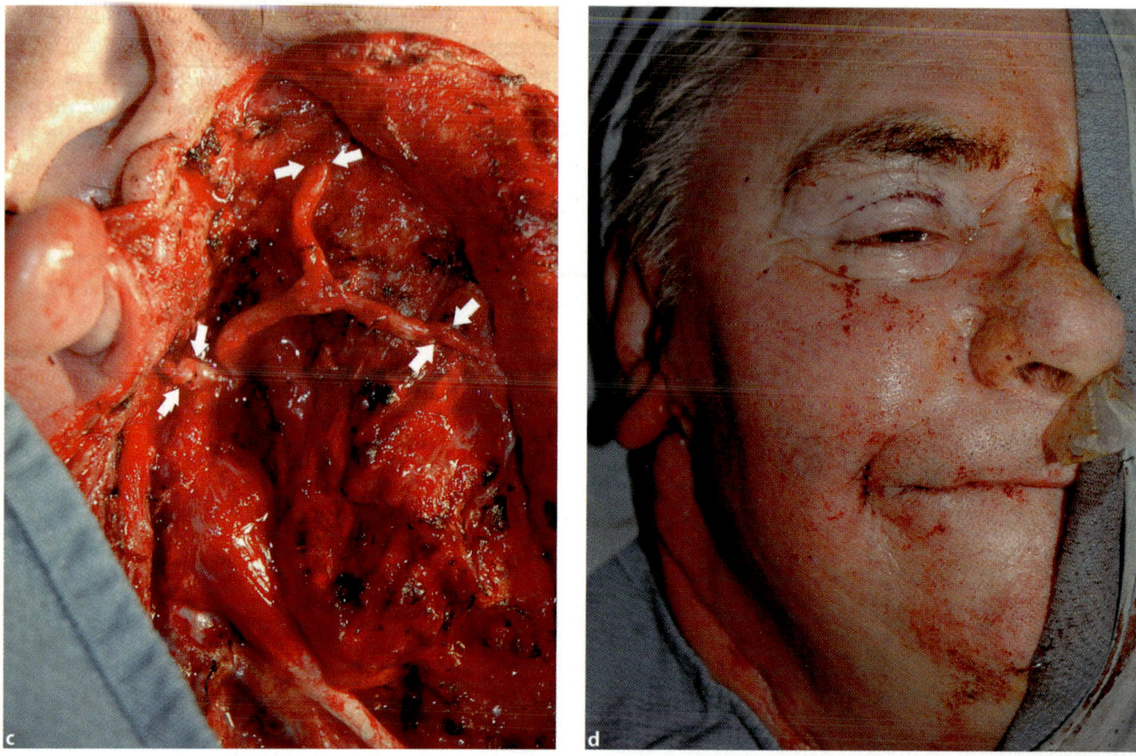

Fig. 26.12a–d: *(continued)* **c** Nerve anastomosis with epineural sutures to the temporal and zygomatic branches. **d** Closure after sural nerve grafting and placement of a fascial lata sling to the midface and upper eyelid gold weight

cases where the surgeon is concerned about the vascularity of the surrounding tissues and the effect of radiotherapy. Several studies have shown better healing in vascularized nerve grafts as compared to conventional nerve grafts, but at the expense of an increased operative time and case complexity. If a free flap is going to be used for a skin, mucosal, or bone defect, a composite flap can be designed to include a vascularized nerve graft, such as the lateral antebrachial cutaneous nerve harvested with an RFFF [35].

Static Reconstruction

A static sling can be used to improve facial symmetry at rest. This is especially helpful in patients in whom nerve regeneration is not expected, due to comorbid conditions or a short life expectancy. In patients who do receive a nerve graft, a static sling can provide support to the midface during reinnervation, which typically takes up to a year [25]. Static slings can be performed using autogenous material, commonly a fascia lata strip or a tendon graft, or alloplastic material such as alloderm. The sling [15] is routinely sewn to modulus, upper and lower lips and fixed either to the deep temporal fascia or the exposed malar bone (Fig. 26.13). Anticipating the relaxation that will occur over time, the surgeon should suspend the patient's oral commissure and lips until the patient's upper canine is exposed (i.e., canine smile).

Upper Eyelid Gold Weight

Complete resection of the facial nerve will result in an immediate flaccid paralysis with the inability to completely close the eye. Prophylactic placement of an upper eyelid gold weight at the time of facial nerve resection

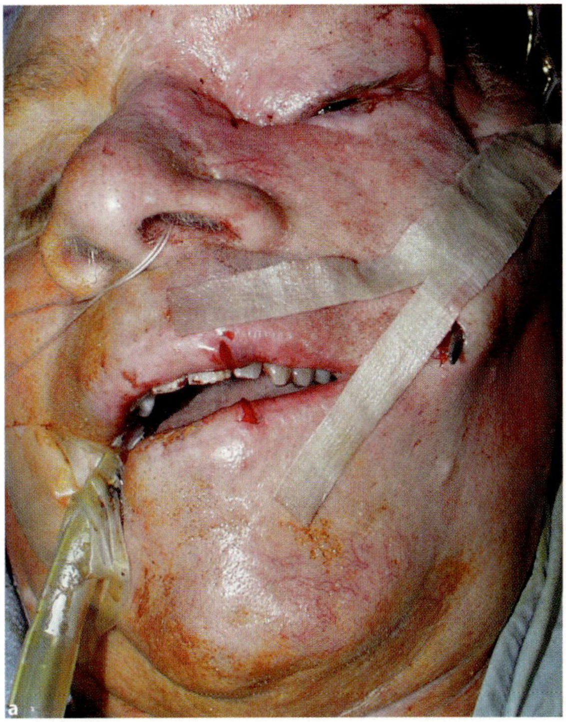

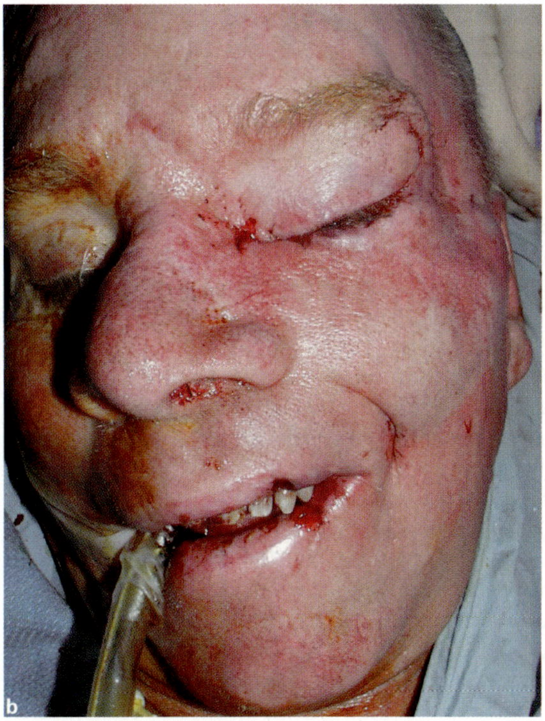

Fig. 26.13: Midface suspension with a fascia lata sling. **a** The fascia lata is sewn into the modiolus and upper and lower lip and suspended to the deep temporalis fascia or malar bone. **b** The midface is suspended to achieve a "canine smile"

can potentially improve eye closure, and thus protection (Fig. 26.14). A 1.2-g gold weight has proved to be the appropriate weight in most of our patients. It is secured to the tarsal plate and can be removed if the patient recovers protective eye function.

Tumors of the Submandibular Gland

Reconstruction after submandibular gland resection only becomes necessary when the tumor has invaded the overlying skin and/or the mandible.

Skin Reconstruction

The cervicofacial flap and cervicodeltopectoral flap are ideal in these cases, due to the proximity and the usual

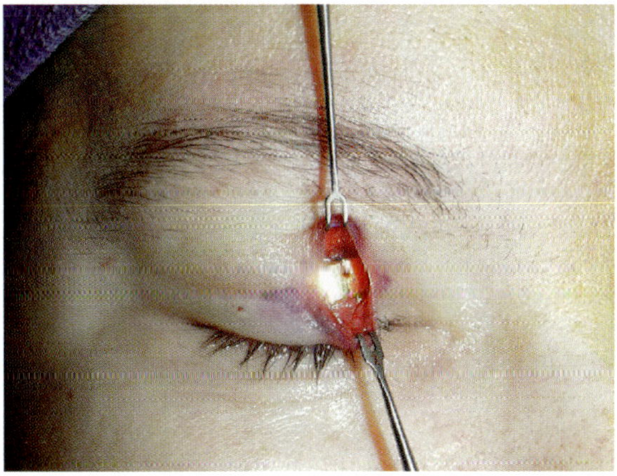

Fig. 26.14: Placement of an upper eyelid gold weight: 1.2 g has proved to be an appropriate weight in most patients receiving a gold weight at the time of facial nerve resection

small size of the cutaneous defect. It is uncommon for these defects to require more complicated reconstruction, but if necessary, the flaps that were described for parotid tumors can be used for these defects. The pectoralis major flap can be especially helpful, due to its easy reach to the submandibular region.

Through and Through Defects

Cancers of the submandibular gland that invade the mandible and overlying skin produce defects classified as type II defects (Fig. 26.10), according to Deleyiannis et al. [17]. These reconstructions require separate skin paddles for reconstruction of the oral mucosa and skin defect. An osteocutaneous free flap (either an RFFF or fibular free flap) with two skin paddles folded over the reconstructed bone defect (Fig. 26.15) or an osteocutaneous flap in conjunction with cervicodeltopectoral flap (CDP) or pectoralis flap is our preferred method for reconstructing a type II defect [11]. The decision to use an osteocutaneous free flap with two skin paddles versus a CDP flap or pectoralis flap is based on anticipating the adequacy of soft tissue coverage provided by folding the cutaneous paddle over the reconstruction plate. The use of a CDP flap for lower face or neck reconstruction provides for a better skin quality match compared to a distant or regional flap. Our decision to use a CDP flap versus a pectoralis myocutaneous flap is based mainly on preoperative planning by marking the anticipated skin defect and determining with a surgical towel cut into a template of the CDP flap whether the flap will rotate sufficiently to close the defect.

Tumors of the Minor Salivary Glands

There are between 450 and 750 minor salivary glands dispersed in the head and neck region. Although it is rare to see tumors in these glands, when they do occur they are more likely to be malignant. Tumors of the minor salivary gland are most common in the hard and soft palate, although they may be seen in the buccal mucosa, tongue, pharynx, nose, maxillary antrum, and other rare sites [4]. Tumors arising in the floor of the mouth and cheek will leave defects that can be covered by a graft (skin or mucosal), local flap, or left to epithelialize spontaneously. The resection of large tumors will leave defects which may include the mandible, through and through cheek defects, or floor of mouth and neck defects. The reconstruction of these defects is very similar to defects arising from parotid and submandibular gland tumors. Reconstruction after glossectomy depends mainly on the extent of resection. Up to one half the tongue can be removed with acceptable functional results without regional or free flap reconstruction; larger resections are best managed by a free muscle flap, such as the rectus abdominis flap [63]. Tumors of the pharynx can be reconstructed by many different methods, ranging from primary closure to free jejunal flaps and fasciocutaneous flaps.

The most common defects after excision of minor salivary glands tumors are those of the palate and maxilla. Recently, Cordeiro and Santamaria proposed a classification system and algorithm for reconstruction of maxillectomy and midfacial structures [12]. The temporalis muscle, soft tissue free flaps (rectus abdominis and radial forearm), nonvascularized bone (rib or calvarium), and vascularized bone flaps (osteocutaneous radial forearm free flap) were used to reconstruct a variety of maxillectomy defects. Palatal defects were closed only with soft tissue. The nonvascularized and vascularized bone was used for the osseous reconstruction of the zygoma, maxilla, and orbital floor. Reconstruction of the orbital floor was done to prevent enophthalmos, vertical dystopia, and diplopia. Other algorithms have been adopted containing many other free flaps and designs [8, 46, 63]. Many have focused on various osteocutaneous flaps such as the fibula and the iliac crest. These latter flaps allow for the osteointegration of implants for dental rehabilitation [22]. In cases of combined midface and lip resection, oral competency can be restored by using local flaps, such as the Abbe lip-switch flap, in combination with free tissue transfer.

► **Fig. 26.15a–d:** Type II defect. Lateral mandibular resection with a through and through defect of the neck after resection of an adenocarcinoma of the submandibular gland: osteocutaneous RFFF with two skin paddles. **a** Skin paddle inset to the floor of mouth. **b** Skin paddle inset to the cervical cutaneous defect. **c** Frontal view: 18 months post-surgery. **d** Oblique view of cutaneous skin paddle: 18 months post-surgery

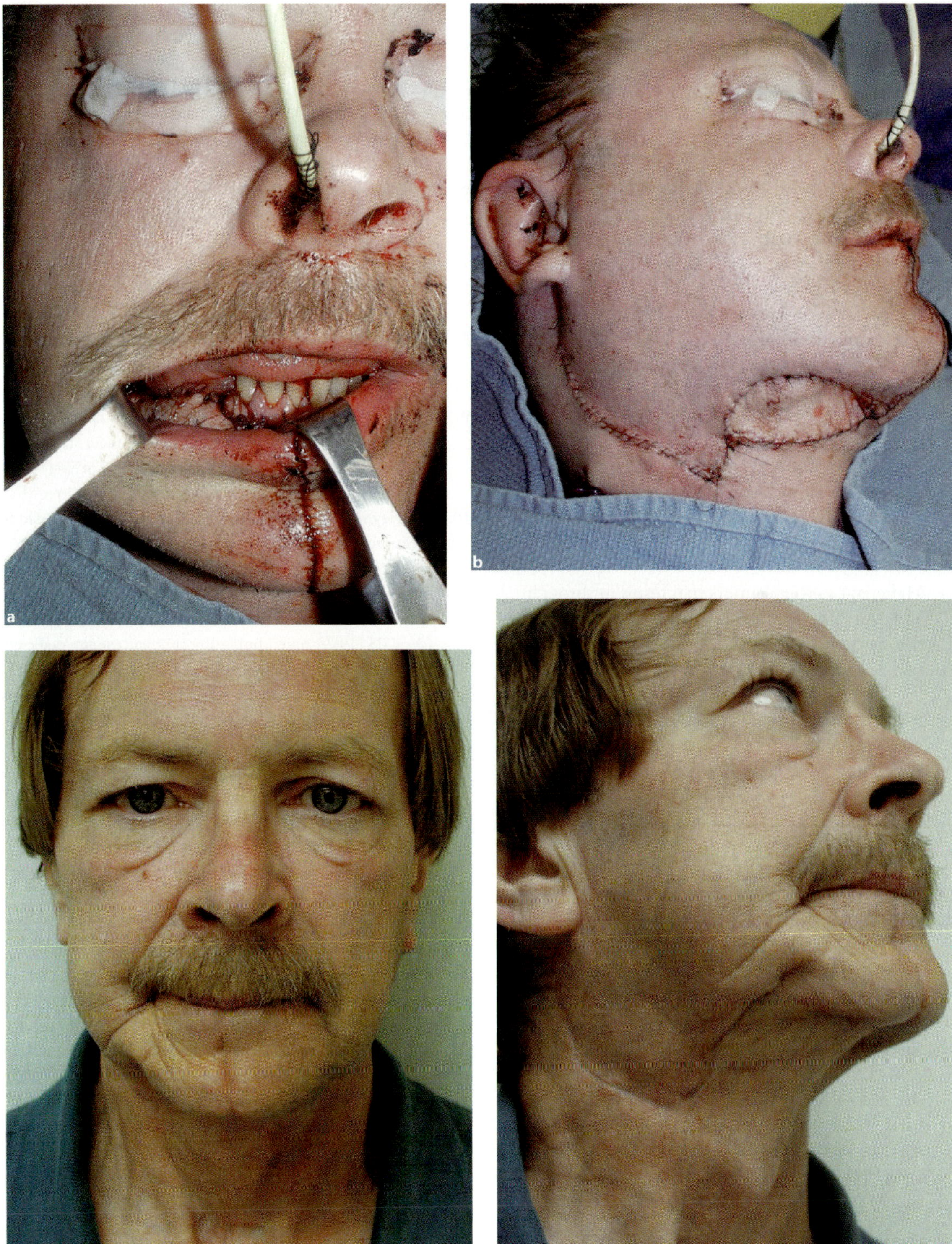
a
b
c
d

26

Take Home Messages

- Alloderm as an onlay graft is the simplest and least morbid option to potentially decrease the risk of Frey's syndrome.
- A cervicofacial or cervicodeltopectoral flap is an ideal option for cheek or neck cutaneous reconstruction after radical resection of a parotid or submandibular tumor.
- For parotidectomy defects which involve a large loss of midface volume (i.e., after resection of cheek skin, parotid, lateral mandible, and muscles of mastication), a rectus abdominis free flap can restore the missing volume.
- For a parotidectomy defect with an extensive skin resection, an anterolateral thigh flap is a reconstructive option with minimal donor site morbidity.
- Malignant salivary tumors that result in through and through mandibular defects can often be reconstructed with a single osteocutaneous free flap designed with two skin paddles.
- In addition to nerve grafting, consider placing a midface static sling and upper eyelid gold weight at the time of facial nerve resection.

References

1. Ahmad QG, Navadgi S, Agarwal R, Kanhere H, Shetty KP, Prasad R (2006) Bipaddle pectoralis major myocutaneous flap in reconstructing full thickness defects of cheek: a review of 47 cases. J Plast Reconstr Aesthet Surg 59(2):166–173
2. Baker DC, Conley J (1979) Facial nerve grafting: a thirty year retrospective review. Clin Plast Surg 6(3):343–360
3. Barton F, Spicer T, Byrd H (1983) Head and neck reconstruction with the latissimus dorsi myocutaneous flap: anatomic observations and report of 60 cases. Plast Reconstr Surg 71:199–204
4. Beckhardt RN, Weber RS, Zane R, Garden AS, Wolf P, Carrillo R, Luna MA (1995) Minor salivary gland tumors of the palate: clinical and pathologic correlates of outcome. Laryngoscope 105(11):1155–1160
5. Bell RB, Dierks EJ, Homer L, Potter BE (2005) Management and outcome of patients with malignant salivary gland tumors. J Oral Maxillofac Surg 63(7):917–928
6. Bonanno PC, Palaia D, Rosenberg M, Casson P (2000) Prophylaxis against Frey's syndrome in parotid surgery. Ann Plast Surg 44(5):498–501
7. Boyd JB, Gullane PJ, Rotstein LE, Brown DH, Irish JC (1993) Classification of mandibular defects. Plast Reconstr Surg 92(7):1266–1275
8. Brown JS, Rogers SN, McNally DN, M Boyle (2000) A modified classification for the maxillectomy defect. Head Neck 22:17–26
9. Casler JD, Conley J (1991) Sternocleidomastoid muscle transfer and superficial musculoaponeurotic plication in the prevention of Frey's syndrome. Laryngoscope 101:95–100
10. Cesteleyn L, Helman J, King S, Van de Vyvere G (2002) Temporoparietal fascia flaps and superficial musculoaponeurotic system plication in parotid surgery reduces Frey's syndrome. J Oral Maxillofac Surg 60(11):1284–1297
11. Chen HC, Demirkan F, Wei FC, Cheng SL, Cheng MH, Chen IH (1999) Free fibula osteoseptocutaneous-pedicled pectoralis major myocutaneous flap combination in reconstruction of extensive composite mandibular defects. Plast Reconstr Surg 103(3):839–845
12. Cordeiro PG, Santamaria E (2000) A classification system and algorithm for reconstruction of maxillectomy and midfacial defects plastic and reconstructive surgery. Plast Reconstr Surg 105:2331–2346
13. Cuono CB, Ariyan S (1980) Immediate reconstruction of a composite mandibular defect with a regional osteomusculocutaneous flap. Plast Reconstr Surg 65:477–483
14. De Vincentiis M, Magliulo G, Soldo P, Manciocco V, Pagliuca G, Del Gaizo R, Gallo A (2005) Extended parotidectomy Acta Otorhinolaryngol Ital 25(3):169–173
15. Deleyiannis FW, Askari M, Schmidt KL, Henkelmann TC, VanSwearingen JM, Manders EK (2005) Muscle activity in the partially paralyzed face after placement of a fascial sling: a preliminary report. Ann Plast Surg 55(5):449–455
16. Deleyiannis FW, Lee E, Gastman B, Nguyen D, Russavage J, Manders EK, Ferris RL, Myers EN, Johnson J (2006) Prognosis as a determinant of free flap utilization for reconstruction of the lateral mandibular defect. Head Neck 28:1061–1068

17. Deleyiannis FWB, Rogers C, Lee E, Russavage J, Gastman B, Dunklebarger J, Lai S, Ferris R, Myers EN, Johnson J (2006) Reconstruction of the lateral mandibulectomy defect: management based on prognosis and the location and volume of the soft tissue resection. Laryngoscope 116:2071–2080
18. Deschler DG, Hayden RE (2000) The optimum method for reconstruction of complex lateral oromandibular-cutaneous defects. Head Neck 22(7):674
19. Dulguerov P, Quinodoz D, Cosendai G, Piletta P, Marchal F, Lehman W (1999) Prevention of Frey syndrome during parotidectomy. Arch Otolaryngol Head Neck Surg 125:833–839
20. Fee WE Jr, Tran LE (2004) Functional outcome after total parotidectomy reconstruction. Laryngoscope 114(2):223–226
21. Forrest C, Boyd B, Manktelow R, Zuker R, Bowen V (1992) The free vascularised iliac crest tissue transfer: Donor site complications associated with eighty-two cases. Br J Plast Surg 45(2):89–93
22. Futran ND, Mendez E (2006) Developments in reconstruction of midface and maxilla. Lancet Oncol 7(3):249–258
23. Garden AS, Weber RS, Morrison WH, Ang KK, Peters LJ (1995) The influence of positive margins and nerve invasion in adenoid cystic carcinoma of the head and neck treated with surgery and radiation. Int J Radiat Oncol Biol Phys 15;32(3):619–626
24. Govindaraj S, Cohen M, Genden EM, Costantino PD, Urken ML (2001) The use of acellular dermis in the prevention of Frey's syndrome Laryngoscope 111:1993–1998
25. Hadlock TA, Greenfield LJ, Wernick-Robinson M, Cheney ML (2006) Multimodality approach to management of the paralyzed face. Laryngoscope 116(8):1385–1389
26. Hanna EY, Suen J (2003) Malignant tumors of the salivary glands. In: Myers EN, Suen JY, Myers JN, Hanna EN (eds) Cancer of the Head and Neck, 4th edn. Saunders, Philadelphia, pp 475–510
27. Harada T, Inoue T, Harashina T, Hatoko M, Ueda K (1993) Dermis-fat graft after parotidectomy to prevent Frey's syndrome and the concave deformity. Ann Plast Surg 31: 450–452
28. Hidalgo DA, Pusic AL (2002) Free-flap mandibular reconstruction: a 10-year follow-up study. Plast Reconstr Surg 110(2):438–449
29. Hoffman HT, Karnell LH, Robinson RA, Pinkston JA, Menck HR (1999) National Cancer Data Base report on cancer of the head and neck: acinic cell carcinoma. Head Neck 21(4):297–309
30. Honig JF (2004) Facelift approach with a hybrid SMAS rotation advancement flap in parotidectomy for prevention of scars and contour deficiency affecting the neck and sweat secretion of the cheek. J Craniofac Surg 15(5):797–803
31. Jones NF, Vogelin E, Markowitz BL, Watson JP (2003) Reconstruction of composite through-and-through mandibular defects with a double-skin paddle fibular osteocutaneous flap. Plast Reconstr Surg 112(3):758
32. Jost G, Guenon P, Gentil S (1999) Parotidectomy: a plastic approach. Aesthetic Plast Surg 23(1):1–4
33. Juri J, Juri C (1979) Advancement and rotation of a large cervicofacial flap for cheek repairs. Plast Reconstr Surg 64(5):692–696
34. Kerawala CJ, McAloney N, Stassen LF (2002) Prospective randomised trial of the benefits of a sternocleidomastoid flap after superficial parotidectomy. Br J Oral Maxillofac Surg 40(6):468–472
35. Kimata Y, Sakuraba M, Hishinuma S, Ebihara S, Hayashi R, Asakage T (2005) Free vascularized nerve grafting for immediate facial nerve reconstruction. Laryngoscope 115(2):331–336
36. Kimata Y, Uchiyama K, Ebihara S, Nakatsuka T, Harii K (1998) Anatomic variations and technical problems of the anterolateral thigh flap: a report of 74 cases. Plast Reconstr Surg 102:1517–523
37. Kroll SS, Robb GL, Miller MJ, Reese GP, Evans GR (1998) Reconstruction of posterior mandibular defects with soft tissue using the rectus abdominis free flap. Br J Plast Surg 51(7):503
38. Kuttner C, Berens A, Troger M, Keil C, Eckardt A (2001) Frey syndrome after lateral parotidectomy. Follow-up and therapeutic outlook. Mund Kiefer Gesichtschir 5(2):144–149
39. Levis C, Hynes N, Archibald S (2005) Through and through defects of the lower face. Clin Plast Surg 32(3):327–337
40. McGuirt WF, Welling B, McCabe BF (1989) Facial nerve function following irradiated cable grafts. Laryngoscope 99:27–34
41. Mehta RP, Deschler DG (2004) Mandibular reconstruction in 2004: an analysis of different techniques. Curr Opin Otolaryngol Head Neck Surg 12(4):288–293
42. Menick FJ (2001) Reconstruction of the cheek. Plast Reconstr Surg 108(2):496–505
43. Meningaud JP, Bertolus C, Bertrand JC (2006) Parotidectomy: assessment of a surgical technique including facelift incision and SMAS advancement. J Craniomaxillofac Surg 34(1):34–37
44. Moore BA, Wine T, Netterville JL (2005) Cervicofacial and cervicothoracic rotation flaps in head and neck reconstruction. Head Neck 27(12):1092–1101
45. Nouraei SA, Hope KL, Kelly CG, McLean NR, Soames JV (2005) Carcinoma ex benign pleomorphic adenoma of the parotid gland. Plast Reconstr Surg 116(5):1206–1213

46. Okay DJ, Genden E, Buchbinder D, Urken M (2001) Prosthodontic guidelines for surgical reconstruction of the maxilla: a classification system of defects. J Prosthet Dent 86: 352–363
47. Osborne RF, Tan JW, Hamilton JS, Calcaterra TC (2004) Bipedicled sternocleidomastoid muscle flap for reconstruction of tail of parotid defects. Laryngoscope 114(11):2045–2047
48. Pohar S, Gay H, Rosenbaum P, Klish D, Bogart J, Sagerman R, Hsu J, Kellman R (2005) Malignant parotid tumors: presentation, clinical/pathologic prognostic factors, and treatment outcomes. Int J Radiat Oncol Biol Phys 1;61(1):112–118
49. Poulsen MG, Pratt GR, Kynaston B, Tripcony LB (1992) Prognostic variables in malignant epithelial tumors of the parotid. Int J Radiat Oncol Biol Phys 23:327–332
50. Reddy PG, Arden RL, Mathog RH (1999) Facial nerve rehabilitation after radical parotidectomy. Laryngoscope 109(6):894–899
51. Savant DN, Patel SG, Deshmukh SP, Gujarati R, Bhathena HM, Kavarana NM (1995) Folded free radial forearm flap for reconstruction of full-thickness defects of the cheek. Head Neck 17(4):293–296
52. Sinha UK, Saadat D, Doherty CM, Rice DH (2003) Use of AlloDerm implant to prevent frey syndrome after parotidectomy. Arch Facial Plast Surg 5(1):109–112
53. Sood S, Quraishi MS, Jennings CR, Bradley PJ (1999) Frey's syndrome following parotidectomy: prevention using a rotation sternocleidomastoid muscle flap. Clin Otolaryngol 24(4):365–368
54. Terhaard CH, Lubsen H, Van der Tweel I, Hilgers FJ, Eijkenboom WM, Marres HA, Tjho-Heslinga RE, de Jong JM, Roodenburg JL; Dutch Head and Neck Oncology Cooperative Group (2004) Salivary gland carcinoma: independent prognostic factors for locoregional control, distant metastases, and overall survival: results of the Dutch head and neck oncology cooperative group. Head Neck 26(8):681–692
55. Tullio A, Marchetti C, Sesenna E, Brusati R, Cocchi R, Eusebi V (2001) Treatment of carcinoma of the parotid gland: the results of a multicenter study. J Oral Maxillofac Surg 59(3):263–270
56. Upton J, Albin RE, Mulliken JB, Murray JE (1992) The use of scapular and parascapular flaps for cheek reconstruction. Plast Reconstr Surg 90(6):959–971
57. Urken ML, Weinberg H, Vickery C, Buchbinder D, Lawson W, Biller HF (1991) The internal oblique-iliac crest free flap in composite defects of the oral cavity involving bone, skin, and mucosa. Laryngoscope 101(3):257
58. Vander Poorten VL, Balm AJ, Hilgers FJ, Tan IB, Loftus-Coll BM, Keus RB, van Leeuwen FE, Hart AA (1999) The development of a prognostic score for patients with parotid carcinoma. Cancer 1;85(9):2057–2067
59. Villaret DB, Futran NA (2003) The indications and outcomes in the use of osteocutaneous radial forearm free flap. Head Neck 25(6):475
60. Wei FC, Celik N, Chen HC, Cheng MH, Huang WC (2002) Combined anterolateral thigh flap and vascularized fibula osteoseptocutaneous flap in reconstruction of extensive composite mandibular defects. Plast Reconstr Surg 109(1):45–52
61. Wei FC, Jain V, Celik N, Chen HC, Chuang DC, Lin CH (2002) Have we found an ideal soft-tissue flap? An experience with 672 anterolateral thigh flaps. Plast Reconstr Surg 109:2219–26; discussion 2227–2230
62. Wei FC, Yazar S, Lin CH, Cheng MH, Tsao CK, Chiang YC (2005) Double free flaps in head and neck reconstruction. Clin Plast Surg 32(3):303–308
63. Wells MD, Edwards AL, Luce EA (1995) Intraoral reconstructive techniques. Clin Plast Surg 22(1):91–108

Chapter 27

Role of Radiotherapy in the Treatment of Tumors of the Salivary Glands

27

George E. Laramore

Contents

Core Features

- Discussion of the role of adjuvant radiotherapy in the treatment of salivary gland tumors
- Definitive conventional radiotherapy for the treatment of salivary gland tumors
- The unique role of neutron radiotherapy in the treatment of salivary gland tumors
- The role of radiotherapy in the treatment of pleomorphic adenomas

Complications to Avoid

- The risk of osteoradionecrosis of the mandible can be reduced with appropriate dental prophylaxis prior to starting radiotherapy.
- The risk of xerostomia can be reduced by using 3D conformal or IMRT techniques to minimize the radiation dose to contralateral salivary glands.
- The risk of normal tissue complications can be minimized by adhering to safe tolerance doses as specified in the literature.

Introduction

The primary treatment for benign and malignant tumors of the salivary gland is usually surgery with radiotherapy being used in an adjuvant setting. Radiotherapy may also be used as the definitive treatment when the patient either presents with an inoperable tumor or when the morbidity associated with a complete surgical extirpation is unacceptable. Like surgery, radiation therapy is a local/regional form of treatment and would be expected to impact survival mainly in circumstances where the tumor has not already metastasized. Local/regional treatments may also impact survival for certain already disseminated tumors where the biological aggressiveness of the metastatic disease is less than that of the primary site. An example of this is adenoid cystic carcinoma where the biological behavior of lung metastases is generally more indolent than that of the primary cancer and hence, aggressive local/regional therapy is warranted even in the setting of disseminated disease.

Tumors of the salivary glands are relatively rare compared to the more common squamous cell tumors of the head and neck and there have been few, if any, randomized trials evaluating the efficacy of adjuvant radiotherapy. Hence, current concepts of the role of radiotherapy in the management of tumors of the salivary glands have evolved over time based upon "comparative analyses" often dealing with patients treated over time spans measured in decades. This introduces a "confounding factor" relating to changes in imaging and diagnostic tumor markers which can result in "stage migration" over time. Technological advances in treatment might also be expected to improve outcomes over time. Series of patients generally include several histological varieties of tumors, a variety of stages, and a multiplicity of sites of origin. Unless there are future, multicenter clinical trials dealing with these tumors, it is unlikely that this situation will change guaranteeing that lively debates will continue at head and neck tumor boards. However, there is an emerging consensus that radiotherapy both improves local/regional control in selected adjuvant settings and is a potentially curative treatment in other settings provided that adequate doses are delivered. In this chapter we will attempt to provide a synopsis of the relevant clinical data and point out their limitations.

Tumors of the salivary glands comprise a diverse spectrum of histological types often with greatly different malignant potential and patterns of spread. For a thorough discussion of their behavior, the reader is referred to earlier chapters in this text. In this chapter when considering specific radiation therapy recommendations, we will generally use the working model of the World Health Organization [41] and group malignant tumors into two categories: (1) low grade consisting of low-grade mucoepidermoid carcinoma, the occasional low-grade adenocarcinoma, and acinic cell carcinoma, and (2) high grade consisting of high-grade mucoepidermoid carcinoma, most adenocarcinomas, carcinoma ex-pleomorphic adenoma, adenoid cystic carcinoma, malignant mixed tumors, and squamous cell carcinoma. In terms of patient survival, low-grade cancer has a more favorable outcome than high-grade cancer [44]. Local/regional forms of cancer spread can be either via direct extension, lymphatic spread, and/or perineural invasion. Different sites and histological types of cancer have varying patterns of spread and thus are treated using individually designed radiotherapy fields. Although this chapter will mainly be concerned with the treatment of malignant neoplasms, we will also include a short section on the role of radiotherapy in the treatment of benign pleomorphic adenomas.

Postoperative Radiotherapy

Often the radiation oncologist is presented with the situation in which the surgeon has operated on the primary site and has not addressed the draining neck nodes. One question to consider is when the neck nodes should be treated? There is some indication as to the risk of nodal metastases for the various histological types from the older surgical literature dealing with parotid tumors [27]. This is summarized in Tables 27.1 and 27.2, respectively, for clinically positive nodes and occult nodal disease as a function of histology. Clearly when positive nodes are found during a neck dissection, treatment of the neck is warranted in the postoperative setting. Perhaps of more interest is the information shown in Table 27.2 which shows the risk of there being occult nodal disease even in the patient with a clinically negative neck. In patients who have squamous cell carcinoma and high-grade mucoepidermoid carcinoma, prophylactic neck irradiation appears warranted whereas it does not appear warranted in patients with adenoid cystic carcinoma, acinic cell carcinoma, and malignant mixed tumors. For adenocarcinomas where the overall incidence of occult disease was about 9%, it seems reasonable to offer this treatment for high-grade cancer and not for low-grade cancer. It should be noted that much of the data in these tables are from the pre-MRI and pre-PET era and so newer imaging modalities may be more effective in identifying nodal metastases from salivary gland cancer just as they have been for the more common cancers of the head and neck of epithelial origin.

While there have been no randomized clinical trials testing the efficacy of pre- or postoperative radiotherapy, there is ample comparative data in the literature arguing for improved local/regional control for postoperative radiotherapy. A selection of such data is shown in Table 27.3. The criteria for patient selection as to who did or did not receive postoperative radiotherapy are often not well specified in the original articles nor are the criteria for follow-up and assessment of outcome. However, it is probably safe to assume that a greater percentage of patients who received postoperative radiotherapy had worrisome prognostic factors than those who did not. It also appears significant that in all of the articles except one, the local/regional control was better in the group of patients treated postoperatively. Summing all of the series together, the net local/regional control rate is 66% for the group treated with surgery alone compared to 82% for the group that also received postoperative radiotherapy. This difference, assuming comparable groups of patients,

Table 27.1. Incidence of clinically positive lymph node metastases at presentation in surgically staged patients as a function of tumor histology for parotid tumors [27]. The total number of patients in this review was 648

Histological subtype	Percent with positive nodes
High-grade mucoepidermoid	44
Adenocarcinoma	25
Adenoid cystic carcinoma	5
Malignant mixed tumor	21
Squamous cell carcinoma	37
Undifferentiated carcinoma	23
Acinic cell carcinoma	13

Table 27.2. Occult nodal disease found at time of surgery as function of tumor histology for parotid tumors [27]. The total number of patients in this review was 177

Histological subtype	Percent with positive nodes
High-grade mucoepidermoid	16
Adenocarcinoma	9
Adenoid cystic carcinoma	0
Malignant mixed tumor	0
Squamous cell carcinoma	40
Acinic cell carcinoma	6

Table 27.3. Comparative local regional control data for patients treated with surgery ± postoperative radiotherapy

	Surgery	Surgery + postoperative radiotherapy
Tran et al. [47]	36/68 (53%)	43/57 (75%)
North et al. [33]	13/23 (58%)	62/67 (92%)
Armstrong et al. [1]	30/46 (66%)	36/46 (73%)
Reddy and Marks [38]	0/12 (0%)	6/8 (75%)
Bisset and Fitzpatrick [5]	9/30 (30%)	37/54 (68%)
Molinari et al. [32]	31/36 (85%)	22/32 (68%)
Frankenthaler et al. [22]	73/91 (80%)	56/64 (88%)
Fitzpatrick and Theriault [21]	30/110 (27%)	174/239 (73%)
Shidnia et al. [42]	22/38 (58%)	21/30 (70%)
Migliancio et al. [31]	17/38 (44%)	33/43 (78%)
Fu et al. [23]	39/52 (75%)	24/29 (83%)
Borthne et al. [6]	51/96 (53%)	34/52 (66%)
Pohar et al. [35]	35/56 (63%)	81/91 (89%)
Terhard et al. [46]	85/112 (76%)	351/386 (91%)
Overall	501/770 (66%)	980/1198 (82%)

would be significant at the $P < 0.0001$ level using a two-sided Fisher exact test.

A selection of comparative survival data is similarly shown in Table 27.4. While not as compelling as the data for improved local/regional control, the summed series seem to show a small improvement in overall survival: 61% for the patients treated with surgery alone compared to 68% for the group treated with surgery and postoperative radiotherapy. Certainly this does not qualify as a meta-analysis but if one where to compare the overall data using a two-sided Fisher exact test, this difference would be significant at the $P = 0.02$ level.

Table 27.4. Comparative survival data for patients treated with surgery ± postoperative radiotherapy

	Surgery	Surgery + postoperative radiotherapy
Tran et al. [47]	49/68 (72%)	47/57 (82%)
North et al. [33]	13/23 (59%)	50/67 (75%)
Armstrong et al. [1]	25/46 (55%)	32/46 (69%)
Bisset and Fitzpatrick [5]	11/30 (37%)	28/54 (52%)
Molinari et al. [32]	30/36 (84%)	21/32 (66%)
Frankenthaler et al. [22]	67/91 (74%)	41/64 (64%)
Fitzpatrick and Theriault [21]	69/110 (63%)	174/239 (73%)
Miglinaico et al. [31]	18/38 (49%)	23/43 (54%)
Eapen et al. [17]	26/35 (76%)	14/19 (75%)
Shidnia et al. [42]	22/38 (58%)	21/30 (70%)
Pohar et al. [35]	21/56 (38%)	50/91 (55%)
Overall	351/571 (61%)	501/742 (68%)

Frankenthaler et al. [22] have analyzed the relative risk factors for local/regional control, survival, and development of distant metastases for patients with cancer of the parotid gland treated with surgery and postoperative radiotherapy. They found that presence of lymph node metastasis, primary tumor size > 3 cm, and deep lobe tumor origin were adverse factors for local/regional control; high-grade histology, presence of lymph node metastasis, primary tumor size > 3 cm, and perineural invasion were adverse factors for survival; while only high-grade histology and primary tumor size > 3 cm were adverse factors for the development of distant metastases.

Garden et al. [24] have specifically addressed the role of postoperative radiotherapy in the treatment of adenoid cystic carcinomas of the parotid. This was a retrospective study on 166 patients who were cleared of gross disease during a surgical resection. For patients with negative or "uncertain" margins the 10-year local control rate was 90%. For patients with microscopically positive margins there was evidence of a dose response with the local control rate being 88% if a radiation dose of greater than 5,600 cGy was given compared to only 40% for doses less than 5,600 cGy. Presence of positive cervical lymph nodes and failure to sacrifice the facial nerve were associated with higher risk of local failure on multivariate analysis. Subgroup analysis by delivered radiation dose showed a crude failure rate of 29% for microscopically positive margins and 60% for invasion of a major "named nerve" if less than 6,000 cGy was given. In spite of their quite good local control rate, the overall rate of distant failures was 37% as is typical for adenoid cystic carcinoma.

An issue of possible concern in considering whether to offer postoperative radiotherapy relates to the risk of damage to a facial nerve graft or to a surgically impaired nerve. Brown et al. [7] have reported retrospectively on 66 patients treated at the Mayo Clinic for parotid tumors and who had a cable nerve graft. Fourteen patients who had a tumor recurrence within a year of treatment were excluded from the analysis. Facial nerve function was scored using the House-Brackmann grading system. Twenty-eight patients received postoperative radiotherapy to a median dose of 6,000 cGy with the median time between nerve grafting and initiation of radiotherapy being 5.1 weeks and 24 patients received no postoperative radiotherapy. Median follow-up time for the entire group of patients was 10.8 years. In spite of the postoperative radiotherapy group having a greater proportion of patients with pathological evidence of perineural invasion and an "unfavorable" type of nerve graft, functional outcome was equivalent between the two groups of patients. The median time to "best" recovery of function was somewhat longer in the irradiated group (13.1 versus 10.8 months) but this was not statistically significant. The general consensus in the radiation oncology community is that while postoperative radiotherapy may delay nerve regeneration, it should not prevent it from ultimately occurring and therefore, facial nerve grafting should not be considered a relative contraindication for delivering postoperative radiotherapy.

Postoperative radiotherapy is indicated whenever: (1) the cancer is high grade (any histology except low-grade mucoepidermoid, low-grade adenocarcinoma, or acinic cell carcinoma with clear margins) regardless of the surgical margins; (2) the surgical margins are "close" or microscopically positive (which will include most deep lobe tumors where the facial nerve was not sacrificed) regardless of the grade of the lesion; (3) the resection has been performed for recurrent disease regardless of the margin status or tumor histology; (4) tumor has invaded skin, bone, nerve, or extraglandular tissue; (5) regional nodes are confirmed positive on a neck dissection; or (6) there is gross residual or unresectable disease.

For any histology except low-grade mucoepidermoid tumors, adenoid cystic carcinoma, acinic cell carcinoma, or low-grade adenocarcinoma, the clinically N0 neck is generally treated to 5,000–5,500 cGy. In the case of adenoid cystic carcinoma which has a propensity to spread along cranial nerves, the initial radiation fields must cover the courses of the cranial nerves adjacent (or traversing) the tumor to the point where they enter the base of the skull and the region treated to a dose appropriate for microscopic disease (5,000–5,400 cGy). Daily fraction size is 180–200 cGy per day. The use of chemotherapy, radiosensitizers, and hyperfractionation or accelerated fractionation schedules must be regarded as investigational at the present time.

Depending upon the radiation fields treated, the critical structures likely to be encountered are the spinal cord, optic nerves and chiasm, retina, and lens. The dose to the spinal cord should be limited to 4,500 cGy, the dose to the optic nerves, chiasm, and retina limited to 5,400 cGy, and the dose to the lens limited to 500 cGy. The major expected late effect is xerostomia relating to irradiation of the parotid glands. This will generally occur at doses between 2,500 and 3,000 cGy and is one reason why aggressive dental prophylaxis should be undertaken prior to initiating radiotherapy. Appropriate choice of radiation fields and the use of intensity modulated radiotherapy (IMRT) may allow one to exclude the contralateral parotid gland from the high radiation dose region and allow for some return of salivary function. There are mixed data on the long-term effectiveness of amifostine as an agent to help prevent xerostomia in the treatment of the more common epithelial tumors of the head and neck but there have been no specific studies using this agent in the treatment of cancer of the salivary glands. On occasion, irradiation of the vestibular apparatus of the inner ear may result in Meniere's syndrome; the radiation dose at which this may occur is not well defined but has been reported to be in the range of 6,000–7,000 cGy.

With modern radiotherapy techniques, the risk of treatment-related sequelae can be minimized. Electron beams have limited penetration and so can be used to lateralize the radiation dose and spare contralateral structures. Newer three-dimensional (3D) conformal and IMRT techniques accomplish this in a more elegant manner. Figure 27.1 shows an IMRT isodose plan for a patient treated postoperatively following resection of an intermediate-grade mucoepidermoid carcinoma of the left parotid gland. The operative bed is shown in red and the isodose lines are as indicated for a transverse cross-section through the center of the parotid bed (Fig. 27.1a) and a coronal cross-section (Fig. 27.1b). Note the lateralization of the isodose lines. Figure 27.2 shows dose volume histograms (DVHs) which are ways of representing the details of the radiation dose distributions through the tumor and selected normal tissues. The mean dose to the primary target volume is 6,515 cGy while the mean dose to the contralateral parotid gland was only 1,337 cGy. The mean mandibular dose was 2,745 cGy with about 10% of the mandible receiving more than 6,000 cGy.

Definitive Radiotherapy with Photons and/or Electrons

With the exception of the randomized trial comparing low linear energy transfer (LET) photon and/or electron radiotherapy with high LET fast neutron radiotherapy (to be discussed in the next section), there have been no programs which deliberately set out to treat a significant number of patients with cancer of the salivary glands with definitive radiotherapy. Rather, in many of the reports primarily concerned with radiotherapy as an adjuvant to surgery, there are reported results for small numbers of patients treated with radiotherapy alone. Often the criteria for this choice in therapy are not well defined but most often this treatment was given in situations where the cancer was too large and/or located such that a cancer operation was not felt to be feasible. For a small number of patients, the cancer may have been technically resectable but medical conditions made the patient a poor operative risk. Table 27.5 summarizes data for definitively treated patients over a wide range of treatment eras. Given the

27

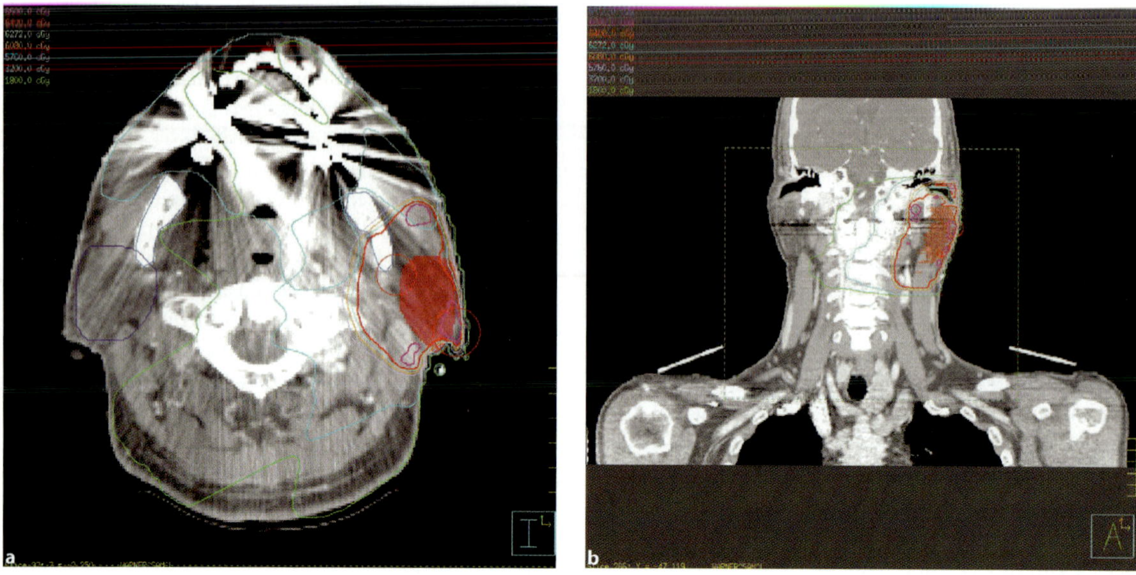

Fig. 27.1: Radiation isodose curves for a patient with a parotid tumor receiving postoperative radiotherapy. **a** Transverse cross-section through the center of the parotid bed. **b** Coronal cross-section. The primary target volume is shown in the red color wash. (Thanks to Thomas Arbuckle RT, RTT, CMD, and Patty Sponseller RT, RTT, CMD, for their help in preparing this figure)

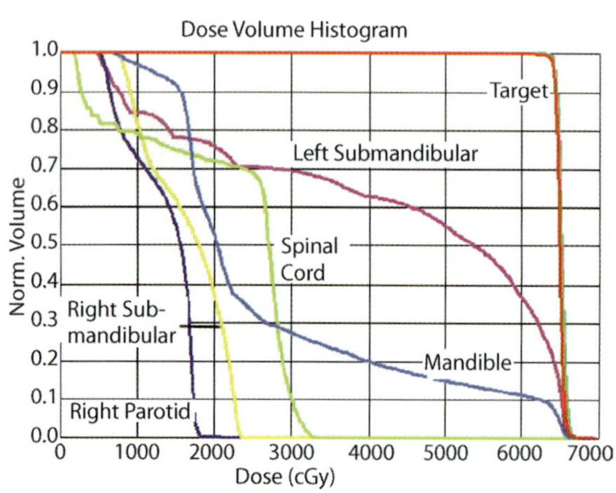

Fig. 27.2: Dose volume histograms for the isodose plan shown in Fig. 27.1. The structures for which the curves were calculated are as indicated. Note the flat curve for the target and the sharp fall off which indicates a homogeneous dose distribution and the low doses achieved for the avoidance structures. (Thanks to Thomas Arbuckle RT, RTT, CMD, and Patty Sponseller RT, RTT, CMD for their help in preparing this figure)

different patient populations, evolution of imaging, and evolution of radiotherapy equipment and techniques it is not possible to compare one series with another. Data from some of the these articles have also been used in Table 27.3 which allows one to make a crude comparison between local control rates for definitively treated patients versus surgery and postoperative radiotherapy for the same institution. The overall local control rate is 30% compared to 82% for the surgery and postoperative radiotherapy group but again it should be noted that these are not comparable patient cohorts. Except for some of the patients reported by Mendenhall et al. [30], all patients were treated using a traditional once-a-day fractionation scheme to doses in the range of 6,500–7,000 cGy. The only publication showing comparable local control rates for the two groups of patients is that of Pohar et al. [35] which shows, respectively, 89% versus 85%.

Mendenhall et al. [30] reported on a group of patients with adenoid cystic carcinomas with 61 patients being treated with surgery and adjuvant radiotherapy and 40 patients being treated with radiation alone. At the 10-year point the local control rate was 43% for the group treated with radiation alone compared to 91% for the group treated with surgery and radiotherapy. The 10-year abso-

Table 27.5. Local control rates for patients treated definitively with low LET photon and/or electron irradiation. The number of patients in each report is indicated in the second column of the table

	Local control
Fitzpatrick and Theriault [21]	6/50 (12%)
Vikram et al. [48]	2/49 (4%)
Borthne et al. [6]	8/35 (23%)
Rafla [36]	9/25 (36%)
Fu et al. [23]	6/19 (32%)
Stewart et al. [45]	9/19 (47%)
Ellis et al. [20]	5/17 (29%)
Dobrowsky et al. [15]	7/17 (41%)
Shidnia et al. [42]	6/16 (38%)
Elkon et al. [19]	2/13 (15%)
Ravasz et al. [37]	3/12 (25%)
Rossman [39]	6/11 (54%)
Mendenhall et al. [30]	22/40 (56%)
Pohar et al. [35]	11/13 (85%)
Overall	102/336 (30%)

lute survival rate was 42% for the radiation along group compared to 55% for the surgery and radiotherapy group. The authors note that the disconnect between local control and survival may be attributable to the high rate of distant metastases for this tumor type, something that has been noted as well by other investigators.

Based upon the available data, it seems preferable to offer surgery rather than standard radiotherapy as the primary treatment when a resection is possible and when the anticipated morbidity is acceptable to the patient.

Neutron Radiotherapy

Unlike high-energy photons and electrons which primarily interact with the electrons in matter, fast neutrons primarily interact with the atomic nuclei producing recoil protons and charged nuclear fragments. These heavy, charged particles create a dense ionization chain as they traverse matter and thus effectively deposit more energy along their paths than do the scattered electrons produced by standard radiotherapy. In particular, fast neutrons effectively deposit in the range of 20–100 kiloelectron volts per micron (keV/μ) whereas the electrons produced by ^{60}Co radiation deposit in the range of 0.2–2 keV/μ. This difference in LET gives rise to different radiobiological properties, a detailed discussion of which is beyond the scope of this chapter; the interested reader is referred to the text by Hall [25]. However, in general the type of radiation damage induced by high LET radiation is less readily repairable than that induced by low LET radiation and therefore certain tumors that are considered to be "radioresistant" may be more susceptible to treatment with fast neutrons. The first radiobiological evidence that fast neutrons offered a therapeutic advantage in the treatment of cancer of the salivary glands is attributed to Battermann et al. [3] who measured the relative biological effectiveness (RBE) of fast neutrons relative to ^{60}Co radiation for human tumors metastatic to lung. Using tumor growth delay as an endpoint, they found that the highest RBE gain occurred for adenoid cystic carcinomas, an RBE of 8.0 compared to 3.0–3.5 as would be expected for late effects in most tissues.

To put this in perspective, if one were to give a dose of 2,000 cGy-neutrons to a parotid tumor, the biological effect in terms of an equivalent photon dose to the temporomandibular joint and mucosa would be in the range of 6,000–7,000 cGy which is well tolerated whereas the equivalent dose to the tumor would be approximately 16,000 cGy. This is a therapeutic gain factor between 2.3 and 2.6. This information, coupled with the relatively poor results of standard radiotherapy (Table 27.5) and the relatively superficial location of cancer of the salivary glands which made them easily treatable with the low energy neutron beams produced by the early treatment facilities, made them a natural tumor system for study. Early neutron single institution data seemed to support this hypothesis. Control rates for inoperable and/or recurrent salivary gland tumors treated on the early, physics laboratory-based facilities is shown in Table 27.6. Patients treated with strictly palliative, low-dose neutron radiotherapy are not included nor are patients treated for microscopic residual disease. What is remarkable is that even with the primitive neutron facilities that were available at that time, the overall local control rate of 67% was more than twice that expected with standard radiotherapy and there is a general consistency to the data.

While intriguing, comparing the data shown in Tables 27.5 and 27.6 is not definitive in terms of the improved efficacy of fast neutron radiotherapy due to the

27

Table 27.6. Local/regional control rates for malignant salivary gland tumors treated using high LET fast neutron radiotherapy. These are early data for patients treated largely on physics laboratory-based facilities published before the RTOG/MRC randomized clinical trial. The number of patients at risk in each series is indicated in the second column

	Control rate
Saroja et al. [40]	71/113 (63%)
Catterall and Errington [9]	50/65 (77%)
Buchholz et al. [8]	40/52 (77%)
Batterman and Mijnheer [4]	21/32 (66%)
Duncan et al. [16]	12/22 (55%)
Maor et al. [29]	6/9 (67%)
Ornitz et al. [34]	3/8 (38%)
Eichhorn [18]	3/5 (60%)
Skolyszewski et al. [43]	2/3 (67%)
Overall	208/309 (67%)

uncontrolled nature of the treated patients in terms of tumor location, histologies, and spectra of follow-up times. Based upon this information in these reported series, the Radiation Therapy Group (RTOG) in the USA and the Medical Research Council (MRC) in UK launched a phase III, randomized clinical trial (80-01) to directly compared fast neutron radiotherapy with conventional photon/electron radiotherapy for patients with inoperable salivary gland tumors [28]. Patients were stratified according to surgical status (inoperable primary versus recurrent unresectable), tumor size (> 5 cm versus < 5 cm), and histology (squamous or malignant mixed versus other). An interim analysis at 2 years showed that the fast neutron group achieved significantly improved local control both at the primary site and in the lymph nodes (67% versus 17%, $P < 0.005$) and there was a trend toward improved survival (62% versus 25%, $P = 0.1$). Hence the study was closed early for ethical reasons after only 25 patients had been enrolled. The final local control and survival curves for this study are shown in Figs. 27.3 and 27.4. These continue to show a statistically-significant benefit to fast neutrons in terms of local/regional control. The suggestion of an improved survival benefit at the 2-year point can still be seen in terms of a difference

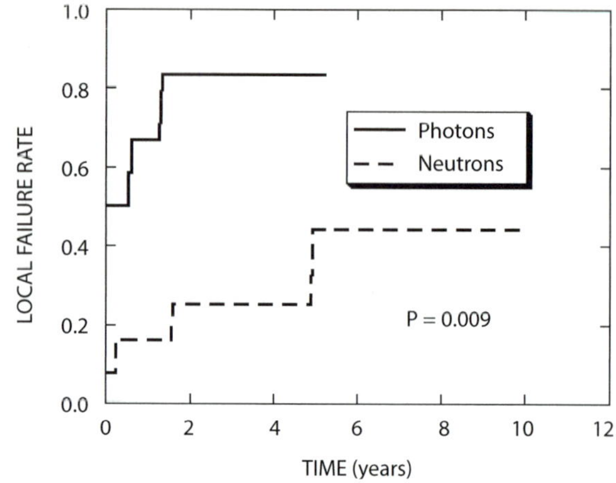

Fig. 27.3: Actuarial local/regional failure curves for patients with unresectable salivary gland tumors who were treated on the randomized clinical trial RTOG/MRC study 80–01. The neutron curve is shown as the *dashed line* and the photon curve is shown as the *solid line*. The difference between the two curves is significant at the $P = 0.009$ level. (Reprinted with permission from Laramore et al. [28])

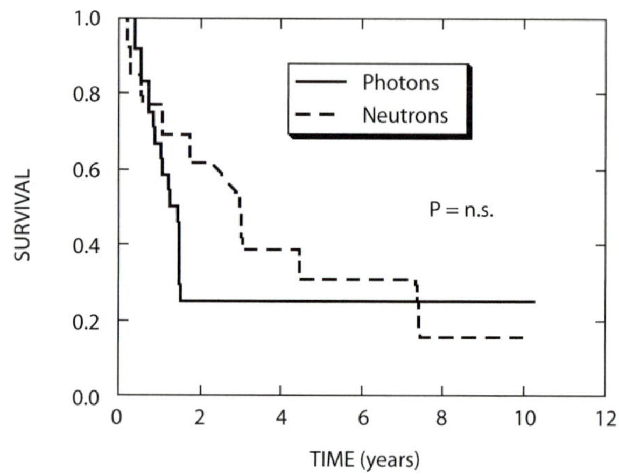

Fig. 27.4: Actuarial survival curves for patients with unresectable salivary gland tumors who were treated on the randomized clinical trial RTOG/MRC study 80–01. The neutron curve is shown as the *dashed line* and the photon curve is shown as the *solid line*. There is no significant difference between the two curves ($P = 0.5$). (Reprinted with permission from Laramore et al. [28])

in median survivals of 2.97 years vs. 1.23 years but at longer times the two curves have come together. It appears that the longer median survival allowed for a greater incidence of distant metastases on the neutron arm and patients succumbed to these distant metastases rather than to local failure. The local control rates of the two patient groups closely approximate the overall control rates for photon and neutron single institutional series shown in Tables 27.5 and 27.6, respectively. There were no fatal complications on either arm. There were two grade 4 toxicities on the neutron arm and 1 on the photon arm.

Modern neutron treatment centers have rotating isocentric gantries, sophisticated field-shaping capabilities through the use of multileaf or multirod collimators. This allows for a 3D conformal approach and has resulted in further improvement of outcome both in terms of tumor control and reduced toxicity. Figure 27.5 shows radiation isodose curves at two different levels for a patient with an adenoid cystic carcinoma of the nasopharynx and paranasal sinuses who was treated with neutron radiotherapy at the University of Washington. The radiation dose distribution is comparable to that which can be delivered with standard 3D conformal radiotherapy.

An analysis of 148 patients with major salivary gland tumors treated at the University of Washington by Douglas et al. [13] showed a local control rate at 9 years of 78% for tumors < 4 cm in size compared with approximately 40% for tumors > 4 cm. All histological types were included in this analysis. Besides size, tumor location (parotid versus submandibular/sublingual) was a factor affecting local control and survival. Results for a different group of 151 patients with adenoid cystic carcinomas of both major and minor salivary glands showed an overall 5-year local control rate of 59% and a 5-year survival rate of 72% [12]. Patients in this series had gross disease present at the time of treatment. Involvement of the base of the skull and biopsy only versus an attempted surgical resection were found to be adverse prognostic factors for both local/regional control and survival. The adverse effect of extension of the cancer through the skull base is understandable in that CNS structures are especially sensitive to high LET irradiation and hence normal tissue tolerance considerations precluded giving a full radiation dose to the most superior extent of tumor.

In an attempt to circumvent this difficulty, the University of Washington group is now advocating a stereotac-

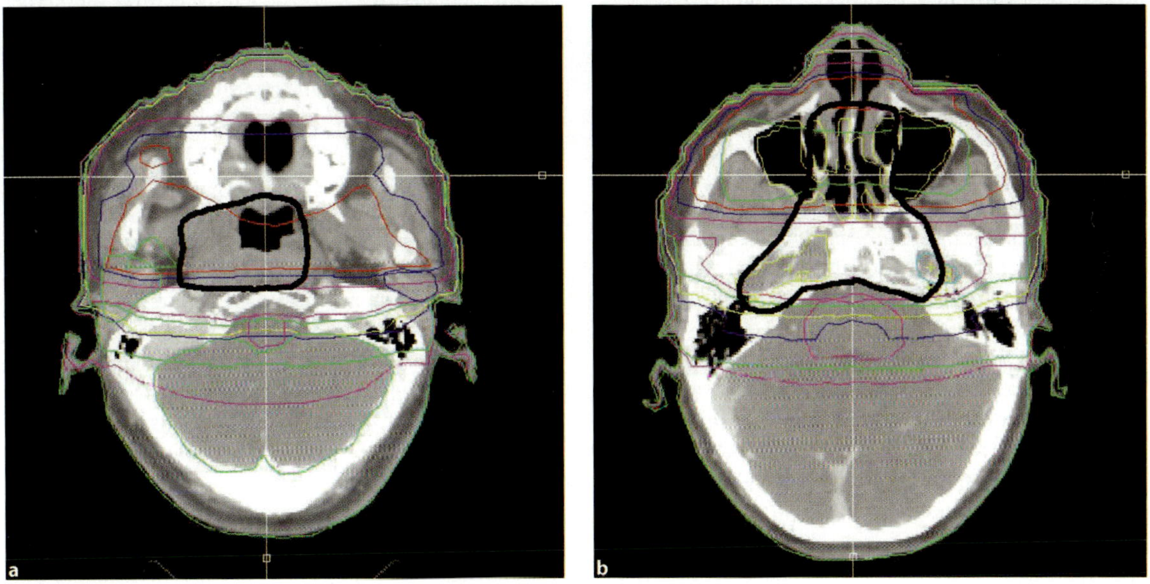

Fig. 27.5: Radiation isodose curves for a patient with an adenoid cystic carcinoma of the nasopharynx and paranasal sinuses who received neutron radiotherapy at the University of Washington. **a** Isodose lines through the nasopharynx. **b** Isodose lines along the skull base. The *heavy black lines* show the extent of gross disease in each transverse section. (Thanks to Thomas Arbuckle, RT, RTT, CMD, for his help in preparing this figure)

27

tic radiosurgery boost to cancer at the skull base following completion of neutron radiotherapy [14]. Although only 8 patients were included in this analysis to date and follow-up time is short, it appears that this procedure is safe and that there is an improved local/regional control of 80% at 2 years compared to patients with skull base disease who did not receive a stereotactic radiosurgery boost. Location of cancer in the trachea was also found to be an adverse factor for local/regional control and retrospectively this is felt due to an inadvertent underdosing of the portion of tumor protruding into the tracheal lumen where the air-tissue interface build-up region resulted in a lower surface dose. In an attempt to rectify this situation, the University of Washington group is now recommending an endotracheal brachytherapy boost to the high-risk regions following completion of neutron radiotherapy. Analysis of the outcome of this procedure is pending. Distant metastases in patients with adenoid cystic carcinoma remains a problem [12]. At the 10-year point approximately 50% of patients had developed distant metastases. It is interesting that median time to development of distant metastases was about 4 years for node-negative patients but only 0.75 years for node-positive patients. It would appear that a reliable form of systemic therapy is needed for this group of patients.

The majority of institutions using neutron radiotherapy to treat cancer of the salivary glands attempt to give as much of the dose with neutrons as possible in order to take advantage of the high RBE gain. However, to reduce the side effects associated with the low-energy neutron beams produced in the early neutron facilities, treatments were often executed using a combination of neutrons and photons (mixed beam). Huber et al. [26] reported on patients with adenoid cystic carcinoma treated at the Heidelberg facility and found a 5-year local control rate of 75% for the neutron-treated group compared to 35% for patients treated with either photons or mixed beam. It thus appears advantageous to use the more effective modality, neutrons, throughout the entire treatment provided that this can be done safely. These investigators also found that a high rate of distant metastases prevented improved local control from being translated into improved survival.

Radiotherapy for Pleomorphic Adenomas

Pleomorphic adenoma is the most common tumor arising in the parotid gland. Fortunately, they rarely infiltrate the facial nerve and so the "treatment of choice" is a nerve-sparing parotidectomy with long-term local control rates being in the range of 95%. There is a role for postoperative radiotherapy in situations where there is either spillage of the tumor or gross disease left behind. The former situation can lead to recurrences in the form of multiple nodules throughout the surgical bed which can be difficult to deal with. Recurrences can be quite late, often in the range of 10–20 years pointing to the need for long-term follow-up. Dawson and Orr [10] have reported on 311 patients with a minimum follow-up of 10 years who were treated with a local excision and postoperative radiotherapy. The majority of these patients were treated with a radium needle implant delivering 5,500–6,000 cGy to a distance of 0.5 cm over 6 days. The recurrence rate was 1% in the 0- to 5-year period, 1.5% in the 5- to 10-year period, and 4% in the 15- to 20-year period. Ten patients had a benign recurrence while four patients developed malignant tumors in the treated parotid bed. One of the malignant tumors was a soft tissue sarcoma and was most likely radiation induced, while the other three tumors were compatible with a malignant degeneration of a pleomorphic adenoma and therefore were only possibly induced by the radiotherapy. Barton et al. [2] report on 187 patients treated postoperatively with the earlier patients in the series being treated with a radium needle implant and the later patients being treated with external beam radiotherapy. One hundred and fifteen patients were treated immediately following their first surgery following an incomplete extirpation or tumor spillage and with a median follow-up of 14 years, there was only one recurrence in this group. Seventy-two patients did not have radiotherapy until one or more recurrences had been surgically treated and there were 9 recurrences in this group with 1 being malignant. There was one radiation-induced second primary occurring 25 years following the radium implant. If radiation is to be given, it is recommended that the fields be closely tailored to the parotid bed and that 6,000–6,500 cGy be given.

There may also be a role for neutron radiotherapy in the setting of very high risk patients. Douglas et al. [11] reported on a group of 16 patients treated with neutron radiotherapy after multiple recurrences. The median number of prior surgical procedures was three (range one to six) and it was felt that additional surgery entailed a high risk of facial nerve dysfunction. The median neutron dose was 1,890 cGy-neutron (range 1,700–2,200 cGy-neutron) and the median period at risk was 96 months from completing neutron radiotherapy to data analysis. At 15 years the local control rate was 100% for patients with microscopic disease versus 76% for patients with gross residual disease at the time of treatment. In terms of the pattern of recurrence, the local control rate at 15 years was 100% for patients with unifocal disease compared to 72% for patients with multinodular disease. Using the joint RTOG/EORTC scoring schema, 2 patients had grade III/IV toxicities (one had an osteoradionecrosis of the mandible and the other developed carotid artery stenosis on the treated side requiring an endarterectomy). In addition 4 patients developed some degree of hearing loss or tinnitus. No malignant tumors developed in the treated region.

Take Home Messages

- The primary treatment for malignant salivary gland tumors is usually surgery with radiotherapy being used in an adjuvant setting.
- Postoperative radiotherapy appears to reduce the risk of local/regional recurrence in many situations and may also offer a small improvement in overall survival.
- Adequate radiation doses and radiotherapy techniques are required to optimize cancer control with acceptable morbidity.
- Postoperative radiotherapy may delay return of facial nerve function but should not preclude it.
- In the patients with gross cancer, fast neutron radiotherapy appears to be more effective than standard radiotherapy and should be considered for selected patients.
- Adjuvant or definitive radiotherapy is warranted for multiply recurrent pleomorphic adenomas or in situations where there is clearly defined spillage of the tumor.

References

1. Armstrong JG, Harrison LB, Spiro RH, et al. (1990) Malignant tumors of major salivary gland origin: A matched pair analysis of the role of combined surgery and postoperative radiation therapy. Arch Otolaryngol Head Neck Surg 116: 290–293
2. Barton J, Slevin NJ, Gleave EN (1992) Radiotherapy for pleomorphic adenoma of the parotid. Int J Radiat Oncol Biol Phys 22: 925–928
3. Battermann JJ, Breur K, Hart GAM, et al. (1981) Observations on pulmonary metastases in patients after single doses and multiple fractions of fast neutrons and cobalt-60 gamma rays. Eur J Cancer 17: 539–548
4. Battermann JJ, Mijnheer BJ (1986) The Amsterdam fast neutron therapy project: A final report. Int J Radiat Oncol Biol Phys 12: 2093–2099
5. Bissett R, Fitzpatrick P (1988) Malignant submandibular gland tumors. A review of 91 patients. Am J Clin Oncol 11: 46–51
6. Borthne A, Kjellevold K, Kaalhus O, et al. (1986) Salivary gland malignant neoplasms: treatment and prognosis. Int J Radiat Oncol Biol Phys 12: 747–754
7. Brown PD, Eshleman JS, Foote RL, et al. (2000) An analysis of facial nerve function in irradiated and unirradiated facial nerve grafts. Int J Radiat Oncol Biol Phys 48: 737–743
8. Buchholz TA, Laramore GE, Griffin BR, et al. (1992) The role of fast neutron radiotherapy in the management of advanced salivary gland malignancies. Cancer 69: 2779–2788
9. Catterall M, Errington RD (1987) The implications of improved treatment of malignant salivary gland tumors by fast neutron radiotherapy. Int J Radiat Oncol Biol Phys 13: 1313–1318
10. Dawson AK, Orr JA (1985) Long-term results of local excision and radiotherapy in pleomorphic adenoma of the parotid. Int J Radiat Oncol Biol Phys 11: 452–455
11. Douglas JD, Finck J, Austin-Seymour M, et al. (2001) Neutron radiotherapy for recurrent pleomorphic adenomas of major salivary glands. Head Neck 23: 1037–1042
12. Douglas JD, Laramore GE, Austin-Seymour M, et al. (2000) Treatment of locally advanced adenoid cystic carcinoma of the head and neck with neutron radiotherapy. Int J Radiat Oncol Biol Phys 46: 551–557
13. Douglas JD, Lee S, Laramore GE, et al. (1999) Neutron radiotherapy for the treatment of locally advanced major salivary gland tumors. Head Neck 21: 255–263

14. Douglas JD, Silbergeld DL, Laramore GE (2004) Gamma knife stereotactic radiosurgical boost for patients treated primarily with neutron radiotherapy for salivary gland neoplasms. Stereotact Funct Neurosurg 82: 84–89
15. Dobrowski W, Schlappack O, Karcher KH, et al. (1986) Electron beam therapy in the treatment of of parotid neoplasm. Radiother Oncol 6: 293–299
16. Duncan W, Orr JA, Arnott SJ, et al. (1987) Neutron therapy for malignant tumors of the salivary glands. A report on the Edinburgh experience. Radiother Oncol 8: 97–104
17. Eapen LJ, Gerig LH, Catton GE, et al. (1988) Impact of local radiation in the management of salivary gland carcinomas. Head Neck Surg 10: 239–245
18. Eichhorn HJ (1981) Pilot study on the applicability of neutron radiotherapy. Radiobiol Radiother 3: 262–292
19. Elkon D, Colman J, Hendrickson FR (1978) Radiation therapy in the treatment of malignant salivary gland tumors. Cancer 41: 502–506
20. Ellis ER, Million RR, Mendenhall WM, et al. (1988) The use of radiation therapy in the management of minor salivary gland tumors. Int J Radiat Oncol Biol Phys 15: 613–617
21. Fitzpatrick PJ, Theriault C (1986) Malignant salivary gland tumors. Int J Radiat Oncol Biol Phys 12: 1743–1747
22. Frankenthaler RA, Luna MA, Lee SS, et al. (1991) Prognostic variables in parotid gland cancer. Arch Otolaryngol Head Neck Surg 117: 1251–1256
23. Fu KK, Leibel AS, Levine ML, et al. (1977) Carcinoma of the major and minor salivary glands: Analysis of treatment results and sites and causes of failures. Cancer 40: 2882–2890
24. Garden AS, El-Nagger AK, Morrison WH, et al. (1997) Postoperative radiotherapy for malignant tumors of the parotid gland. Int J Radiat Oncol Biol Phys 37: 79–85
25. Hall EJ (1992) Radiobiology for the Radiologist, 4th edn. Lippincott, Philadelphia. (See in particular Chapters 9 and 14)
26. Huber PE, Debus J, Latz D, et al. (2001) Radiotherapy for advanced adenoid cystic carcinoma: neutrons, photons, or mixed beam? Radiother Oncol 59: 161–167
27. Kaplan MJ, Johns ME (1993) Malignant neoplasms. In: Cummings CW, Frederickson JM, Harker LA, et al. (eds) Otolaryngology – Head and Neck Surgery. Mosby, St. Louis, pp 1043–1078
28. Laramore GE, Krall JM, Griffin TW, et al. (1993) Neutron versus photon irradiation for unresectable salivary gland tumors: Final report of an RTOG-MRC randomized clinical trial. Int J Radiat Oncol Biol Phys 27: 235–240
29. Maor MH, Hussey DH, Fletcher GH, et al. (1981) Fast neutron radiotherapy for locally advanced head and neck tumors. Int J Radiat Oncol Biol Phys 7: 155–163
30. Mendenhall WM, Morris CG, Amdur RJ, et al. (2003) Radiotherapy alone or combined with surgery for adenoid cystic carcinoma of the head and neck. Head Neck 26: 154–162
31. Migliancio L, Eschwege F, Marandas P, et al. (1987) Cervico-facial adenoid cystic carcinoma: Study of 102 cases. Int J Radiat Oncol Biol Phys 13: 673–678
32. Molinari R, Guzzo M, Mattavelli F, et al. (1993) Indications and efficacy of postoperative radiation therapy for salivary gland cancer. In: Johnson JT, Didolkar MS (eds) Head and Neck Cancer, Vol. III. Elsevier Press, Amsterdam, pp 607–617
33. North CA, Lee DJ, Piantadosi S, et al. (1990) Carcinoma of the major salivary glands treated by surgery or surgery plus postoperative radiotherapy. Int J Radiat Oncol Biol Phys 18:1319–1326
34. Ornitz R, Herskovic A, Bradley E, et al. (1979) Clinical observations of early and late normal tissue injury and tumor control in patients receiving fast neutron irradiation. In: Barendsen GW, Broerse J, Breur K (eds) High LET Radiations in Clinical Radiotherapy. Pergamon Press, New York, pp 43–50
35. Pohar S, Gay H, Rosenbaum P, et al. (2005) Malignant parotid tumors: Presentation, clinical/pathologic prognostic factors, and treatment outcomes. Int J Radiat Oncol Biol Phys 61: 112–118
36. Rafla S (1977) Malignant parotid tumors: natural history and treatment. Cancer 40: 136–144
37. Ravasz LA, Terhaard CHJ, Hordijk GJ, et al. (1990) Radiotherapy in epithelial tumors of the parotid gland: Case presentation and literature review. Int J Radiat Oncol Biol Phys 19: 55–59
38. Reddy SP, Marks JE (1988) Treatment of locally advanced, high-grade, malignant tumors of major salivary glands. Laryngoscope 98: 450–454
39. Rossman KJ (1975) The role of radiation therapy in the treatment of parotid carcinomas. Am J Roentgenol Radium Ther Nucl Med 123: 492–499
40. Saroja KR, Mansell J, Hendrickson FR, et al. (1987) An update on malignant salivary gland tumors treated with neutrons at Fermilab. Int J Radiat Oncol Biol Phys 13: 1319–1325
41. Seifert G, Sobin LH (1991) Histological Typing of Salivary Gland Tumours. WHO International Histological Classification of Tumours, 2nd edn. Springer, Berlin New York Heidelberg

42. Shidnia H, Hornback NB, Hamaker R, et al. (1980) Carcinoma of major salivary glands. Cancer 45:693–697
43. Skolyszewski J, Bryski E, Chrzanowska A, et al. (1982) A preliminary report on the clinical application of fast neutrons in Krakow. Int J Radiat Oncol Biol Phys 8: 1781–1786
44. Spiro RH (1998) Management of malignant tumors of the salivary glands. Oncology 12: 671–680
45. Stewart JG, Jacksopn AS, Chew MK (1968) The role of radiation therapy in the management of malignant tumors of the salivary glands. Am J Roentgenol 102: 100–108
46. Terhard CHJ, Lubsen H, Rasch CRN, et al. (2005) The role of radiotherapy in the treatment of malignant salivary gland tumors. Int J Radiat Oncol Biol Phys 61: 103–111
47. Tran L, Sadeghi A, Hanson D, et al. (1986) Major salivary gland tumors: Treatment results and prognostic factors. Laryngoscope 96: 1139–1144
48. Vikram B, Strong EW, Shah JP, et al. (1984) Radiation therapy in adenoid cystic carcinomas. Int J Radiat Oncol Biol Phys 10: 221–223

Chapter 28

Chemotherapy in the Management of Malignant Tumors of Salivary Gland Origin

28

Scott A. Laurie and Athanassios Argiris

Contents

Core Features

- There are insufficient data to support the routine use of adjuvant or neoadjuvant chemotherapy.
- Chemotherapy should be reserved for the palliation of disease-related symptoms and for patients at risk of developing such symptoms due to rapid progression of locally recurrent or metastatic disease.
- In patients with indolent disease and without symptoms, watchful waiting is acceptable, and may be the preferred approach.
- The different histological subtypes of malignant tumors of salivary gland origin may have differing responsiveness to chemotherapeutic agents.
- The published literature on the role of systemic therapy in malignancies of the salivary glands is inadequate and limits the generation of evidence-based recommendations.
- All patients should be considered for participation in clinical trials to help define the role of systemic therapies in these tumors.
- As the understanding of the underlying molecular abnormalities of these tumors grows, there will be opportunities for the development and testing of novel, targeted agents.

Complications to Avoid

- Ensure a definitive histological diagnosis
- Weigh the potential benefits of symptom improvement against the potential risks and toxicities of therapy
- Consider measures other than chemotherapy to control symptoms
- There appears to be little likelihood of benefit of additional chemotherapy in those patients who have received first-line treatment
- Avoid empiric use of targeted agents outside a clinical trial, given their unproven benefit, potential toxicities, and cost
- Avoid assuming disease stabilization is an indication of effectiveness of therapy

Introduction

Malignant tumors originating in the salivary glands are diverse and are classified into over twenty recognized histological subtypes [10]. These rare tumors vary widely in their molecular phenotypes, biological behavior, and responsiveness to chemotherapy. The vast majority of patients for whom systemic therapy is usually considered will have either adenoid cystic carcinoma (ACC), mucoepidermoid carcinoma (MEC), or adenocarcinoma, as these are the most common histologies and are the ones which, along with salivary ductal carcinoma (SDC), have the greatest tendency to recur and/or metastasize. Accordingly, most of the data regarding the role of chemotherapy in advanced salivary gland cancers relates to these subtypes.

At the present time, chemotherapy is reserved for the palliation of patients with metastatic disease or with locoregional recurrence that is not amenable to further surgery and/or radiation. There is no established role for chemotherapy in the adjuvant or neoadjuvant setting. This chapter will provide a review of the evidence for the role of classic cytotoxic chemotherapy in the treatment of salivary gland cancer, as well as an overview of the potential of newer agents that target specific molecular abnormalities which may be of relevance in these malignancies (Fig. 28.1, Fig. 28.2).

Histological and Molecular Characteristics of Malignant Tumors of Salivary Gland Origin

Cancers of the salivary glands can be divided into those believed to arise from the intercalated ducts (such as ACC and adenocarcinoma) and those believed to originate from the secretory ducts (which include MEC and SDC). A higher tumor grade appears to correlate with more aggressive behavior in MEC and adenocarcinoma not otherwise specified [36, 67, 78], but the relevance of grade to other subtypes, such as ACC, is unclear [64, 79, 94].

As agents targeting the molecular abnormalities present in other, more common, malignancies have shown promise, there has been an interest in evaluating salivary gland cancers for the presence of these targets. Table 28.1 lists the molecular abnormalities that have been described in salivary gland malignancies, along with agents targeting these abnormalities that have been studied in these cancers (Fig. 28.2). Possible explanations for the wide variation in reported rates of expression of the various targets between studies of the same histological subtype include small numbers, different methodologies, use of archival tissue and problems with antigen retrieval, and intrinsic biological variability.

Given the histological similarities between certain salivary malignancies, in particular SDC, and carcinoma of the breast, and given the observation that ACC may occasionally arise in the breast, many investigators have evaluated salivary gland cancers for the presence of hormonal receptors. In general, the majority of salivary gland cancers are negative for androgen, estrogen, and progesterone receptors. Positivity is seen in less than 10% cases of ACC [19, 21, 44, 56, 62, 63, 65, 73] and of MEC [44, 63, 65], and usually the staining is weak. SDC, while usually not expressing estrogen or progesterone receptors [9, 40, 49, 63, 93], commonly strongly expresses androgen receptors [28, 63, 65]. There are reports of expression of hormonal receptors in other histological subtypes of salivary gland cancers [56, 65], but the number of cases in the literature is too small to determine the true frequency of positivity. Although there are anecdotal reports of the use of antiandrogen therapies in SDC and adenocarcinomas, no prospective clinical studies with antiandrogens have been performed (see section on Adenocarcinoma).

The epidermal growth factor receptor (EGFR), a transmembrane receptor involved in signal transduction, is commonly overexpressed and/or constitutively activated

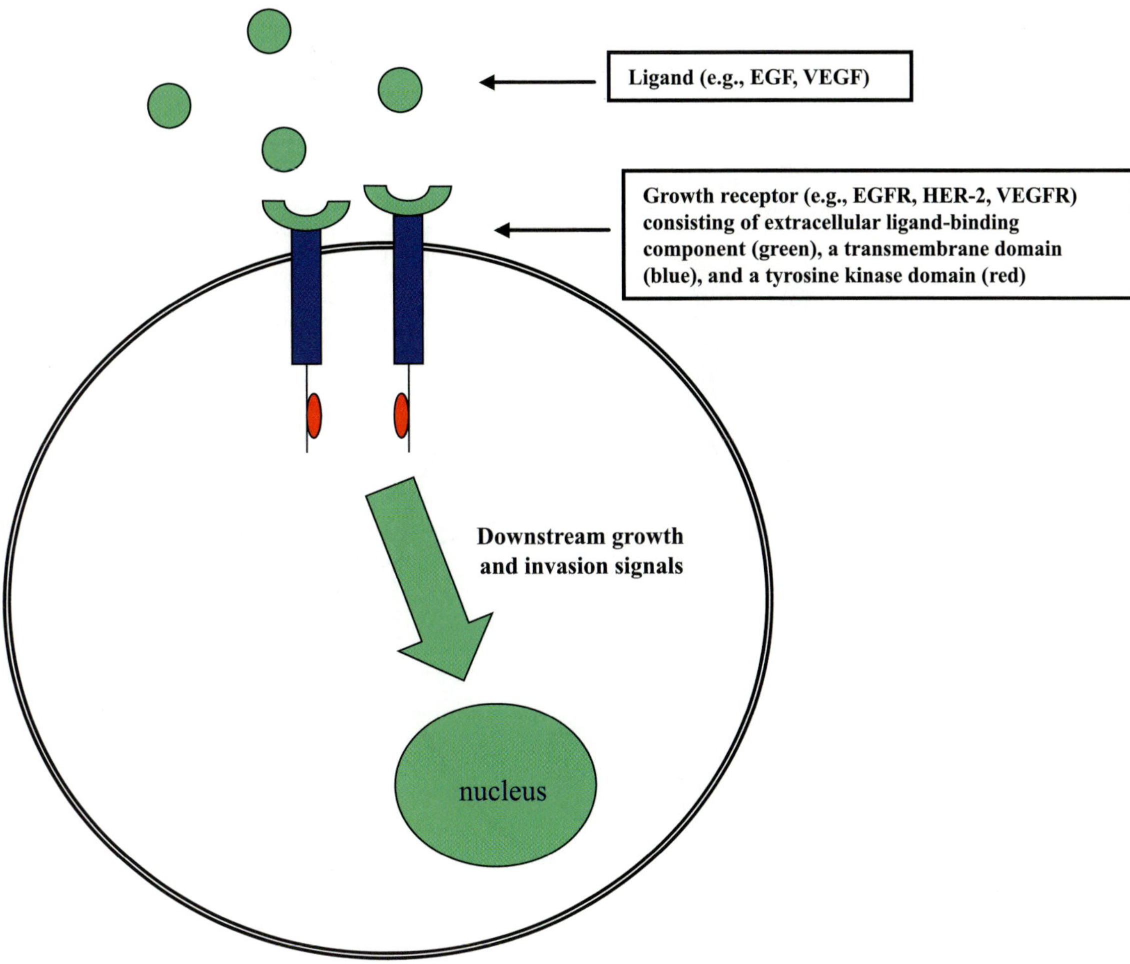

Fig. 28.1: Schematic drawing of a transmembrane growth receptor, which has an extracellular ligand-binding domain, a transmembrane domain, and an intracellular tyrosine kinase domain. When bound by its ligand, a receptor dimerizes with another of the same receptor (homodimerization) or another member of the same receptor family (heterodimerization), leading to phosphorylation of the tyrosine kinase domain, which in turn activates downstream members of the signal transduction pathway, ultimately leading to growth and survival signals delivered to the cells nucleus

in a number of malignancies, and has been associated with aggressive malignant behavior. Agents which inhibit this receptor, both monoclonal antibodies that compete for ligand binding at the extracellular domain and small molecule inhibitors of the intracellular tyrosine kinase domain, have shown benefit in the treatment of a variety of cancers, including non-small cell lung cancer [72] and squamous cell carcinoma of the head and neck [12, 13]. Expression of EGFR is common (> 50% frequency) in both MEC [32, 47] and SDC [29, 56], but less common in ACC [32, 47, 56, 74].

HER-2, another member of the EGFR family of receptors, is also expressed or overexpressed in a variety of malignancies. Although having no known natural ligand,

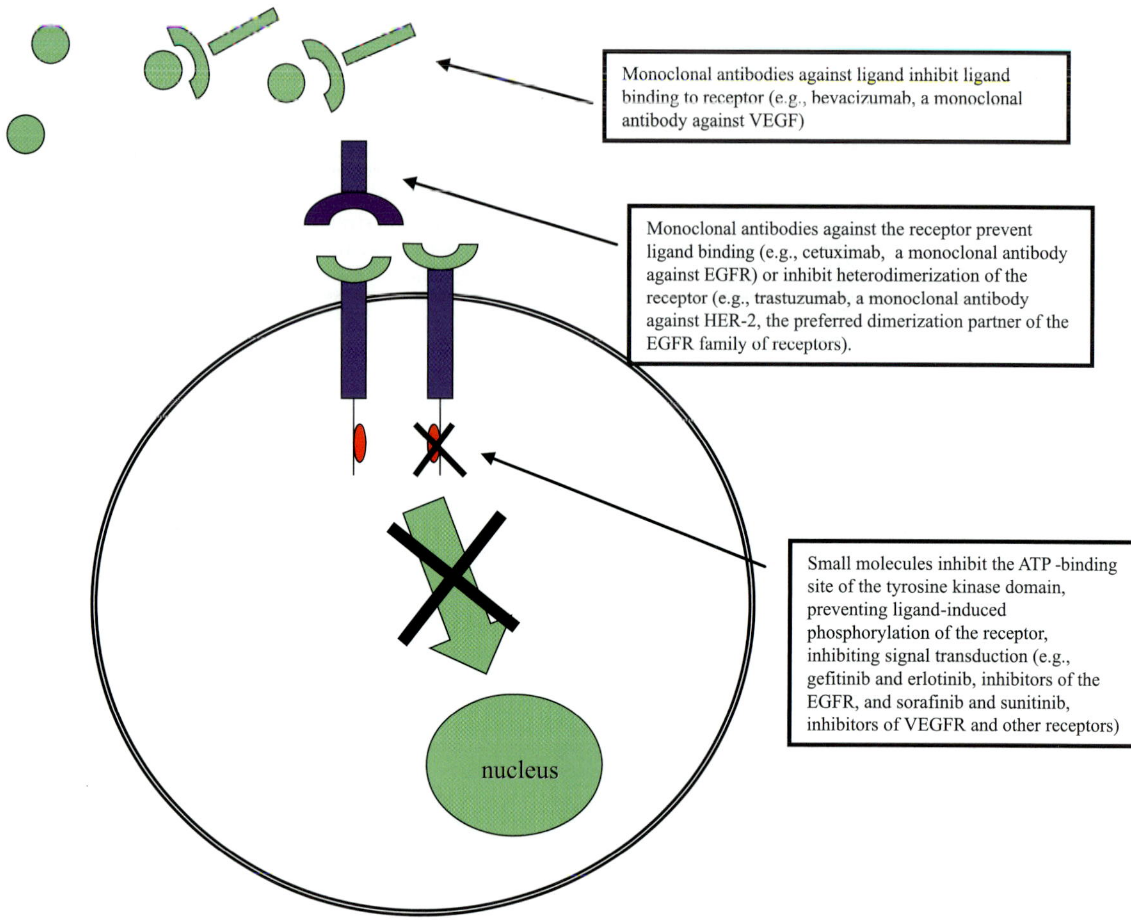

Fig. 28.2: Schematic drawing of mechanisms of action of targeted therapies that have been studied in salivary gland cancers

the receptor may undergo heterodimerization with other members of the EGFR family of receptors, including EGFR, and in this way is involved in signal transduction. Trastuzumab, a monoclonal antibody targeting the HER-2 receptor, is effective in breast cancer that overexpresses HER-2 [75]. Overexpression of HER-2 is more likely in cancers of excretory duct origin. It is commonly observed in SDC [25, 34, 40] and occasionally seen in MEC [32, 34, 67], with some suggestion that overexpression may be negatively prognostic in these subtypes [31, 67]. Overexpression is rare in tumors originating in the intercalated ducts, including ACC [34, 56].

The c-kit proto-oncogene encodes a transmembrane cell surface receptor (KIT) that is related to platelet-derived growth factor receptor [57]. When bound by its ligand, stem cell factor, KIT is involved in transduction of signals which regulate cell growth and development. Activating mutations of c-kit have been described in gastrointestinal stromal tumors (GIST), and imatinib, a small molecule inhibitor of KIT, has demonstrated significant activity in this malignancy [18]. KIT is commonly expressed or overexpressed in ACC [7, 23, 42, 45, 56], but gain-of-function mutations have not been detected [42, 45]. KIT protein expression is rare in other histological subtypes, including MEC [7, 45], with the exception of polymorphous low-grade adenocarcinoma [7, 23], a tumor with a very low risk of recurrence and metastasis.

Table 28.1. Potential molecular targets and agents for salivary gland cancers

Molecular target			Agents	
Name	Postulated function	Rates of expression in salivary cancers	Name	Mechanism of action
c-kit	Signal transduction	ACC: common Other histologies: rare	Imatinib	TKI
EGFR	Signal transduction; promotes growth, survival	MEC and SDC: common Other histologies: rare	Gefitinib Lapatinib Cetuximab	TKI TKI MoAb
HER-2	Dimerizes with other EGFR members for signal transduction	SDC: common Other histologies: rare	Trastuzumab Lapatanib	MoAb TKI
VEGF	Angiogenesis, increases vascular permeability	ACC: overexpression common Other histologies: no data	Bevacizumab	MoAb
VEGF receptor	Transduces signals from VEGF	No data	Sunitinib Sorafenib	TKI TKI
Proteasome	Diverse effects due to inhibition of protein degradation	No data	Bortezomib	Proteasome inhibition

VEGF vascular endothelial growth factor, *EGFR* epidermal growth factor receptor, *TKI* tyrosine kinase inhibitor, *MoAb* monoclonal antibody, *ACC* adenoid cystic carcinoma, *MEC* mucoepidermoid carcinoma, *SDC* salivary ductal carcinoma

As the molecular understanding of salivary cancers grows, the number of potential targets and therapies increases. For example, it has recently been reported that MEC often displays the specific chromosomal rearrangement t(11;19), that results in a fusion gene product [24, 84]. This fusion product is felt to mediate tumorigenicity by altering NOTCH signaling pathways and aberrantly activating cyclic-AMP-responsive element binding protein (CREB) signaling pathways [14]; inhibitors of this fusion product may be a future target in MEC. In ACC, both microvessel density, a measure of tumor angiogenesis, and tumor levels of vascular endothelial growth factor (VEGF) [54, 96] and nuclear factor κB (NF-κB) [96], potent pro angiogenic factors, have been shown to be prognostic of survival. Inhibitors of angiogenesis may therefore have a role in the treatment of salivary gland cancers. Other described molecular abnormalities include occasional mutations in H-ras in MEC [95], as well as altered expression of members of the retinoblastoma gene family [26, 68].

Overview of the Evidence for the Role of Systemic Therapies

Due to the rarity of these tumors, there is little published literature on the role of chemotherapy in their management. The greatest amount of data is available for ACC, for which there are clinical trials specific to this histological subtype. However, a review of all reports of chemotherapy in advanced ACC spanning over 20 years revealed less than 300 patients [48]. There are no trials in the literature specific to any of the other histological types.

Many reports include case series and/or retrospective reviews of institutional experience with heterogeneous treatments, rather than prospectively performed clinical trials [48]. Published case reports are inherently biased toward positive results (i.e., responses to treatment), leading to a likely overestimation of the benefit of a therapy. Objective response criteria in many reports are poorly defined. Many studies report rates of stabilization of disease, but do not state whether clear evidence of disease progression was a criterion for study entry. Disease stabilization may reflect only the variable biology of these often indolent tumors, rather than efficacy of therapy. Moreover, most studies are small and have included patients who are often heterogeneous with respect to histology, the number and type of prior therapies, and the proportion of patients with only locoregionally recurrent disease without distant metastasis. Often, the results of therapy are not reported separately for the different histological subtypes. Additionally, there have been revisions of the classification of salivary gland cancers [10, 70], leading to difficulties in determining which histological subtype is being described in older trials; this is especially relevant to adenocarcinoma and its variants. All of these issues hinder the ability to interpret the results and to compare across trials. Finally, the methodological quality of trials is often suboptimal [48], and there is some suggestion that clinical trials of poorer methodological quality may be more likely to produce positive results than those of more rigorous design [58]. Both the evidence for the role of any treatment and the true effectiveness of that treatment need to be interpreted bearing in mind these limitations.

Systemic Therapy for Metastatic or Unresectable Locoregionally Recurrent Disease

The majority of patients referred for consideration of palliative chemotherapy will have one of three histological types: ACC, MEC, or high-grade adenocarcinoma. Aggregate response rates of these histological types to different chemotherapeutic agents and regimens from patients in the published literature are summarized in Tables 28.2 (single agents) and 28.3 (combination regimens), and for novel agents targeting molecular abnormalities in Table 28.4.

The natural history of recurrent or metastatic cancer of the salivary glands can be highly variable, and many patients will have indolent disease with few or no symptoms. For example, the median survival following the development of metastatic ACC is 3 years [59, 61, 80, 88], and 10% will live for more than 10 years from the development of metastases [80, 83]. Patients with lung metastases only from ACC have a longer survival than those with other sites of disease [81, 88]. Others, however, will have a more rapidly progressive course, with one third dying within 2 years [61, 80, 83].

As there are no data as to whether chemotherapy alters the natural history of these cancers or prolongs survival, the goal of therapy is the palliation of disease-related symptoms. Consideration should be given to local measures (either surgery or radiation) for patients with single sites of symptomatic metastases. Asymptomatic patients at risk for the development of symptoms due to rapid disease progression, or due to the presence of metastases that are threatening important organ function, could be considered for chemotherapy. Attempts should be made to review prior radiological imaging for a retrospective assessment of rate of disease progression. For those without symptoms and slowly progressive, indolent disease, watchful waiting is an appropriate recommendation. Finally, the participation of patients with salivary gland malignancies in clinical trials should be strongly encouraged.

Adenoid Cystic Carcinoma

Standard cytotoxics that have been studied as single agents in adequate numbers of patients with ACC are mitoxantrone, vinorelbine, epirubicin, paclitaxel, and cisplatin; the studies of cisplatin, vinorelbine, and paclitaxel also enrolled patients with other histological subtypes. Mitoxantrone has been studied in a total of 54 patients with ACC in two studies [60, 92]. The European Organization for the Research and Treatment of Cancer (EORTC) group conducted a trial that enrolled 36 chemotherapy-naïve patients with symptomatic and/or progressive ACC not suitable for surgery or radiotherapy. Mitoxantrone was administered at a dose of 14 mg/m^2 every 3 weeks [92]. Toxicity was generally mild. There were four partial responses (objective response rate 12%, 95% confidence interval (CI) 4–29%) with a response duration of 3–13 months; an additional 22 patients (69%) had stabilization of disease for a median of 7.6 months (range 2.5–30.5 months). Less activity was seen in a second study that used a somewhat lower dose of mitoxantrone of 12 mg/m^2 in a cohort of 18 patients, the majority of whom had previously received chemotherapy [60]. Only one major objective response was seen (response rate 6%) in a patient who had not previously received cytotoxic chemotherapy. Twelve of 18 patients had stable disease for a median of 6 months, but it is not stated whether evidence of progression of disease was required for study entry, and so the contribution of the therapy to this disease stabilization is unclear.

Table 28.2. Single-agent cytotoxics in patients with advanced salivary gland cancers (selected studies)

Reference	Agent	Dose/schedule	Response data by histology					
			ACC		MEC		Adenocarcinoma	
			Total number of patients	Number of patients responding/(ORR)	Total number of patients	Number of patients responding/(ORR)	Total number of patients	Number of patients responding/(ORR)
Vermorken (1993) [91]	Epirubicin	30 mg/m²/week 90 mg/m²/q3w	20	2 (20%)	–	–	–	–
Verweij (1996) [92]	Mitoxantrone	14 mg/m²/q3w	32	4 (12%)	–	–	–	–
Mattox (1990) [60]	Mitoxantrone	12 mg/m²/q3w	18	1 (6%)	–	–	–	–
Gilbert (2006) [33]	Paclitaxel	200 mg/m²/q3w	14	0 (0%)	14	3 (21%)	17	5 (29%)
Airoldi (2001) [4]	Vinorelbine	30 mg/m²/week	13	2 (15%)	–	–	9	2 (22%)
Licitra (1991) [50]	Cisplatin[a]	100 mg/m²/q3w	13	2 (15%)	5	1 (20%)	5	0 (0%)
De Haan (1992) [17]	Cisplatin[b]	50–120 mg/m²/q4w	10	0 (0%)	–	–	–	–
Schramm (1981) [69]	Cisplatin[b]	80–100 mg/m²/q4-6w	10	7 (70%)	–	–	–	–

ACC adenoid cystic carcinoma, *MEC* mucoepidermoid carcinoma, *ORR* objective response rate
[a]Prospective phase II clinical trial
[b]Data from a retrospective case series

Table 28.3. Combination cytotoxic regimens in patients with advanced salivary gland cancers (selected studies)

References	Regimen	Doses/ schedule	Response data by histology					
			ACC		MEC		Adenocarcinoma	
			Total number of patients	Number of patients responding/ (ORR)	Total number of patients	Number of patients responding/ (ORR)	Total number of patients	Number of patients responding/ (ORR)
Licitra (1996) [52] Creagan (1988)[a] [15]	Cyclophos-phamide	400–500 mg/m²/q3-5w	36	9 (25%)	11	5 (45%)	24	14 (58%)
Dreyfuss (1987) [22] Belani (1988)[a] [11]	Doxorubicin	40-50 mg/ m²/q3-5w						
Alberts (1981) [5]	Cisplatin (CAP regimen)	40-60 mg/ m²/q3-5w						
Venook (1987) [89] Airoldi (1989) [2] Tsukuda (1993) [86] Dimery (1990) [20]	Anthracycline Cisplatin ± 5-fluorouracil	Various	23	10 (43%)	3	2 (67%)	19	8 (42%)
Creagan (1993)[a] [16] Hill (1997) [41] Airoldi (2001) [4] Posner (1982)[a] [66]	Cisplatin-based, no anthracycline	Various	25	5 (20%)	3	2 (67%)	11	5 (45%)

ACC adenoid cystic carcinoma, *MEC* mucoepidermoid carcinoma, *ORR* objective response rate
[a]Data from a retrospective case series

Table 28.4. Phase II trials with novel molecular targeted agents in salivary gland malignancies

Reference	Agent	Molecular target	Number of evaluable patients enrolled			Efficacy		
			Total	ACC	Others	PR	SD	Comments
Haddad (2003) [37]	Trastuzumab	HER-2	14	2	12	1 (MEC)	2 (SDC)	
Glisson (2005) [35]	Gefitinib	EGFR	28	19	9	0	10/19 ACC	In ACC: 5/19 had stable disease for > 6 months
Hotte (2005) [43]	Imatinib	c-kit	15	15	0	0	9/15	Six-month PFS 12.5%; median PFS 2.3 months
Slevin (2004) [76]	Imatinib	c-kit	12	12	0	0	10/12	One PR with the addition of cisplatin at cycle 3
Agulnik (2006) [1]	Lapatinib	EGFR and HER-2	39	20	19	0	15/20 ACC 9/19 other	7/20 (35%) of ACC patients had SD ≥ 6 months; in ACC, median PFS 3.5 months[a]
Licitra (2006) [53]	Cetuximab	EGFR	30	23	7	0	20/23 ACC	9/20 (45%) of patients ACC had SD ≥ 6 months; 6-month PFS 43%[a]
Argiris (2006) [8]	Bortezomib	Proteasome	25	25	0	0	17/25	Six-month PFS 67%; median PFS 8.4 months

ACC adenoid cystic carcinoma, *MEC* mucoepidermoid carcinoma, *SDC* salivary duct carcinoma, *PR* partial response, *SD* stable disease, *EGFR* epidermal growth factor receptor, *PFS* progression-free survival

[a]Time to progression reported in the abstract

The EORTC has also performed a phase II trial of epirubicin in 20 eligible patients with advanced or recurrent ACC [91]. Only three patients had received prior chemotherapy. Epirubicin was administered at a starting dose of 30 mg/m^2 per week; non-responders were switched to a dose of 90 mg/m^2 or higher given once every 3 weeks. Overall, treatment was well tolerated, with no evidence of clinical cardiotoxicity in any patient. There were two objective responses (ORR 10%, 95% CI 4.5–35.5%), but several patients without an objective response had improvement in disease-related symptoms. No data on disease stabilization were reported.

The activity of cisplatin in ACC has been reported in three manuscripts, including a prospective phase II trial in which all patients received 100 mg/m^2 every 3 weeks [50], and two retrospective case series of patients treated at doses ranging from 50 to 120 mg/m^2 every 3–6 weeks [17, 69]. Two objective responses were observed in 13 patients in the prospective trial, lasting 5 and 8 months, respectively; several other patients had disease stabilization, however, disease progression was not a requirement for treatment on study. Responses were reported in 7 of 10 patients in one case series [69], and in none of 10 in the second [17]. This highlights the risk of relying on retrospective series in attempting to determine the true activity of an agent. Minimal toxicity data are presented in these manuscripts, however, cisplatin is known to be associated with significant nausea, neurotoxicity, ototoxicity, and renal toxicity.

The Eastern Cooperative Oncology Group (ECOG) conducted a phase II trial in which paclitaxel, administered at 200 mg/m^2 over 3 h every 3 weeks, was given to patients with advanced, chemotherapy-naïve salivary gland cancers [33]. No objective responses were observed in the 14 patients with ACC that were enrolled, while 7 patients had stable disease as their best response. Despite the lack of responses, the 5-year survival for these patients was 32%, and the median survival 25 months. However, disease progression was not a requirement for enrollment and no details are available on subsequent therapies, and so the exact contribution of paclitaxel to these results is unclear.

Single-agent vinorelbine, administered at 30 mg/m^2 weekly, was assessed in 14 patients with progressive ACC as part of a randomized phase II trial (discussed in greater detail below) [4]. Treatment was well tolerated, with no significant toxicities seen. Two patients, both previously treated with chemotherapy, had an objective response (ORR 15%, 95% CI 4.7–43%). Moreover, symptom relief was observed even in the absence of an objective response.

In a brief report of a prospective phase II trial, single-agent gemcitabine did not lead to any responses in 16 patients with salivary gland cancers, of which 8 had ACC [37]. Retrospective reviews and/or single case reports have suggested that both 5-fluorouracil and doxorubicin, given as monotherapy, have induced responses in patients with metastatic ACC [46, 82, 90]. However, there are no prospective data of the effectiveness of these agents, and the true rate of efficacy cannot be determined.

Taken together, these data suggest that some antitumor activity and symptom palliation are seen with single agents, including mitoxantrone, vinorelbine, and epirubicin in previously untreated patients. There are no data showing that patients previously treated with chemotherapy derive any benefit from further chemotherapy.

A number of studies have reported results with combination chemotherapy regimens in ACC. The most commonly studied combination regimens include cisplatin and/or anthracycline; the combination of cisplatin and doxorubicin has been examined in seven reported trials, together with cyclophosphamide (the "CAP" regimen) [11, 15, 22, 52], 5-fluorouracil [89], both [20], or bleomycin [17]. The dose and schedule of administration of the CAP regimen varied between studies (see Table 28.3). The aggregate response rate for CAP in these studies was 9 of 36 patients (ORR 25%, 95% CI 11–39%). Expected toxicities for cisplatin and doxorubicin were common and occasionally severe. There are no data on the role of this (or any) combination regimen in previously treated patients. Other regimens containing cisplatin and an anthracycline other than doxorubicin have also reported objective responses, but these trials have enrolled 6 or fewer patients with ACC [2, 86].

As both single-agent vinorelbine and cisplatin may have activity in salivary gland malignancies, the combination of cisplatin (80 mg/m^2 day 1) and vinorelbine (25mg/m^2 days 1 and 8, both recycled every 3 weeks) was compared with single-agent vinorelbine in a randomized phase II trial that enrolled 36 patients with salivary gland malignancies (22 with ACC), the majority of which had not received any prior chemotherapy [4]. Documentation of progressive disease was a requirement for study entry. Toxicity, in particular nausea/vomiting and myelosuppression, was more frequent in the combination arm. In patients with ACC, vinorelbine resulted in a 15%

response rate (2/13) versus 44% (4/9) for cisplatin plus vinorelbine. No previously treated patient responded. Relief of symptoms was reported, even in some patients who did not have objective tumor shrinkage.

Antitumor activity in ACC has been observed with other, but not all, platinum-based, non-anthracycline-containing regimens tested in small numbers of patients [3, 30, 41]. Overall, the response rate for cisplatin-based combination regimens in published reports is approximately 25%, with a very wide range of reported response durations. However, due to small sample sizes, the reported response rates to any agent or combination regimen have wide, overlapping confidence intervals. Therefore, there is no conclusive evidence that combination therapy is superior to single-agent therapy. The likelihood of additional toxicities of a cisplatin-based regimen, over a single agent, also needs to be considered when choosing a therapy. If combination therapy is chosen, the greatest amount of data exists for a CAP regimen.

Targeted agents, including gefitinib [35], trastuzumab [38], imatinib [43, 76], lapatinib [1], cetuximab [53], and bortezomib [8], have been studied in prospective clinical trials in patients with ACC (see Table 28.4). Many patients enrolled in these trials had been previously treated with cytotoxic chemotherapy. Two clinical studies evaluated imatinib, an agent that targets KIT which is frequently expressed in ACC [43, 76]. Nevertheless, no objective responses were observed in a total of 27 patients who received imatinib alone [43, 76]. There are, however, case reports of patients with ACC responding to doses of this agent similar to those used in the above-mentioned studies [6, 27]. Possible explanations for these disparate findings include the degree of overexpression of KIT and the proliferative rate of the tumors of the enrolled patients [27]; additional study of this agent in selected patients appears warranted, but its routine use outside of a clinical trial is not supported by the data at this time.

No objective responses have been observed with agents targeting EGFR or HER-2 [1, 35, 38, 53]. Overexpression of HER-2 is extremely unusual in ACC [34], suggesting that this is unlikely to be a relevant target in this histological type.

Bortezomib, a selective inhibitor of the 26S proteasome which is central for the ubiquitin-proteasome degradation pathway, was investigated in a phase II clinical trial that has reported preliminary results [8]. Twenty-five patients with advanced, incurable ACC who had evidence of disease progression within the previous 9 months and had received any number of prior therapies were treated with bortezomib 1.3 mg/m^2 intravenously on days 1, 4, 8, and 11 every 21 days until disease progression, at which time doxorubicin at 20 mg/m^2 given intravenously on days 1 and 8 was added to the bortezomib. There were no objective responses to single-agent bortezomib, but 17 patients (68%) had stabilization of disease with a median duration of 8.2 months. The progression-free survival (PFS) at 6 months was 67% and the median PFS was 8.4 months. Preliminary data showed that one of 4 evaluable patients had a partial response with the addition of doxorubicin. Overall, bortezomib therapy was well tolerated with rare occurrence of serious neuropathy and fatigue.

Although recent phase II trials with a number of novel agents including gefitinib [35], trastuzumab [38], imatinib [43, 76], lapatinib [1], cetuximab [53], and bortezomib [8] in salivary gland malignancies, predominantly ACC, reported no objective response rates, the rate of stable disease generally exceeded 50%. For example, Hotte et al. reported that 60% (9/15) of patients with ACC treated with imatinib had stable disease as best response [43]; Glisson et al. reported that 53% (10/19) patients with adenoid cystic carcinoma treated with gefitinib had stable disease which was maintained for 16 weeks or more in 26% (5/19) [35]; and Argiris et al. observed that 68% (17/25) of patients with ACC treated with bortezomib had stable disease [8]. Moreover, the median PFS of 8.4 months with single-agent bortezomib was encouraging. It is possible that PFS is a more meaningful endpoint than the objective response rate for the evaluation of novel, non-cytotoxic agents in ACC. However, whether prolonged stable disease represents a true drug effect or a manifestation of the natural history of an indolent malignancy is difficult to discern. A randomized study of a novel agent versus no therapy has yet to be performed in patients with cancer of the salivary gland.

In conclusion, there are no data to support the routine use of any targeted agent outside of a clinical trial. Too few patients have been studied, and much of the data has been presented only in abstract form. The trials suffer from many of the concerns discussed above that limit their evaluation. Nevertheless, the evaluation of novel agents should continue in patients with incurable ACC. Indeed, a number of clinical trials are ongoing or planned. For example, the ECOG has proposed a phase II trial of sorafenib, an inhibitor of multiple kinases, including VEGFR, in incurable ACC.

28

Mucoepidermoid Carcinoma

Although not explicitly stated in published reports, most patients with MEC likely have high-grade lesions, as these are much more likely to recur and/or metastasize [36, 77]. There are no trials specific to this histological type, and there are less than 50 patients in the literature for which the outcome of treatment in those with MEC is reported separately [11, 20, 33, 38, 46, 51, 66, 89]; only one trial has enrolled more than 5 patients with this histology.

The largest reported experience of patients treated with the same chemotherapy regimen is from a phase II study with single-agent paclitaxel 200 mg/m^2 administered over 3 h every 21 days, conducted by the ECOG [33]. In a total of 14 patients with MEC, 3 patients (21%) had objective responses, and 4 additional patients had stable disease. Most other patients have received cisplatin-based combination chemotherapies, either in conjunction with an anthracycline [11, 15, 20, 52, 89] or bleomycin and methotrexate [16, 66], and objective responses have been reported. However, the regimens used are variable, many are case reports not prospective clinical trials, and so the true response rate cannot be determined. Of five patients with MEC enrolled to a trial of single-agent cisplatin, only one patient had an objective response [50]. Based on the above data, if single-agent therapy is chosen, paclitaxel is a reasonable choice.

There have been only two and three reported patients treated with the targeted agents gefitinib [35] and trastuzumab [34, 38], respectively. One patient with a tumor strongly overexpressing HER-2 had a durable partial response to trastuzumab. No responses were seen with gefitinib. Clearly there are insufficient data regarding the role of these agents in MEC, and further study is required. An ongoing phase II study by the Southwest Oncology Cooperative Group examines the role of trastuzumab in high-grade, non-ACC salivary gland cancers (including MEC and adenocarcinoma) that overexpress HER-2 by immunohistochemistry and/or gene amplification as assessed by fluorescence in situ hybridization.

Adenocarcinoma

It is likely that most reported cases of adenocarcinoma are high-grade lesions not otherwise specified, as these are most likely to recur and metastasize. Other lesions classified as subtypes of adenocarcinoma (such as basal cell carcinoma or polymorphous low-grade adenocarcinoma) are exceedingly rare and/or highly unlikely to metastasize. In a phase II study with single-agent paclitaxel that included other histological subtypes of salivary gland malignancies and was also discussed in previous sections [33], 5 objective responses were observed in 17 enrolled patients with adenocarcinoma (29%). Vinorelbine, administered as a single-agent, led to two responses in five patients [4]; while reportedly well tolerated, further study of this agent is needed given the small number of patients. Cisplatin-anthracycline-based combination regimens have also been utilized, in particular CAP, with a number of objective responses reported. This is similar to the situation for MEC, discussed above, and the same caveats apply: small numbers of patients treated with heterogeneous regimens preclude a true estimate of the effectiveness of therapy. Outside of a clinical trial, both single-agent paclitaxel and cisplatin-anthracycline combination chemotherapy are acceptable options, with the choice determined by the patient's medical and functional status and acceptance of potential toxicities.

With respect to targeted agents, it has been noted that these cancers often express the androgen receptor [56, 65]. While there are no prospective clinical trials of anti-androgens, there have been two case reports of significant objective responses to androgen-deprivation therapy [55, 87], indicating that this is worthy of further study. Overexpression of HER-2 is uncommon in these tumors [34, 56], and no patient (of three enrolled) with adenocarcinoma responded to trastuzumab in a small phase II trial [38]; as mentioned above, there is an ongoing phase II trial of this agent in HER-2-overexpressing salivary gland cancers. It is reported that two patients treated with gefitinib had stabilization of their disease [35], but as the information is only in abstract form to date, details regarding duration of stabilization and whether the disease was progressing prior to initiation of study therapy, are not available.

Other Histological Types

Reports of outcomes with chemotherapy in other histological types are scarce, relating to both their rarity and, for most subtypes, the infrequency of recurrence. In addition, several of these subtypes are variants of adenocarcinoma, and are not separated out from this histology. These reports include poorly differentiated carcinoma

(12 patients), acinic cell carcinoma (7 patients), malignant myoepithelioma (3 patients), malignant mixed tumor/carcinoma ex-pleomorphic adenoma (13 patients), and salivary duct carcinoma (2 patients) [2, 3, 5, 46, 50, 52, 66]. As cyclophosphamide-doxorubicin-cisplatin is the regimen most commonly studied in salivary gland cancers, most reports of objective responses in these histological types have been obtained with this combination, and in the absence of a clinical trial, it would be reasonable to offer this regimen to suitable patients.

As salivary duct carcinoma commonly overexpresses both EGFR and HER-2, studies of agents targeting these receptors should be considered. To date there are only three patients enrolled in a trial of gefitinib and all had progression of disease as their best response [35], while two patients treated with trastuzumab had stabilization of disease for 24 and 40 weeks [34]. There are no reports of the use of any other targeted agents in this histological type.

Neoadjuvant and Adjuvant Systemic Therapy

There are very few data regarding the role of chemotherapy given before or after definitive local therapy, either surgery or radiation, in the management of salivary gland malignancies. There are case reports of patients with bulky, unresectable tumors who responded to chemotherapy and subsequently underwent a complete surgical resection. Regimens to which such responses have been reported in case reports include cyclophosphamide and doxorubicin [66], cyclophosphamide, doxorubicin, cisplatin [11, 22], and intra-arterial cisplatin [71]. There is only one reported prospective trial of neoadjuvant chemotherapy in patients with locally advanced salivary gland cancer [89]. This study enrolled patients with bulky tumors that were felt to be technically difficult to resect, and administered a regimen of cisplatin-doxorubicin-5-fluorouracil. Of nine patients, there were three with ACC, three with adenocarcinoma, two with MEC, and one with a poorly differentiated carcinoma. Objective responses were observed only in those with adenocarcinoma histology, although several of the other patients received only one cycle of therapy. Surgery was performed in eight of nine patients, with two patients having incomplete resections; the remaining patient received radiotherapy. With relatively short follow-up, ranging from 2 to 26 months, all but two patients had recurrent disease. The authors themselves caution that it is unclear if the chemotherapy impacted on the course of the disease.

Similarly, there is only one reported trial in which adjuvant chemotherapy was administered to patients with ACC [85]. Subjects were eligible if they had no clinical evidence of disease following postoperative radiotherapy for an incomplete resection of either a first presentation or a locoregional recurrence. Fourteen patients were enrolled; 11 had tumors that originated in the minor salivary glands. Six cycles of chemotherapy consisting of 5-fluorouracil, cyclophosphamide, and vincristine were administered. While chemotherapy was reported to be well tolerated, when these 14 patients were compared to 15 matched historical controls from the same institution who did not receive adjuvant chemotherapy, no difference in the median time to recurrence was observed. Given the lack of evidence, and the uncertainty regarding the benefit of systemic therapy in the setting of metastatic cancer, patients with localized disease who undergo definitive therapy of their primary site should not receive adjuvant chemotherapy. Due to the rarity of these cancers, their protracted natural course, and the intrinsic variability in their natural history, it would be very difficult to conduct a trial to determine if adjuvant chemotherapy improved survival in these patients.

In resectable patients, clinical trials of neoadjuvant therapy, particularly newer, targeted agents, would offer a valuable opportunity to perform translational studies on the surgical specimen following exposure to the investigational agent. Paired, pre- and post-treatment biopsy samples would then be available, as many patients would have a diagnostic biopsy. Enrolling patients with earlier stage, resectable disease would also increase the number of potential subjects for study, and therefore help to identify active agents for use in the palliation of patients with advanced disease. Routine administration of chemotherapy to patients with resectable disease outside the setting of a clinical trial is not recommended.

Concurrent Chemoradiation

Radiotherapy as primary treatment for localized salivary gland malignancies is usually reserved for those patients with locally advanced, unresectable disease. As such, there is a significant selection bias and as one would expect these patients to do worse, with higher rates of locoregional recurrence. As concurrent chemotherapy and radiation has become a standard primary or postoperative treatment for squamous cell carcinomas of the head and neck, there is a potential interest in applying similar principles in the management of salivary gland malignancies. Postoperative chemoradiotherapy for high-risk patients is sometimes employed in clinical practice but without supporting literature, whereas the role of concurrent chemotherapy and radiation as primary therapy for locally advanced cancer of the salivary gland has not been studied prospectively. A case series of five patients with advanced, unresectable ACC treated with radiation with concurrent weekly paclitaxel and carboplatin has been reported [39]. Four patients had extension into the base of the skull from a primary cancer in the paranasal sinus. All patients have had a radiographic response to therapy, and no patient has had a local failure, with a median duration of follow-up of 36 months. These data, while encouraging, require confirmation in future studies. A prospective clinical trial of chemoradiation in patients with locally advanced, unresectable ACC is warranted.

Conclusions and Future Directions

Chemotherapy has a potential role in the palliation of symptomatic patients with advanced locoregionally recurrent and/or metastatic disease that is not amenable to local therapies. At present the greatest amount of experience is with cisplatin or anthracycline-based combination regimens, especially in ACC, which result in objective responses in up to one third of patients. However, single-agent therapy is an acceptable option for those patients who cannot tolerate or who wish to avoid the potential toxicities associated with cisplatin-based regimens. To date, there are insufficient data to support the routine use of any molecularly targeted agent. For patients with asymptomatic, indolent disease, watchful waiting is the preferred approach, with the option of chemotherapy reserved until symptoms are imminent due to progression. Adjuvant or neoadjuvant chemotherapy is not recommended outside of a prospective clinical trial.

The lack of high-quality data regarding the role of systemic therapy in the management of cancer of the salivary gland emphasizes the importance of conducting clinical trials in these rare tumors. The different histological subtypes of salivary gland malignancies need to be considered and studied separately, as there is evidence that responsiveness to therapies, biology, and underlying molecular abnormalities differ considerably. Studies of neoadjuvant therapy, particularly in the more aggressive histological subtypes, should be considered, and this will require the close collaboration between surgical and medical oncologists. It is encouraging that in recent years there have been a number of reports of multi-institutional clinical trials of novel agents in the treatment of cancer of the salivary glands, demonstrating that there is the ability and interest to study this disease.

Take Home Messages

- Watchful waiting is an appropriate recommendation for some patients; reserve chemotherapy for palliation of those patients with progressive, symptomatic disease for whom local therapy is not an option.
- Single-agent therapy is a reasonable option for patients who wish to minimize potential toxicities, as combination regimens are not clearly superior in terms of response rates; the choice of single agent will vary with the histological subtype.
- If combination therapy is chosen, the greatest amount of data exists for the regimen of cisplatin-doxorubicin-cyclophosphamide.
- There are no data to support the use of systemic therapy in previously treated patients.
- Enrollment in prospective clinical trials should be considered for all patients with cancer of the salivary glands, including those patients with resectable, early-stage disease.

References

1. Agulnik M, Cohen EE, Cohen RB, et al: A phase II study of lapatinib in recurrent or metastatic EGFR and/or ErbB2 expressing adenoid cystic (ACC) and non-ACC malignant tumors of the salivary glands (MSGT). J Clin Oncol 24:296s (abstract 5566), 2006

2. Airoldi M, Pedani F, Brando V, et al: Cisplatin, epirubicin and 5-fluorouracil combination chemotherapy for recurrent carcinoma of the salivary gland. Tumori 75:252–256, 1989
3. Airoldi M, Fornari G, Fedani F, et al: Paclitaxel and carboplatin for recurrent salivary gland malignancies. Anticancer Res 20:3781–3784, 2000
4. Airoldi M, Pedani F, Succo G, et al: Phase II randomized trial comparing vinorelbine versus vinorelbine plus cisplatin in patients with recurrent salivary gland malignancies. Cancer 91:541–547, 2001
5. Alberts DS, Manning MR, Coulthard SW, et al: Adriamycin/cis-Platinum/Cyclophosphamide combination chemotherapy for advanced carcinoma of the parotid gland. Cancer 47:645–648, 1981
6. Alcedo JC, Fabrega JM, Arosemena JR, et al: Imatinib mesylate as treatment for adenoid cystic carcinoma of the salivary glands: report of two successfully treated cases. Head Neck 26:829–831, 2004
7. Andreadis D, Epivatianos A, Poulopoulos A, et al: Detection of c-kit (CD117) molecule in benign and malignant salivary gland tumours. Oral Oncol 42:57–65, 2006
8. Argiris A, Goldwasser MA, Burtness B, et al: Phase II trial of PS-341 (bortezomib) followed by the addition of doxorubicin at progression in incurable adenoid cystic carcinoma of the head and neck: an Eastern Cooperative Oncology Group study. J Clin Oncol 24:298s (abstract 5573), 2006
9. Barnes L, Rao U, Contis L, et al: Salivary duct carcinoma. Part II. Immunohistochemical evaluation of 13 cases for estrogen and progesterone receptors, cathepsin D, and c-erbB-2 protein. Oral Surg Oral Med Oral Pathol 78:74–80, 1994
10. Barnes L, Everson JW, Reichart P, et al: World Health Organization classification of tumours. Pathology and genetics of head and neck tumours. Lyon, IARC Press, 2005
11. Belani CP, Eisenberger MA, Gray WC: Preliminary experience with chemotherapy in advanced salivary gland neoplasms. Med Pediatr Oncol 16:197–202, 1988
12. Bonner JA, Harari PM, Giralt J, et al: Radiotherapy plus cetuximab for squamous-cell carcinoma of the head and neck. N Engl J Med 354:567–578, 2006
13. Cohen EE, Kane MA, List MA, et al: Phase II trial of gefitinib 250 mg daily in patients with recurrent and / or metastatic squamous cell carcinoma of the head and neck. Clin Cancer Res 11:8418–8424, 2005
14. Coxon AB, Rozenblum E, Park Y-S, et al: Mect1-Maml2 fusion oncogene linked to the aberrant activation of cyclic AMP/CREB regulated genes. Cancer Res 65:7134–7144, 2005
15. Creagan ET, Woods JE, Rubin J, et al: Cisplatin-based chemotherapy for neoplasms arising from salivary glands and contiguous structures in the head and neck. Cancer 62:2313–2319, 1988
16. Creagan ET, Schutt AJ, Richardson RL, et al: Phase II trial of VP-16, bleomycin, and cisplatin in patients with advanced non-squamous cell head and neck neoplasms. Am J Clin Oncol 16:291–294, 1993
17. de Haan LD, de Mulder PHM, Vermorken JB, et al: Cisplatin-based chemotherapy in advanced adenoid cystic carcinoma of the head and neck. Head Neck 14:273–277, 1992
18. Demetri GD, von Mehren M, Blanke CD: Efficacy and safety of imatinib mesylate in advanced gastrointestinal stromal tumors. N Engl J Med 347:472–480, 2002
19. Dimery IW, Jones LA, Verjan RP, et al: Estrogen receptors in normal salivary gland and salivary gland carcinoma. Arch Otolaryngol Head Neck Surg 113:1082–1085, 1987
20. Dimery IW, Legha SS, Shirinian M, et al: Fluorouracil, doxorubicin, cycolphosphamide, and cisplatin combination chemotherapy in advanced or recurrent salivary gland carcinoma. J Clin Oncol 8:1056–1062, 1990
21. Dori S, Trougouboff P, David R, et al: Immunohistochemical evaluation of estrogen and progesterone receptors in adenoid cystic carcinoma of salivary gland origin. Oral Oncol 36:450–453, 2000
22. Dreyfuss AI, Clark JR, Fallon BG, et al: Cyclophosphamide, doxorubicin, and cisplatin combination chemotherapy for advanced carcinomas of salivary gland origin. Cancer 60:2869–2872, 1987
23. Edwards PC, Bhuiya T, Kelsch RD: C-kit expression in the salivary gland neoplasms adenoid cystic carcinoma, polymorphous low-grade adenocarcinoma, and monomorphic adenoma. Oral Surg Oral Med Oral Pathol 95:586–593, 2003
24. Enlund F, Behboudi A, Andren Y, et al: Altered Notch signaling resulting from expression of a WAMTP1-MAML2 gene fusion in mucoepidermoid carcinomas and benign Warthin's tumors. Exp Cell Res 292:21–28, 2004
25. Etges A, Pinto DS, Kowalski LP, et al: Salivary duct carcinoma: immunohistochemical profile of an aggressive salivary gland tumour. J Clin Pathol 56:914–918, 2003
26. Etges A, Nunes FD, Ribeiro KC, et al: Immunohistochemical expression of retinoblastoma pathway proteins in normal salivary glands and in salivary gland tumours. Oral Oncol 40:326–331, 2004
27. Faivre S, Raymond E, Casiraghi O, et al: Imatinib mesylate can induce objective response in progressing, highly expressing KIT adenoid cystic carcinoma of the salivary glands. J Clin Oncol 23:6271–6273, 2005

28. Fan CY, Wang J, Barnes EL: Expression of androgen receptor and prostatic specific markers in salivary duct carcinoma: an immunohistochemical analysis of 13 cases and review of the literature. Am J Surg Pathol 24:579–586, 2000
29. Fan CY, Melhem MF, Hosal AS, et al: Expression of androgen receptor, epidermal growth factor receptor, and transforming growth factor alpha in salivary duct carcinoma. Arch Otolaryngol Head Neck Surg 127:1075–1079, 2001
30. Gedlicka C, Schull B, Formanek M, et al: Mitoxantrone and cisplatin in recurrent and/or metastatic salivary gland malignancies. Anticancer Drugs 13:491–495, 2002
31. Giannoni C, El-Naggar AK, Ordonez NG, et al: c-erbB-2/neu Oncogene and Ki-67 analysis in the assessment of palatal salivary gland neoplasms. Otolaryngol Head Neck Surg 112:391–398, 1995
32. Gibbons MD, Manne U, Carroll WR, et al: Molecular differences in mucoepidermoid carcinoma and adenoid cystic carcinoma of the major salivary glands. Laryngoscope 111:1373–1378, 2001
33. Gilbert J, Li Y, Pinto HA, et al: Phase II trial of Taxol in salivary gland malignancies (E1394): a trial of the Eastern Cooperative Oncology Group. Head Neck 28:197–204, 2006
34. Glisson B, Colevas AD, Haddad R, et al: HER2 expression in salivary gland carcinomas: dependence on histologic subtype. Clin Cancer Res 10:944–946, 2004
35. Glisson B, Blumenschein G, Francisco M, et al: Phase II trial of gefitinib in patients with incurable salivary gland cancer. J Clin Oncol 23, 2005
36. Goode RK, Auclair PL, Ellis GL: Mucoepidermoid carcinoma of the major salivary glands. Clinical and histopathological analysis of 234 cases with evaluation of grading criteria. Cancer 82:1217–1224, 1998
37. Haddad R, Posner MR: Palliative chemotherapy in patients with salivary gland neoplasms and preliminary reports of 2 recent phase II studies with trastuzumab and gemcitabine. Clin Adv Hematol Oncol 1:226–228, 2003
38. Haddad R, Colevas AD, Krane JF, et al: Herceptin in patients with advanced or metastatic salivary gland carcinomas. A phase II study. Oral Oncol 39:724–727, 2003
39. Haddad R, Posner MR, Busse PM, et al: Chemoradiotherapy for adenoid cystic carcinoma. Am J Clin Oncol 29:153–157, 2006
40. Hellquist HB, Karlsson MG, Nilsson C: Salivary duct carcinoma – a highly aggressive salivary gland tumour with overexpression of c-erb-B2. J Pathol 172:35–44, 1994
41. Hill ME, Constenla DO, A'Hern RP, et al: Cisplatin and 5-fluorouracil for symptom control in advanced salivary adenoid cystic carcinoma. Oral Oncol 33:275–278, 1997
42. Holst VA, Marshall CE, Moskaluk CA, et al: KIT protein expression and analysis of c-kit gene mutation in adenoid cystic carcinoma. Mod Pathol 12:956–960, 1999
43. Hotte S, Winquist E, Lamont E, et al: Imatinib mesylate in patients with adenoid cystic cancers of the salivary glands expressing c-kit: a Princess Margaret Hospital phase II consortium study. J Clin Oncol 20:585–590, 2005
44. Jeannon J-P, Soames JV, Bell H, et al: Immunohistochemical detection of oestrogen and progesterone receptors in salivary tumours. Clin Otolaryngol 24:52–54, 1999
45. Jeng Y-M, Lin C-Y, Hsu H-C: Expression of the c-kit protein is associated with certain subtypes of salivary gland carcinoma. Cancer Lett 154:107–111, 2000
46. Kaplan MJ, Johns ME, Cantrell RW: Chemotherapy for salivary gland cancer. Otolaryngol Head Neck Surg 95:165–170, 1986
47. Katopodi E, Patsouris E, Papanikolaou V, et al: Immunohistochemical detection of epidermal growth factor and its receptor in salivary gland carcinomas. Oral Surg Oral Med Oral Pathol 95:266–268, 2003
48. Laurie SA, Su YB, Pfister DG: Chemotherapy in the management of metastatic adenoid cystic carcinoma: a systematic review. J Clin Oncol 2005 ASCO Annual Meeting Proceedings 23:5581, 2005
49. Lewis JE, McKinney BC, Weiland LH, et al: Salivary duct carcinoma: clinicopathological and immunohistochemical review of 26 cases. Cancer 77:223–230, 1996
50. Licitra L, Marchini S, Spinazze S, et al: Cisplatin in advanced salivary gland carcinoma. Cancer 68:1874–1877, 1991
51. Licitra L, Bonafonte V, Spinazze S, et al: Cyclophosphamide, doxorubicin, and cisplatin (CAP) for advanced salivary gland carcinomas. Proc Ann Meet Am Soc Clin Oncol 10:204, 1991
52. Licitra L, Cavina R, Grandi C, et al: Cisplatin, doxorubicin and cyclophosphamide in advanced salivary gland carcinoma. Ann Oncol 7:640–642, 1996
53. Licitra L, Locati LD, Potepan P, et al: Cetuximab (C225) in recurrent and/or metastatic salivary gland caricnomas (RMSGCs): a monoinstitutional phase II study. J Clin Oncol 24 (18S):291s (abstract 5547), 2006
54. Lim JJ, Kang S, Lee MR, et al: Expression of vascular endothelial growth factor in salivary gland carcinomas and its relation to p53, Ki-67 and prognosis. J Oral Pathol Med 32:552–561, 2003
55. Locati LD, Quattrone P, Bossi P, et al: A complete remission with androgen-deprivation therapy in a recurrent androgen receptor-expressing adenocarcinoma of the parotid gland. Ann Oncol 14:1327–1328, 2003

56. Locati LD, Perrone F, Losa M, et al: Treatment relevant immunophenotyping of 139 salivary gland carcinomas. Ann Oncol (in press)
57. Longely BJ, Reguera MJ, Ma Y: Classes of c-KIT activating mutations: proposed mechanisms of action and implications for disease classification and therapy. Leuk Res 25:571–576, 2001
58. Mariani L, Marubini E: Content and quality of currently published phase II cancer trials. J Clin Oncol 18:429–436, 2000
59. Matsuba HM, Thawley SE, Simpson JR, et al: Adenoid cystic carcinoma of major and minor salivary gland origin. Laryngoscope 94:1316–1318, 1984
60. Mattox DE, Von Hoff DD, Balcerzak SP: Southwest Oncology Group study of mitoxantrone for treatment of patients with advanced adenoid cystic carcinoma of the head and neck. Invest New Drugs 8:105–107, 1990
61. Miglianico L, Eschwege F, Marandas P, et al: Cervico-facial adenoid cystic carcinoma: study of 102 cases. Influence of radiation therapy. Int J Radiation Oncology Biol Phys 13:673–678, 1987
62. Miller AS, Hartman GG, Chen S-Y, et al: Estrogen receptor assay in polymorphous low-grade adenocarcinoma and adenoid cystic carcinoma of salivary gland origin. Oral Surg Oral Med Oral Pathol 77:36–40, 1994
63. Moriki T, Ueta S, Takahashi T, et al: Salivary duct carcinoma. Cytologic characteristics and application of androgen receptor immunostaining for diagnosis. Cancer (Cancer Cytopathol) 93:344–350, 2001
64. Nascimento AG, Amaral ALP, Prado LAF, et al: Adenoid cystic carcinoma of salivary glands: a study of 61 cases wth clinicopathologic correlation. Cancer 57:312–319, 1986
65. Nasser SM, Faquin WC, Dayal Y: Expression of androgen, estrogen and progesterone receptors in salivary gland tumors. Frequent expression of androgen receptor in a subset of malignant salivary gland tumors. Am J Clin Pathol 119:801–806, 2003
66. Posner MR, Ervin TJ, Weichslebaum RR, et al: Chemotherapy of advanced salivary gland neoplasms. Cancer 50:2261–2264, 1982
67. Press MF, Pike MC, Hung G, et al: Amplification and overexpression of HER-2/neu in carcinomas of the salivary gland: correlation with poor prognosis. Cancer Res 54:5675–5682, 1994
68. Russo G, Zamparelli A, Howard CM, et al: Expression of cell cycle-regulated proteins pRB2/p130, p107, E2F4, p27, and pCNA in salivary gland tumors: prognostic and diagnostic implications. Clin Cancer Res 11:3265–3273, 2005
69. Schramm VL, Srodes C, Myers EN: Cisplatin therapy for adenoid cystic carcinoma. Arch Otolaryngol 107:739–741, 1981
70. Seifert G, Sobin LH: The World Health Organization's histological classification of salivary gland tumors. A commentary on the second edition. Cancer 70:379–385, 1992
71. Sessions RB, Lehane DE, Smith RJH, et al: Intra-arterial cisplatin treatment of adenoid cystic carcinoma. Arch Otolaryngol 108:221–224, 1982
72. Shepherd FA, Rodrigues Pereria J, Ciuleanu T, et al: Erlotinib in previously treated non-small-cell lung cancer. N Engl J Med 353:123–132, 2005
73. Shick PC, Riordan GP, Foss RD: Estrogen and progesterone receptors in salivary gland adenoid cystic carcinoma. Oral Surg Oral Med Oral Pathol 80:440–444, 1995
74. Shintani S, Funayama T, Yoshihama Y, et al: Expression of C-erbB family gene products in adenoid cystic carcinoma of salivary glands: an immunohistochemical study. Anticancer Res 15:2623–2626, 1995
75. Slamon DJ, Leyland-Jones B, Shak S, et al: Use of chemotherapy plus a monoclonal antibody against HER2 for metastatic breast cancer that overexpresses HER2. N Engl J Med 344:783–792, 2001
76. Slevin NJ, Mais KL, Bruce I, et al: Imatinib with cisplatin in recurrent and / or metastatic salivary adenoid cystic carcinoma – response assessed by FDG-PET scanning. Proc Ann Meet Am Soc Clin Oncol 40:512, 2004
77. Spiro RH, Huvos A, Berk R, et al: Mucoepidermoid carcinoma of salivary gland origin: a clinicopathologic study of 367 cases. Am J Surg 136:461–468, 1978
78. Spiro RH, Huvos AG, Strong EW: Adenocarcinoma of salivary origin: clinicopathologic study of 204 patients. Am J Surg 144:423–431, 1982
79. Spiro RH, Huvos AG: Stage means more than grade in adenoid cystic carcinoma. Am J Surg 164:623–628, 1992
80. Spiro RH: Distant metastasis in adenoid cystic carcinoma of salivary origin. Am J Surg 174:495–498, 1997
81. Sur RK, Donde B, Levin V, et al: Adenoid cystic carcinoma of the salivary glands: a review of 10 years. Laryngoscope 107:1276–1280, 1997
82. Tannock IF, Sutherland DJ: Chemotherapy for adenocystic carcinoma. Cancer 46:452–454, 1980
83. Terhaard CHJ, Lubsen H, Van der Tweel I, et al: Salivary gland carcinoma: independent prognostic factors for locoregional control, distant metastases and overall survival: results of the Dutch Head and Neck Oncology Cooperative Group. Head Neck 26:681–693, 2004

84. Tonon G, Modi S, Wu L, et al: t(11;19)(q21;p13) translocation in mucoepidermoid carcinoma creates a novel fusion product that disrupts a Notch signaling pathway. Nat Genet 33:208–213, 2003
85. Triozzi PL, Brantley A, Fisher S, et al: 5-fluorouracil, cyclophosphamide, and vincristine for adenoid cystic carcinoma of the head and neck. Cancer 59:887–890, 1987
86. Tsukuda M, Kokatsu T, Ito K, et al: Chemotherapy for recurrent adeno- and adenoidcystic carcinomas in the head and neck. J Cancer Res Clin Oncol 119:756–758, 1993
87. van der Hulst RWM, van Krieken JHJM, van der Kwast TH, et al: Partial remission of parotid gland carcinoma after goserelin. Lancet 344:817, 1994
88. Van Der Waal JE, Becking AG, Snow GB, et al: Distant metastases of adenoid cystic carcinoma of the salivary glands and the value of diagnostic examinations during follow-up. Head Neck 24:779–783, 2002
89. Venook AP, Tseng J, Alexander, Meyers FJ, et al: Cisplatin, doxorubicin, and 5-fluorouracil chemotherapy for salivary gland malignancies: a pilot study of the Northern California Oncology Group. J Clin Oncol 5:951–955, 1987
90. Vermeer RJ, Pinedo HM: Partial remission of advanced adenoid cystic carcinoma obtained with adriamycin. Cancer 43:1604–1606, 1979
91. Vermorken JB, Verweij J, de Mulder PHM, et al: Epirubicin in patients with advanced or recurrent adenoid cystic carcinoma of the head and neck: A phase II study of the EORTC Head and Neck Cancer Cooperative Group. Ann Oncol 4:785–788, 1993
92. Verweij J, de Mulder PHM, de Graeff A, et al: Phase II study on mitoxantrone in adenoid cystic carcinomas of the head and neck. Ann Oncol 7:867–869, 1996
93. Wick MR, Ockner DM, Mills SE, et al: Homologous carcinomas of the breasts, skin, and salivary glands. Am J Clin Pathol 109:75–84, 1998
94. Witt RL: Adenoid cystic carcinoma of the minor salivary glands. Ear Nose Throat J 70:218–222, 1991
95. Yoo J, Robinson RA: H-ras gene mutations in salivary gland mucoepidermoid carcinomas. Cancer 88:518–523, 2000
96. Zhang J, Peng B, Chen X: Expression of nuclear factor kB, inducible nitric oxide synthase, and vascular endothelial growth factor in adenoid cystic carcinoma of salivary glands: correlations with the angiogenesis and clinical outcome. Clin Cancer Res 11:7334–7343, 2005

Chapter 29

Quality of Life in Patients with Disease and Tumors of Salivary Gland Origin

29

Yoav P. Talmi

Core Features

- Current definitions of quality of life (QOL)
- QOL instruments and challenges in QOL evaluation and measurement
- Effects, sequelae, and complications of salivary gland surgery
- Influence of the above on QOL
- Effects of surgery on salivary flow
- The changing approach with use of sialoendoscopy
- Advantages of cosmetically oriented incision lines

Quality of life (QOL) generally refers to the patient's perception of the effects of the disease and treatment, and their impact on daily functioning and general feeling of well being. QOL has two fundamental foundations. First, it is multidimensional, incorporating physical, psychological, social, emotional, and functional domains. Secondly, it is subjective and must be based on self-reporting, according to the patient's own experiences.

Quality of life is recognized as an important endpoint in clinical research, in addition to the conventional endpoints such as disease-related and global survival. QOL is particularly relevant for patients with tumors of the head and neck because social interaction and expression depend largely on the structural and functional integrity of the head and neck area.

Thus, data from QOL questionnaires are becoming an important supplement to information pertaining to the treatment outcome. There are now a variety of well-validated QOL instruments available for use in the field of head and neck surgery and oncology. These include the generic type such as the Short Form-36 (SF-36), the cancer-specific type, such as the Functional Assessment of Cancer Treatment (FACT-G) and the European Organization for Research and Treatment of Cancer Quality of Life Questionnaire (EORTC QLQ-C30), and the cancer site-specific type, such as the University of Washington Quality of Life (UW-QOL) questionnaire or the FACT-HN, EORTC Head and Neck Module (QLQ-H&N35) [1, 10, 19, 26].

Initially, QOL studies were problematic in numerous respects [26]. QOL is not universally defined and may vary among cultures and even among patients of different socioeconomic levels. Not only are there dozens of suggested head and neck related QOL questionnaires but they also vary to an extent in domains assessed. Overall in the literature, many studies are cross-sectional rather than longitudinal and most are retrospective. Few reports include a sample size of over 100 patients, fewer yet were interventional and many contain information pertaining to survivors only. Another inherent drawback in most global QOL questionnaires stems from what was defined by Weymuller et al. [31] as the "cancellation effect." This relates to the lack of effect on the total score if one domain improved while another deteriorated. Moreover, results are subjectively compared to the pretreatment phase during which function is obviously hampered by pain, tumor mass, swelling, trismus, etc. although these symptoms may be mild. The focal point is on recording the subjective experience of the patient and indeed, surprisingly high levels of QOL may be seen despite significant functional impairment [24]. Good relationship with the treating physician along with support of family and friends can also favorably influence results of QOL studies. Furthermore, patients with poor QOL are less likely to cooperate in filling out questionnaires and even when complying, the quality of their replies is affected [28, 31]. Further confounding the issue of data accumulation is that results have been shown to significantly vary between what patients define as "good" versus "bad" days [6].

In recent years, however, more and more longitudinal studies are published with larger patient cohorts using well-validated instruments and some of the drawbacks described are minimized or eliminated altogether. The number of QOL-related papers in the literature has nearly doubled in the past five years compared to the previous five. One must bear in mind that while the measurement of QOL is evolving, the importance of QOL is "here to stay" even when addressing benign disease or tumors. Assessing QOL is beneficial not only in having advance knowledge of the course of treatment and post-treatment patient-related well being, but also is helpful in deciding which treatment regimen or even which surgical approach is preferable when outcome is similar.

Naturally, as a majority of salivary gland procedures are for benign disease, a shift in considerations regarding QOL may ensue. Factors that may seem insignificant to a person with malignant disease even after deemed cured, may appear important to a basically healthy individual. This was not however found to be the case in a QOL study of parotidectomy [22].

Salivary gland tumors comprise approximately 2% of head and neck neoplasms; 80% of these tumors are encountered in the parotid gland. Parotidectomy is performed for benign or malignant primary or metastatic disease and for selected benign inflammatory and autoimmune conditions. Excision of the submandibular salivary glands is performed for benign and malignant tumors, as part of neck dissection, for some inflammatory and autoimmune conditions, for sialadenitis not amenable to endoscopic treatment, for sialorrhea, and for purposes of access. Excision of the sublingual glands is uncommon and may be performed for tumor removal or excision of ranula.

Sialorrhea adversely influences QOL in affected individuals by distancing them from their immediate social circle. Chronic sialadenitis or sialolithiasis may also influence QOL prior to surgery.

Complete excision of one or both submandibular glands and superficial, total, or radical parotidectomy may be performed with possible consequential morbidity and associated complications. Other than transient immediate or perioperative complications, recognized complications or sequelae of parotidectomy are facial nerve paralysis, scarring with possible keloid formation and depression where glandular tissue is removed, salivary fistula, auriculotemporal syndrome (gustatory sweating or Frey's syndrome), and anesthesia of the ear from severing the greater auricular nerve. Recurrent tumor is clearly a major complication. Recognized complications of surgery of the submandibular and sublingual glands are trauma to the hypoglossal and lingual nerves or to the mandibular branch of the facial nerve. Scarring and change in facial contour are also a concern.

By meticulous technique, the majority of complications can be minimized or avoided altogether. Other sequelae associated with parotidectomy may be obviated by specific techniques. Scarring may be minimized by modification of the incision [11, 29] and depression at the operative site can be prevented to an extent by transposition of the sternocleidomastoid muscle [4, 11]. Terris et al. [29] described a modified face-lift incision that resulted in improved patient satisfaction compared to the modified Blair incision. A retrotragal incision curving posteriorly, close to the hairline and curving back if necessary along a skin crease is far more cosmetically pleasing than the modified Blair incision (Fig. 29.1a, b). A standard face-lift incision is even more cosmetic although wide access may be limited.

Reducing the incidence of Frey's syndrome by natural or synthetic implants with good results was suggested Dulguerov et al. [7] although in a commentary on this report, Kornblut [13] strongly contested the use of implants. While the sternocleidomastoid muscle (SCM) flap was useful for preventing the depression in the face created by the parotid surgery [14], it was shown in one study to be ineffective in preventing the occurrence of gustatory sweating [15]. Only 23 of the 70 patients in this study had subjective complaints related to Frey's syndrome, none of whom were incapacitated or required additional care [15]. Gooden et al. [9] stated that the use of the SCM flap does not alter the incidence of Frey's syndrome that was 31% in their series, and further; it did not significantly improve facial contour.

The face is the center of expression and any defect or dysfunction are readily observed and noted. Despite preventive techniques, complications and sequelae do occur and may affect patients' QOL. We have retrospectively studied QOL in patients following parotidectomy for benign and malignant disease [22]. A QOL instrument was created specifically for the purpose of this study, conceptually based on the University of Washington QOL in-

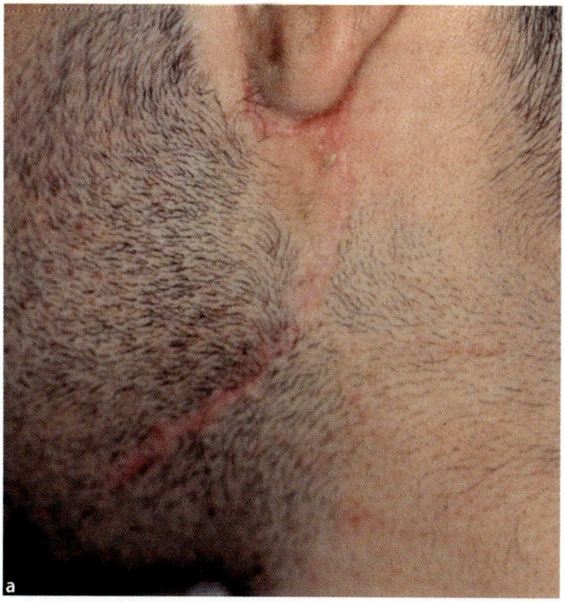

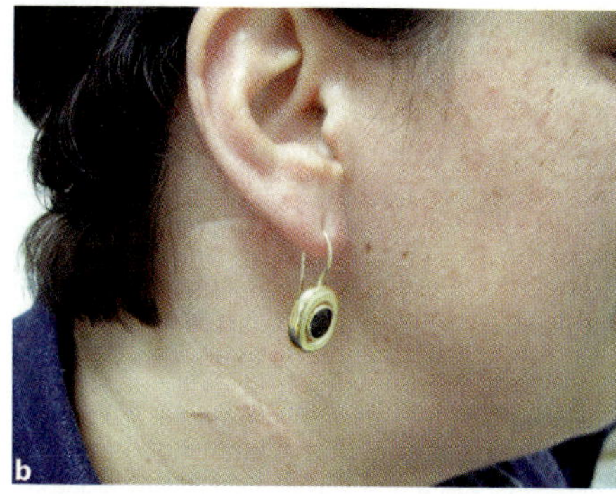

Fig. 29.1: **a** Modified Blair incision. **b** Retrotragal posteriorly curving incision

strument [30] with domain importance ratings and free text options. The UW-QOL is short, simple, and can easily be completed by the patient. Scoring for importance of each domain is a key issue and the option of free text allows for patient comments addressing concerns.

While the concept and scoring system of the UW-QOL was preserved, the content was adapted to specific, parotid surgery oriented questions. In addition to general QOL domains, it included questions which addressed recognized complications of parotid surgery that can affect patient well being, function, and QOL. These included appearance addressing both scarring and changes in facial contour and asymmetry, local sensation, symptoms associated with Frey's syndrome, salivary fistula, and facial nerve function. A computerized database search identified 173 patients who underwent parotidectomy during the study period. One hundred and twenty-five patients met the study criteria and had questionnaires mailed to their known address. Nine patients could not be located and 53 of 116 (46%) fully replied to the questionnaire. Global health score was 3.5 in a scale of 1–5 corresponding with "good" to "very good" and compared to one year formerly the mean was between "the same" and "better." Except for local sensation with a score of 50, all other domains scored above 76. The highest score was 85.4 indicating near lack of significance of pain and 80 signifying a low importance of salivary fistulae. Pain was reported by 16 patients (30%) and 37 patients (70%) reported change in their appearance although specific scarring and local indentation were reported by 60%. Long-term pain was not formerly reported nor expected following parotidectomy. As in other instances, responding to QOL questionnaires may raise to the surface formerly unnoted or unforeseen issues. It may be considered to inform patients undergoing parotidectomy of the possibility of prolonged albeit mild pain. Pain following parotidectomy after the acute early stage could be attributed to neuroma formation of the greater auricular nerve stump [27]. While rarely seen after neck dissection with nerve sacrifice, we have several patients with a neuroma of the greater auricular nerve after parotidectomy and these, possibly affecting QOL, should be treated including by resection if indicated. Importance attributed to all domains except facial function was low. Loss of sensation was noted in all but three patients. Two patients defined loss of sensation as "unbearable" and the overall score was lowest at 50 with importance of 3.1. It should be noted however, that these patients did not complain of their own accord, nor were so determined during routine follow-up visits.

Fourteen patients reported facial nerve impairment. Four patients had facial paralysis independent of the index procedure. This was noted either prior to the procedure in three or one year following surgery due to recurrent tumor in one patient. Overall, including these four patients, facial nerve function scored 76.3 with an importance level of 4.2 (high). Three of the remaining ten patients had parotidectomy for malignant disease with intentional sacrifice of one or more branches of the facial nerve, one had surgery for recurrent pleomorphic adenoma and two others were referred to our service for revision parotidectomy for a second recurrence of pleomorphic adenoma.

According to follow-up notes, three of the seven patients with primary or recurrent benign tumor had minimal mandibular or temporal branch paresis. In three patients, records explicitly note normal facial function although some paresis was noted in two patients in the early postoperative period. These patients conceived their postoperative facial function more critically or at least, differently from the follow-up team. This concept of facial function led us to now indicate in the charts not only our findings but also the patient's perception. These findings are in support of Kahn et al. who developed and validated a patient-based instrument to measure both facial impairment and disability, the Facial Clinimetric Evaluation (FaCE) Scale [12]. Overall, the FaCE Scale showed significant correlation with the House-Brackmann Grading System and the Facial Grading System. The FaCE Scale contains domains that allow for separation and analysis of aspects of facial dysfunction that are not available from physician-graded scales or from more global health status QOL instruments.

Kwok et al. [17] studied QOL after parotid and temporal bone surgery for cancer. Global QOL in 23 patients with cancer of the parotid gland or temporal bone correlated with communication difficulty, physical symptoms, and social disturbances but surprisingly, not with impaired facial nerve function or facial disfigurement. In this study, the cosmetic variables correlated with the UW-QOL disfigurement item but not with the EORTC instrument. The authors speculate that a possible explanation for this may be due to the fact that on the one hand the UW-QOL item leans toward objectivity while on the other hand the EORTC item leans toward subjectivity by asking the patients to rate how much they are bothered by their appearance. This paper coauthored by Morton, a pioneer in QOL research in head and neck surgery, serves well to indicate the different perception between the objective findings and patients' perception of their appearance.

Thirty of our patients (57%) reported local erythema and/or sweating during eating. Overall score was 77 and importance was 2.7 only. Two patients defined these symptoms as intolerable but no patient received treatment nor was interested in seeking treatment of this problem with Botox.

Scores for appearance were significantly better for the younger age group compared with those over 45 years of age. As incisions are similar, we would have expected the younger patients to be more concerned with changes in their appearance. Perhaps reduced facial tone in the older age group serves to amplify the effect of scarring.

There was no significant difference between QOL scores in patients with benign versus malignant disease except for a trend in general health as may be expected.

Reduced salivary flow expressed as xerostomia is known to adversely affect QOL. While complaints regarding this issue are common due to disease processes or treatment affecting the major salivary glands, such complaints related to salivary gland tumors are uncommon. Chaushu et al. [3] studied salivary flow dynamics and sialochemistry in patients undergoing parotidectomy. None of the patients complained of "dry mouth" before or after surgery. Analysis of the individual results revealed three patterns of pre- and postoperative response, compatible with an either preoperative or postoperative compensatory mechanism in the contralateral gland. The postoperative decrease in flow rate corresponded with the amount of parotid gland removed. Salivary electrolyte composition was unchanged. Severely reduced salivary flow may lead to severe symptomatology including candidiasis and pain [2] but even if there is temporary flow reduction, no such problems are incurred even after removal of more than one major salivary gland. Some patients show concern regarding the effect of removal of the parotid gland on salivary flow and should be assured that this is not expected.

Nahlieli is one of the pioneers of the use of sialoendoscopy for treatment of salivary gland disease. In a study of salivary gland sialolithiasis [21] the authors found 189 of the 217 patients followed for 40 months with sialolithiasis to be completely symptom- and stone-free, both endoscopically and by radiographs (overall success rate, 87%) with an 89% and 83% success in the submandibular gland and the parotid, respectively. No severe complications were noted. This technique is successfully used for sialadenitis as well [20]. Obviating the need for removal of the salivary gland in many cases of sialolithiasis and sialadenitis is naturally contributory to QOL and should be used whenever applicable.

While global QOL issues in parotid surgery have largely been overlooked, individual sequelae or complications have been selectively addressed.

Faber and Pedersen [8] reported in the Danish literature a study of 114 patients with parotid tumors, 95 of whom completed a questionnaire. Twenty-four reported various degrees of pain at the time of the investigation, and 57 reported numbness or uncomfortable sensations of the skin. Twenty patients with clinically significant complaints were interviewed and examined. Five patients had a neuroma in the parotid region and hypoesthesia was found in 18. The authors suggest sparing of the posterior branch of the great auricular nerve. Patel et al. [23] studied the effect of greater auricular nerve sacrifice during parotidectomy in 53 patients. Thirty patients (57%) reported experiencing at least one abnormal symptom decreasing significantly with time. Even among patients experiencing symptoms, 23 (77%) reported only a little or no bother caused by the symptoms, and 27 (90%) reported no interference or almost none with their daily activities. The authors conclude that their results indicate no significant effect on QOL. Preservation of the posterior branch of the greater auricular nerve was advocated and reported as "successful" in 70.5% of procedures [5] and Yokoshima et al. [32] preserved the posterior branch of the great auricular nerve in 65% of cases. This was reported to favorably affect QOL assessed at two and six months postoperatively. Ryan and Fee [25] found that the impact of sacrifice of the greater auricular nerve on patient quality of life is tolerable and improves during the first postoperative year although patients did have difficulty using the telephone, shaving, combing their hair, wearing earrings, and sleeping on the operative side because of both anesthesia and paresthesia. The authors feel that greater auricular nerve morbidity may be bothersome enough to warrant efforts to preserve the posterior branch.

Laccourreye et al. [18] reviewed their 25- year experience with 229 parotidectomies for benign pleomorphic adenoma. The overall incidence of Frey's syndrome was 66%. Immediate complications listed were hemorrhage, hematoma, wound infection, seroma, partial skin necrosis, and phlebitis while long-term complications included keloid scar in 8.3% and neuroma formation in 16%. A 62% incidence of Frey's syndrome in a cohort of 69 patients was reported by Kuttner et al. [16]. Nineteen patients felt their QOL had been decreased by the symptoms. Botulinum toxin was shown to be effective in treating these symptoms.

Other than intracutaneous injections of botulinum toxin, a number of noninvasive methods are suggested for symptomatic patients who require treatment. These include topical applications of scopolamine or glycopyrrolate, aluminum chloride hexahydrate, or diphemanil methylsulfate [13].

Quality of life studies related to surgery of the submandibular and sublingual gland have not been reported. Prevention of associated complications and cosmetically oriented incisions will probably minimize QOL changes following these procedures. The classic curved incision "two finger breadths" under the mandible should be replaced by a non-curved incision along a nearly present neck crease that even if is a bit lower than the original suggested line will be more pleasing cosmetically (Fig. 29.2a–c). Utilization of endoscopic procedures reduces the indications for open procedures and further will prevent deleterious effects on QOL.

Take Home Messages

- Quality of life (QOL) is a subjective measure not necessarily corresponding with performance status.
- Health-related QOL reflects an individual's overall sense of well being reflecting in essence a person's overall enjoyment of life.
- In medical studies, QOL is measured using standardized questionnaires to rating factors as pain, treatment side effects, mood, energy level, family and social interactions, sexual function, ability to work, and ability to keep up with routine daily activities.
- Salivary gland surgery and parotid surgery in particular may have potentially devastating effects on QOL mainly, facial nerve paralysis.
- Other factors to consider are damage to the hypoglossal and lingual nerves, local contour changes and scarring, loss of sensation, pain, and gustatory sweating (Frey's syndrome).
- Overall salivary flow is not affected by removal of one parotid gland and no xerostomia is expected following excision of a major salivary gland.
- Postoperative sequelae were noted in a majority of patients undergoing parotidectomy. The dominant were altered sensation, change in appearance, Frey's syndrome, and pain. A degree of permanent postoperative facial nerve impairment was reported by some. Yet, overall, parotidectomy does not seem to severely affect QOL.

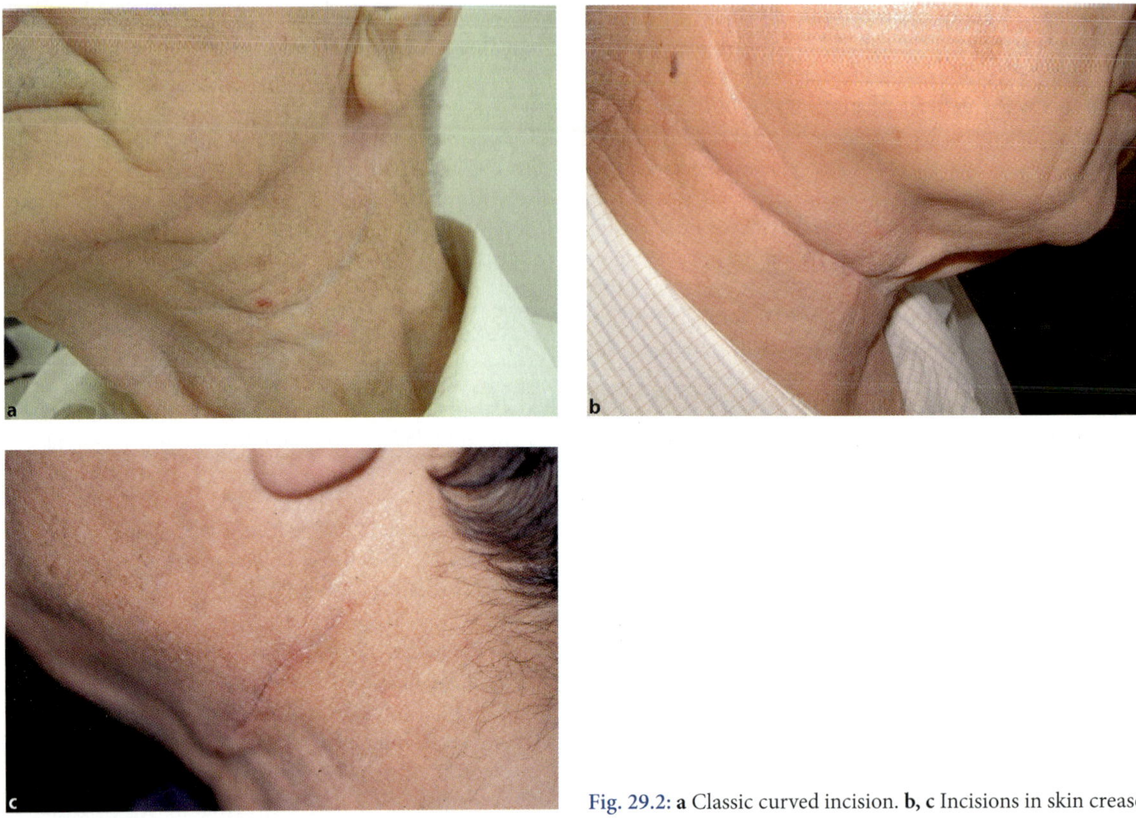

Fig. 29.2: **a** Classic curved incision. **b, c** Incisions in skin crease

References

1. Bjordal K, Hammerlid E, Ahlner-Elmqvist M, de Graeff A, Boysen M, Evensen JF, Biorklund A, de Leeuw JR, Fayers PM, Jannert M, Westin T, Kaasa S (1999) Quality of life in head and neck cancer patients: validation of the European Organization for Research and Treatment of Cancer Quality of Life Questionnaire-H&N35. J Clin Oncol 17: 1008–1019
2. Chaushu G, Bercovici M, Dori S, Waller A, Taicher S, Kronenberg J, Talmi YP (2000) Salivary flow and its relation with oral symptoms in terminally ill patients. Cancer 88: 984–987
3. Chaushu G, Dori S, Sela BA, Taicher S, Kronenberg J, Talmi YP (2001) Salivary flow dynamics after parotid surgery: a preliminary report. Otolaryngol Head Neck Surg 124: 270–273
4. Chow TL, Lam CY, Chiu PW, Lim BH, Kwok SP (2001) Sternomastoid-muscle transposition improves the cosmetic outcome of superficial parotidectomy. Br J Plast Surg 54: 409–411
5. Christensen NR, Jacobsen SD (1997) Parotidectomy. Preserving the posterior branch of the great auricular nerve. J Laryngol Otol 111: 556–559
6. Cohen SR, Mount BM (2000) Living with cancer: good days and bad days—what produces them? Can the McGill quality of life questionnaire distinguish between them? Cancer 89: 1854–1865
7. Dulguerov P, Quinodoz D, Cosendai G, Piletta P, Marchal F, Lehmann W (1999) Prevention of Frey syndrome during parotidectomy. Arch Otolaryngol Head Neck Surg 125: 833–839
8. Faber CE, Pedersen AT (1996) Pain and sensory impairment following parotidectomy. A descriptive study. Ugeskr Laeger 158: 270–273
9. Gooden EA, Gullane PJ, Irish J, Katz M, Carroll C (2001) Role of the sternocleidomastoid muscle flap preventing Frey's syndrome and maintaining facial contour following superficial parotidectomy. J Otolaryngol 30: 98–101
10. Hassan SJ, Weymuller-EA J (1993) Assessment of quality of life in head and neck cancer patients. Head Neck 15: 485–496

11. Jost G, Guenon P, Gentil S (1999) Parotidectomy: a plastic approach. Aesthetic Plast Surg 23: 1–4
12. Kahn JB, Gliklich RE, Boyev KP, Stewart MG, Metson RB, McKenna MJ (2001) Validation of a patient-graded instrument for facial nerve paralysis: the FaCE scale. Laryngoscope 111: 387–398
13. Kornblut AD (2000) The fallacy of preventing Frey syndrome during parotidectomy. Arch Otolaryngol Head Neck Surg 126: 556–557
14. Kornblut AD, Westphal P, Miehlke A (1974) The effectiveness of a sternomastoid muscle flap in preventing post- parotidectomy occurrence of the Frey syndrome. Acta Otolaryngol 77: 368–373
15. Kornblut AD, Westphal P, Miehlke A (1977) A reevaluation of the Frey syndrome following parotid surgery. Arch Otolaryngol 103: 258–261
16. Kuttner C, Troger M, Dempf R, Eckardt A (2001) Effectiveness of botulinum toxin A in the treatment of gustatory sweating. Nervenarzt 72: 787–790
17. Kwok HC, Morton RP, Chaplin JM, McIvor NP, Sillars HA (2002) Quality of life after parotid and temporal bone surgery for cancer. Laryngoscope 112: 820–833
18. Laccourreye H, Laccourreye O, Cauchois R, Jouffre V, Menard M, Brasnu D (1994) Total conservative parotidectomy for primary benign pleomorphic adenoma of the parotid gland: a 25-year experience with 229 patients. Laryngoscope 104: 1487–1494
19. Morton RP, Izzard ME (2003) Quality-of-life outcomes in head and neck cancer patients. World J Surg 27: 884–889
20. Nahlieli O, Bar T, Shacham R, Eliav E, Hecht-Nakar L (2004) Management of chronic recurrent parotitis: current therapy. J Oral Maxillofac Surg 62: 1150–1155
21. Nahlieli O, Shacham R, Bar T, Eliav E (2003) Endoscopic mechanical retrieval of sialoliths. Oral Surg Oral Med Oral Pathol Oral Radiol Endod 95: 396–402
22. Nitzan D, Kronenberg J, Horowitz Z, Wolf M, Bedrin L, Chaushu G, Talmi YP (2004) Quality of Life following Parotidectomy for Malignant and Benign Disease. Plast Reconstr Surg 114: 1060–1067
23. Patel N, Har-El G, Rosenfeld R (2001) Quality of life after great auricular nerve sacrifice during parotidectomy. Arch Otolaryngol Head Neck Surg 127: 884–888
24. Ruhl CM, Gleich LL, Gluckman JL (1997) Survival, function, and quality of life after total glossectomy. Laryngoscope 107: 1316–1321
25. Ryan WR, Fee WE Jr. (2006) Great auricular nerve morbidity after nerve sacrifice during parotidectomy. Arch Otolaryngol Head Neck Surg 132: 642–649
26. Talmi YP (2002) Quality of Life Issues in Cancer of the Oral Cavity. J Laryngol Otol 116: 785–790
27. Talmi YP, Bedrin L, Dori S, Horowitz Z, Wolf M, Yahalom R, Peleg M, Teicher S, Kronenberg J (2003) Amputation neuromas after neck dissection. Otolaryngol Head Neck Surg 128: 196–199
28. Talmi YP, Roth Y, Waller A, Chesnin V, Adunski A, Lander MI, Kronenberg J (1995) Care of the terminal head and neck cancer patient in the hospice setting. Laryngoscope 105: 315–318
29. Terris DJ, Tuffo KM, Fee WE Jr. (1994) Modified facelift incision for parotidectomy. J Laryngol Otol 108: 574–578
30. Weymuller EA Jr., Alsarraf R, Yueh B, Deleyiannis FW, Coltrera MD (2001) Analysis of the performance characteristics of the University of Washington Quality of Life instrument and its modification (UW-QOL-R). Arch Otolaryngol Head Neck Surg 127: 489–493
31. Weymuller EA, Yueh B, Deleyiannis FW, Kuntz AL, Alsarraf R, Coltrera MD (2000) Quality of life in patients with head and neck cancer: lessons learned from 549 prospectively evaluated patients. Arch Otolaryngol Head Neck Surg 126: 329–335
32. Yokoshima K, Nakamizo M, Ozu C, Fukumoto A, Inai S, Baba S, Yagi T (2004) Significance of preserving the posterior branch of the great auricular nerve in parotidectomy. J Nippon Med Sch 71: 323–327

Subject Index

D

E

Q

R